DETERMINANTS OF NEURONAL IDENTITY

DETERMINANTS OF NEURONAL IDENTITY

EDITED BY

Marty Shankland

Department of Anatomy and Cellular Biology
Harvard Medical School
Boston, Massachusetts

Eduardo R. Macagno

Department of Biological Sciences
Columbia University
New York, New York

ACADEMIC PRESS, INC.
Harcourt Brace Jovanovich, Publishers
San Diego   New York   Boston   London
Sydney   Tokyo   Toronto

Cover photograph legends

Inset: In the leech nervous system, the set of neuronal cell bodies stained by antibodies to the neuropeptide SCP differs from one segmental ganglion to the next. The most prominently labeled cells are the CAS neurons, which are here shown to lie on alternate right and left sides of successive ganglia. See Chapter 2 by M. Shankland and M.Q. Martindale for more details. Photo courtesy of M. Shankland. *Background:* In the kitten, subplate neurons pioneer the axonal pathway between the cerebral cortex and thalamus. The subplate neurons are here shown retrogradely labeled by DiI, which was injected into the internal capsule near the end of fetal development. See Chapter 12 by S.K. McConnell for more details. Photo courtesy of S.K. McConnell.

This book is printed on acid-free paper. ∞

Academic Press, Inc.
1250 Sixth Avenue, San Diego, California 92101

United Kingdom Edition published by
Academic Press Limited
24–28 Oval Road, London NW1 7DX

Library of Congress Cataloging-in-Publication Data

Determinants of neuronal identity / [edited by] Marty Shankland,
   Eduardo R. Macagno.
        p.   cm.
     Includes bibliographical references and index.
     ISBN 0-12-638280-8
     1. Developmental neurophysiology.   2. Nerves--Differentiation.
   3. Nerves--Differentiation.   4. Nerves--Growth.   I. Shankland,
   Marty.   II. Macagno, Eduardo R.
       [DNLM: 1. Neurons--cytology.   WL 102.5 D479]
   QP356.25.D47 1992
   591.1'88--dc20
   DNLM/DLC
   for Library of Congress   91-41218
                                                                    CIP

PRINTED IN THE UNITED STATES OF AMERICA
  92 93 94 95 96 97   EB   9 8 7 6 5 4 3 2 1

Contents

3

Control of Central Neurogenesis in the Leech

Thomas Becker and Eduardo R. Macagno

4

Intrinsic and Extrinsic Factors Influencing the Development of Retzius Neurons in the Leech Nervous System

Kathleen A. French and William B. Kristan, Jr.

The Generation of Neuronal Diversity in the *Drosophila* Embryonic Central Nervous System

Chris Q. Doe

Initial Determination of the Neurectoderm in *Drosophila*

Ralph J. Greenspan

Cell Choice and Patterning in the *Drosophila* Retina

Ross Leigh Cagan and S. Lawrence Zipursky

Development of the Peripheral Nervous System in *Drosophila*

Alain Ghysen and Christine Dambly-Chaudière

Endocrine Influences on the Postembryonic Fates of Identified Neurons during Insect Metamorphosis

Janis C. Weeks and Richard B. Levine

Neuron Determination in the Ever-Changing Nervous System of Hydra

Hans R. Bode

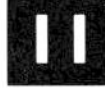

Cell Lineage Segregation in the Vertebrate Neural Crest

Marianne Bronner-Fraser

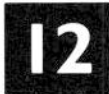

The Determination of Neuronal Identity in the Mammalian Cerebral Cortex

Susan K. McConnell

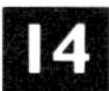

Generation of Neuronal Diversity in the Vertebrate Retina

Thomas A. Reh

Development of Motoneuronal Identity in the Zebrafish

Judith S. Eisen

Cellular and Molecular Mechanisms Determining Neurotransmitter Phenotypes in Sympathetic Neurons

Story C. Landis

Contributors

Numbers in parentheses indicate the pages on which the authors' contributions begin.

Thomas Becker (79)
Department of Biological Sciences,
Columbia University
New York, New York 10027

Hans R. Bode (323)
Developmental Biology Center
Department of Developmental
  and Cell Biology
University of California, Irvine
Irvine, California 92717

Marianne Bronner-Fraser (359)
Developmental Biology Center
University of California, Irvine
Irvine, California 92717

Ross Leigh Cagan (189)
Department of Molecular Biology
Howard Hughes Medical Institute
School of Medicine
University of California, Los Angeles
Los Angeles, California 90024

Helen M. Chamberlin (1)
Howard Hughes Medical Institute
Division of Biology
California Institute of Technology
Pasadena, California 91125

Christine Dambly-Chaudière (225)
Laboratoire de Génétique
Département de Biologie Moléculaire
Université Libre de Bruxelles
1640 Rhode-Saint-Genèse, Belgium

Chris Q. Doe (119)
Department of Cell and Structural Biology
University of Illinois
Urbana, Illinois 61801

Judith S. Eisen (469)
Institute of Neuroscience
University of Oregon
Eugene, Oregon 97403

Kathleen A. French (97)
Department of Biology
University of California, San Diego
La Jolla, California 92093

Alain Ghysen (225)
Laboratoire de Neurobiologie
Département de Biologie Moléculaire
Université Libre de Bruxelles
1640 Rhode-Saint-Genèse, Belgium

Ralph J. Greenspan (155)
Department of Neurosciences
Roche Institute of Molecular Biology
Nutley, New Jersey 07110

William B. Kristan, Jr. (97)
Department of Biology
University of California, San Diego
La Jolla, California 92093

Story C. Landis (497)
Department of Neurosciences
Case Western Reserve University
School of Medicine
Cleveland, Ohio 44106

Richard B. Levine (293)
Arizona Research Laboratories
Division of Neurobiology
Department of Physiology
University of Arizona
Tucson, Arizona 85721

Katharine Liu (1)
Howard Hughes Medical Institute
Division of Biology
California Institute of Technology
Pasadena, California 91125

Eduardo R. Macagno (79)
Department of Biological Sciences
Columbia University
New York, New York 10027

Mark Q. Martindale (45)
Department of Organismal
   Biology and Anatomy
University of Chicago
Chicago, Illinois 60637

Susan K. McConnell (391)
Department of Biological Sciences
Stanford University
Stanford, California 94305

Thomas A. Reh (433)
Department of Biological Structure
University of Washington
Seattle, Washington 98195

Marty Shankland (45)
Department of Anatomy and
   Cellular Biology
Harvard Medical School
Boston, Massachusetts 02115

Paul W. Sternberg (1)
Howard Hughes Medical Institute
Division of Biology
California Institute of Technology
Pasadena, California 91125

Janis C. Weeks (293)
Department of Biology
Institute of Neuroscience
University of Oregon
Eugene, Oregon 97403

S. Lawrence Zipursky (189)
Department of Molecular Biology
Howard Hughes Medical Institute
School of Medicine
University of California, Los Angeles
Los Angeles, California 90024

Preface

One of the most fundamental problems in developmental neurobiology is the determination of neuronal identities. This topic lies at the interface between the traditional domains of the developmental biologist, who strives to understand how the developing organism generates cells of differing specificity, and the neurobiologist, who tries to determine how that cellular specificity results in a functional nervous system capable of shaping itself to the demands of the environment. In formulating this book, we sought to bring together current reviews from a number of experimental systems in which it has been feasible to understand one or more aspects of the problem of neuronal specification.

The biologist is faced with a thorny predicament, in that generalizable principles must be extracted from a natural world that is most remarkable for its organismal diversity. We have chosen to bring together here studies from a wide range of organisms, vertebrate and invertebrate, and to challenge both our contributors and the reader to confront that diversity in search of common themes. Some of the organisms discussed in this volume control the cellular composition of their nervous systems by tightly constraining the cell lineages that generate neurons, while others create order secondarily through patterns of postmitotic cell interaction—yet all of the species use one or another means of regulating the number, kind, and distribution of mature neuronal phenotypes. Thus, the diversity of cellular and molecular mechanisms to be found within these assembled chapters should serve to remind the reader that no single organism is a paragon for the complex process of nervous system formation, and that the specifics of any one system must be appreciated within a larger scheme that takes into account the evolutionary history of the particular organism as well as the organizational principles of the nervous system as a whole.

Different organisms have proven amenable to differing types of analysis, and as a result there is also considerable diversity in the experimental techniques employed in the various chapters. The 1980s brought an explosive growth in the cellular and molecular technologies that are available to the developmental neurobiologist, and in the use of those technologies to re-examine and redefine many of the long-standing issues in the field. We have tried to assemble articles that emphasize a variety of different approaches. Some species are suitable for genetic analysis, and the traditional mutational approach is herein complemented by more recently developed methodologies, such as the establishment of enhancer-trap lines and the expression of transgenes in tissue culture cells. Other organisms are preferable for the experimental analysis of morphogenesis, and many of the articles rely upon state-of-the-art techniques for labeling single cells and tracing the developmental fate of cell lineages in both normal and experimentally manipulated embryos. Both approaches are feasible in some systems, for instance, by physically transplanting cells of known genotype between mutant and wild-type backgrounds to assay the morphogenetic role of the gene product.

In order to focus this book on the problem of neuronal specification, we felt obliged to eschew other exciting areas of research in neural development, such as axon guidance, synaptogenesis, and plasticity. For the most part, these phenomena occur secondary to the establishment of the neuron's identity, and are more related to the process of differentiation than they are to the present discussion of determination. What we have sought to provide is a format in which the reader can consider how neurons are generated, how their developmental identities are specified, and to what degree those identities can be subsequently modified to meet the changing needs of the organism. We hope that the ideas presented will help currently active researchers to synthesize a conceptual framework for future studies, and will inspire in the reader some of the intellectual challenge and excitement of discovery that continues to draw young scientists into this particular field of inquiry.

Marty Shankland
Eduardo R. Macagno

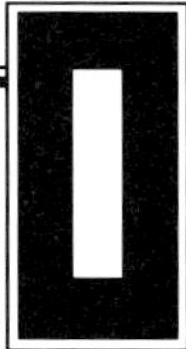

Specification of Neuronal Identity in *Caenorhabditis elegans*

Paul W. Sternberg, Katharine Liu,
and Helen M. Chamberlin
Howard Hughes Medical Institute
Division of Biology
California Institute of Technology
Pasadena, California

I. Introduction

Caenorhabditis elegans is a free-living nematode whose invariant anatomy, hermaphroditic self-fertilization, and short (3.5-day) generation time readily allow genetic and developmental studies. Embryos, larvae, and adult *C. elegans* are transparent and can grow on a microscope slide; thus every cell can be visualized in the light microscope using Nomarski DIC optics.

Thus, it is possible to follow the division, migration, differentiation, and/or death of each cell. By such direct observation, the entire cell lineage—the series of divisions a cell and its progeny undergo before terminal differentiation—has been determined for both the hermaphrodite and the male. The cell lineage is essentially invariant among individuals (Sulston and Horvitz, 1977; Kimble and Hirsh, 1979; Sulston *et al.*, 1980, 1983).

Detailed light and electron microscopy has enabled researchers to reconstruct the entire hermaphrodite nervous system, including axonal branches and synapses, and produce a "circuit diagram" (e.g., White *et al.*, 1986). Of the 959 somatic nuclei that are eventually produced during the development of the *C. elegans* hermaphrodite, 302 are neurons, and an additional 56 are glial and support cells. Most of the neurons are in the circumpharyngeal nerve ring in the anterior of the animal or in the ventral nerve cord. The male possesses 79 additional neurons, most of which are located in the copulatory structures of the tail. There is relatively little branching of neuronal processes; the 302 hermaphrodite neurons make a total of roughly 5000 chemical synapses, 2000 neuromuscular junctions, and 600 gap junctions.

Nematodes, although evolutionarily diverged from arthropods and vertebrates, are nonetheless useful for the study of general aspects of neurobiology. The *C. elegans* nervous system has been shown by immunological and biochemical assays to possess classical neurotransmitters [acetylcholine (Ach), γ-amino butyric acid (GABA), 5-hydroxytryptamine (5-HT), dopamine, octopamine] and neuropeptides (e.g., FMFRamide-like neuropeptides), as well as enzymes that synthesize and catabolize them (e.g., acetylcholinesterase) (reviewed by Chalfie and White, 1988). Several of the genes encoding these enzymes have been identified. Genes have also been identified that control cell migration, axon outgrowth, and synaptogenesis (Hedgecock *et al.*, 1985, 1987, 1990; Manser and Wood, 1990). Since the general features of the *C. elegans* nervous system are common to all metazoa, its simplicity and the facility for developmental and behavioral genetics have allowed researchers to address the problem of how neuronal cell fate is specified during development.

The determinants of neuronal identity are the genes and their products that instruct a cell to a specific fate. Such genes must function at four levels: (1) generation of the cell; (2) specification—assigning a specific identity; (3) differentiation—acquiring the characteristic traits; and (4) proper function. For purposes of this discussion, we have divided the specification of neuronal fate into two sections corresponding to "early" and "late" neurogenesis. Genes or processes that are involved in choices among different neuronal precursors (the generation of alternative "sublineages;" see subsequent text) are considered "early." Genes or processes that govern differentiation of a particular cell are considered "late." Although these subdivisions may prove artificial, they form a useful framework for discussing different experimental techniques and developmental issues.

A. Neuronal Cell Lineage

At each division of a cell lineage, the fates of the daughter cells often become different from those of their mothers and sometimes from those of other daughter cells. In some organisms, some segregation of neuronal fate appears to occur relatively early in development, for example, the formation of the neural tube in mammals and the segregation of neural ectoderm in *Drosophila*, which generates the neuroblasts. In *C. elegans*, one might expect to find a similar point of divergence, that is, all neurons or at least all of one type of neuron should be generated from one branch of the lineage. Instead, one finds that neurons are generated from many branches of the cell lineage (Sulston and Horvitz, 1977; Sulston *et al.*, 1980, 1983). For example, of the 8 classes of ventral motor neurons that control locomotion, only 3 arise during embryogenesis. The remaining 5 classes are generated postembryonically from a total of 13 different precursors, W and the Pn.a cells (Sulston and Horvitz, 1977).

Another example of the relationship of cell lineage and neuronal fate is provided by the lineal histories of the many sensilla in *C. elegans.* A sensillum generally consists of one or more neurons surrounded by support cells, the sheath and socket cells. Some sensilla consist of cells that are closely related in the lineage. In postdeirid development, the neuron and neuronal support cells are all generated postembryonically by the cell V5.pa. (This cell also generates an interneuron and another cell that undergoes programmed cell death; Fig. 1A.) The cells of most of the male-specific sensilla, which are also generated postembryonically, exhibit close lineal relationships (e.g., Fig. 1B). These *C. elegans* sublineages are similar to the cell lineages that generate the sensory organs in the *Drosophila* peripheral nervous system (e.g., Bodmer *et al.*, 1989; Hartenstein and Posakony, 1989; reviewed in Chapter 8). For example, the four cells of the *Drosophila* external sense organ arise from a single precursor cell. The tormogen and trichogen cells (structural and support cells functionally analogous to the *C. elegans* socket cells) are sisters, and the thecogen (sheath analog) cell and neuron of the sensillum are sisters. In contrast, close lineal relationships are not seen in the cells of the amphid and phasmid sensilla. For instance, the cells that make up the left amphid arise from both ABa and ABp (Fig. 1C). Thus AB, the anterior blastomere in a 2-cell embryo, is the last ancestral cell common to all amphid cells. In addition, the cells that constitute these sensilla are not closely related (i.e., sisters or cousins). Close lineal relationship is also lacking among the cells of the phasmids,

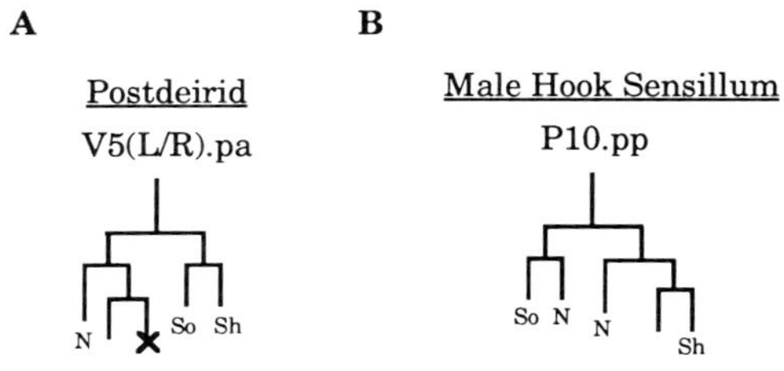

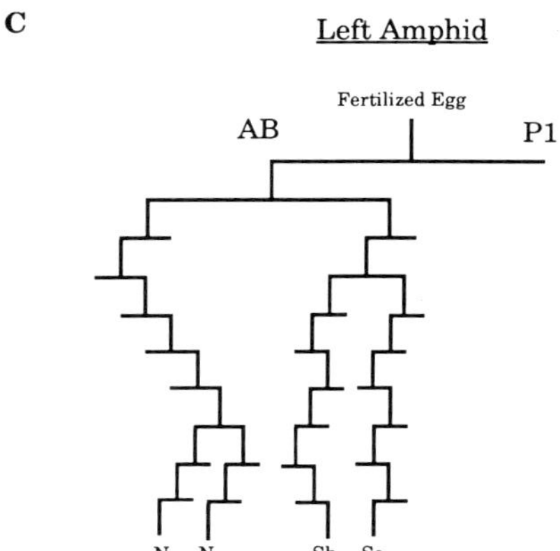

Figure 1. Origin of sensilla. A. Postdeirid. B. Male hook sensillum. C. Amphid. The diverse origins of the cells that constitute the left amphid are shown in this abbreviated embryonic lineage. N, neuron; Sh, sheath cell; So, socket cell; X, programmed cell death. Data of Sulston and Horvitz (1977) and Sulston *et al.* (1980, 1983).

which are generated in two distinct developmental phases. In the embryo, the neurons and sheath cells are generated from distant branches of the AB lineage; the adult socket cells are then generated in the larva by two bilaterally symmetric blast cells (TR and TL, derivatives of the AB blastomere).

These and other examples indicate that development of the nervous system occurs in a fragmented fashion throughout the worm. Because neurons are generated in many diverse ways, several mechanisms probably act to specify neuronal identities. As revealed by extensive developmental genetic analysis, general aspects of specification of neuronal identity are very similar to specification of other cell fates; thus, information can often be generalized from one cell type to another.

In addition to the piecemeal production of neuronal cell type, the reproducibility of cell generation and specification in *C. elegans* might suggest that development in this animal is mostly mosaic, that is, the fate of most cells is based solely on their lineal history (by factors that are segregated in their precursors) rather than on environmental cues. This would seem to contrast with vertebrate development in which intercellular signalling is known to play a dominant role (see Chapter 11). However, a variety of cell ablation studies and other experiments, discussed in detail in this chapter, have revealed many examples of cell interactions that are critical to cell fate determination in the nematode. The invariant lineage is as much caused by highly reproducible cell interactions as by mosaic development. The position of each cell with respect to its neighbors is invariant; consequently, the positional cues and intercellular signals are invariant. The invariance of *C. elegans* development, rather than being unique, makes the nematode a useful experimental system in which to study how cell interactions specify cell fate.

Considering the importance of cell interactions, the relative positions of cells in the developing animal become as important as their lineage histories. Neuronal precursors, when viewed in the context of the cell lineage, arise from divergent locations; however, when viewed anatomically, they occupy a common position in the animal. For example, the Pn.a cells that generate the postembryonic motor neurons sit evenly spaced along the anterior–posterior axis at the most ventral part of the animal. In fact, most neuronal precursor cells occupy the position of the ventral ectoderm. Anatomically, neuroblasts are segregated in the same manner as their counterparts in other animals are (see Hedgecock and Hall, 1990, for a discussion of comparative neurogenesis). These unrelated neuroblasts then generate neurons via similar patterns of cell divisions or sublineages (see subsequent text). Therefore, although the neurons generated are not related, their lineal histories are similar.

Although many examples of cell interactions are now characterized in *C. elegans* (see, for example, Section II,A), most researchers assume that, in the absence of contradictory evidence, lineage plays a primary role in determining the fate of a particular cell. In this framework, one can describe precursor cells as undergoing sublineage choice, that is, genes that act early in neuronal development govern switches (triggered either externally or internally) that distinguish between alternative sublineages. Once such a decision has been made, a relatively short, apparently intrinsically specified developmental program is executed, resulting in the generation of a stereotypical set of progeny cells.

B. Intrinsic versus Extrinsic Specification

A cell lineage can be thought of as a series of decisions between alternative cell fates. This divergence in fate can result either from the lineage history of the cell and its inherited internal constituents (asymmetric cell divisions) or from environmental cues (cell interactions). In molecular terms, one can imagine that asymmetric cell divisions result from particular gene products acting in or on one of the daughters, making it different from its sibling. Thus, molecules that are differentially segregated to one daughter and molecules that establish asymmetry in the parent might be components of the mechanism underlying an autonomous asymmetric division. On the other hand, cell-signaling molecules, receptor molecules, and extracellular matrix molecules might be components involved in cell fate specification, enabling the two daughter cells to respond to differences in their environment. Transcriptional regulators could be involved in any mode of cell fate specification.

Both autonomous and nonautonomous cell-factors play a role in establishing cell fates in the *C. elegans* embryo and larva. A particularly good example of a combination of these factors in the development of a single structure is seen in the specification of pharyngeal muscles. The pharynx consists of several cell types, including muscles, neurons, and glands (Albertson and Thomson, 1976). Priess and Thomson (1987) used a pharyngeal-muscle-specific antibody to characterize cell fate specification in the cells of this organ. Like the amphids, the cells that make up the pharynx are generated at diverse points in the cell lineage. Pharyngeal muscle nuclei are derived from ABa, the anterior daughter of AB, as well as from EMS, the anterior daughter of P1. Thus, in the second round of cell division, two cells are produced that will eventually produce pharynx muscle, and two are produced that will not. To distinguish ABa and EMS from their posterior sisters, Priess and Thomson (1987) removed early blastomeres from the *C. elegans* egg and observed the remaining cell(s) for differentiation of their progeny. Pharyngeal-muscle-specific staining was seen in progeny of isolated P1 blastomeres and in partial embryos with P2 (posterior daughter of P1) removed, indicating autonomous development. In contrast, no staining was seen in the progeny of isolated AB cells and in partial embryos with EMS removed, suggesting that inductive interactions were required. From these experiments, Priess and Thomson concluded that (1) the P1 blastomere does not require AB-derived cells to generate pharyngeal muscle cells, but AB does require P1-derived cells to generate pharyngeal muscle cells, and (2) the abilities of P1 to produce pharynx muscles and to induce pharynx muscles are properties of EMS and/or its progeny. Finally, if ABa and ABp are manipulated with a micropipette so the two blastomeres exchange relative positions, the embryo nevertheless develops into a normal fertile animal. Thus, the ABa and ABp blastomeres are probably initially equivalent, and the position of ABa in the embryo, through interaction with EMS or its progeny, induces pharyngeal muscle formation. It is not known whether the pharyngeal neurons are specified in the same manner as the muscles. However, it is evident from this example that both cell interactions and autonomous specification can play a role in embryonic cell fate specification in nematodes.

Another example of the fundamental importance of cell interactions in nematode development is provided by the origin of bilateral asymmetry. The bilateral asymmetry of the nematode includes the asymmetric migrations of the Q neuroblasts (Sulston and Horvitz, 1977; see Section III,A). The general aspects of bilateral asymmetry of *C. elegans* can be reversed by manipulation of blastomeres at the 6-cell stage, indicating that cell interactions are involved in determining differences in the fates of cells on the left and right sides of the animal (Wood, 1991).

C. Methodology

The methods used to study cell-type specification in nematodes are cell ablation, developmental and behavioral genetics, and molecular biology. In cell ablation experiments, individual cells are killed with a laser microbeam and the resulting effects on related and surrounding cells are observed. These experiments allow an assessment of the relative contributions of environmental and autonomous components in cell fate specification (Sulston and White, 1980). Ablation studies have shown that, in the lab environment, only two neuronal cell types (a total of three neurons) are essential for a minimal form of viability (Avery and Horvitz, 1989; J. Sulston, personal communication). Thus, mutations affecting the nervous system can be isolated and propagated (Brenner, 1974). Animals with these mutations are analyzed morphologically, anatomically, behaviorally, and genetically. Such analysis allows the identification of genes that are necessary for the normal processes. The phenotypes of mutations that lower or eliminate activity of a particular gene allow its wild-type function to be inferred: if elimination of the function of a gene results in misspecification of a cell, the normal function of that gene must be to promote specification of that cell. Such genetic analysis allows an understanding of the effect of one particular gene in the context of the normal functioning of all other genes. One thus deals with a very large number of controlled variables. Other types of mutations—including ones that result in a hyperactive gene product, a novel function of a gene product, or a function antagonistic to the normal gene product—are known and can also be useful for interpreting the wild-type function of a gene product. Molecular cloning strategies based on "transposon tagging" and correlation of genetic and physical maps allow the isolation of genes defined solely by mutations (e.g., Moerman *et al.*, 1986; Ruvkun *et al.*, 1989) and the creation of reagents necessary to elucidate biochemical functions and cellular locations of those gene products (e.g., Costa *et al.*, 1988; Ruvkun and Guisto, 1989; Way and

Chalfie, 1989). Additional molecular and genetic analysis allows the deduction of pathways of gene action.

II. Early Neurogenesis

In the following sections, we discuss mechanisms of cell fate specification involved in the production of specified cell types. We focus on the experimental evidence for exemplary cases. First we will discuss cell interactions; then we will focus on asymmetric cell divisions.

A. Establishment of Postembryonic Blast Cell Fates

The fates of blast cells during postembryonic development have been analyzed more extensively than other precursor cells whose fates are established by cell interactions. Primarily, this is because alternative cell fates can easily be discovered for these cases. The role of cell interactions in specifying blast cell fates in the developing nematode larva has been demonstrated through use of cell ablation with a laser microbeam. If ablation of a cell or a subset of cells causes other cells to behave differently, then the ablated cells or their progeny are involved in the specification of the fate of the affected cells. However, if ablation of one cell does not produce a change in the fate of the other, then, at least by the time of ablation, interactions between these cells are not required to specify fate. This technique does not rule out the possibility that cell interactions are involved in cell fate specification earlier in the lineage that produces that cells, nor the possibility that cellular debris remaining from the killed cell is able to function in the interactive process. Other methods, such as genetic mosaic analysis (reviewed by Herman, 1989), can also reveal hitherto unsuspected or untestable cell interactions. For example, the possible role of a third tissue during hermaphrodite vulval induction has been suggested by the nonautonomy of the *lin-15* gene (Herman and Hedgecock, 1990); in this case, the presumed cell is a large syncytium that cannot be ablated without killing the animal. However, cell ablation experiments have provided many examples of nonautonomous specification of cell fate.

I. EQUIVALENCE GROUPS

In some cases, specific sets of cells that normally have different fates have been shown to be equally capable of adopting the fate of a specific cell destroyed by ablation. Such ablation experiments have helped to characterize the specification of the fates of 11 ventral cord precursor cells, P1.p–P11.p, in both males and hermaphrodites (Sulston and Horvitz, 1977). In particular, P9.p, P10.p, and P11.p in the male form an equivalence group (Sulston and White, 1980); although in the intact animal their fates are invariant, these cells are of equal developmental potential. In the wild-type male, the cells P1.p–P9.p fuse with a large hypodermal syncytium called hyp7 (Sulston *et al.*, 1980). P10.p divides to produce nine cells, three of which also fuse with hyp7; one differentiates into a male-specific motor neuron and the remainder make up a structure called the hook, necessary for male mating, and its associated sensillum. The hook sensillum consists of two neurons, a sheath cell, a socket cell, and the cell that makes the hook. In contrast, P11.p divides to produce seven cells: four male-specific interneurons and three cells associated with, but not part of, the hook sensillum. Ablation experiments demonstrate that the fates of P9.p, P10.p, and P11.p result from cell interactions (Sulston and White, 1980). If P11.p is ablated, P10.p will migrate posteriorly and adopt the fate of P11.p; P9.p will, in turn, adopt the fate of P10.p (Fig. 2), that is, P9.p will divide with the timing and axes of cell division normally associated with P10.p and produce a normal hook sensillum. If both P11.p and P10.p are ablated, then P9.p will adopt the fate of P11.p. If all three are ablated, however, none of the more anterior cells (P1.p–P8.p) will adopt a different fate. Thus, the three more posterior cells (P9.p–P11.p) are considered to be an equivalence group because these cells are equivalent in potential, although each adopts a different fate depending on its position in the animal. The P11.p fate is considered primary (1°), indicating that each of the three cells can adopt that fate if it is the only cell present or if it is the most posterior of the cells. If two cells are present, the more anterior one adopts the P10.p fate, which is thus secondary (2°). The 2° fate will only be expressed if a 1° cell already exists. Finally, if all three cells are present, then the most posterior (P11.p) adopts the 1° fate, the middle cell (P10.p) adopts the 2° fate, and the remaining cell (P9.p) adopts the tertiary (3°) fate.

The *lin-12* gene controls aspects of cell fate specification in the hook equivalence group; in other sets of equivalent cells, activity of *lin-12* also can distinguish one cell from its neighbors (Greenwald *et al.*, 1983). (Nematode genes are given a three letter name followed by a number; *lin* stands for "cell *lin*eage abnormal;" *lin-12* is the twelfth such gene identified.) Two major classes of mutations at the *lin-12* locus reveal its role in fate specification: recessive loss-of-function *(lf)* mutations have phenotypic effects opposite from those of semidominant gain-of-function *(gf)* mutations. Genetic evidence indicates that high *lin-12* activity specifies one cell fate, whereas low *lin-12* activity specifies an alternative fate. Many of the cells affected by *lin-12* have common features. For instance, *lin-12* mutations affect several equivalence groups the fate of which is specified by cell interactions. Thus, *lin-12* is

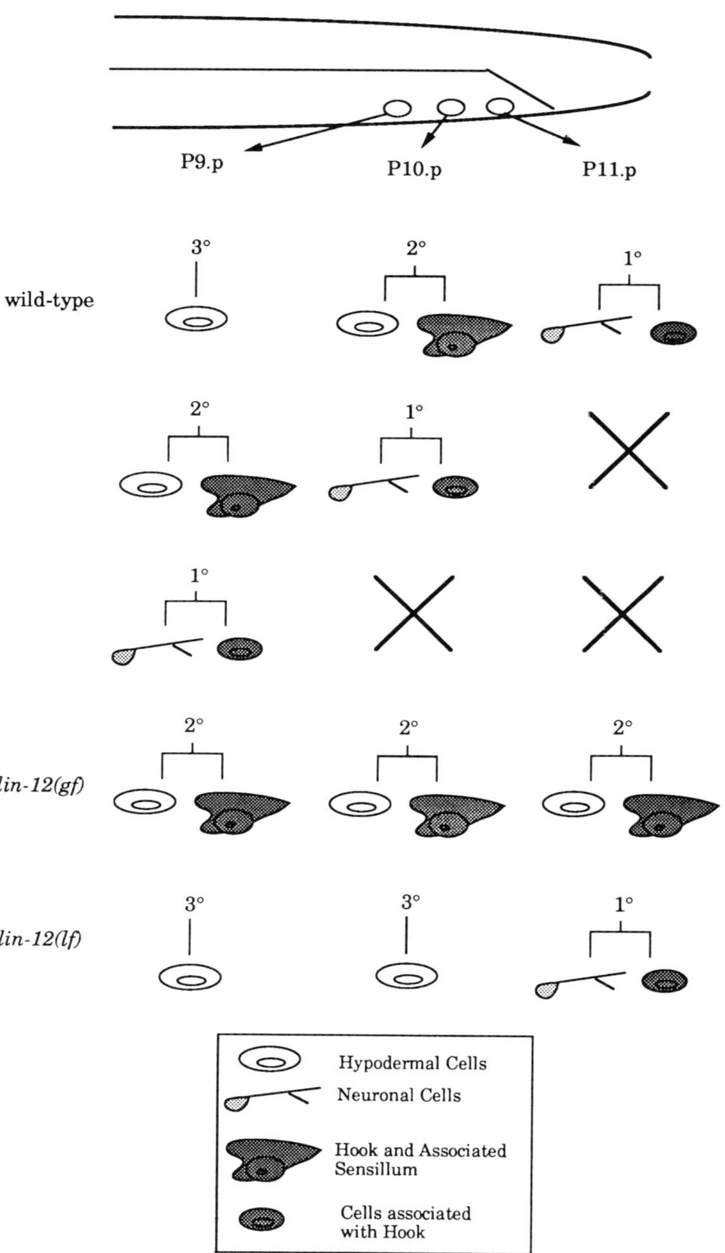
P9.p
P10.p
P11.p
3°
wild-type
2°
1°
2°
1°
1°
lin-12(gf)
2°
2°
2°
lin-12(lf)
3°
3°
1°
Hypodermal Cells
Neuronal Cells
Hook and Associated
Sensillum
Cells associated
with Hook

a strong candidate for being an important molecule in intercellular signaling. In the male hook equivalence group, *lin-12* controls whether a cell will have the 2° fate: *lin-12(gf)* mutations result in all three cells adopting the 2° fate and generating the sublineage of the wild-type P10.p (Fig. 2). Thus, three hooks are produced. In contrast, *lin-12(lf)* mutations result in all three cells adopting non-2° fates: P9.p and P10.p adopt the 3° fate and P11.p adopts the 1° fate. In these animals, no 2° sublineage is generated; thus, no hook is formed. There must be another mechanism that determines the 1° and 3° fates.

Another role of *lin-12* is in hermaphrodite vulval induction (Greenwald *et al.*, 1983). In this case, the pathway that distinguishes 1° from 3° is known. During hermaphrodite vulval induction, *lin-12* specifies 2° fates in the vulval equivalence group consisting of the cells P3.p–P8.p. Like those of P9.p–P11.p in the male, the fates of these cells are set by cell interactions (Sulston and White, 1980). An inductive signal from the anchor cell in the gonad acts to promote 1° and 2° fates (Kimble, 1981; Sternberg and Horvitz, 1986; see Horvitz and Sternberg, 1991, for review). This inductive signal has been proposed to act via the receptor tyrosine kinase encoded by the *let-23* gene and the Ras protein encoded by *let-60 ras* (*let*hal, Aroian *et al.*, 1990; Han and Sternberg, 1990). A lateral signal, probably acting via *lin-12*, promotes a 2° at the expense of 1° fate (Sternberg, 1988; Sternberg and Horvitz, 1989). Studies of the vulval and male hook equivalence groups indicate that, in three-fate equivalence groups, at least two fate-specifying pathways operate. *lin-12* plays an analogous role, the specification of the 2° fate, in both groups. Therefore, *lin-12* is involved in specifying alternative cell fates rather than in promoting the differentiation of particular cell types.

The independence of these two pathways is further evidenced by analysis of other equivalence groups. *lin-12* controls the fates of cells in many but not all equivalence groups (Greenwald *et al.*, 1983). P11, the parent of P11.p, and its homolog P12 constitute a 2-cell equivalence group; the P12 fate is 1° in this case (Sulston and White, 1980). The fates of the two members of this group are controlled not by *lin-12*, but by the genetic pathway defined by *let-23* and *let-60 ras* (Fixsen *et al.*, 1985; Beitel *et al.*, 1990; Han *et al.*, 1990; Aroian and Sternberg, 1991; M. Han and P. W. Sternberg, unpublished observations).

Figure 2. Specification of sublineages in the hook equivalence group. The three tripotent precursor cells are shown in their posterior position in the ventral cord. The 3° fate is to fuse with the large hypodermal syncytium (hyp7). The 2° fate is to generate the hook sensillum and other hypodermal cells. The 1° lineage generates neurons and hypodermal cells. An "X" represents a cell ablated by laser microbeam irradiation. In mutants with hyperactive *lin-12* protein [*lin-12(gf)V*], all three precursor cells are 2°, and three hook sensilla are formed. In mutants with inactive *lin-12* [*lin-12(lf)*], no 2° lineages are generated; P10.p either adopts a 3° or a 1° fate. Data of Sulston and White (1980), Sulston *et al.* (1980), and Greenwald *et al.* (1983).

let-23 and *let-60 ras* appear to be required for the 1° fate, P12. Thus, each of the two fate-specifying pathways involved in the hook equivalence group can act independently to specify cell fates in simpler equivalence groups.

lin-12 mutations also affect cells that are not known to be part of an equivalence group, that is, that show no lineage disruption or fate regulation after ablation of neighbors. One example is a pair of lineal homologs in the tail called Y and DA9. In the hermaphrodite, both of these cells become motor neurons. In the male, the Y cell divides to produce an anterior motor neuron (homologous to the hermaphrodite Y or PDA neuron) and a posterior neuroblast that divides to produce most of the cells for the male postcloacal sensilla. The fates of these cells do not appear to depend on cell interactions (Sulston *et al.*, 1983). However, in animals carrying *lin-12(gf)* mutations, both cells behave like a normal Y cell (in males, both divide with a Y-like lineage), whereas in animals carrying *lin-12(lf)* mutations, both behave like DA9 (Greenwald *et al.*, 1983). Therefore, *lin-12* specifies the fates of multipotent cells in response to cell interactions (as in the male hook equivalence group), but also specifies the fates of homologous cells that appear to have only a single potential in the wild type (DA9/Y pair).

Mosaic analysis was used to determine the cells in which *lin-12* gene function is required. In general, mosaic animals are generated through the use of free duplications, chromosome fragments that are semi-stably maintained at cell division with loss of the fragment about once in every 200 cell divisions (reviewed by Herman, 1989). If the duplication carries a wild-type copy of a gene, and the chromosomes carry two recessive mutant copies, loss of the duplication results in cells with a mutant genotype. If a gene product functions autonomously, either as an autonomously segregated factor or on the receiving side of a cell interaction, a mutant genotype (loss of the duplication) will result in a mutant phenotype in that cell. In contrast, if a gene product function is required on the signaling side of a cell interaction, the receiving cell can have a mutant genotype but produce a normal phenotype as long as the signaling cell is genotypically wild type. Seydoux and Greenwald (1989) have shown by mosaic analysis that *lin-12* acts autonomously in the one equivalence group examined. Since *lin-12* is already shown to be involved, at least in some examples, in specification that results from cell interactions, the mosaic results suggest that *lin-12* functions are on the receiving end of these interactions

The inferred product of *lin-12* is consistent with a role in cell interactions. The *lin-12* locus encodes a putative transmembrane product similar in overall structure to the *Drosophila Notch* gene and the *C. elegans glp-1* gene (germ line proliferation), both of which are also important in cell interactions (reviewed by Greenwald, 1989; see Chapter 6 for a discussion of the action of this family). This gene family has motifs similar to those found in a variety of cell-surface and extracellular molecules: EGF-like repeats (for review, see Davis, 1990). Mutations that produce the dominant *lin-12* phenotype have been localized to the *lin-12* coding region, indicating that the dominant effect is due to a protein that is hyperactive rather than to a protein that is over-expressed (Greenwald and Seydoux, 1990).

2. POSITIONAL SPECIFICATION OF CELL FATES ALONG THE BODY AXIS

Cell fate specification can show added complexity beyond that described for the male hook or hermaphrodite vulva. For instance, the *C. elegans* larva hatches with a row of seven cells, V1–V6 and T, that are located in an anterior to posterior array along each lateral midline (Fig. 3A). In both males and hermaphrodites, V1–V4 divide to produce hypodermal cells and "seam cells" that secrete characteristic cuticular ridges (lateral alae) on the sides of L1 and adult animals. V5 divides to produce a specialized sensory structure of unknown function called a postdeirid, and T divides to produce socket cells for another sensory structure of unknown function called a phasmid. In the male, V5, V6, and T progeny also include the cells of the 18 (9 on each side) male-specific "rays" necessary for male copulatory behavior. Sulston and White (1980) demonstrated that cell interactions specify the lineages generated by these cells. Sulston and White performed a series of ablation experiments in which they destroyed particular sets of cells and observed which cells generated sensory ray cell groups (RCGs, which generate individual sensilla) and which generated postdeirid cell groups. On each side of the wild-type male, T generates three RCGs, V6 generates five RCGs, and V5 generates one RCG and one postdeirid. Ablation of T does not affect the fates of V1–V6, which produce essentially the same complement of neuronal sensilla as they would in the wild type. However, ablation of V6 and T results in a posterior migration of V5 and its generation of 4–5 RCGs but no postdeirid. Ablation of T, V5, and V6 (or V5 and V6 only) results in V4 producing up to four RCGs, thereby partially compensating for the loss of V6.

These experiments reveal two aspects of the mechanism that specifies the fates of these cells. First, unlike in the hook equivalence group, no distinct division between recruitable and nonrecruitable V cells was detected. More anterior V cells appear to have a graded ability to replace V6 (i.e., to make an RCG), which may be a function inherent to the cells or a function of their distance from the posterior of the animal (the V6 environment). Second, the ability to make a postdeirid cell group is a function inherent only to V5. If V6 is missing, V5 can make V6-like rays at the expense of the postdeirid, but in no case can another cell replace V5 and make a postdeirid (Fig. 3B). Thus, cell fate specification in the V5 lineage, for example, involves the interplay of

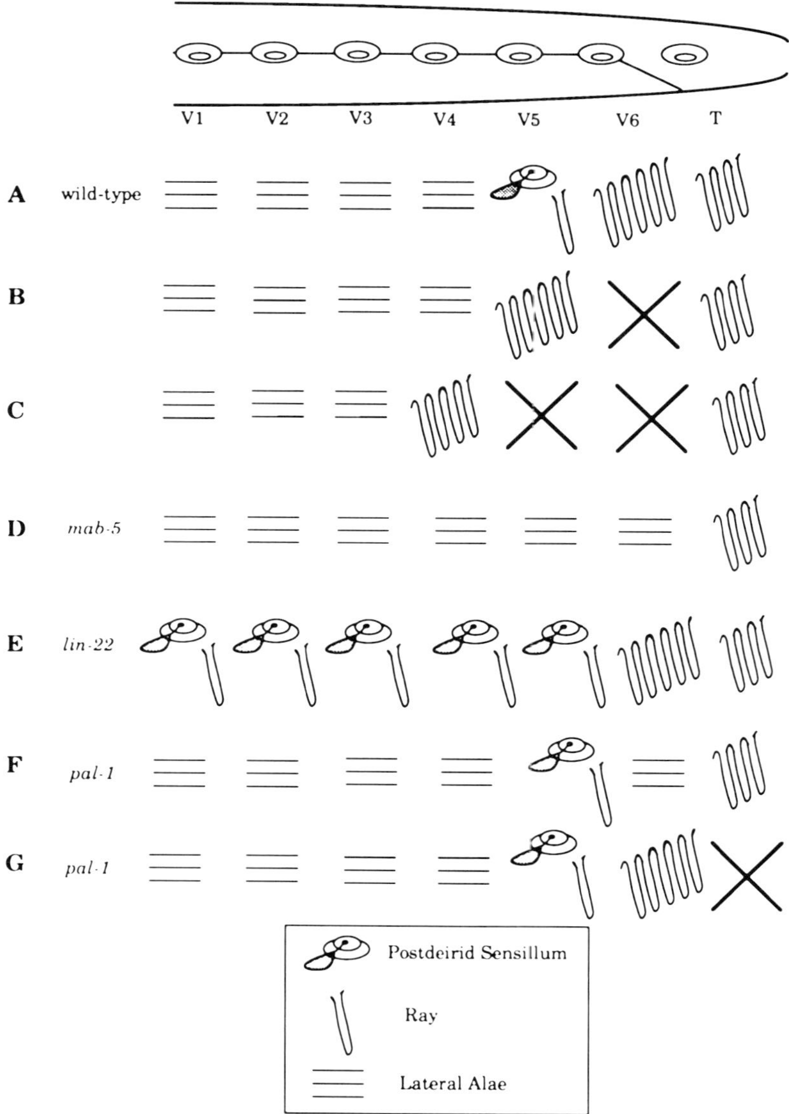

Figure 3. Specification of the postdeirid and ray sublineages. An "X" represents a cell ablated by laser microbeam irradiation. Data of Sulston and White (1980), Sulston *et al.* (1980), Fixsen *et al.* (1985), Kenyon (1986), and Waring and Kenyon (1990).

environmental (formation of rays) and autonomous (formation of postdeirid) factors.

Several genes affect positional specification among the V1–V6 cells. Mutations in *lin-22* cause V1–V4 as well as V5 to generate postdeirid cell groups (Fixsen *et al.*, 1985). In males, these more anterior cells also can produce a RCG, resulting in anterior ectopic rays (Fig. 3E). Thus, the wild-type *lin-22* gene product functions to make V1–V4 different from their posterior neighbor V5, and inhibits their production of postdeirid and ray cell groups. In contrast, mutations in *mab-5* (*m*ale *ab*normal) prevent V5 and V6 generation of rays; instead, V5 and V6 generate seam cells and lateral alae. *mab-5* mutations result in several abnormalities in cell lineage and behavior of cells in the posterior of the animal, suggesting that the wild-type *mab-5* product function distinguishes posterior cells, including V5 and V6, from their anterior homologs and neighbors (Kenyon, 1986).

Gene dosage experiments, in which the number of functional copies of *mab-5* were varied from zero to three in a *lin-22* mutant background, suggest that these two genes interact to specify the distinction between "anterior" and "posterior" neighbors (Kenyon, 1986). A double mutant defective in both *lin-22* and *mab-5* has a phenotype closer to the wild-type phenotype than a mutant of either *lin-22* or *mab-5* alone. However, these animals display no distinct delineation between cells that produce ray precursors and those that produce seam cells. Thus, *lin-22* functions to distinguish V1–V4 from their posterior neighbors, and *mab-5* functions to distinguish V5 and V6 from their anterior neighbors. *mab-5* encodes a homeodomain-containing protein (Costa *et al.*, 1988) and acts autonomously in V cells (Kenyon, 1986). These observations suggest that *mab-5* is a transcription factor that, if active in a cell, can activate functions necessary for ray production and repress functions necessary for alae production. The *mab-5* product appears to be spatially restricted: *mab-5* mRNA is found only in the posterior region of the body (Costa *et al.*, 1988). Thus, *mab-5* plays a key role in specification of the region-specific utilization of sublineages (in this case, the RCG).

Characterization of the genes *lin-22* and *mab-5* has provided only partial understanding of the cell interaction process elucidated by cell ablation experiments. Another gene, *pal-1* (*p*osterior *al*ae), provides more information about this process (Fig. 3F). Mutations in *pal-1* result in a phenotype similar to *mab-5*; in *pal-1* mutant males, V6 fails to make ray sensilla and instead produces alae (Waring and Kenyon, 1990; Fig. 3). V5, however, can generate a RCG. In contrast to the results in *mab-5* mutants, ablation of the T cell in *pal-1* mutant animals (the posterior neighbor of V6) results in V6 forming its full complement of rays (Fig. 3G). Waring and Kenyon (1990) suggest that, in wild-type animals, the T cell (and, by analogy, the other posterior V cells) inhibits production of rays by its anterior neighbor. Wild-type *pal-1* gene product, however, overrides this inhibition and allows V6 to make rays. This inhibition–counter–inhibition system of cell interactions is consistent with the ablation results discussed earlier. For instance, ablation of V5, V6, and T results in V4 producing up to 4 rays. From this perspective, V5 inhibits V4 production of rays, but removal of the inhibitor (V5 and V6) allows V4 division and production of rays. The *pal-1* gene encodes a homeodomain-containing protein and acts cell autonomously (Waring and Kenyon, 1991), suggesting that it acts in V6 to prevent a response to a negative signal from T. Analysis of these signaling pathways has identified putative transcription factors that play key roles in the regulation of cell fate, presumably by regulating or responding to the intercellular signals involved.

3. TEMPORAL CUES

lin-22, mab-5, and *pal-1* are components of a system that specifies the *position-specific* utilization of sublineages. In general, the *sex-specific* utilization of sublineages is under the control of the major sex-determining pathway (reviewed by Villeneuve and Meyer, 1990). Another set of genes controls the *stage-specific* utilization of sublineages (Ambros and Horvitz, 1984). *C. elegans,* like most nematodes, undergoes four larval stages (L1, L2, L3, and L4) prior to reaching adulthood. The postdeirid sublineage is generated during the L2 stage, and the RCG during the L3 and L4 stages. In mutants defective in any of the heterochronic genes, the temporal regulation of a variety of stage-specific events, including the use of sublineages (Ambros and Horvitz, 1984), is disrupted. For example, a *lin-14(lf)* mutation results in the use of the postdeirid sublineage by V5.a during the L1 stage instead of by V5.pa during the L2 stage as in wild type (Fig. 1A). A *lin-14* mutation also causes the generation of a ray sublineage during L2 and L3, one stage early. *lin-14* encodes a nuclear protein whose level decreases during development (Ambros and Horvitz, 1987; Ruvkun and Guisto, 1989). Defects in *lin-28,* another heterochronic gene, similarly cause V5, V6, and T to generate ray sublineages earlier than in wild type, during the L2 and L3 stages. The heterochronic genes thus provide information regarding the use of sublineages at relative times during development. Since the execution of the postdeirid and ray sublineages is normal although it occurs at an incorrect time, any necessary positional cues must be present normally at that time, or are produced by the cells generated by the sublineage.

B. Execution of a Sublineage

Once a blast cell is specified to generate a particular sublineage by genes such as those described earlier, the products of other genes are required for proper execution of that sublineage. Such genes specify the number, orientation, timing, and symmetry of cell division, and the types of progeny cells produced. Mutations in several genes disrupt the normal asymmetric cell divisions that are key aspects of the execution of particular sublineages. (It is impossible to rule out the possibility that rapid or very local cell interactions— for example, between sister cells—are responsible for the apparent autonomy of cell fate specification; even if such interactions do occur, it would not affect the general conclusions stated here.)

Mutations in the *lin-26* gene affect the asymmetric division of the 12 Pn cells (Ferguson and Horvitz, 1985; Fixsen *et al.*, 1985). During development of the *C. elegans* ventral cord, each of the 12 Pn cells divides to produce an anterior neuroblast (Pn.a) and a posterior cell (Pn.p); the Pn.p cells are either hypodermal or undergo regional and sex-specific divisions (see previous text). In *lin-26* mutants, the Pn.p cells differentiate into neurons or are neuroblasts. Therefore, both sisters are neuronal, like the wild-type Pn.a cells (Fig. 4). The *lin-26* gene could act in the parent cell (Pn) to establish the asymmetry of the cell division, or in one of the progeny cells to regulate neuronal as opposed to hypodermal cell type in response to the asymmetry of the division. Although the role of *lin-26* in asymmetric cell division is not known, the roles of two other genes necessary for execution of sublineages have been analyzed in more detail. The *lin-17* gene appears to establish the asymmetry of a parent cell and the *unc-86* gene appears to act in response to the asymmetry of a cell division.

Mutations in *lin-17* affect the asymmetric first division of several blast cells that divide postembryonically (Ferguson *et al.*, 1987; Sternberg and Horvitz, 1988). For example, in a wild-type male, the B blast cell divides to produce a larger anterior cell and a smaller posterior cell. The anterior cell divides further to produce a large number of cells, many of which make up the male spicules (Fig. 5). The posterior cell divides to produce a smaller number of progeny that primarily differentiate into proctodeal cells. *lin-17* mutations result in B.a and B.p cells of equal size; both cells then undergo multiple rounds of cell division. In effect, the wild-type asymmetric division of B becomes symmetrical, with both daughter cells behaving like B.a in the wild type. Since *lin-17* affects the cytokinesis of the B cell, it must act at or prior to the B cell division.

lin-17 mutations also affect the asymmetric division of the two T cells in the tail (Sternberg and Horvitz, 1988; E. Hedgecock, personal communication). In the hermaphrodite, T normally divides to produce an anterior daughter that gives rise primarily to hypodermal cells, and a posterior cell that gives rise to several neurons and the adult phasmid socket cells (Fig. 5). In *lin-17* mutant animals, T divides to produce two cells that have identical lineage and give rise to hypodermal cells, both behaving like the wild-type T.a daughter. Although mutations in *lin-17* affect the genesis of neuronal tissue and structures, *lin-17* is not promoting neural differentiation *per se.* The defect in the B cell division results in both progeny behaving like B.a, which in wild type gives rise to the complex neuronal sensory structures, the spicules, at the expense of B.p lineage, which normally produces primarily proctodeal and hypodermal cells. On the other hand, the transformation in the T cell results in both cells adopting the T.a hypodermal lineage at the expense of the T.p

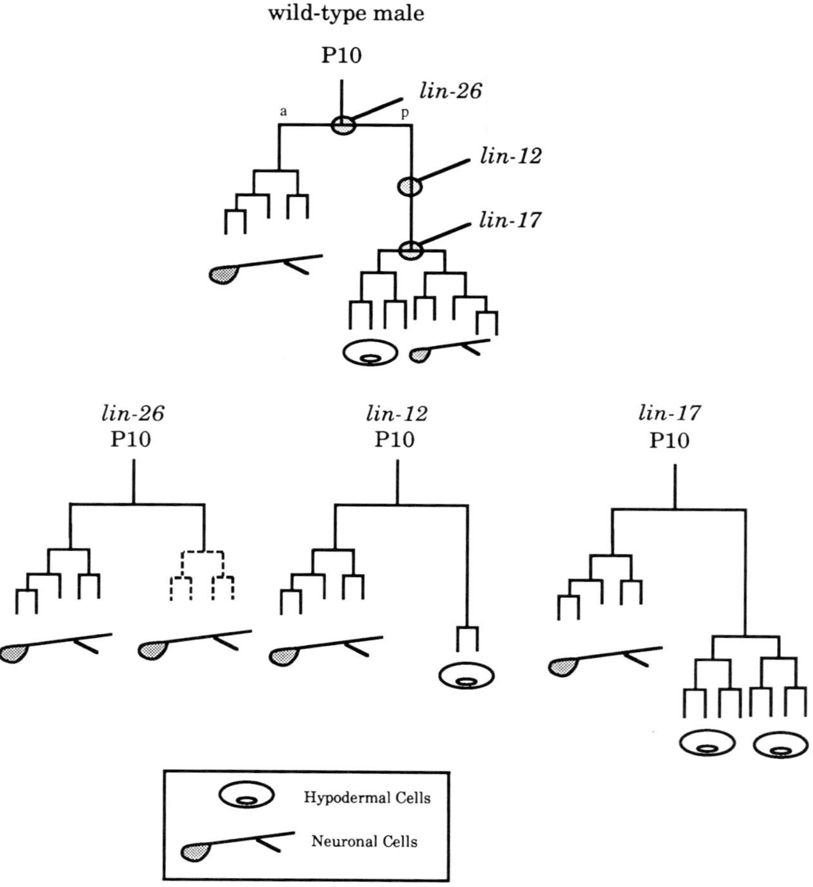

Figure 4. Sequential action of genes in nested sublineages. During the first larval stage, P10 generates an anterior (a) daughter that is a neuroblast and a posterior (p) daughter that is a member of the hook equivalence group. In the wild-type intact male, P10.p has the 2° fate and generates an anterior daughter that produces hypodermal cells and a posterior daughter that produces neurons. In a *lin-26* mutant, P10.p also can generate neurons; the number of neurons generated is variable (dashed lines). In a *lin-12* mutant, P10.p becomes either 3° (as shown) or 1°. In a hypodermal cells. Data of Greenwald *et al.* (1983), Fixsen *et al.* (1985), and Sternberg and Horvitz (1988).

neural lineage. In other words, *lin-17* activity does not, on its own, define a cell as a neuroblast. It is involved, however, in establishing asymmetrical cell division that contributes to the systematic generation of cells, including neurons, that will differentiate with specific unique fates.

Mutations in the *unc-86* gene (*unc*oordinated movement) cause abnormalities in some sublineages, but the result is not the transformation of asymmetric to symmetric division (Chalfie *et al.,* 1981). Instead, one of the progeny cells, rather than adopting its normal fate, appears to retain the fate of the parent. An *unc-86* mutation thus transforms the normal lineage to one

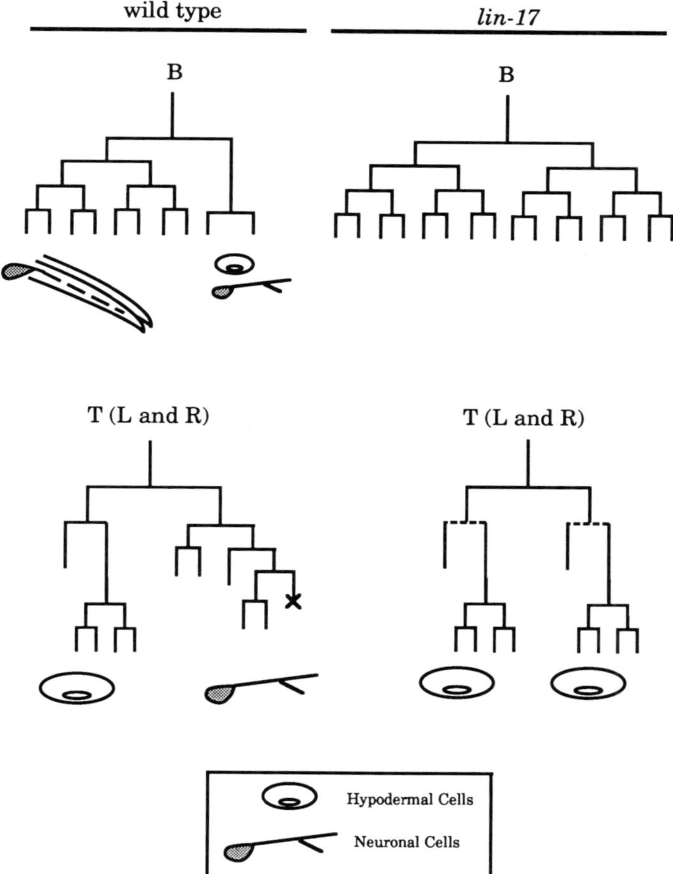

Figure 5. *lin-17* and asymmetric cell divisions. The anterior daughter of the male-specific ectoblast B generates spicule cells. The posterior daughter generates fewer cells. *lin-17* disrupts the asymmetry of this cell division. Data of Sulston and Horvitz (1977) and Sternberg and Horvitz (1988).

that has the characteristics of a stem cell lineage (see Fig. 6). One lineage that is affected by an *unc-86* mutation is the postdeirid sublineage of V5. During generation of the postdeirid in a wild-type animal, the V5.paa neuroblast generates an anterior neuron that is histochemically positive for dopamine and a posterior cell that produces a dopamine-negative neuron and a cell that undergoes programmed cell death (Fig. 1A). In animals mutant for *unc-86*, however, the anterior daughter is produced normally, but the posterior daughter divides to produce yet another anterior dopamine-positive neuron and a posterior cell that can often divide yet again. This reiteration can result in the production of not just one neuron, but a cluster of up to four neurons that are dopamine-positive. To interpret the *unc-86* phenotype, Chalfie *et al.* (1981) suggest that there may be latent cell lineage reiterations involved in the development of *C. elegans,* and that the wild-type activity of *unc-86* modifies and perhaps masks the underlying stem-cell-like lineage. *unc-86* encodes a product similar to mammalian transcription factors of the *pit-1* and *oct-1* family (Finney *et al.,* 1988; see Ruvkun and Finney, 1991, for review). Finney and Ruvkun (1990) demonstrated that *unc-86* protein accumulates in the nuclei of the affected daughter cells minutes after cell division. Thus, *unc-86* must respond to the asymmetry of the V5.paa cell division, and then act to specify an aspect of cell identity.

The distinction between utilization and execution of sublineages is nicely illustrated by the interactions of *lin-22* and *unc-86* mutations that affect utilization and execution, respectively. In a double mutant defective in both *unc-86* and *lin-22,* V1–V5 can all be specified to produce a postdeirid lineage due to the *lin-22* mutation, but the execution is abnormal due to the *unc-86* mutation (Horvitz *et al.,* 1983b). Thus, the double mutant can have a series of dopamine-positive clusters of neurons running along its length. In general, such observations suggest that the same genes are required for the execution of a sublineage wherever and whenever it is utilized. Mutation of *lin-22* overrides some of the positional controls over the utilization of the postdeirid sublineage. Since these sublineages are executed normally at their ectopic position, no positional information generated from outside the sublineage is needed, unless it is ectopically produced in the mutant.

III. Cell Type Specification and Differentiation (Late Neurogenesis)

Thus far we have discussed the specification of precursor cell fates via early acting genes that govern switches that distinguish between alternative sublineages or fates. These decisions eventually lead to the generation of cells, at the termini of the lineage, that, under normal circumstances, do not divide but differentiate into a specific cell type. This process requires two steps: specification and differentiation. Genes involved in specification function to make one cell different from its sister or neighbors. Differentiation refers to the acquisition of the characteristics of the cell once cell fate is already assigned; thus it might include genes that regulate the process (e.g., genes that act in regulatory pathways, for example, transcription factors and protein kinases) and those that execute it (e.g., genes necessary for the synthesis of neurotransmitters or microtubules). A major consequence of specification is the regulation of the genes involved in the specialized characteristics of each cell type. That is, specification genes normally regulate differentiation genes. Specification and differentiation are not always distinguishable; for example, a transcription factor might be involved in either specification or differentiation, depending on how much of cellular phenotype it controls and on our ability to assay its properties.

In this section, we will focus on these two steps in the context of the acquisition of three neuronal cell types: the touch cell, the hermaphrodite-specific neuron (HSN), and programmed cell death, which can be thought of as a differentiated state.

A. Touch Cell Developmental Pathway

The touch cells are a set of six neurons that extend their processes along the length of the animal. They are characterized by electron-dense large (15 protofilament) microtubules, specific to the touch cells, and an extracellular adaptation called the mantle, which serves to secure the cells to the cuticle (Chalfie *et al.*, 1985). At hatching the animal possesses four lateral touch cells—an anterior bilateral pair (the ALMs) and an analogous posterior pair (the PLMs). Two ventral cells (AVM and PVM) are generated later by post-embryonic divisions. The ALMs and AVM are electrically coupled and synapse via interneurons onto motor neurons of the body wall muscle (Chalfie *et al.*, 1985). The PLMs form a similar circuit. The structure and position of these cells make them likely candidates for mechanoreceptors. Cell ablation experiments indicate that these cells mediate a reflexive response to fine touch (Chalfie and Sulston, 1981). A wild-type animal, when stroked across the head or tail with an eyelash, will reflexively move backward or forward, respectively. Ablation of both ALMs in the young larvae result in animals that fail to respond to touch to the head, but still move in response to a harsher stimulus such as prodding with a platinum wire. These animals begin to respond variably to a gentle touch (about 30% of the time) 40 hr after hatching. This effect is mediated by AVM, which is forming functional synapses at about that time. When the ALMs and AVM are ablated, the variable response disappears. Ablation of both PLMs results in animals that fail to respond to touch to the tail. The function of PVM is unknown: ablation of PVM alone or in combination with any of the other neurons results in no observable behavioral defect.

Mutants defective in the touch cells were obtained by identifying animals that do not respond to the eyelash but do respond to a prod with a platinum wire (Chalfie and Sulston, 1981; Chalfie and Au, 1989). Such mutants are specifically defective in the touch response, in contrast with more general mutants such as uncoordinated mutants that are unable to move and, thus, unable to respond. From the mutants studied, 18 genes were identified whose products are necessary for proper touch cell generation, specification, and function (Fig. 6).

Mutations in two genes, *lin-32* and *unc-86,* prevent the generation of the touch cells by altering the lineages of their progenitors. *unc-86* mutants lack all the touch cells (Chalfie *et al.,* 1981), whereas in *lin-32* mutants the two ALM touch cells are formed normally, as evidenced by touch sensitivity of the head (Chalfie and Au, 1989). One lineage defect in *lin-32* animals affects the generation of the two ventral cells (AVM and PVM; see Fig. 6), which are generated from the Q neuroblasts on the right and left sides of the developing larva, respectively. In *lin-32* mutants, the initial precursor never divides. In *unc-86* mutants, the posterior daughter, which should give rise to a ventral cell, reiterates the fate of its mother (Fig. 6). Thus, AVM and PVM are not formed in either mutant. Mutations in these genes affect the lineages of several other cells and are not specific to the touch cells.

As discussed earlier, *unc-86* is a putative transcription regulator. The wild-type gene product, after generation of the proper cell, may activate (directly or indirectly) genes involved in the proper specification of that cell. One possible target gene is *mec-3.* Loss of *mec-3* function results in cells that fail to take on their normal touch cell fate. Since *mec-3* mutations confer no observable pleiotropic effects on other cell types, *mec-3* activity seems specific to the touch cells (however, see *mec-3* expression results discussed subsequently). In *mec-3* mutants, these cells lack the characteristics of the differentiated touch cells such as the 15-protofilament microtubules and the mantle. These cells do not fail to differentiate, but differentiate into a different type of neuron instead. Thus, although *mec-3* is required to specify touch cell identity, these cells are already constrained to a neuronal fate. Consistent with this observation, the posterior sisters of the touch cells are also neurons.

mec-3 contains both a homeodomain and a novel cysteine-rich motif, designated LIM *(lin-11, isl-1,* and *mec-3),* that is shared by *lin-11,* another *C. elegans* gene, and *isl-1,* which encodes the rat insulin I gene enhancer binding protein (Freyd *et al.,* 1990; Karlsson *et al.,* 1990). This motif, in conjunction

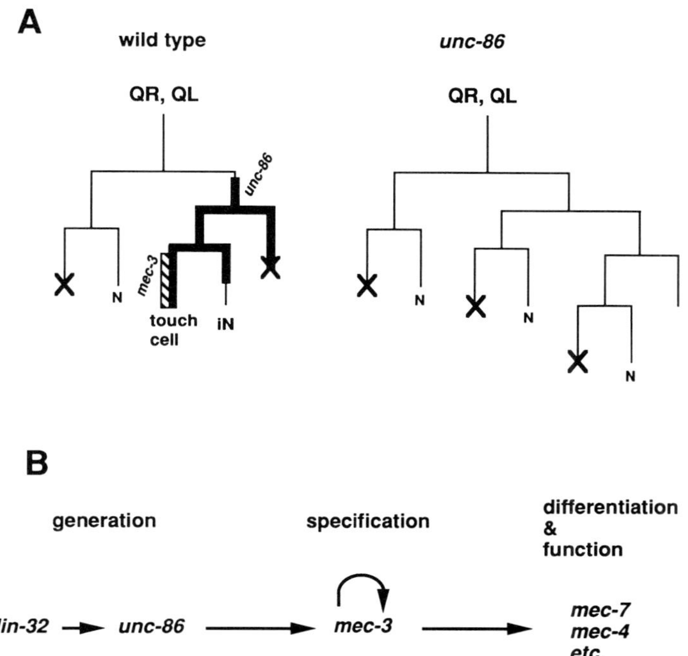

Figure 6. Specification of the touch cell. A. Two of the six touch cells, AVM and PVM, are generated by the postembryonic blast cells QR and QL, respectively. The heavy black lines indicate *unc-86* expression. The striped line indicates *mec-3* expression. In wild-type animals, only the posterior daughter expresses *unc-86;* Q.paa later expresses *mec-3* and differentiates as a touch cell. In an *unc-86* mutant, no *mec-3*-expressing cells are produced and no touch cells are formed. N, ciliated sensory neuron (AQR, PQR); TC, touch cell (AVM, PVM); iN, interneuron (SDQR, SDQL); X, programmed cell death. The ALM and PLM cells are formed embryonically, while the AVM and PVM cells are formed postembryonically. B. Genetic pathway for touch cell development. The generation of touch cells depends on *lin-32* and *unc-86*. *mec-3* is a key specifier of touch cell identity. Differentiation and function of the touch cells involve a number of genes. Data of Sulston and Horvitz (1977), Chalfie *et al.* (1981), White *et al.* (1986), Chalfie and Au (1989), Way and Chalfie (1989), and Finney and Ruvkun (1990).

with the homeodomain, suggests that *mec-3* could be a DNA-binding protein involved in transcription regulation. Since both *mec-3* and *lin-11* are thought to specify cell fate in asymmetric cell divisions, the *mec-3* protein product may be expressed only in the potential touch cells (anterior daughters) due to the action of some other, differentially segregated factor. Once expressed in an anterior daughter, the *mec-3* protein is proposed to activate its own transcription as well as that of other genes not activated in the posterior cells.

Consistent with its role in specification of the touch cells, the *mec-3* gene is expressed in the touch cells, as evinced by the expression of a *mec-3:lacZ* fusion (the *Echerichia coli lacZ* gene encoding β-galactosidase fused to the regulatory region of *mec-3*) in transgenic animals (Way and Chalfie, 1989). In addition, no β-galactosidase staining was observed in an *unc-86* mutant background, indicating that *mec-3* expression depends on *unc-86*. However, the *unc-86* protein is expressed in a total of 57 neurons, not all of which express *mec-3*, indicating that *unc-86* is not sufficient to activate *mec-3* (Finney and Ruvkun, 1990). Since the *mec-3:lacZ* fusion lacks *mec-3* activity, the possibility of autoregulation of *mec-3* could be examined. In a *mec-3* mutant background, β-galactosidase staining is initially normal, but gradually disappears after hatching. This observation indicates that the *mec-3* gene product is necessary for the maintenance of its own transcription, a feature common to many cell-type regulators (e.g., *myoD1;* Thayer *et al.,* 1989).

mec-3 is also expressed in two pairs of neurons called the PVDs and the FLPs (Way and Chalfie, 1989). The PVDs are known to be mechanoreceptors that mediate harsh touch. Further examination reveals that specification of the PVDs is also *mec-3* dependent, since *mec-3* mutants are harsh-touch insensitive. The function of the FLPs is not known; thus their dependence on *mec-3* cannot be tested. Because of their structure, however, they are also likely to be mechanosensory in nature. Thus, *mec-3* seems to specify 10 mechanoreceptors—the touch cells, PVDs, and FLPs. Other genes not regulated by *mec-3* must distinguish between these three neuronal types. Indeed, two genes known to affect touch cell differentiation (*mec-4* and *mec-17;* see subsequent text) affect *mec-3* expression in the touch cells but not in the PVDs and FLPs (Way and Chalfie, 1989).

Fifteen genes are candidates for acting downstream of *mec-3*. Five of these genes affect visible characteristics of the touch cells and are thus involved in touch cell differentiation. Mutations in three genes—*mec-7, mec-12,* and *mec-17*—affect the 15-protofilament microtubules. Mutations in two genes—*mec-1* and *mec-5*—affect the mantle. *mec-7* encodes a tubulin predicted to be touch-cell specific (Savage *et al.,* 1989). Mutations in the remaining 10 genes (except the dominant alleles of *mec-4*) result in touch cells that appear normal yet fail to function. These genes are thought to mediate touch cell function. The relatively late temperature-sensitive periods of mutations in several of these genes (after the cells differentiate) (Chalfie and Au, 1989) are consistent with their involvement in function of the touch cells. Also, a *mec-3* mutation is epistatic to a mutation in one putative function gene, *mec-4*. Dominant alleles of *mec-4* (*mec-4(d)*) cause the touch cells to degenerate, probably because of an abnormal function of a protein normally expressed in the touch cells (see Section III,C). In a double mutant carrying both *mec-3* and *mec-4(d)* mutations, the cells that would become the touch cells do not die, suggesting that *mec-3* is necessary for *mec-4* function and might be a transcriptional activator of *mec-4* (Fig. 6).

Our current understanding of touch cell specification is that *mec-3* is activated in a subset of cells generated from *unc-86*-dependent lineages. *mec-3* then acts intrinsically to regulate a battery of downstream genes specific to the touch cells. However, it is not known what causes the four types of touch cells to differentiate from one another. As Chalfie and Au (1989) point out, no genes found to date affect only a subset of the touch cells. One possibility is that specific genes are not needed for this stage of differentiation, and that differentiation relies solely on positional cues. Evidence for such non-autonomous cues comes from Chalfie *et al.* (1983), who used mutant phenotypes and ablations to study the differences between the two ventral touch cells, AVM and PVM. These cells are generated from homologous lineages. Q2 generates AVM on the right and Q1 generates PVM on the left. In the wild-type animal, Q1 and Q2 are generated close together. However, Q2 migrates a long distance anteriorly, whereas Q1 migrates a short distance posteriorly, leaving their progeny physically quite separated. AVM sends its axon anteriorly, where it enters the nerve ring and branches onto neurons there. In contrast, the PVM axon never reaches the nerve ring. In *mab-5* mutants, the migration of Q1 is abnormal and it moves anteriorly instead, resulting in a PVM that is more anterior than usual. In this background, the PVM axon sometimes reaches the nerve ring and forms the same synapses that AVM does. In these animals, PVM is capable of mediating a weak touch response in the absence of AVM and the two ALMs, similar to the response mediated by AVM in the absence of the ALMs. Conversely, ablation of cells that lie in the migratory path of Q2 prevents the cell from migrating as far forward as it normally does. In these cases, AVM develops in a way similar to PVM. Thus, the difference between these two neurons could be determined environmentally. However, this conclusion must be drawn cautiously, since *mab-5,* as already discussed, can transform cells from posterior to anterior fates. Thus, another interpretation is that PVM is transformed to the AVM fate in the *mab-5* background; thus it becomes capable of making connections to the nerve ring. This interpretation implies that the cell's identity, not its position, enables it to make the connections. The ablation experiment makes the former interpretation more likely, since the ability of AVM to make synapses seems to be determined by positional cues. The same is likely to be true for PVM.

Another example of external influences necessary for proper touch cell differentiation is seen in studies in which a pair of interneurons, the BDUs, are ablated in the young larva (Walthall and Chalfie, 1988). In the absence of these neurons, AVM does not make the proper connections in the nerve ring, as evinced by a lack of touch sensitivity in the absence of the ALMs. Ablation of the interneurons afterward has no effect, suggesting that the BDUs are only necessary while AVM is making its connections. These cells might serve to guide AVM to its proper target.

B. Hermaphrodite-Specific Neuron Developmental Pathway

The essential components of the egg-laying system in the hermaphrodite are the vulval muscles and a bilateral pair of neurons called the hermaphrodite-specific neurons (HSNs) that innervate the vulval muscles (Trent *et al.*, 1983). The HSNs are generated during embryogenesis in the tail (Sulston *et al.*, 1983). About 10 min after their birth, they begin migrating toward the middle of the animal where, in the hermaphrodite, they remain until the L4 stage, at which time they begin to differentiate. In the male, these neurons die about 0.5 hr after the migration begins, an example of sexual dimorphism generated by specific cell death. During the L4 stage in the hermaphrodite, the HSNs undergo maturation: the nucleus and nucleolus enlarge, a "hood" forms around the nucleus, and the cell sends out a single axon that grows ventrally to innervate the vulval (and uterine) muscles and then anteriorly to the nerve ring (White *et al.*, 1986).

Mutants that fail to lay eggs under normal laboratory culture conditions, but that have normal vulvae, could be defective in the vulval muscles or in the HSNs. Desai and Horvitz (1989) screened preferentially for HSN-defective mutants by looking for egg-laying defective mutants that would lay eggs in the presence of serotonin but not in the presence of imipramine. Since exogenous serotonin can bypass HSN function, responsiveness to serotonin demonstrates that the muscles are functional; since imipramine blocks serotonin reuptake and therefore potentiates the effects of endogenous serotonin, serotonin-responsive but imipramine-insensitive animals are likely to lack the source of serotonin—the HSNs. Nonfunctional HSNs presumably would not release any serotonin to potentiate; thus mutants with nonfunctional HSNs would fail to lay eggs in imipramine. Desai *et al.* (1988) also screened existing mutants for HSNs that were missing or looked abnormal under Nomarski optics. This screen identified mutants that failed the criteria of the first screen but were nonetheless abnormal. For example, some of the mutants in neural migration were identified only by such anatomical screening.

From these screens, Desai *et al.* (1988) identified many (but probably not all) of the genes involved in HSN development, and were able to deduce a genetic pathway for the development of the HSNs (Fig. 7). In a manner similar to the touch cell studies, genes were identified by mutations that affected HSN specification, differentiation, and function. No mutations, however, were

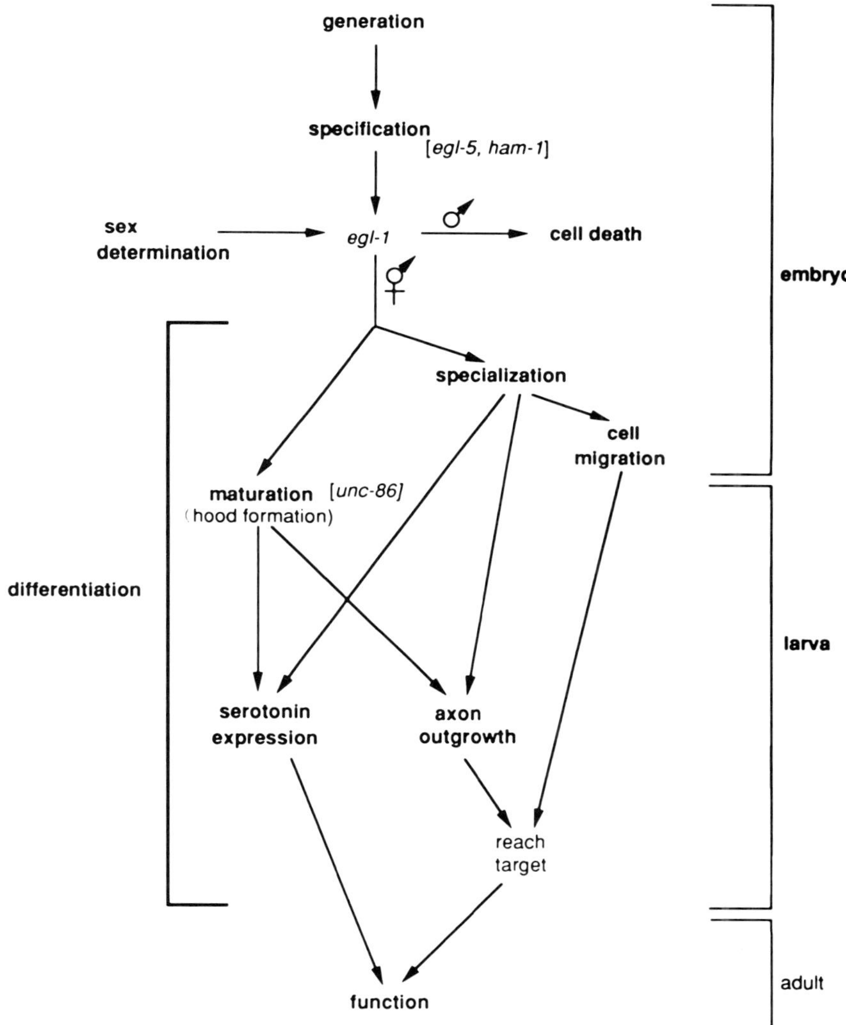

Figure 7. Specification of the HSN. Solid lines reflect the steps in the pathway as indicated by genetic evidence. No genes have been identified that affect hood formation specifically. Thus, one possibility is that the maturation step controls hood formation, which then allows serotonin expression and axonal outgrowth, and thereby allows function. Another possibility is that hood formation, serotonin expression, and axonal outgrowth are controlled independently by the maturation step, and allow function independently. Data of Desai *et al.* (1988).

found that affected HSN generation, possibly due to lethality or redundancy in the pathway.

Two genes are thought to specify the acquisition of the HSN identity. In *egl-5* mutants, the neurons are defective in all aspects of HSN development. Desai *et al.* proposed that *egl-5* initiates the HSN developmental program. In the absence of the wild-type gene product, the cells have an alternative fate, as do touch cells in a *mec-3* mutant. In *ham-1* mutants, the animal forms from zero to four HSN-like cells. The HSNs fail to exhibit some of their characteristic properties, and another pair of neurons (thought to be sisters of the HSNs, the PHBs) displays some HSN properties. Thus, the *ham-1* gene might distinguish the fates of these sister cells. As for the touch cells, in the absence of HSN specification by these two genes, the alternative cell fate is still neuronal.

Once the identity of the HSNs is specified, the neurons are subject to direction from the sex determination pathway. The decision whether or not to die is made in response to the major sex-determining pathway. Hermaphrodites defective in the genes *tra-2, her-1, egl-41,* and *egl-1* lack HSNs (Trent *et al.,* 1983; Desai *et al.,* 1988), which are generated but die like the HSNs in the male. However, in a *ced-3* double mutant background, which prevents cell death (see Section III,C), the HSNs survive and differentiate normally, suggesting that the genes in question cause a sexual transformation of the cells to the male fate, which in this case is cell death. Indeed, the first two genes *(tra-1* and *her-1)* are known to act in the sex determination pathway (Hodgkin, 1987) and the third *(egl-41)* is suspected to, since it affects many aspects of sexual morphology. *egl-1,* however, appears to affect only the HSNs. Thus, the initiation of programmed death in these cells appears to require two conditions: specification of HSN identity and determination of male sex. *egl-1* might be a gene that links these two decisions. It might function specifically in the HSNs to allow them to respond to the sex determination pathway and take on the hermaphrodite-specific fate of survival.

Once the HSNs have been specified and determined to survive, a series of genes acts downstream in the process of differentiation. Although mutations in some genes affect a single aspect of the differentiated neuron (e.g., serotonin expression), three classes of mutations affect multiple traits. These pleiotropic effects could arise by a defect in a regulatory protein or a non-regulatory protein required for the execution of more than one function.

Three genes (including *unc-86*) affect HSN hood formation, serotonin expression, and axonal outgrowth (Desai *et al.,* 1988). In mutants defective in any of these genes, the presumptive HSNs appear normal until the L4 stage, at which time they fail to undergo the normal process of nuclear growth and hood formation. This is the first of a series of developmental steps that begin after a period of quiescence. Genes that control this step, termed "maturation," might regulate a transition from early to late HSN differentiation; *unc-86* may play a role in the initiation of differentiation. In doing so, it activates the genes necessary for a number of traits—hood formation, serotonin expression, and axon outgrowth.

Both migration and serotonin expression are affected by mutations in five genes (Desai *et al.*, 1988). At least two genes also affect axonal outgrowth. (Results for the others are inconclusive, since failure to stain for serotonin makes axon outgrowth difficult to score.) Since the defects are specific to the HSNs, these pleiotropies are probably due to a defect in another regulatory step rather than due to a defect in proteins common to the three processes. This additional step in the developmental pathway, termed "specialization," is common to migration, serotonin expression, and axonal outgrowth. The five genes involved probably act to turn on necessary downstream genes for these processes. Unlike maturation, specialization is not temporally specific since it acts both early (in cell maturation) and late (in serotonin expression).

Downstream of these putative regulatory genes are genes involved in specific aspects of differentiation—cell migration (six genes), axonal outgrowth (six genes), and transmitter expression (two genes). Three other genes affect both cell migration and axon outgrowth. With the exception of four genes involved in migration *(egl-18, egl-20, egl-21,* and *mig-1)*, mutations in all of these genes affect other neuronal cell types. Defects in the serotonin-expression genes, *cat-1* and *cat-4,* result in decreased serotonin staining throughout the animal. The remaining genes are thought to act in global cell–axon guidance rather than in specific guidance of particular cells (as evinced by their uncoordinated phenotypes). For example, *unc-6,* which affects both HSN migration and outgrowth of AVM and PVM axons, appears necessary for dorsal–ventral migration in general (Hedgecock *et al.,* 1990). *unc-6* encodes laminin B2, a major component of basal lamina, to which these neurons have access (Ishii *et al.,* as cited in Hedgecock *et al.,* 1990).

Six genes have been identified that act downstream of those just discussed. Mutations in these genes result in neurons that appear normal by all criteria yet fail to drive egg-laying. The temperature-sensitive period of one of these genes is after HSN differentiation. For these reasons, the genes are thought to be involved in HSN function rather than development.

A proposed pathway for HSN development is outlined in Fig. 7. The pathway is based on the assumption that these mutations reduce or eliminate the function of the genes they define; thus, the normal function of the gene can be inferred from the defect. Each gene will have to be analyzed in detail to verify this assumption. The characteristic of migration, axonal outgrowth, and serotonin expression can be specified independently since mutations can be found that selectively affect each trait. However, four classes of genes have multiple effects and are thus thought to be regulatory genes for reasons discussed previously. Initially, the cells are determined to take on the HSN identity. These cells are then subject to the sex determination pathway: only hermaphrodite HSNs continue to differentiate. The pathway then branches. The two steps of "maturation" and "specialization," which were added solely because of genetic evidence, control partially overlapping functions. Maturation affects hood formation, axonal outgrowth, and serotonin expression. Specialization affects cell migration, axonal outgrowth, and serotonin expression. These latter steps ultimately control the function of the HSNs.

As for the touch cells, some aspects of HSN differentiation are likely to be environmentally influenced rather than intrinsically specified. In lineage mutants defective in ventral cord development, the HSNs, while apparently normal at hatching, are often displaced or missing in older animals (Sulston and Horvitz, 1981). This observation suggests that some of the ventral cord neurons might be necessary for proper HSN development. Cell ablation experiments done by Li and Chalfie (1990) have shown that proper branching of the HSNs is partly dependent on the presence of the vulval cells (as opposed to vulval muscle). Abnormal branching is also seen in mutants in which the vulva is missing. Finally, in mutants with more than one cluster of vulval tissue, ectopic branching is observed. In a complementary set of experiments, Thomas *et al.* (1990) have demonstrated that the HSN branches follow the position of the vulva in a mutant in which the entire egg-laying system is displaced. Thus, although other aspects of differentiation may be under intrinsic control, axonal branching appears to require external cues.

C. Cell Death

During the course of development of the wild-type *C. elegans* hermaphrodite, 131 cells are generated that ultimately die. As in other animals, cell death figures prominently in *C. elegans* neural development: of the 131 cells that undergo programmed cell death (see subsequent text), 107 are in lineages that lead only to neurons or neuronal support cells. The systematic nature of the process, and the fact that uncontrolled cell death could be devastating to the animal, leads one to believe that cell death is a tightly regulated process.

I. TYPES OF CELL DEATH

Three types of cell death have been identified in *C. elegans* (Fig. 8). Cell degeneration occurs in some mutant backgrounds. This type of cell death, not seen in wild-type animals, is thought to be due to toxicity of an altered gene product (Chalfie and Wolinsky, 1990). Chalfie and Wolinsky (1990) have shown that a mutation in the *deg-1* gene, which encodes a putative membrane

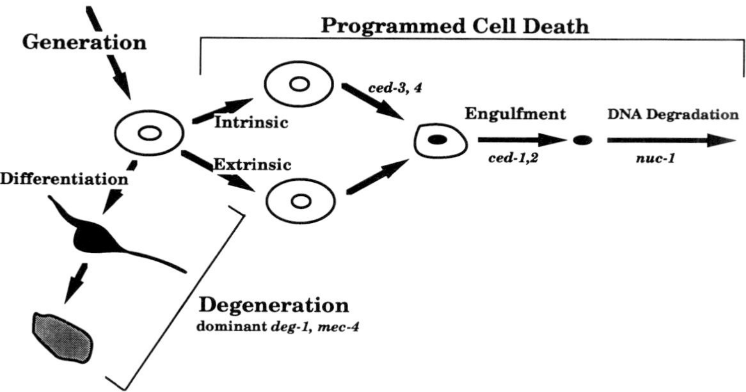

Figure 8. Programmed and degenerative cell death. Three types of cell death in nematodes are summarized. Programmed cell death occurs during development of wild-type *C. elegans* by mechanisms intrinsic to the doomed cell or by extrinsic mechanisms in "murder" of a neighboring cell; these pathways converge on a common pathway involving the destruction of the cell. Degeneration occurs in mutant animals carrying rare dominant mutations in particular genes. Data of Ellis and Horvitz (1986), Hedgecock *et al.* (1983; cited in Horvitz, 1988), and Chalfie and Wolinsky (1991).

protein, results in degeneration of touch cells and other neurons. The late onset of the *deg-1* mutant phenotype and the genetic properties of the *deg-1* mutation suggest that degeneration is a consequence of a poisonous gene product that is expressed in differentiated touch cells. *mec-4(d)* is another mutation defining a second gene that can mutate to cause a phenotype like that of *deg-1*. Driscoll and Chalfie (1991) have shown that *mec-4* encodes a product similar to the *deg-1* product. These genes thus define a family of proteins, dubbed "degenerins," that can mutate to caused a dominant degenerative death of the cells in which they are expressed. *mec-6* mutations disrupt touch cell function, and also block the degeneration caused by a *deg-1* or a *mec-4(d)* mutation (Chalfie and Wolinsky, 1990). *mec-6* might regulate the synthesis or localization of *deg-1* and *mec-4,* or be a target or co-factor of their actions. Study of these genes might well illuminate not only the mechanisms of touch cell differentiation, but also one mechanism of neuronal degeneration.

A second type of cell death is represented by two cases in the development of the male tail in which "murder" is thought to be responsible for a cell death (Sulston and White, 1980; Sulston *et al.,* 1980). In these cases, if a particular neighboring cell is ablated, the cell that normally dies is able to survive.

A third, much more common, type of cell death is intrinsically programmed cell death. From their birth, affected cells appear specified to die:

they have small compact nuclei and do not show the differentiated characteristics of their neighbors (Sulston and Horvitz, 1977). The cells die in a stereotypical process that includes an increased refractility of the nucleus, engulfment by a neighboring cell, and enzymatic breakdown (Robertson and Thomson, 1982; Hedgecock *et al.,* 1983). Removal of neighboring cells, including the cell that normally engulfs the dying cell, does not result in their survival. Thus, it appears that these cells follow a cell autonomous program of death.

2. ROLES OF CELL DEATH

Programmed cell death can play an important role in the development of an animal in several ways. First, lineages might be programmed so some unnecessary cells must be generated along with the necessary cells. These unnecessary cells can then be eliminated via programmed cell death, which can serve to modify a sublineage locally. Many of the cell deaths observed in *C. elegans* may be of this class. For instance, in the hermaphrodite, P(3–8).aap differentiate as motor neurons, whereas the lineage homologs, P(1,2,9–12).aap, undergo programmed cell death instead. Mutations in the gene *lin-39* result in a regional transformation of cell death fate, in which P(3–8).aap adopt the fate of their lineal homologs and undergo programmed cell death (Fixsen *et al.* 1985). Thus the *lin-39* gene product is likely to be involved in specifying regional differences in cell death among the P(1–12).aap homologs.

Second, over the course of evolution, cells that are present or even necessary in one species at one time may not be necessary for its descendants in a different time or environment. Elimination of specific cells can be a fairly simple mode of rapid change in the morphology of an animal during the course of evolution. For instance, specific cell death early in the development of the somatic gonad of the nematode *Panagrellus redivivus* contributes to the production of its characteristic single-arm gonad, which contrasts with the two-arm gonad of *C. elegans* (Sternberg and Horvitz, 1981).

Third, cell death also can be used to eliminate cells that function transiently but are no longer needed [e.g., eclosion muscles and motor neurons in *Drosophila* (Kimura and Truman, 1990) and *Manduca sexta* (Truman, 1983); Mauthner cells in ascidians (Zottoli, 1978)]. In *C. elegans,* the linker cell in the male somatic gonad functions to guide the developing gonad as it migrates toward the tail, and to link the gonad to the cloaca. Once this function has been completed, the linker cell's death is induced by another cell (Kimble and Hirsh, 1979; Sulston and White, 1980; Sulston *et al.,* 1980).

Finally, another function of cell death is to generate sexual dimorphism in the animal. Neurons are generated in both sexes and undergo cell death in one sex. This has been established in song bird song nuclei (Konishi and Akutagawa, 1985), rat bulbocavernosus nucleus (Breedlove, 1984), and rat preoptic area (Murakami and Arai, 1989). In *C. elegans,* two types of neurons are generated that undergo this fate. The CEMs (cephalic companion neurons) die in the hermaphrodite and the HSNs die in the male (Sulston *et al.,* 1983). However, this process of creating sexual dimorphism is only used for embryonically generated neurons. Further sexual dimorphism in the post-embryonic lineages is generated by differential generation of cells rather than differential elimination (e.g., division of the B and Y blast cells in the male).

3. GENETIC CONTROL OF PROGRAMMED CELL DEATH

Mutations in several genes have been identified that disrupt different steps of the normal cell death process. For instance, mutations in the genes *ced-3* and *ced-4* disrupt cell death, so the cells do not appear to initiate the cell death program (Ellis and Horvitz, 1986). These genes affect only programmed cell deaths, since "murders" and neuronal degeneration are not blocked by these mutations (Ellis and Horvitz, 1986; Chalfie and Wolinsky, 1990). Mutations in the genes *ced-1* and *ced-2* result in cells that die but remain in the refractile stage for tens of hours, failing to undergo normal engulfment and breakdown (Hedgecock *et al.,* 1983). Mutations in the gene *nuc-1* result in reduced endodeoxyribonuclease activity (Albertson *et al.,* 1978), so targeted cells undergo cell death, but their condensed chromatin persists in the cells that engulf them because the DNA cannot be fully degraded. Unlike *ced-3* and *ced-4,* these last three genes also function in cell "murders," since mutations also block the engulfment and degradation of "murdered" cells (Fig. 7). Finally, a number of mutations have been isolated that block cell death in a subset of the cells normally affected. These mutations define the *ces* genes (reviewed by Horvitz, 1988). Double mutant analysis has shown that (1) *ces* function is required for *ced* function, (2) *ced-3* and *ced-4* function is required for *ced-1* and *ced-2* function (i.e., they act upstream in the pathway), and (3) *ced-1* and *ced-2* function is required for *nuc-1* function (Ellis and Horvitz, 1986).

The results are consistent with the idea that programmed cell death is an actively chosen cell fate. Cells die as a result of the activation of genes that set into motion a program of self-destruction. Programmed cell death in nematodes is similar to cell death in vertebrates. For example, macromolecular synthesis is required for the rapid death of nerve growth factor (NGF)-dependent cells deprived of NGF (Martin *et al.,* 1988; Wallace and Johnson, 1989). The nematode studies suggest that initiation of the death program might occur by different mechanisms (intrinsic *ced-3,4*-dependent as opposed to extrinsic *ced-3,4*-independent), but that later steps in the pathway are common (Fig. 8). It is unlikely that *ced-3* and *ced-4* actually specify the cell death fate, since they have been shown to act downstream of other genes (*ces* genes and *egl-1;* see Section III,B) that seem to perform the function of specification. *ced-3* or *ced-4* may act to regulate cell death by initiating the process once the cell death fate is specified, possibly by regulating downstream genes. Alternatively, they could simply act directly to kill the cell.

The fact that ablation of neighboring cells in a wild-type animal does not disrupt programmed cell death suggests that this type of cell death is a cell autonomous process. In keeping with this idea, mosaic analysis experiments by Yuan and Horvitz (1990) suggest that both *ced-3* and *ced-4* act autonomously to result in the death of the cell. These results are consistent with the hypothesis that programmed cell death is cell autonomous; however, they do not rule out the possibility that *ced-3* and *ced-4* are receptors on transducers (and, thus, cell autonomous) in a process that involves cell interaction. It is also possible that *ced-3* and *ced-4* act in the parent of the dying cell (see Yuan and Horvitz, 1990, for discussion).

Although *ced-3* and *ced-4* mutant animals have extra cells, since they retain those that normally would have died, the presence of these extra cells does not appear to be detrimental to the animals, since there is no gross phenotype (for example, excessive cell division) in *ced* mutants. There is compelling circumstantial evidence that many of these spared cells are capable of differentiation. Some of the cells that die are derived from sublineages that generate serotonergic and dopaminergic neurons. In *ced-3* and *ced-4* mutants, additional cells stain for these transmitters (Ellis and Horvitz, 1986). Avery and Horvitz (1987) have demonstrated conclusively that a specific surviving cell can differentiate into a functional neuron. The M4 neuron innervates part of the pharynx and is necessary for feeding. If this cell is ablated in a newly hatched larva, the animal cannot move food from the anterior part of its pharynx to its intestine, and its growth is arrested. In wild-type animals, no other cell can function in the place of M4. However, if this cell is ablated in a *ced-3* mutant, the animal can often grow into a fertile, if slightly stunted, adult. Thus, a cell that has survived because of the *ced-3* mutation can functionally replace (at least in part) the ablated cell. The sister of the normal M4, which dies in wild-type animals, is likely to be the cell that can function as M4 in the ablated animal. The fact that only partial replacement is seen might indicate that only some of the spared cells can differentiate properly; if so, the presence of additional undifferentiated cells might have no phenotypic consequence.

D. Comparisons

The systems discussed—touch cell and HSN development and, to a certain extent, programmed cell death—illustrate the common process by which cell fates are attained (Fig. 9). In touch cell and HSN development,

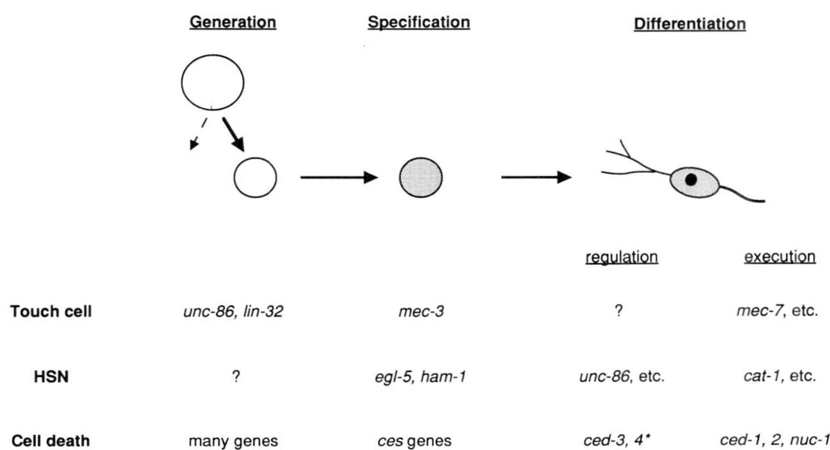

	Generation	Specification	Differentiation	
			regulation	execution
Touch cell	*unc-86, lin-32*	*mec-3*	?	*mec-7*, etc.
HSN	?	*egl-5, ham-1*	*unc-86*, etc.	*cat-1*, etc.
Cell death	many genes	*ces* genes	*ced-3, 4* *	*ced-1, 2, nuc-1*

Figure 9. Comparison of three examples of cell fate specification. See text and Figures 6, 7, and 8 for details. It is possible that *ced-3* and *ced-4* are involved in early steps of execution.

genes can be identified that appear to be responsible for specifying their unique cell fates (*mec-3* and *egl-5,* respectively). Downstream of these genes are those that act to regulate or carry out the process of differentiation. In the case of the touch cells, these genes are easy to categorize since they directly control the expression of touch-cell-specific traits. The HSNs, on the other hand, also require genes that, although not directly responsible for the expression of HSN-specific traits, serve to coordinate their expression. These genes have been categorized under the terms maturation and specialization. For cell death, the *ces* genes appear to specify which cells will die, whereas *ced-3* and *ced-4* might act as regulatory genes to initiate and coordinate the program of death.

Although analogous genes have been identified that direct specific neuronal fates, few genes have been identified that have a function common to the touch cell and the HSN developmental pathways, that is, genes that direct cells to become neurons in general. The one common regulatory gene is *unc-86.* However, it appears to have different roles in the two developmental pathways. In HSN development, it is involved in the transition of immature neurons to mature HSNs. In contrast, in touch cell development *unc-86* acts in the precursors to promote correct generation of the cells. Thus, this regulatory protein seems to act in different ways at different times. This is reminiscent of the homeotic and segmentation genes in *Drosophila* (see Chapter 5), which also specify cell fate in both precursor cells and postmitotic neurons.

Clearly, the final decision that leads to a specific cell fate is not made in isolation of previous decisions. Specification of a particular cell type, such as the HSNs, is the result of every cell division (cell fate choice) leading to its generation, with a reduction in potential cell fates along the way. This process can be seen by looking at the alternative fates these cells adopt in the absence of the ultimate regulatory decision. For example, in touch cell development, the lack of *mec-3* function results in cells that fail to differentiate as touch cells, but are neurons nonetheless. Similarly, in HSN development, mutations in the genes *ham-1* and *egl-5* result in non-HSN cells that still appear to be neuronal in nature. No mutations have been found in which these cells are generated yet fail to take on a neuronal fate. In this context, it is interesting that the cells generated from neuronal lineages that normally undergo cell death take on a neuronal appearance when allowed to live in a *ced-3* mutant background. These cells, failing their normal fate, still appear constrained by their ancestry to the neuronal fate.

A few conclusions can be drawn concerning the complexity of cell-type specification and differentiation. Genes acting in these pathways "instruct" the cells to their fates rather than to alternative fates. The more genes that participate, the greater the information provided, which increases the potential for both specificity and plasticity in the system.

The HSN genetic pathway is more complex than that of the touch cells (compare Figs. 6B and 7): the HSNs have an additional step of maturation (which corresponds to their undifferentiated state) for a period of time after specification. In contrast, the touch cells begin differentiation soon after migrating to their final positions. Thus, the additional regulatory step of maturation is necessary to initiate the process of differentiation in the HSNs (beginning with hood formation) after a period of quiescence. In the touch cells, no such step is required.

The divergence of HSN differentiation into two pathways ("maturation" and "specialization") also seems to confer a degree of plasticity in this system that is absent in the touch cell system, since it allows some aspects of differentiation to be regulated independent of each other. For example, serotonin expression and axonal outgrowth appear to be dependent on hood formation but can occur independent of cell migration. Thus the HSNs in cell migration mutants are still functional, since increased axon outgrowth is capable of compensating for the migration defect. Such compensation is not seen in the touch cells: if AVM is prevented from assuming its normal position in the ventral cord, the posteriorly displaced cell fails to make its connections to nerve ring (Chalfie *et al.,* 1983). Presumably, axonal outgrowth in the touch cells is programmed by intrinsic mechanisms to proceed to a specific distance and cannot compensate for alterations in cell migration.

IV. Prospects

Our understanding of cell-type specification in *C. elegans* has reached an exciting phase. The powerful genetics of this organism has led to the identification of hundreds of genes involved in the generation, specification, and differentiation or programmed death of individual neurons. Functional relationships among these genes have been inferred from genetic studies. With the advent of the genome mapping project (Coulson *et al.,* 1986, 1988) and techniques for rapid production of transgenic animals (Fire, 1986; Mello *et al.,* 1991), the facility of molecular biological analysis has caught up with genetics and developmental biology. Thus, most genes can now be cloned readily, and their roles can begin to be understood mechanistically. Conserved classes of gene products, such as transcription factors [*unc-86* (Finney *et al.,* 1988); *lin-11* (Freyd *et al.,* 1990); *mec-3* (Way and Chalfie, 1988); *mab-5* (Costa *et al.,* 1988)] and protein kinases [*daf-1* (Georgi *et al.,* 1990); *let-23* (Aroian *et al.,* 1990)] have been found to be encoded by genetically defined genes. As in all organisms, the introduction of polymerase chain reaction (PCR)-based technology has allowed the rapid cloning of homologous genes. PCR or low-stringency hybridization has helped identify *C. elegans* genes encoding such potential cell regulatory proteins as homeodomain-containing transcription factors (Burglin *et al.,* 1989), G protein subunits (Fina Silva and Plasterk, 1990; Lochrie *et al.,* 1990; van der Voorn *et al.,* 1990), and protein kinases (Kamb *et al.,* 1989; Gross *et al.,* 1990; Hu and Rubin, 1990; Lu *et al.,* 1990). This type of study indicates the universality of such gene families. Clearly, each intensively studied organism can now contribute to the effort to elucidate general mechanisms of cell regulation according to its strength as an experimental system. For *C. elegans,* these strengths are based on the small genome, rapid generation time, small cell number, and invariant development, and hold out the promise of understanding entirely the specification of all 302 hermaphrodite and 381 male neurons. Such intensive analysis might reveal the full spectrum of mechanisms that specify neuronal identity in all organisms.

Acknowledgments

We thank Nancy Bonini, Chand Desai, Gregg Jongeward, Linda Huang, Min Han, and Jamie Mazer for discussions and editorial comments, and Mike Finney, Bob Herman, and Ron Plasterk for preprints. H. M. C. is an NSF predoctoral fellow. K. L. is a Hansen graduate fellow. P. W. S. is a Presidential Young Investigator of the National Science Foundation (NSF) and an investigator of the Howard Hughes Medical Institute.

References

Albertson, D. G., Sulston, J. E., and White, J. G. (1978). Cell cycling and DNA replication in a mutant blocked in cell division in the nematode *Caenorhabditis elegans*. *Dev. Biol.* **63**, 165–178.

Albertson, D. G., and Thomson, J. N. (1976). The pharynx of *Caenorhabditis elegans*. *Phil. Trans. R. Soc. Lond. B.* **274**, 299–325.

Ambros, V., and Horvitz, H. R. (1984). Heterochronic mutants of the nematode *Caenorhabditis elegans*. *Science* **226**, 409–416.

Ambros, V., and Horvitz, H. R. (1987). The *lin-14* locus of *C. elegans* controls the time of expression of specific postembryonic developmental events. *Genes Devel.* **1**, 398–414.

Aroian, R. V., Koga, M., Mendel, J. E., Ohshima, Y., and Sternberg, P. W. (1990). The *let-23* gene necessary for *C. elegans* vulval induction encodes a tyrosine kinase of the EGF receptor subfamily. *Nature (London)* **348**, 693–699.

Aroian, R. V., and Sternberg, P. W. (1991). Multiple functions of *let-23*, a *C. elegans* receptor tyrosine kinase gene required for vulval induction. *Genetics* **128**, 251–267.

Avery, L., and Horvitz, H. R. (1987). A cell that dies during wild-type *C. elegans* development can function as a neuron in a *ced-3* mutant. *Cell* **51**, 1071–1078.

Avery, L., and Horvitz, H. R. (1989). Pharyngeal pumping continues after laser killing of the pharyngeal nervous system of *C. elegans*. *Neuron* **3**, 473–485.

Beitel, G., Clark, S., and Horvitz, H. R. (1990). The *Caenorhabditis elegans ras* gene *let-60* acts as a switch in the pathway of vulval induction. *Nature (London)* **348**, 503–509.

Bodmer, R., Caretto, R., and Jan, Y.-N. (1989). Neurogenesis of the peripheral nervous system in *Drosophila* embryos: DNA replication patterns and cell lineages. *Neuron* **3**, 21–32.

Breedlove, S. M. (1984). Androgen forms sexually dimorphic spinal nucleus by saving motorneurons from programmed death. *Soc. Neurosci. Abstr.* **10**, 927.

Brenner, S. (1974). The genetics of *Caenorhabditis elegans*. *Genetics* **77**, 71–94.

Burglin, T. R., Finney, M., Coulson, A., and Ruvkun, G. (1989). *Caenorhabditis elegans* has scores of homeobox-containing genes. *Nature (London)* **341**, 239–243.

Chalfie, M., and Sulston, J. E. (1981). Developmental genetics of the mechanosensory neurons of *Caenorhabditis elegans*. *Dev. Biol.* **82**, 358–370.

Chalfie, M., Horvitz, H. R., and Sulston, J. E. (1981). Mutations that led to reiterations in the cell lineages of *Caenorhabditis elegans*. *Cell* **24**, 59–69.

Chalfie, M., Thomson, J. N., and Sulston, J. E. (1983). Induction of neuronal branching in *Caenorhabditis elegans*. *Science* **221**, 61–63.

Chalfie, M., Sulston, J. E., White, J. G., Southgate, E., Thomson, J. N., and Brenner, S. (1985). The neural circuit for touch sensitivity in *Caenorhabditis elegans*. *J. Neurosci.* **5(4)**, 956–964.

Chalfie, M., and White, J. (1988). The nervous system. *In* "The Nematode *Caenorhabditis elegans*," (W. B. Wood, ed.), pp. 337–392. New York: Cold Spring Harbor Laboratory Press.

Chalfie, M., and Au, M. (1989). Genetic control of differentiation of the *Caenorhabditis elegans* touch receptor neurons. *Science* **243**, 1027–1033.

Chalfie, M., and Wolinsky, E. (1990). The identification and suppression of inherited neurodegeneration in *Caenorhabditis elegans*. *Nature (London)* **345**, 410–416.

Costa, M., Weir, M., Coulson, A., Sulston, J., and Kenyon, C. (1988). Posterior pattern formation in *C. elegans* involves position-specific expression of a gene containing a homeobox. *Cell* **55**, 747–756.

Coulson, A. R., Sulston, J., Brenner, S., and Karn, J. (1986). Toward a physical map of the genome of the nematode *Caenorhabditis elegans. Proc. Natl. Acad. Sci. U.S.A.* **83**, 7821–7825.

Coulson, A., Waterston, R., Kiff, J., Sulston, J., and Kohara, Y. (1988). Genome linking with yeast artificial chromosomes. *Nature (London)* **335**, 184–186.

Davis, C. G. (1990). The many faces of epidermal growth factor repeats. *New Biol.* **2**, 410–419.

Desai, C., Garriga, G., McIntire, S. L., and Horvitz, H. R. (1988). A genetic pathway for the development of the *Caenorhabditis elegans* HSN motor neurons. *Nature (London)* **336**, 638–646.

Desai, C., and Horvitz, H. R. (1989). *Caenorhabditis elegans* mutants defective in the functioning of the motor neurons responsible for egg laying. *Genetics* **121**, 703–721.

Driscoll, M., and Chalfie, M. (1991). The *mec-4* gene is a member of a family of *Caenorhabditis elegans* genes that can mutate to induce neuronal degeneration. *Nature (London)* **349**, 588–593.

Ellis, H. M., and Horvitz, H. R. (1986). Genetic control of programmed cell death in the nematode *C. elegans. Cell* **44**, 817–829.

Ferguson, E. L., and Horvitz, H. R. (1985). Identification and characterization of 22 genes that affect the vulval cell lineages of *Caenorhabditis elegans. Genetics* **110**, 17–72.

Ferguson, E. L., Sternberg, P. W., and Horvitz, H. R. (1987). A genetic pathway for the specification of the vulval cell lineages of *Caenorhabditis elegans. Nature (London)* **326**, 259–267.

Fino Silva, I. F., and Plasterk, R. H. A. (1990). Characterization of a G-protein α subunit gene from the nematode *Caenorhabditis elegans. J. Mol. Biol.* **215**, 483–487.

Finney, M., Ruvkun, G., and Horvitz, H. R. (1988). The *C. elegans* cell lineage and differentiation gene *unc-86* encodes a protein containing a homeodomain and extended sequence similarity to mammalian transcription factors. *Cell* **55**, 757–769.

Finney, M., and Ruvkun, G. (1990). The *unc-86* gene product couples cell lineage and cell identity in *Caenorhabditis elegans. Cell* **63**, 895–905.

Fire, A. (1986). Integrative transformation of *Caenorhabditis elegans. EMBO J.* **5**, 2675–2680.

Fixsen, W., Sternberg, P., Ellis, H., and Horvitz, R. (1985). Genes that affect cell fates during the development of *Caenorhabditis elegans. Cold Spring Harbor Symp. Quant. Biol.* **50**, 99–104.

Freyd, G., Kim, S. K., and Horvitz, H. R. (1990). Novel cysteine-rich motif and homeodomain in the product of the *Caenorhabditis elegans* cell lineage gene *lin-11. Nature* **344**, 876–879.

Georgi, L. L., Albert, P. S., and Riddle, D. R. (1990). *daf-1,* a *C. elegans* gene controlling dauer larva development, encodes a novel receptor protein kinase. *Cell* **61**, 635–645.

Greenwald, I. S. (1985). *lin-12,* a nematode homeotic gene, is homologous to a set of mammalian proteins that includes epidermal growth factor. *Cell* **43**, 583–590.

Greenwald, I. (1989). Cell–cell interactions that specify certain cell fates in *C. elegans* development. *Trends Genet.* **5**, 237–241.

Greenwald, I. S., Sternberg, P. W., and Horvitz, H. R. (19830. *lin-12* specifies cell fates in *C. elegans. Cell* **34**, 435–444.

Greenwald, I., and Seydoux, G. (1990). Analysis of gain-of-function mutations of the *lin-12* gene of *Caenorhabditis elegans. Nature (London)* **346**, 197–199.

Gross, R. E., Bagchi, S., Lu, X., and Rubin, C. S. (1990). Cloning, characterization, and expression of the gene for the catalytic subunit of cAMP-dependent protein kinase in *Caenorhabditis elegans. J. Biol. Chem.* **265**, 6896–6907.

Han, M., Aroian, R., and Sternberg, P. W. (1990). The *let-60* locus controls the switch between vulval and nonvulval cell types in *C. elegans. Genetics* **126**, 899–913.

Han, M., and Sternberg, P. W. (1990). *let-60,* a gene that specifies cell fates during *C. elegans* vulval induction, encodes a *ras* protein. *Cell* **63,** 921–931.

Hartenstein, V., and Posakony, J. (1989). Development of adult sensilla on the wing and notum of *Drosophila melanogaster. Development* **107,** 389–405.

Hedgecock, E., Sulston, J. E., and Thomson, J. N. (1983). Mutations affecting programmed cell death in the nematode *Caenorhabditis elegans. Science* **220,** 1277–1280.

Hedgecock, E. M., Culotti, J. G., Thomson, J. N., and Perkins, L. A. (1985). Axonal guidance mutants of *Caenorhabditis elegans* identified by filling sensory neurons with fluorescein dyes. *Devel. Biol.* **111,** 158–170.

Hedgecock, E. M., Culotti, J. G., Hall, D. H., and Stern, B. D. (1987). Genetics of cell and axon migrations in *Caenorhabditis elegans. Development* **100,** 365–382.

Hedgecock, E. M., Culotti, J. G., and Hall, D. H. (1990). The *unc-5, unc-6,* and *unc-40* genes guide circumferential migrations of pioneer axons and mesodermal cells on the epidermis in *C. elegans. Neuron* **2,** 61–85.

Hedgecock, E. M., and Hall, D. H. (1990). Homologies in the neurogenesis of nematodes, arthropods and chordates. *Sem. Neurosi.* **2,** 159–172.

Herman, R. K. (1989). Mosaic analysis in the nematode *Caenorhabditis elegans. J. Neurogenetics* **5,** 1–24.

Herman, R. K., and Hedgecock, E. M. (1990). Limitation of the size of the vulval primordium of *Caenorhabditis elegans* by *lin-15* expression in surrounding hypodermis. *Nature (London)* **348,** 169–171.

Hodgkin, J. (1987). A genetic analysis of the sex-determining gene, tra-1, in the nematode *Caenorhabditis elegans. Genes. Dev.* **1,** 731–745.

Holstein, T. W. and David, C. N. (1990). Putative intermediates in the nerve cell differentiation pathway in hydra have properties of multipotent stem cells. *Developmental Biology* **142,** 401–405.

Horvitz, H. R. (1988). The nematode *Caenorhabditis elegans. In* "Genetics of cell lineage" (W. B. Wood, ed.). Cold Spring Harbor, New York: Cold Spring Harbor Laboratory.Horvitz, H. R., and Sulston, J. E. (1980). Isolation and genetic characterization of cell lineage mutants of the nematode *Caenorhabditis elegans. Genetics* **96,** 435–454.

Horvitz, H. R., Ellis, H. M., and Sternberg, P. W. (1983a). Programmed cell death in nematode development. *Neurosci. Comm.* **1,** 56–65.

Horvitz, H. R., Sternberg, P. W., Greenwald, I. S., Fixsen, W., and Ellis, H. M. (1983b). Mutations that affect neural cell lineages and cell fates during the development of the nematode *Caenorhabditis elegans. Cold Spring Harbor Symp. Quant. Biol.* **48,** 453–463.

Horvitz, H. R., and Sternberg, P. W. (1991). Multiple intercellular signalling pathways control *C. elegans* vulval development. *Nature (London)* **351,** 535–541.

Hu, E., and Rubin, C. S. (1990). Casein kinase II from *Caenorhabditis elegans. J. Biol. Chem.* **265,** 5072–5080.

Kamb, A., Weir, M., and Rudy, B., Varmus, H., and Kenyon, C. (1989). Identification of genes from pattern formation, tyrosine kinase, and potassium channel families by DNA amplification. *Proc. Natl. Acad. Sci. U.S.A.* **86,** 4372–7376.

Karlsson, O., Thor, S., Norberg, T., Ohlsson, H., and Edlund, T. (1990). Insulin gene enhancer binding protein lsl-1 is a member of a novel class of proteins containing both a homeo- and a Cys–His domain. *Nature (London)* **344,** 879–882.

Kenyon, C. (1986). A gene involved in the development of the posterior body region of *C. elegans. Cell* **46,** 477–487.

Kimble, J. (1981). Lineage alterations after ablation of cells in the somatic gonad of *Caenorhabditis elegans. Dev. Biol.* **87,** 286–300.

Kimble, J., and Hirsh, D. (1979). Postembryonic cell lineages of the hermaphrodite and male gonads in *Caenorhabditis elegans. Dev. Biol.* **70,** 396–417.

Kimura, K., and Truman, J. W. (1990). Postmetamorphic cell death in the nervous and muscular systems of *Drosophila melanogaster. J. Neurosci.* **10,** 403–411.

Konishi, M., and Kutagawa, A. (1985). Neuronal growth, atrophy and death in a sexually dimorphic song nucleus in the zebra finch brain. *Nature* **315,** 145–147.

Li, C., and Chalfie, M. (1990). Organogenesis in *C. elegans:* Positioning of neurons and muscles in the egg-laying system. *Neuron* **4,** 681–695.

Lochrie, M. A., Mendel, J. E., Sternberg, P. W., and Simon, M. I. (1991). Homologous and unique G protein alpha subunits in the nematode *Caenorhabditis elegans. Cell Reg.* **2,** 135–154.

Lu, X., Gross, R. E., Bagchi, S., and Rubin, C. S. (1990). Cloning, structure, and expression of the gene for a novel regulatory subunit of cAMP-dependent protein kinase in *Caenorhabditis elegans. J. Biol. Chem.* **265,** 3293–3303.

Manser, J., and Wood, W. B. (1990). Mutations affecting embryonic cell migrations in *Caenorhabditis elegans. Dev. Genet.* **11,** 49–64.

Martin, D. P., Schmidt, R. E., DiStefano, P. S., Lowry, O. H., Carter, J. G., and Johnson, E. M., Jr. (1988). Inhibitors of protein synthesis prevent neuronal death caused by nerve growth factor deprivation. *J. Cell Biol.* **106,** 829–844.

Mello, C. C., Kramer, J. M., Stinchcomb, D., and Ambros, V. (1991). Efficient gene transfer in *C. elegans* after microinjection of DNA into germline cytoplasm: extrachromosomal maintenance and integration of transforming sequences. *EMBO J.,* in press.

Moerman, D. G., Benian, G. M., and Waterston, R. H. (1986). Molecular cloning of the muscle gene *unc-22* in *Caenorhabditis elegans* by Tc1 transposon tagging. *Proc. Natl. Acad. Sci. U.S.A.* **83,** 2579–2583.

Murakami, S., and Arai, Y. (1989). Neuronal death in the developing sexually dimorphic periventricular nucleus of the preoptic area in the female rat—Effect of neonatal androgen treatment. *Neurosci. Lett.* **102,** 185–190.

Pilar, G., Landmesser, L., and Burstein, L. (1980). Competition for survival among developing ciliary ganglion cells. *J. Neurophysiol.* **43,** 233–254.

Priess, J. R., and Thomson, J. N. (1987). Cellular interactions in early *C. elegans* embryos. *Cell* **48,** 241–250.

Robertson, A. M. G., and Thomson, J. N. (1982). Morphology of programmed cell death in the ventral nerve cord of *Caenorhabditis elegans* larvae. *J. Embryol. Exp. Morphol.* **67,** 89–100.

Ruvkun, G., Ambros, V., Coulson, A., Waterston, R., Sulston, J., and Horvitz, H. R. (1989). Molecular genetics of the *Caenorhabditis elegans* heterochronic gene *lin-14. Genetics* **121,** 501–516.

Ruvkun, G., and Guisto, J. (1989). The *Caenorhabditis elegans* heterochronic gene *lin-14* encodes a nuclear protein that forms a temporal developmental switch. *Nature (London)* **338,** 313–319.

Ruvkun, G., and Finney, M. (1991). Regulation of transcription and cell identity by POU domain proteins, *Cell* **64,** 475–478.

Savage, c., Hamelin, M., Culotti, J. G., Coulson, A., Albertson, D. G., and Chalfie, M. (1989). *mec-7* is a β-tubulin gene required for the production of 15-protofilament microtubules in *Caenorhabditis elegans. Genes Devel.* **3,** 870–881.

Seydoux, G., and Greenwald, I. (1989). Cell autonomy of *lin-12* function in a cell fate decision in *C. elegans. Cell* **57,** 1237–1245.

Sternberg, P. W. (1988). Lateral inhibition during vulval induction in *Caenorhabditis elegans. Nature (London)* **335,** 551–554.

Sternberg, P. W., and Horvitz, H. R. (1981). Gonadal cell lineages of the nematode *Panagrellus redivivus* and implications for evolution by the modification of cell lineage. *Dev. Biol.* **88,** 147–166.

Sternberg, P. W., and Horvitz, H. R. (1986). Pattern formation during vulval development in *Caenorhabditis elegans. Cell* **44,** 761–772.

Sternberg, P. W., and Horvitz, H. R. (1988). *lin-17* mutations of *C. elegans* disrupt asymmetric cell divisions. *Dev. Biol.* **130,** 67–73.

Sternberg, P. W., and Horvitz, H. R. (1989). The combined action of two intercellular signalling pathways specifies three cell fates during vulval induction in *C. elegans. Cell* **58,** 679–693.

Sulston, J., and Horvitz, H. R. (1977). Postembryonic cell lineages of the nematode *Caenorhabditis elegans. Dev. Biol.* **56,** 110–156.

Sulston, J. E., Albertson, D. G., and Thomson, J. N. (1980). The *Caenorhabditis elegans* male: Postembryonic development of nongonadal structures. *Dev. Biol.* **78,** 542–576.

Sulston, J. E., and White, J. G. (1980). Regulation and cell autonomy during postembryonic development of *Caenorhabditis elegans. Dev. Biol.* **78,** 577–597.

Sulston, J., and Horvitz, H. R. (1981). Abnormal cell lineages in mutants of the nematode *Caenorhabditis elegans. Dev. Biol.* **82,** 41–55.

Sulston, J. E., Schierenberg, E., White, J. G., and Thomson, J. N. (1983). The embryonic cell lineage of the nematode *Caenorhabditis elegans. Dev. Biol.* **100,** 64–119.

Thayer, M. J., Tapscott, S. J., Davis, R. L., Wright, W. W., Lassar, A. B., and Weintraub, H. (1989). Positive autoregulation of the myogenic determination gene *MyoD1. Cell* **58,** 241–248.

Thomas, J. H., Stern, M. J., and Horvitz, H. R. (1990). Cell interactions coordinate the development of the *C. elegans* egg-laying system. *Cell* **62,** 1041–1052.

Trent, C., Tsung, N., and Horvitz, H. R. (1983). Egg-laying defective mutants of the nematode *Caenorhabditis elegans. Genetics* **104,** 619–647.

Truman, J. W. (1983). Programmed cell death in the nervous system of an adult insect. *J. Comp. Neurol.* **216,** 445–452.

van der Voorn, L., Gebbink, M., Plasterk, R. H.A., and Ploegh, H. L. (1990). Characterization of a G-protein β-subunit gene from the nematode *Caenorhabditis elegans. J. Mol. Biol.* **213,** 17–26.

Villeneuve, A. M., and Meyer, B. J. (1990). The regulatory hierarchy controlling sex determination and dosage compensation in *Caenorhabditis elegans. In* "Genetic Regulatory Hierarchies in Development" (T. R. F. Wright, ed.), Advances in Genetics Vol. 27, pp. 117–188. San Diego: Academic Press.

Wallace, T. L., and Johnson, E. M., Jr. (1989). Cytosine arabinoside kills postmitiotic neurons: Evidence that deoxycytidine may have a role in neuronal survival that is independent of DNA synthesis. *J. Neurosci.* **9,** 115–124.

Walthall, W., and Chalfie, M. (1988). Cell–cell interactions in the guidance of late-developing neurons in *Caenorhabditis elegans. Science* **239,** 643–645.

Waring, D., and Kenyon, C. (1990). Selective silencing of cell communication influences anteroposterior pattern formation in *C. elegans. Cell* **60,** 123–131.

Waring, D., and Kenyon, C. (1991). Regulation of cellular responsiveness to inductive signals in the developing *C. elegans* nervous system. *Nature* **350,** 712–715.

Way, J., and Chalfie, M. (1988). *mec-3,* a homeobox-containing gene that specifies differentiation of the touch receptor neurons in *C. elegans. Cell* **54,** 5–16.

Way, J. C., and Chalfie, M. (1989). The *mec-3* gene of *Caenorhabditis elegans* requires its own product for maintained expression and is expressed in three neuronal cell types. *Genes Dev.* **3,** 1823–1833.

White, J. G. (1988). The anatomy. *In* "The Nematode *Caenorhabditis elegans*" (W. B. Wood, ed.), pp. 81–122. Cold Spring Harbor, New York: Cold Spring Harbor Laboratory.

White, J. G., Southgate, E., Thomson, J. N., and Brenner, S. (1986). The structure of the nervous system of the nematode *Caenorhabditis elegans*. *Phil. Trans. Soc. Lond. B.* **314,** 1–340.

Wood, W. B. (1991). Evidence from reversal of handedness in *C. elegans* embryos for early cell interactions determining cell fates. *Nature (London)* **349,** 536–539.

Yochem, J., Weston, K., and Greenwald, I. (1988). *C. elegans lin-12* encodes a transmembrane protein similar to *Drosophila Notch* and yeast cell cycle gene products. *Nature (London)* **335,** 547–550.

Yochem, J., and Greenwald, I. (1989). *glp-1* and *lin-12,* genes implicated in distinct cell–cell interactions in *C. elegans,* encode similar transmembrane proteins. *Cell* **58,** 553–563.

Yuan, J., and Horvitz, H. R. (1990). The *Caenorhabditis elegans* genes *ced-3* and *ced-4* act cell autonomously to cause programmed cell death. *Dev. Biol.* **138,** 33–41.

Zottoli, S. J. (1978). Comparative morphology of the mauthner cell in fish and amphibians. *In* "Neurobiology of the Mauthner Cells" (D. Faber and H. Korn, eds.), pp. 13–45. New York: Raven.

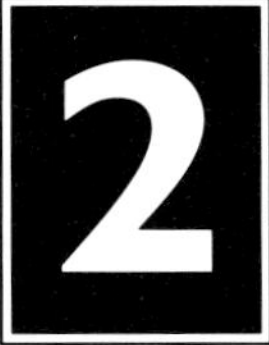

Segmental Differentiation of Lineally Homologous Neurons in the Central Nervous System of the Leech

Marty Shankland
Department of Anatomy and Cellular Biology
Harvard Medical School
Boston, Massachusetts

Mark Q. Martindale
Department of Organismal Biology and Anatomy
University of Chicago
Chicago, Illinois

I. Introduction

Individual neurons express a precisely coordinated constellation of morphological, biochemical, and physiological features that defines their phenotypic identities. Neuronal isolation experiments (Fuchs *et al.*, 1981) indicate that such identities are the manifestation of stable, intrinsically determined programs of cell differentiation; one of the central problems in developmental neurobiology is to understand the sequence of cellular and molecular events that specifies and defines different neuronal phenotypes.

At the heart of this problem lies the fundamental paradigm of developmental biology, namely, the idea that each individual cell has an intrinsic potential that determines its developmental fate as a function of its extrinsic environment. The relative degree to which intrinsic and extrinsic factors contribute to neuronal cell fate can vary dramatically. The development of all neurons is conditional on their environment, since the cell relies on its surroundings to provide substrates for axonal outgrowth and partner cells for synapse formation. However, some postmitotic neurons seem to have autonomous identities that allow them to manifest many aspects of their normal fates, even in grossly abnormal environments (Huff *et al.*, 1989; Torrence *et al.*, 1989), whereas others respond to instructive environmental cues by choosing between two or more terminal phenotypes of striking dissimilarity (Patterson, 1978; Kuwada and Goodman, 1985; Reinke and Zipursky, 1988). It appears likely that intrinsic properties must play a pivotal role in determining to what degree individual neurons depend on their environment for instructive signals, and to which of these signals a given neuron will respond.

This distinction between intrinsic and extrinsic determinants is complicated by the cumulative nature of the developmental process, since a cell's intrinsic properties are a reflection of developmental commitments made following its own birth, as well as commitments made by and inherited from its lineal progenitors. Such inherited commitments implicate cell lineage as a determinative factor, yet the progenitor cell may itself have been specified to a particular developmental pathway by positional cues (Shankland and Weisblat, 1984; Doe and Goodman, 1985b). Thus, the experimental demonstration that the fate of a particular cell is autonomously determined in accordance with its lineage history does not necessarily mean that there are no conditional steps among the events that lead to its formation.

In order to unravel the sequence of events that leads to the formation and differentiation of particular neurons, some biologists have turned to experimental organisms such as the nematode or leech, which normally develop from egg to adult via a spatiotemporally invariant pattern of cell divisions. This sort of developmental stereotypy offers conceptual and experimental advantages. In particular, both the postmitotic neurons and their lineal progenitors can be uniquely identified by cell lineage history; as a result, both pre- and postmitotic commitment events can be studied at the level of single, experimentally identifiable cells. This situation is in stark contrast to vertebrate organisms, which construct their nervous system from highly variable cell lineages, so differences between neuronal progenitors must be inferred from experimental analysis of their developmental potential (see Chapter 11).

In this chapter we will discuss the specification of neuronal phenotypes in the nervous system of the leech, an annelid worm. The leech is segmented, and its nervous system is largely composed of identified neuronal phenotypes that are periodically repeated from one segment to the next. In particular, we will focus on the process by which lineally homologous neurons situated in different body segments obtain their unique identities, and consider how homologous neurons become specified to undertake distinct segment-specific patterns of differentiation.

II. Leech Neuroanatomy

A. Segmental Organization

The leech's central nervous system (CNS) consists of a ganglionated nerve cord composed of 32 segmentally repeating units. The rostral ganglion encircles the esophagus, and is traditionally divided into supra- and subesophageal components (Fig. 1). The subesophageal ganglion represents the fused contributions of 4 embryological segments, but cell lineage studies have shown that the supraesophageal ganglion is of a separate nonsegmental origin (Weisblat *et al.,* 1984). Posterior to the head ganglion is a chain of 21 unfused midbody ganglia, which are attached to one another by longitudinal connective nerves. At the posterior end of the nerve cord is a compound caudal ganglion that is composed of 7 fused segmental neuromeres and innervates the rear sucker. The leech's peripheral nervous system is also segmental in its organization, but in this chapter we will focus exclusively on the development of the CNS.

Several anatomical conventions have been used to define and number the segmental repeats of the leech body plan. This chapter will adhere to the widely accepted "neurocentric" convention, in which individual segments are defined according to the ganglia and neuromeres of the CNS (Sawyer, 1986).

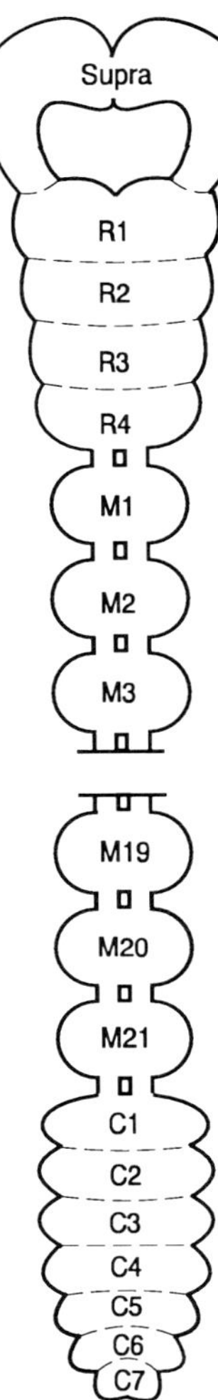

Figure 1. Schematic diagram of the leech CNS, with anterior toward the top. The compound rostral ganglion consists of a nonsegmental supraesophageal component as well as four fused segmental neuromeres (R1–R4). Each of the 21 midbody segments is innervated by a single unfused segmental ganglion (M1–M21). The rear sucker is innervated by a compound caudal ganglion that consists of seven fused segmental neuromeres (C1–C7).

However, the number of leech segments is more problematic, since most classical schemes assumed that the supraesophageal ganglion was segmental, whereas the more recent neurophysiological literature suffers from a failure to include the fused segments in the numbering system. In this chapter, we will number the segments in anteroposterior order; the rostral segments are designated R1–R4, the midbody segments M1–M21, and the caudal segments C1–C7 (Fig. 1).

The segmental ganglia of the leech CNS are for the most part quite similar to one another in cellular composition (for an overview, see Muller *et al.*, 1981). A typical ganglion contains the cell bodies of roughly 400 neurons (Macagno, 1980), including all the known motor neurons and interneurons as well as a small number of sensory neurons. Many or all of these central neurons have unique, experimentally verifiable identities. Indeed, some central neurons can be reliably identified solely by their cell body size and position within the ganglion. A similar set of neurons is found in every body segment— including the fused neuromeres of the rostral and caudal ganglia (Yau, 1976)—and the majority of neurons are present as bilaterally symmetric pairs. Thus, most leech neurons have a contralateral homolog within the same ganglion that is of nearly identical phenotype, and phenotypically similar homologs in many or all of the other segments.

B. Segmental Specificity

Although most neuronal phenotypes are represented by a segmentally repeated set of similar homologs, the individual neurons in this set are often specialized in a manner that correlates with their segmental location along the anteroposterior (AP) body axis. For example, the Retzius neurons in different segments are initially similar in their morphogenesis and neurotransmitter expression. However, in all leech species examined, the Retzius cells in the reproductive segments begin to manifest pronounced and segment-specific differences in cell body size and axonal projection by the end of embryonic life (Glover and Mason, 1986), and eventually develop distinct patterns of pharmacological sensitivity (Loer and Kristan, 1989a) and synaptic connectivity (Wittenberg *et al.*, 1990). In a similar manner, the dorsolateral serotonin (DLS) neurons initially express serotonin at a comparable level in every segment of the embryonic nerve cord but, during postembryonic development of the leech *Haementeria ghilianii,* the DLS neurons in the reproductive segments (M5 and M6) cease to store detectable levels of serotonin, although they nonetheless survive and presumably take part in the functioning of the adult CNS (Glover, 1987).

However, the majority of segment-specific neuronal phenotypes is known only from descriptions of the later developmental stages; it is often unclear how that particular phenotype came to be associated only with certain segments. For instance, the leech nervous system has been stained with antibodies to a variety of peptide and amine neurotransmitters—as well as monoclonal antibodies to unknown antigens—and many segmental differences have been reported in the number and distribution of immunoreactive neurons (Zipser and McKay, 1981; Kuhlman *et al.*, 1985; Li and Calabrese, 1985; Loer *et al.*, 1986; Stuart *et al.*, 1987; Evans and Calabrese, 1989; Shankland and Martindale, 1989). In addition, some of the mature neurons that have been characterized by electrophysiological techniques do not have readily identifiable homologs in other segments (Shafer and Calabrese, 1981; Weeks, 1982). In this situation, one cannot know *a priori* whether the segment-specific phenotype has arisen by the divergent differentiation or differential survival of segmentally homologous neurons (as described in the preceding paragraph), or if some neurons have arisen by segment-specific cell divisions and therefore do not have strict lineal homologs in other body segments (see Chapter 3).

In addition to differences among segments, the leech CNS also displays differences in the differentiation of homologous neurons in right and left hemisegments. The neurogenic cell lineages of the leech are bilaterally symmetric (Zackson, 1984; Shankland, 1987a,b), yet each segmental ganglion of the mature nerve cord contains a small cluster of medially situated interneurons that are traditionally designated "unpaired" because of the apparent singularity of their phenotypes (Weeks, 1982). Embryological studies have shown that at least two of these unpaired medial neurons arise as bilaterally homologous cell pairs of which one homolog undergoes an embryonic cell death (Stuart *et al.*, 1987; Macagno and Stewart, 1987; Shankland and Martindale, 1989). Such asymmetries are not restricted to the medial unpaired neurons, since certain of the laterally situated neurons have been shown to develop a striking asymmetry of neuropeptide expression (Shankland and Martindale, 1989; Evans and Calabrese, 1989). We will include these lateral asymmetries in our discussion of segmental differentiation, since they likewise arise by the diversification of homologous cells situated in segmentally repeated subunits.

III. Neurogenesis and Segmental Homology

The leech embryo develops via a stereotyped cell lineage, and lineal relationships have been studied extensively in the developing CNS (Kramer and

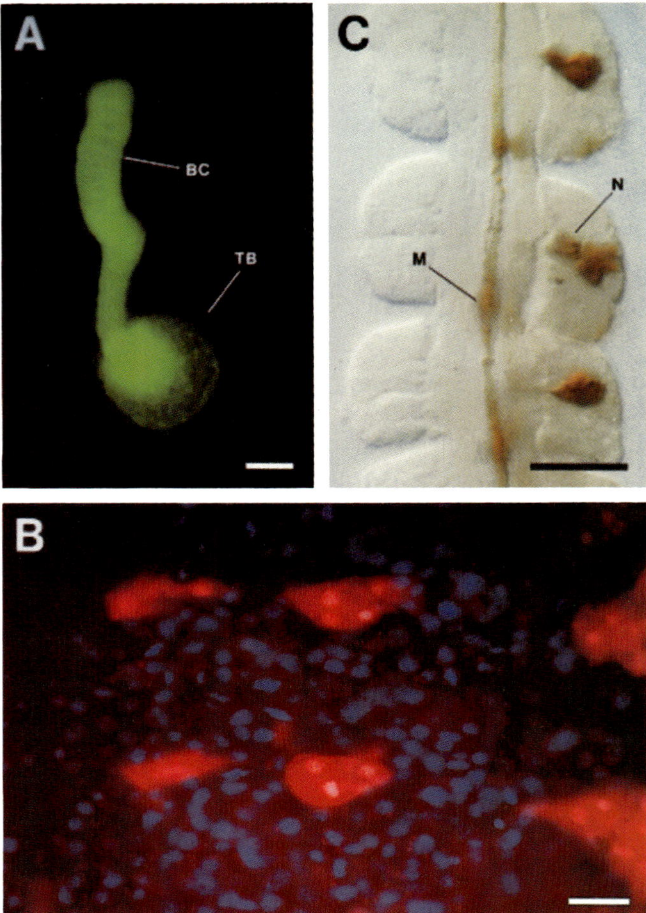

FIGURE 2. Selective labeling of individual cell lineages by intracellular injection of vital cell lineage tracers. A. A single teloblast (TB) generates a linear chain of primary blast cell daughters (BC). In this fluorescence photomicrograph of a *Helobdella triserialis* embryo, a single teloblast was injected with fluorescein–dextran one day earlier and produced a total of 20 labeled blast cell daughters during the intervening period. Note that this tracer compound is partially excluded from the yolky cytoplasm at the perimeter of the teloblast and from the blast cell nuclei. B. Blast cell clones that have been labeled by injection of the ancestral teloblast can be traced through the course of embryonic morphogenesis. In this fluorescence photomicrograph of a *Theromyzon rude* embryo, segmentally repeating groups of rhodamine-dextran-labeled neuroblasts and glioblasts can be seen migrating toward the nascent CNS, which is situated to the left. The nuclei of both labeled and unlabeled cells have been stained fluorescent blue with the dye Hoechst 33258. Photograph kindly provided by Steve Torrence. C. Tracer compounds injected in the early embryo can be visualized in the postmitotic neurons of the CNS. This Nomarski photomicrograph shows three abdominal ganglia of a *H. triserialis* embryo in which the right M teloblast lineage was labeled by injection of biotin–dextran, then visualized in fixed tissue by avidin:peroxidase staining and diaminobenzidine reaction. Note that the M teloblast gives rise to a segmentally repeating cluster of four neuronal cell bodies (N) as well as muscle fibers (M) in the neural sheath. Bars: 20 μm.

Weisblat, 1985; Weisblat and Shankland, 1985). In the leech, cell lineage has been described both by direct observation of cell divisions, and by the intracellular injection of lineage tracing compounds into identified embryonic blastomeres (Weisblat *et al.*, 1978; Gimlich and Braun, 1985). Following such injections, the labeled descendent clone can be examined and the constituent cells enumerated at progressively later developmental stages (Fig. 2). Such tracers persist over several rounds of mitosis, and there is little increase in cellular volume until postembryonic life. Nearly all of the leech's central neurons are generated embryonically (Stewart *et al.*, 1986); thus, tracer compounds injected in the early embryo can be readily visualized in the postmitotic neurons of the late embryo or juvenile leech (Fig. 2C).

Although different leech species show a high degree of similarity in the cellular organization of the nervous system and the overall pattern of segmentation, there are some pronounced differences in their developmental life history (Sawyer, 1986). Microinjection studies have focused almost exclusively on the glossiphoniid leeches (Stent *et al.*, 1982), because their eggs are much larger than those of other leeches and develop directly into the mature form without passing through an intervening larval stage. We will discuss only those aspects of the glossiphoniid leech's embryonic cell lineage that are directly pertinent to the segmental patterning of nervous system differentiation; for a more complete description, see Sandig and Dohle (1988) or Bissen and Weisblat (1989).

A. Formation of the Embryonic Stem Cells

The segmental tissues of the adult leech derive from a set of embryonic stem cells known as teloblasts (Fig. 2A). These teloblasts are formed by the early embryonic cleavages, and are arranged on either side of the embryo as five bilaterally symmetric cell pairs. The individual teloblasts can be uniquely identified by their cell lineage history—with one noteworthy exception (Weisblat and Blair, 1984)—and are thereby designated as cells M, N, O, P, and Q.

Lineage trace injection has shown that each identified teloblast generates a stereotyped and distinct set of descendent tissues in the mature leech (Kramer and Weisblat, 1985; Weisblat and Shankland, 1985). These teloblast clones are segmentally iterated and restricted to one side of the body midline (Fig. 2B,C). Each clone is essentially identical in cellular composition to that produced by the symmetric teloblast on the contralateral side. The process by which these 10 segmented cell lineages come together to form the mature body plan has been amply described elsewhere (Stent *et al.*, 1982; Weisblat and Shankland, 1985). In this article we will focus exclusively on the question of how each individual teloblast lineage generates its own periodic array of descendent cell phenotypes. This reductionist approach is warranted by the way in which the organism develops, since experimental studies suggest that each teloblast lineage establishes its own segmental periodicity independent of the rest (reviewed by Shankland, 1991).

B. Formation of the Segmental Founder Cells

Each teloblast produces a segmentally organized descendent lineage by generating an iterative sequence of similar daughter cells. These much smaller daughters are known as primary blast cells (Fig. 2A), and are designated by the same letter as their parent teloblast in lower case (m, n, etc.). Blast cell daughters of the same teloblast form a linear chain, or bandlet, and their spatial organization in the bandlet reflects the temporal order of their birth (Figs. 2A,3). Each bandlet will eventually become aligned along the AP body axis of the developing embryo, so the firstborn blast cell contributes its descendent clone to the most anterior body segments and later blast cells contribute their clones to progressively more posterior segments.

The primary blast cells of the leech embryo serve as segmental founder cells, since each one generates a segmentally defined subunit of the tissues produced by its particular bandlet (Fig. 3). Cell lineage analysis has shown that blast cells in the same bandlet undergo very similar sequences of cell division (Zackson, 1984) to produce descendent clones of roughly 10^2 cells apiece that are nearly identical in cellular composition, although situated in different segments (Weisblat and Shankland, 1985; Shankland, 1987a,b). Thus, the segmental periodicity of the mature leech body plan has its origin in the fact that successive blast cells in the bandlet undergo the same basic developmental program in a tandem array (Fig. 3).

This relationship between cell lineage and segmentation is most obvious for the M, O, and P lineages. In each of these three bandlets, all the blast cells are homologous to one another, and their descendent clones become arrayed along the body axis with a spatial frequency of one blast cell clone per segment (Fig. 3A). The N and Q lineages exhibit a slightly more complicated arrangement, since they produce two primary blast cells per segment; thus, their bandlets are composed of two alternating types of blast cell clone (Fig. 3B).

The observation that different blast cells in the same bandlet give rise to descendent clones of nearly identical cellular composition explains why most leech neurons are arrayed as a set of bilaterally symmetric and segmentally iterated homologs. Homologous neurons situated in different segments on the same side of the nerve cord derive from different blast cells in the same bandlet, whereas the homologous neurons situated on the contralateral side derive from the blast cells of the contralaterally homologous bandlet.

C. Cell Lineage and Homology

Before exploring the developmental events that lead to the diversification of homologous neurons, it first seems warranted to examine the meaning of cellular homology. The concept of homology requires that the entities under consideration share a common or similar origin. In developmental biology, this term is frequently used to characterize cells that have arisen through similar formative mechanisms. For instance, two cells can be considered homologous because they have arisen from the same developmental pathway in two different individuals of the same or closely related species, or in different but comparable spatial domains of the same individual.

Cellular homology is easily understood in an organism such as the leech, because cells of individually identifiable phenotype arise from fixed cell lineage histories, and the same module of cell lineages is segmentally repeated along the body's length. Thus, different hemisegments contain a developmentally homologous set of postmitotic cells. Each cell in that set can be deemed the lineal homolog of a cell that arose from the same sequence of cell divisions in any other hemisegment. [It should, however, be noted that sister cells cannot be distinguished by ancestry, and that cells at any point in the embryonic genealogy can be *uniquely* identified on the basis of cell lineage history only if their formative cell divisions have a fixed asymmetry or spatial orientation. This has been shown to be the case for the early part of the blast cell lineages (Zackson, 1984; Shankland, 1987a,b; Bissen and Weisblat, 1989), and is herein assumed to be true of the later cell divisions as well.]

A similar relationship between cell lineage and segmentation is found in the insect nervous system, which also arises by fixed cell lineage from a segmentally repeated set of neuronal precursors (Doe and Goodman, 1985a). It would, however, be incorrect to assume that cellular homologies can only be assigned in the context of fixed lineage relationships. For example, the zebrafish nervous system arises from a variable cell lineage, but nonetheless contains a segmentally repeating array of uniquely identifiable neurons (Kimmel and Warga, 1986). In this latter organism, phenotypically similar neurons in different body segments cannot be said to be lineal homologs, yet they can be viewed as homologous nonetheless in the sense that they are specified to

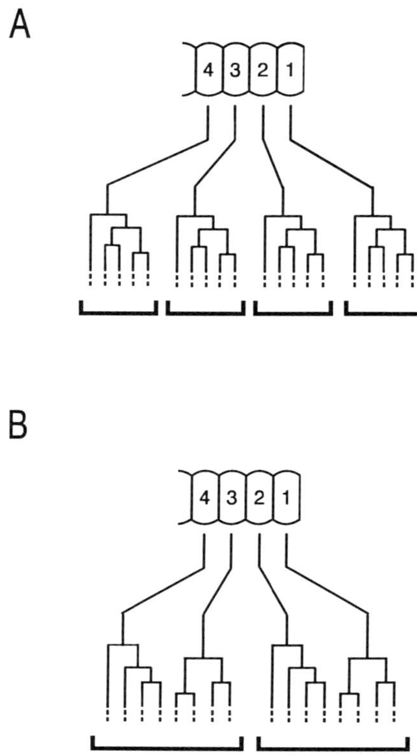

Figure 3. Primary blast cells in the same bandlet undergo nearly identical lineages, and produce descendent clones that are tandemly oriented repeats. In this way, each blast cell bandlet gives rise to a segmentally periodic array of mature tissues. Numbers represent blast cell birth ranks, and brackets demarcate segmental repeats. A. In the M, O, and P lineages, every blast cell undergoes the same bandlet-specific sequence of cell divisions. The final pattern of descendent tissues is composed of one blast cell clone per segment. B. In the N and Q lineages, the odd- and even-numbered blast cells undergo distinct lineages. One type of blast cell produces the anterior half of the segmental repeat, and the other produces the posterior half. Thus, the N and Q lineages are composed of two blast cell clones per segment.

utilize a common program of differentiation by the same segmentally repeated set of extracellular cues (see Chapter 14). A somewhat similar phenomenon is observed in the head segments of the leech, where certain neuronal phenotypes are generated by a sequence of cell divisions that is genealogically distinct from the pattern of cell divisions that generates those same phenotypes in the other body segments (Shankland, 1987c).

IV. Determination of Neuronal Phenotype by Cell Lineage History

In principle, segmentally homologous neurons could develop unique properties as a response to their differing segmental environments, or because they already possess distinct identities at the time of their birth. Cell-intrinsic segmental identities might directly lead homologous neurons to undertake dissimilar patterns of differentiation, or might bias their response to environmental cues that are common to the various segments. In this section we will focus on the role such intrinsic differences play in the segmental differentiation of the leech CNS, and will discuss experiments that indicate that at least some aspects of segmental identity are conveyed to the postmitotic neurons as a result of their differing cell lineage histories.

A. Correlation of Cell Lineage and Segmental Location

The stereotyped cell lineages of the leech embryo occur in concert with a highly regular pattern of morphogenesis. Each bandlet is a linear array of primary blast cells whose spatial order mirrors their sequence of birth and predicts the anteroposterior positioning of their descendent clones in the mature leech. Thus, a blast cell daughter of any given teloblast has a birth rank—determined by the number of blast cells previously generated by that teloblast—and its descendent clone comes to lie a corresponding number of segments posterior to the animal's head. This numerical correspondence may be either 1:1 or 2:1, depending on whether the parent teloblast generates 1 or 2 blast cells per segment (Weisblat and Shankland, 1985).

The correlation between birth rank and segmental fate has been deduced from a number of experimental observations (Weisblat *et al.,* 1978; Weisblat and Shankland, 1985). First, lineage tracer injection of newly born teloblasts indicates that the first blast cell daughter consistently contributes its descendent clone to a specific segmental location in the animal's head (Ho and Weisblat, 1987; M. Shankland, unpublished observations). Second, there is no evidence of primary blast cell death or variability in clonal size in the main portion of the bandlet, indicating an orderly progression of blast cell clones along the body's length (Zackson, 1984; Shankland, 1987a,b). Finally, timed injection of teloblasts that are in the midst of blast cell production demonstrates an exceedingly high degree of spatiotemporal coordination in the segmental fate of blast cells produced by symmetric teloblasts (Shankland, 1984; Martindale and Shankland, 1988), as could only occur if each individual teloblast follows a very rigid timetable of blast cell production. All of these findings suggest that the actual relationship between a blast cell's birth rank and the segmental location of its descendent clone is exact, although a definitive demonstration of this point will require that the birth rank of individual blast cells be determined by directly counting teloblast cell divisions prior to lineage tracer injection.

B. Bandlet Slippage

Our current understanding of segmental differentiation comes in large part from an experimental technique known as "bandlet slippage," in which blast cells are relocated so their descendent clones take part in the formation of segments that are inappropriate for their birth rank (Shankland, 1984; Martindale and Shankland, 1988, 1990a; Gleizer and Stent, 1990). In this way, it is possible to test the relative importance of cell lineage and segmental environment in the differentiation of the blast cell clone.

During normal development, the five ipsilateral blast cell bandlets come together in parallel to form a unified germinal band in which they assume a common segmental registration (Fig. 4). This merger begins at the anterior end of the bandlets (Sandig and Dohle, 1988) and proceeds posteriorly at a fairly constant rate. However, if a bandlet breaks during this merger, the trailing fragment will often fall out of register with the flanking bandlets, particularly if the break occurs near the point of entry into the band (Shankland, 1984). In this situation, the trailing fragment enters the germinal band with some delay; as a result, its constituent blast cells slip posteriorly with respect to the overall pattern of body segmentation (Fig. 4).

In the glossiphoniid leech *Helobdella,* such rearrangements can be routinely induced by photolesioning 2–3 blast cells from a single bandlet that has been labeled by injection of its parent teloblast with a photosensitizing lineage tracer (Shankland, 1984). The slipped blast cells in the trailing fragment of the lesioned bandlet generate descendent clones that integrate readily with the other unslipped bandlets to form segmental tissues, but they are frameshifted so their descendent clones take part in the formation of segments posterior to those they would normally have occupied. Slippage tends to occur uniformly along the bandlet's length; thus, a single slippage experiment can be used to simultaneously test the segmental specificity of nearly all the primary blast cell clones in the bandlet.

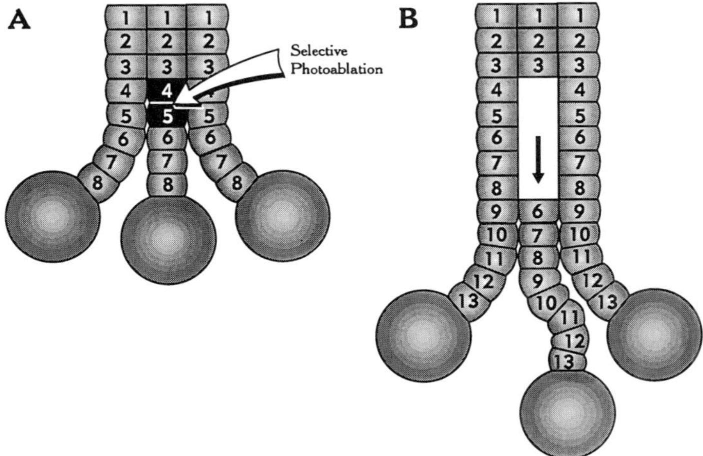

Figure 4. The blast cells of one bandlet can be selectively relocated by a process known as bandlet slippage into segments that are inappropriate for their cell lineage history. Numbers represent blast cell birth ranks. A. Blast cells destined for the same segment come together during the normal course of morphogenesis, but abnormal alignments can be induced by photoablating a small number of cells at the point at which the bandlets merge. B. The lesion produced by photoablation results in a gap that widens as development proceeds. Blast cells in the trailing fragment of the broken bandlet fail to keep up with the flanking bandlets and, as a result, take part in the formation of segments that are inappropriate for their birth ranks.

C. Differentiation of Neurons in Ectopic Segments

Slippage experiments have shown that some leech neurons will develop their normal segment-specific characteristics even if they are forced to differentiate in segments that are inappropriate for their cell lineage history. This phenomenon has been most thoroughly studied for the N lineage (Martindale and Shankland, 1990a), which gives rise to approximately two-thirds of the leech's central neurons (Kramer and Weisblat, 1985). The degree to which blast cells are relocated by bandlet slippage can be measured with an accuracy equivalent to the dimensions of a single blast cell clone (Shankland, 1984). In the case of the n bandlet this means that the slippage can be measured with an accuracy of ± ½ segment, so it is possible to assess the pattern of blast cell rearrangement with great precision.

The nz4 neurons are N-derived cells that initially express SCP-like immunoreactivity over a wide range of segments (Shankland and Martindale,

1989). During normal development, only those nz4 neurons situated in segments R4–M3—the future RAS neurons—will continue to express this immunoreactivity into maturity (Fig. 5). (As discussed in Section V,A, only one of the two nz4 neurons in each of these segments will take on the mature RAS phenotype.) Following slippage of the right or left n bandlet, the pattern of immunoreactive RAS neurons on the experimental side is shifted posteriorly

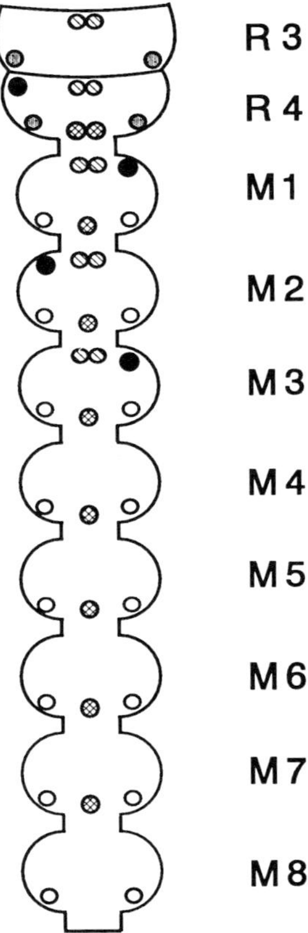

Figure 5. Segmental distribution of four neuronal phenotypes in the CNS of the glossiphoniid leech. The RAS, AMS, and PMS neurons have only been observed in certain body segments of the mature leech. In addition to segmental specificity, the RAS and PMS neurons exhibit an asymmetric or unpaired distribution. The PLS1 neuron is present in all of these segments, but stains more intensely with anti-SCP (⊚) in the fused rostral ganglion. The distribution of the RAS neuron (●) was determined by Shankland and Martindale (1989); the distribution of the PLS1 neuron (○) was determined by Martindale and Shankland (1990a); the distribution of AMS (◑) and PMS (⊚) neurons was determined by Stuart et al. (1987) and confirmed by D. Stuart (personal communication).

by a corresponding distance (Fig. 6A,B), whereas slippage of the other bandlets has no effect on the distribution of these cells. There is a strong correlation between the observed location of RAS neurons on the experimental side of the operated embryos and the location predicted solely on the basis of blast cell rearrangement, assuming that only those n blast cells that normally occupy segments R4–M3 have the potential to generate mature RAS neurons (Fig. 7A). Thus, the data suggest that those nz4 neurons that—on the basis of cell lineage—normally occupy those segments possess the ability to maintain neuropeptide expression in segmental environments that do not support that same phenotype in other nz4 neurons.

Other segment-specific derivatives of the n bandlet show similar redistributions following bandlet slippage (Martindale and Shankland, 1990a). The PLS1 neuron also expresses an SCP-like immunoreactivity (Shankland and Martindale, 1989). In the *Helobdella* embryo, the PLS1 neurons in the fused rostral ganglion show much stronger antibody staining than do their midbody homologs (Fig. 6A). Following n bandlet slippage, the boundary between intensely and faintly immunoreactive PLS1 neurons is shifted posteriorly on the experimental side (Fig. 6B), and the magnitude of this shift corresponds very closely to the experimental displacement of the ancestral blast cells (Fig. 7B). The n bandlet also gives rise to two segment-specific serotonergic cells (Stuart *et al.*, 1987), whose distributions are also shifted posteriorly by a corresponding distance following n bandlet slippage (Figs. 6C, 7C,D).

However, bandlet slippage does not alter the segmental pattern of all neuronal phenotypes in the descendent cell lineage. The Retzius neuron is another serotonergic descendent of the N lineage; during normal development the Retzius cells in the reproductive segments undergo a distinctive pattern of morphological differentiation (Glover and Mason, 1986). Following slippage of the n bandlet, we observe that at least one of these attributes—a smaller cell body—is still restricted to the reproductive segments (Fig. 8), even though the Retzius neurons that occupy those segments would in the absence of experimental intervention have been located in more anterior segments. This observation is consistent with studies in the leech *Hirudo medicinalis,* in which it has been shown that the Retzius cells that occupy the reproductive segments choose an alternative pathway of differentiation as a result of innervating the genitalia (Macagno *et al.,* 1986; Loer *et al.,* 1987; Loer and Kristan, 1989a,b, see also Chapter 4).

Together, these findings suggest that the process of segmental diversification occurs in multiple steps. The primary step involves the specification of segmental identity at the level of the primary blast cells, so many neurons are born with a commitment to undertake a pattern of differentiation that is appropriate for their normal segment of destiny. However, other segmental differences are not specified until later stages, and involve cell interactions in which pre-existing differences in one cell lineage serve as a template for the segmental patterning of other cells or tissues (Martindale and Shankland, 1988).

D. Role of Cell Lineage in Neuronal Differentiation

Each primary n blast cell generates approximately 70 descendent neurons; thus, segmental identities established at the level of the primary blast cell must be handed down over roughly six rounds of cell division before they become manifest in the neurotransmitter or peptide phenotype of the postmitotic neuron. The slippage experiments do not directly address the means by which segmental identity is conveyed from the primary blast cell to its postmitotic descendants, since the blast cell clone is relocated as a whole. Different neurons might receive their segment-specific developmental instructions by different mechanisms. For instance, one could imagine that only a subset of the blast cell's lineal descendants directly inherit its segmental identity, yet these lineally differentiated sublineages could then act in the blast cell clone to induce segmental differences in other sublineages. Thus, the slippage experiments emphasize the developmental significance of lineage history without precluding the coexistence of determinative cell interactions in either the formation or differentiation of those same neurons. Indeed, there is not a perfect correlation between blast cell slippage and neuronal differentiation following bandlet slippage (Fig. 7), and it is possible that the occasional discrepancies seen in these studies reflect cell interactions that are (in a minority of cases) sufficient to override a neuron's lineal propensities.

Figure 6. Altered segmental distribution of neuronal phenotypes in leech embryos *(Helobdella robusta)* that have been subjected to unilateral n bandlet slippage. These micrographs represent photonegatives of nerve cords stained by indirect immunofluorescence. Numbers denote the segmental identity of the midbody ganglia. A. Anti-SCP staining of nerve cord from an embryo in which the right n bandlet was slipped posteriorly by 1 ± ½ segment. The pattern of SCP-immunoreactive neurons is normal on the left, but shifted posteriorly by one segment on the right, as evinced by a RAS neuron (R) in the fourth midbody ganglion and an intensely immunoreactive PLS1 neuron (P) in the first midbody ganglion. An arrow marks the normally positioned contralateral PLS1 neuron. B. Anti-SCP staining of nerve cord from an embryo in which the left n bandlet was slipped 3 ± ½ segment posteriorly. A comparable shift is observed in the distribution of neuronal phenotypes, including an immunoreactive PLS1 neuron (P) in ganglion 3 and immunoreactive RAS neurons (R) in ganglia 4 and 5. C. Antiserotonin staining of nerve cord from an embryo in which the right n bandlet was slipped posteriorly by 1 ± ½ segment. The anteromedial serotonin neuron (AM) is a paired cell that is not normally found posterior to midbody segment 3. However, unilateral posterior slippage of the ancestral cell lineage results in the formation of a single neuron of this phenotype in the fourth midbody ganglion as well. Bars: 10 μm.

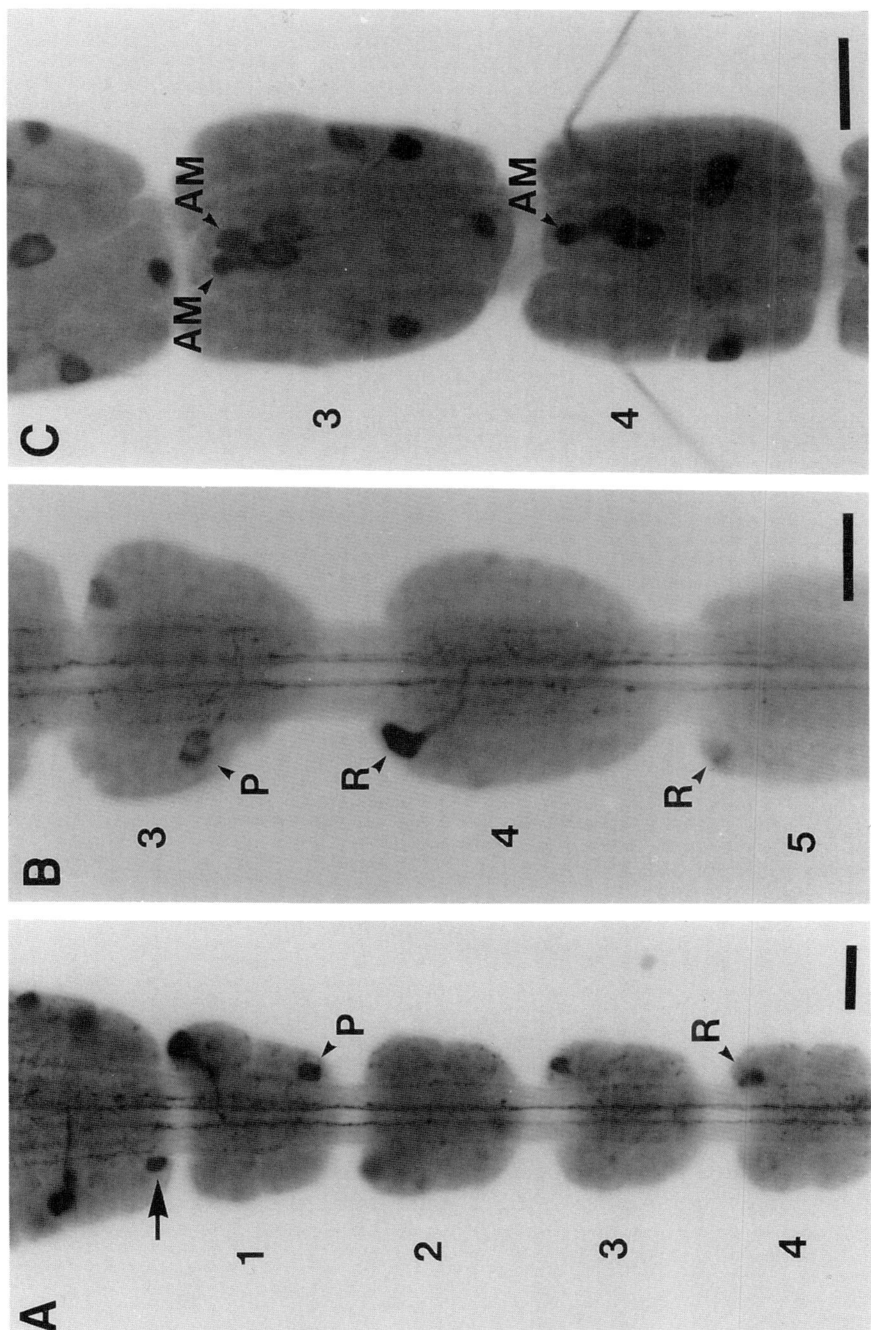

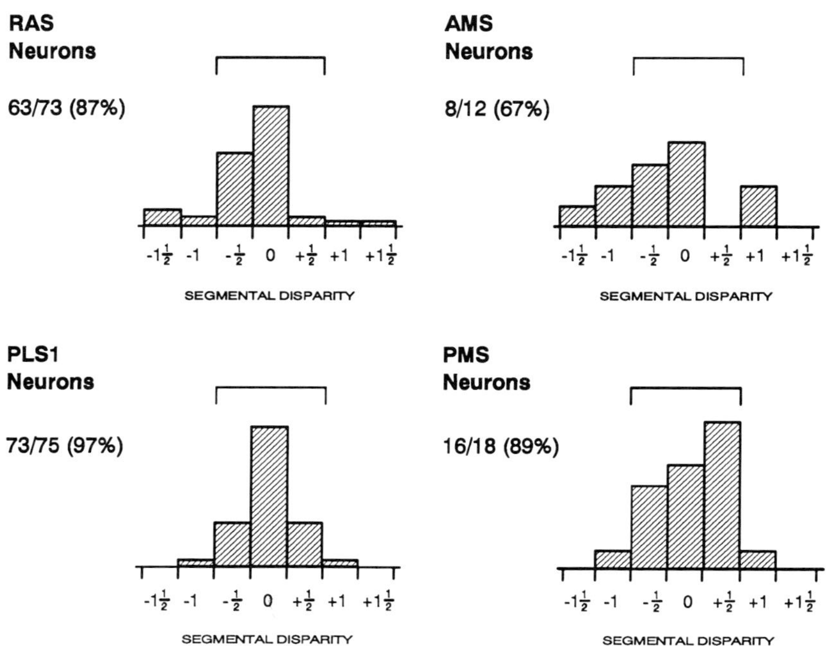

Figure 7. Histograms showing the close correlation between cell lineage and segmental specificity following n bandlet slippage for each of four neuronal phenotypes. Data were obtained in *H. robusta* embryos in which either the right or left n bandlet was slipped posteriorly by a measured distance of 1–7 segments. If the birth rank of an n blast cell were the sole determinant of its developmental fate, then descendent neurons should be relocated posteriorly by the same number of segments. Each histogram depicts the observed disparities between the actual and predicted location of the most posterior immunoreactive neuron of a given phenotype. Slippage measurements have an uncertainty of ± ½ segment (marked by brackets); percentages indicate how often the most posterior immunoreactive neuron was located in the predicted range of segments. The findings support the idea that the segmental specificity of these particular neuronal phenotypes is determined largely by the cell lineage identity of the relocated blast cell progenitors.

E. Specification of Blast Cell Identity

The close correlation between each n blast cell's lineal identity and the developmental fate of its descendent clone argues that segmental identity has already been determined at the time slippage occurs, that is, prior to the onset of subsidiary cell divisions, and before the blast cells come into segmental registration with the other blast cell bandlets (Weisblat and Shankland, 1985). Bandlet slippage experiments involving two of the other blast cell bandlets

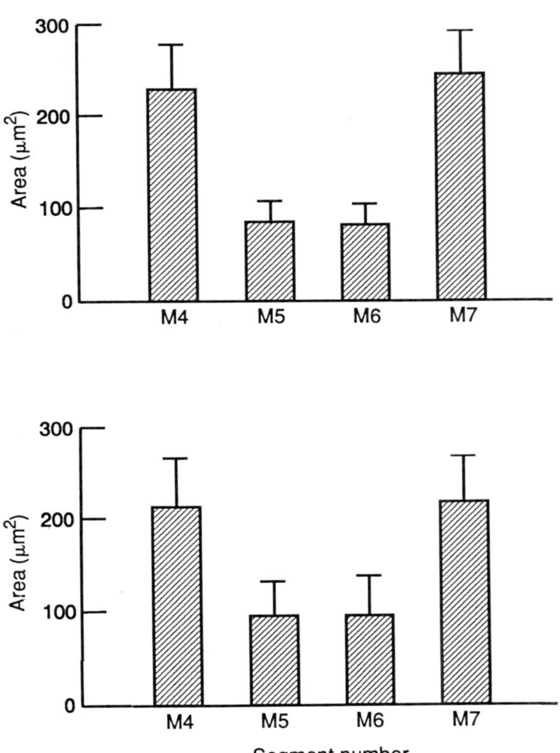

Figure 8. Cell body size of the Retzius neuron is dependent on its own location relative to the reproductive segments (M5 and M6), whether or not the ancestral n blast cells are relocated by bandlet slippage. The cross-sectional area of the Retzius cell body was measured in antibody-stained nerve cords mounted under cover slips and viewed from the dorsal side in 8 normal *H. robusta* embryos *(top)* and 51 embryos in which either the right or left n bandlet had slipped by ≥ 1 segment *(bottom)*. Error bars denote standard deviations. We were unable to reliably determine the right or left origin of Retzius neurons based on their cell body position; therefore, right and left neurons are included in both samples. Thus, the data presented for experimental embryos includes both the relocated neuron on the operated side and the normally located neuron on the control side.

have led to similar conclusions. The blast cells of the p bandlet also seem predetermined to produce a segment-specific pattern of SCP-like immunoreactive neurons (M. Q. Martindale, unpublished observations), and the blast cells of the mesodermal m bandlet generate nephridia and/or genitalia in accordance with their lineage histories, even when they are frameshifted with respect to the ectodermal bandlets (Gleizer and Stent, 1990).

It could be that the blast cell's segmental identity is specified by its environment some time prior to slippage, or that the primary blast cells are already endowed with segmental identities at the time of their birth. Two lines of evidence support this latter view. First, no cell interactions have been shown to play a consistent role in specifying the segmental identity of the blast cell. The persistence of blast cell identity following bandlet slippage eliminates the possibility of instructive cues from other bandlets. In addition, blast cell identity is not altered by ablation of more anterior blast cells in the same bandlet (Martindale and Shankland, 1990a) or by ablating the parent teloblast to prevent the formation of more posterior blast cells (M. Shankland, unpublished observations). There is experimental evidence that the n_s and n_f blast cells are differentially determined from one another at a similarly early stage in development. This distinction is correlated with specific differences in the successive cell cycles by which the N teloblast generates these two subclasses of n blast cell (Bissen and Weisblat, 1987). Thus, sequential blast cell daughters of a given leech teloblast may be endowed with a different set of intrinsic determinants from the time of their respective births.

If the segmental identity of the primary blast cells is determined at birth, it would imply that the teloblast effectively "counts" its mitotic cycles (Martindale and Shankland, 1990a), and specifies the identity of its progeny accordingly. A very similar pattern of stem cell behavior and a dependence of cell determination on mitotic cycle number has also been described for the neuroblasts that give rise to the insect CNS (Doe and Goodman, 1985b; Huff *et al.*, 1989). It is clear that many other determinative events are also associated with specific mitotic cycles, both in organisms with stereotyped cell lineages (Edgar and McGhee, 1988; Finney and Ruvkun, 1990) and in the variable cell lineages that give rise to the neurons of the vertebrate CNS (see Chapter 12). However, the nature of this link between the cell cycle and the activation of particular development programs is, for the most part, a matter of conjecture. One could envision that the differential specification of successive blast cell daughters by the leech teloblast might involve an orderly packaging of regulatory molecules that are present over many cell cycles, or a differential expression of regulatory molecules by the teloblast as it proceeds through each successive cell cycle.

F. Genetic Basis of Segmental Identity

Segmental identity arises in the embryo of the fruitfly *Drosophila* in a manner that has some intriguing parallels to the results described here.

Although leech and fruitfly generate their segmental founder cells by a decidedly different sequence of events (compare Akam, 1987, and Shankland, 1991), the founder cells of both species possess discrete segmental identities from the time of their formation, and long before the onset of organogenesis. As in the leech, different segments of the insect embryo undergo a similar pattern of organogenesis, including the detailed cell lineages of the CNS (Doe and Goodman, 1985a). Overt segmental differences become progressively more apparent as development proceeds; it is interesting to note that this final period of neuronal diversification is accompanied by segment-specific patterns of regulatory gene expression within the CNS of both *Drosophila* (Doe *et al.*, 1988) and the leech (Wysocka-Diller *et al.*, 1989).

The genes that are responsible for establishing segmental identity in the *Drosophila* embryo are very well characterized, and are generically referred to as the "homeotic genes," in reference to the fact that their mutation results in a loss of the normally occurring segmental differences (Akam, 1987; Morata *et al.*, 1990). The homeotic genes are not required for the establishment of segmental periodicity (Struhl, 1981). Rather, each of the fruitfly's homeotic genes is responsible for the development of segment-specific characteristics in a single domain of several contiguous body segments (Akam *et al.*, 1988).

Molecular studies indicate that the homeotic genes of *Drosophila* represent a gene complex that is highly conserved throughout much of the animal kingdom and may be involved in the establishment of segmental identity in phyletically diverse organisms (Akam, 1989). Several apparently homologous genes have now been isolated from the leeches *Hirudo medicinalis* (Wysocka-Diller *et al.*, 1989) and *Helobdella robusta* (Shankland *et al.*, 1991). Their further analysis may eventually yield insight into the molecular basis of the cellular events just described. By analogy with the fruitfly, one could envision that these particular leech genes may be activated in various combinations to determine the identity of individual blast cells or segments. Consistent with this idea, Wysocka-Diller *et al.* (1989) have found that *Lox2*—an apparent homolog of the homeotic genes *Ultrabithorax* and/or *Abdominal A*—is expressed in a striking segment-specific pattern in the developing leech CNS. However, there is, as yet, no evidence that any of these leech genes is expressed at earlier stages of embryogenesis, when the experimental studies indicate that segmental identities are first established. We would anticipate that gene products that are involved in the initial establishment of segmental identity should be expressed either in the teloblast or in the newly born blast cell; attempts to demonstrate such expression will be a major object of future research in this area.

V. Determination of Neuronal Phenotype by Postmitotic Cell Interactions

Although cell lineage plays an important role in determining some aspects of neuronal differentiation, there is also ample evidence that the postmitotic neurons of the leech CNS manifest considerable plasticity in the course of their terminal differentiation (Gao and Macagno, 1987a,b; Loer *et al.,* 1987; Stuart *et al.,* 1987; Blair *et al.,* 1990; Martindale and Shankland, 1990b). In this section we will recount evidence that certain bilateral pairs of neuronal homologs undergo postmitotic cell interactions that result in asymmetric patterns of differentiation.

A. Neuronal Competition

The RAS and CAS cells are asymmetric interneurons that can be readily visualized in the mature CNS by their intense anti-SCP staining (Fig. 6). Embryological studies have shown that the RAS neurons arise from a bilaterally symmetric set of immature nz4 neurons through a selective process of asymmetric differentiation. The CAS neurons arise in a similar manner from a bilaterally symmetric set of immature mz3 neurons, which are descendants of the M teloblast lineage (Shankland and Martindale, 1989). In both cases, the future RAS/CAS neuron and its contralateral homolog begin to express SCP-like immunoreactivity at roughly the same time, but this immunoreactivity disappears from the contralateral homolog several days before the end of the embryonic life. It is difficult to follow the fate of the contralateral homolog neuron after it loses detectable immunoreactivity; it is currently unclear whether or not this loss of peptide expression is a prelude to cell death (Shankland and Martindale, 1989).

The asymmetric differentiation of homolog neurons on the right and left sides of the ganglion is under the control of extrinsic determinants, and appears to depend in large part upon interactions between the neurons themselves. Unilateral ablation of cell lineages that give rise to these neurons causes the contralaterally homologous cell to take on the persistently immunoreactive phenotype in nearly every case (Blair *et al.,* 1990; Martindale and Shankland, 1990b). Since each neuron has a 50% chance of taking on the nonimmunoreactive fate during normal development, such ablations must therefore lead to a change in the fate of roughly half the homolog neurons contralateral to the lesion. In contrast, patterns of RAS or CAS neuron differentiation are largely unaffected by ablation of embryonic cell lineages that do not give rise to their homolog, although such ablations remove large portions of the CNS (Martindale and Shankland, 1990b). These findings suggest that the transiently immunoreactive neuron loses its neuropeptide expression largely because of interactions with its contralateral homolog, that is, the future RAS or CAS neuron. Stuart *et al.* (1987) have drawn similar conclusions for one of the leech's serotonergic interneurons, whose unilateral cell death can be prevented by selective ablation of the cell lineage that would normally give rise to its contralateral homolog.

This sequence of cellular events has been explained with reference to the idea of developmental equivalence groups (Kimble, 1981). The right and left homolog neurons can be viewed as initially equivalent cells that have the same potential to take on the immunoreactive or nonimmunoreactive cell fates. Right and left homolog in the same ganglion would compete for the immuno-reactive phenotype, and an inherent instability in this interaction would insure that one or the other cell gains the upper hand and forces its contralateral homolog into the nonimmunoreactive pathway. Many developmental equiva-lence groups are composed of cells that share some degree of lineal homology (Weisblat and Blair, 1984; Kuwada and Goodman, 1985). In the nematode *C. elegans,* there are several cases of bilaterally homologous cells diversifying through a process of cell interaction (Sulston and White, 1980; Kimble, 1981). Such interactions are inherently competitive in nature, since one cell excludes the other from selecting the same developmental pathway.

The leech CNS displays several other developmental cell interactions that are also demarcated by patterns of neuronal homology. The N or nociceptive neurons have been shown to compete with segmental homologs in their formation of mutual axosomatic connections (Gu and Muller, 1990). There is evidence of competition between their extraganglionic axons for territories of peripheral innervation (Blackshaw *et al.,* 1982). In addition, several leech neurons extend interganglionic axons that halt their growth and subsequently retract after encountering the axons of homologs from the next segment in the interganglionic connectives (Gao and Macagno, 1987a,b). In these ex-amples, neurons interact via their axons, and the interaction has a local effect on axonal growth or synaptogenesis. Thus, the interaction may not be altering the cell's intrinsic identity, but producing a local and reversible modulation of its behavior.

The competitive interactions between the differentiating neurons of the nz4 (RAS) and mz3 (CAS) equivalence groups also occur at a distance from the cell body and may very well involve axonal contacts (Blair *et al.,* 1990). However, this interaction must generate an intracellular signal that is con-veyed back to the cell body in order to influence neuropeptide expression. It is not previously known whether this regulation of neuropeptide expression is a selective event, or if the putative retrograde signal coordinately governs a number of differentiative processes. For example, studies of Retzius neuron transformation in the leech's reproductive segments indicate that peripheral axon contacts can coordinately modify the processes of growth, synaptogenesis, and the expression of neurotransmitter receptors on distant parts of a cell (Loer and Kristan, 1989a). If it can be shown that retrograde signal generated from growth cone or synapse can profoundly and permanently alter the internal workings of an entire cell, then it would seem both biologically and semantically reasonable to refer to this alteration as a change in cell identity.

B. Critical Period for Neuronal Interaction

An important feature of those determinative events that depend on extrinsic cues is that they provide an opportunity to selectively examine each phase in the commitment process. With respect to RAS/CAS neuron determination, the process of cellular commitment has been studied in *Helobdella* embryos by unilaterally ablating the nz4 or mz3 neurons at progressively later stages in embryonic life (Martindale and Shankland, 1990b). Such ablations were accomplished by labeling the relevant cell lineage with a photosensitizing tracer compound, and selectively ablating the labeled cell lineage in the intact embryo at various times by illumination at the photosensitizer's excitation wavelength (Shankland, 1984).

Figure 9 summarizes the results obtained by timed unilateral ablation of the mz3 neurons. Ablation of the newly formed mz3 neurons or their precursor cell lineage has a pronounced effect on the pattern of CAS neuron differentiation among the contralateral neurons (Martindale and Shankland, 1990b). This finding suggests that all of the mz3 neurons in the appropriate segmental domain are still competent at the time of their birth to select either the immunoreactive CAS neuron phenotype or the alternative nonimmunoreactive phenotype. In contrast, ablations performed several days later in development did not alter the contralateral pattern of CAS neuron differentiation, suggesting that the individual mz3 neurons had become committed to one or the other phenotype by that stage. Unilateral ablation of the nz4 neuron revealed a similar time-course of RAS neuron determination (Martindale and Shankland, 1990b).

Our interpretation of these results is that the postmitotic neuron has at least two potential fates, and that it becomes committed to one or the other developmental pathway as a result of interactions with its contralateral homolog. Once the cell is committed to a particular pathway, its neuropeptide phenotype is unaffected by any subsequent ablation of the contralateral homolog. The data suggest that this commitment occurs approximately 2–3 days after the nz4 and mz3 neurons initiate axonogenesis, and around the time at which they begin to express immunologically detectable levels of the SCP-like neuropeptide (Fig. 9).

A major issue in developmental neurobiology is to learn whether the determinative cell interactions that govern neuronal identity are mediated by molecular mechanisms that are dedicated to that purpose, or whether they are a byproduct of those synaptic or hormonal cell interactions that are involved in the functioning of the mature CNS. In this context, it is interesting to note that the decision of the nz4 and mz3 neurons to cease or continue expressing the SCP-like neuropeptide is associated with a relatively late period of differentiation when the postmitotic neurons have already generated many of the morphological and biochemical features required for intercellular communication.

C. **Intersegmental Interactions**

The establishment of neuronal asymmetry exhibits a degree of indeterminacy that is otherwise unusual for the development of the leech CNS. All of the asymmetric neurons that have been examined show an equal likelihood of developing either a right- or left-handed orientation in any given body segment (Stuart *et al.,* 1987; Macagno and Stewart, 1987; Evans and Calabrese, 1989; Shankland and Martindale, 1989). There is no apparent correlation in the asymmetry developed by different nonhomologous neurons in the same ganglion (Shankland and Martindale, 1989). However, homologous neurons in adjacent ganglia show a pronounced tendency to develop asymmetries of opposite orientation (Macagno and Stewart, 1987; Shankland and Martindale, 1989). Depending on the identity of the neuron and the segments under consideration, there is a likelihood of 80% to nearly 100% that homologous cells in adjacent segments will manifest an asymmetry of opposite orientation, leading to a segmentally alternating pattern of neuronal phenotypes in the mature CNS (Fig. 10).

Experimental studies indicate that this segmentally alternating pattern of differentiation depends on interaction of the homolog neurons in adjacent ganglia. In the *Helobdella* embryo, asymmetry can be forced on a particular ganglion by unilateral ablation of a single nz4 or mz3 neuron, with the result that the homologous neurons in neighboring ganglia show a pronounced and statistically significant tendency to develop the opposite asymmetry (Blair *et al.,* 1990). The nz4 and mz3 neurons have interganglionic axons (Blair *et al.,* 1990); in the much larger embryos of the duck leech *Theromyzon rude,* it has been possible to interfere with some of these interganglionic interactions by surgical transection of the intervening connectives (Martindale and Shank-

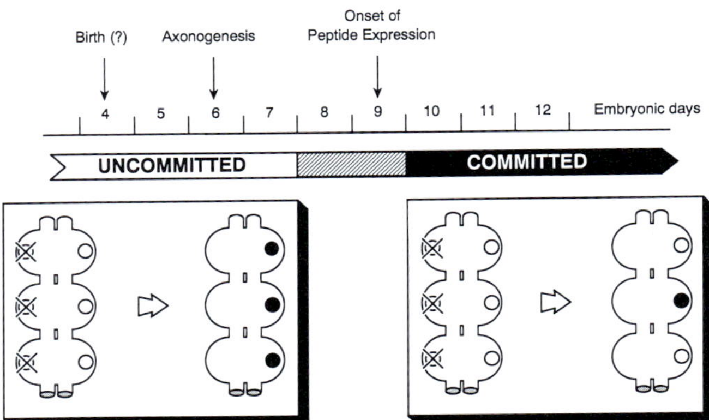

Figure 9. In *Helobdella,* the mz3 neurons become committed to their alternative CAS or non-CAS phenotypes on embryonic days 8–9. This commitment occurs around the onset of neuropeptide expression, and several days after the neuron is first known to be postmitotic. Panels *(bottom)* show the result of ablation experiments performed before and after commitment. Before commitment, unilateral elimination of the mz3 neurons results in all their contralateral homologs acquiring the persistently immunoreactive CAS phenotype (●). After commitment, the same experiment does not alter the segmentally alternating pattern of CAS and non-CAS (○) phenotypes in their contralateral homologs. Similar results have also been obtained for the RAS neurons (Martindale and Shankland, 1990b).

land, 1990b). Thus, one of the differences between segments—the right- or left-handedness of neuronal asymmetry—is also determined by postmitotic cell interactions.

VI. Spatial Patterning of Neuronal Differentiation

In this chapter we have addressed the process of cell type specification in the developing leech nervous system by focusing on a single aspect of neuronal identity, namely, the positional diversification of segmentally homologous neurons. Diversification occurs by modification of a common developmental program; it is therefore feasible to study the origin of particular differences without undertaking explication of the phenotype as a whole. This latter problem has been addressed in *C. elegans* by compiling catalogues of genes whose disruption influences the phenotype of particular neurons. Indeed, the results of such studies support the idea that there is a multiplicity of developmental events that leads to the birth, specification, and ultimate differentiation of single cells (Desai *et al.,* 1988; Chalfie and Au, 1989).

The origin of segmental differences in the leech nervous system can be broken down into several steps. In this concluding section we will exemplify this process by reviewing the development of the nz4 (RAS) neurons. The first step is the generation of a single nz4 neuron per hemisegment. The leech embryo displays a bilaterally symmetric and segmentally repeated cell lineage; thus, the formation of a similar set of postmitotic neurons in each hemisegment of the CNS reflects spatial iterations in the process of neurogenesis. It is not known how the nz4 neuron becomes differentially specified from the other postmitotic neurons in its hemisegment, although such specification clearly must occur before expression of the SCP-like neuropeptide, since the nz4 neuron is the only cell in its region of the ganglion to do so at that early stage. The stereotyped nature of the formative cell divisions suggests that lineage history may play a critical role in nz4 specification, but this observation alone does not exclude determinative cell interactions. For instance, the neurons of the insect CNS arise by strict lineage histories, yet pairs of sibling neurons interact with one another to bring about the differential specification of their final phenotypes (Kuwada and Goodman, 1985).

Segmentally homologous nz4 neurons show the same initial pattern of axonal projection and neuropeptide expression (Shankland and Martindale, 1989), but only those homologs that are situated in segments R4–M3 will become RAS neurons. Moreover, the bandlet slippage experiments suggest that the potential to become a RAS neuron is intrinsic to those nz4 neurons that occupy this segmental domain, and is not a property of the cellular environment in that domain. Thus, although the postmitotic neurons of the leech CNS show a segmentally repeated distribution, the experimental studies indicate that they already possess a cryptic pattern of segment-specific commitments at the time of their birth. Indeed, one interpretation of our results is that the segmental identity of the postmitotic neuron reflects a developmental commitment that is in effect at the level of its distant ancestor, the primary blast cell, and is conveyed to the neuron as a consequence of its cell lineage history.

The final step in RAS neuron differentiation is the competitive interaction of the postmitotic nz4 neurons in the domain that is circumscribed by this prior specification of segmental identity (Fig. 10). Interactions cause the eight nz4 neurons in these segments to diverge into alternative RAS and non-RAS developmental pathways; the outcome of these events shows both random and nonrandom components. The numerical outcome is precise: four nz4 neurons choose the RAS phenotype while the other four become committed to the non-RAS fate. However, the spatial patterning of these decisions varies from one animal to the next. The intraganglionic competition appears to be quite strong, so only a single mature RAS neuron is formed on either the right or left side in each of the four ganglia. However, the interganglionic interac-

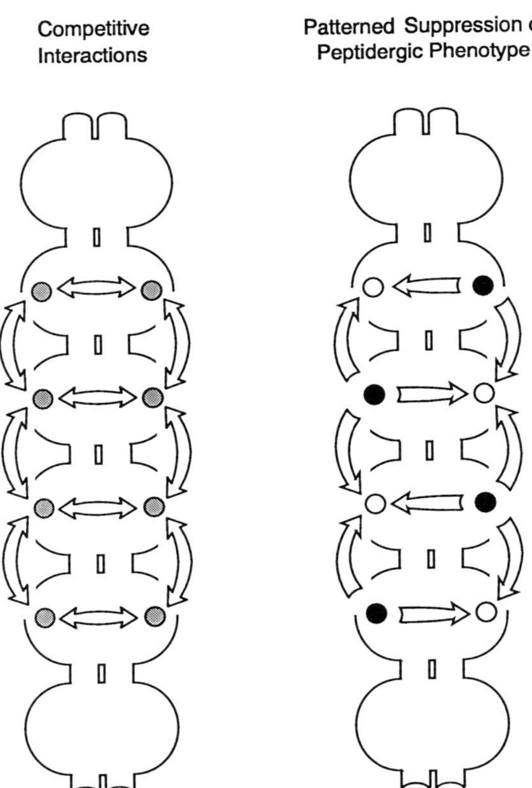

Figure 10. Segmentally alternating patterns of neuronal differentiation appear to be an emergent property of a patterned array of postmitotic cell interactions. The example shown here is meant to represent the development of nz4 (RAS) neurons. Initially, homolog neurons (◉) situated over a span of four consecutive segments have the potential to take on the mature RAS phenotype. The immature neurons compete for the RAS phenotype (bidirectional arrows), both with their contralateral homologs in the same ganglion and with homologs in neighboring ganglia. The typical outcome is for four mature RAS neurons (●) to develop on alternate right and left sides in successive ganglia and to suppress the peptidergic phenotype (unidirectional arrows) in the other four homologs (○).

tions must have a weaker influence on the decision to be RAS or non-RAS, since (1) the right–left alternation of RAS neurons in adjacent segments is not perfect, and (2) experimental studies have shown that RAS neurons are unable to turn off the RAS phenotype in ipsilateral homologs in neighboring ganglia if the latter cells are deprived of the intraganglionic competition (Martindale and Shankland, 1990b). As was first suggested by Macagno and Stewart (1987) for the posteromedial serotonin neuron, we envision that each intraganglionic competition has a stochastic outcome, and that the first ganglion to establish a significant asymmetry coordinates the asymmetry of homolog pairs in neighboring segments through interganglionic cell interactions.

Thus, the final outcome of these determinative cell interactions is to generate a nervous system in which there is a precisely regulated number of RAS neurons, but in which the spatial distribution of these neurons varies to some degree. From an evolutionary standpoint, this variability indicates that natural selection has not constrained the exact positioning of the RAS neuron cell bodies, perhaps because the positioning of these particular cells is of little functional consequence in the workings of the mature nervous system. From a developmental standpoint, these findings indicate that the final pattern of neuronal differentiation is an emergent property of a network of cell interactions.

This latter issue is not only relevant to those animals that develop via stereotyped cell lineages, but also to vertebrate organisms, which construct their nervous systems through variable cell lineages (Kimmel and Warga, 1986; Turner and Cepko, 1988). In the vertebrate retina, the specification of different neuronal phenotypes occurs in large part at the level of the postmitotic neuron or its immediate precursors. Cell interactions are required as a feedback mechanism to insure the correct proportioning of cells into the various differentiative pathways (Reh and Tully, 1986; Reh, 1987). This parallel suggests that competitive cell interactions may be of general importance as a means for assigning the appropriate number of neurons to each of several alternative developmental pathways.

Acknowledgments

The authors would like to thank Eduardo Macagno for a critical reading of this manuscript. The original work discussed here was supported by NIH grant RO1-HD21735, March of Dimes grants 5-593 and 1-1190, and NSF grant BNS-8718045 (to M. S. and Seth Blair).

References

Akam, M. (1987). The molecular basis for metameric pattern in the *Drosophila* embryo. *Development* **101**, 1–22.

Akam, M. (1989). *Hox* and HOM: Homologous gene clusters in insects and vertebrates. *Cell* **57**, 347–349.

Akam, M., Dawson, I., and Tear, G. (1988). Homeotic genes and the control of segment diversity. *Devel. Suppl.* **104,** 123–133.

Bissen, S. T., and Weisblat, D. A. (1987). Early differences between alternate n blast cells in leech embryo. *J. Neurobiol.* **18,** 251–269.

Bissen, S. T., and Weisblat, D. A. (1989). The durations and compositions of cell cycles in embryos of the leech, *Helobdella triserialis. Development* **106,** 105–118.

Blackshaw, S. E., Nicholls, J. G., and Parnas, I. (1982). Expanded receptive fields of cutaneous mechanoreceptor cells after single neurone deletion in leech nervous system. *J. Physiol.* **326,** 261–268.

Blair, S. S., Martindale, M. Q., and Shankland, M. (1990). Interactions between adjacent ganglia bring about the bilaterally alternating differentiation of RAS and CAS neurons in the leech nerve cord. *J. Neurosci.* **10,** 3183–3193.

Chalfie, M., and Au, M. (1989). Genetic control of differentiation of the *Caenorhabditis elegans* touch receptor neurons. *Science* **243,** 1027–1033.

Desai, C., Garriga, G., McIntire, S. L., and Horvitz, H. R. (1988). A genetic pathway for the development of the *Caenorhabditis elegans* HSN motor neurons. *Nature (London)* **336,** 638–646.

Doe, C. Q., and Goodman, C. S. (1985a). Early events in insect neurogenesis. I. Development and segmental differences in the pattern of neuronal precursor cells. *Dev. Biol.* **111,** 193–205.

Doe, C. Q., and Goodman, C. S. (1985b). Early events in insect neurogenesis. II. The role of cell interactions and cell lineage in the determination of neuronal precursor cells. *Dev. Biol.* **111,** 206–219.

Doe, C. Q., Hiromi, Y., Gehring, W. J., and Goodman, C. S. (1988). Expression and function of the segmentation gene *fushi tarazu* during *Drosophila* neurogenesis. *Science* **239,** 170–175.

Edgar, L. G., and McGhee, J. D. (1988). DNA synthesis and the control of embryonic gene expression in *C. elegans. Cell* **53,** 589–599.

Evans, B. D., and Calabrese, R. L. (1989). Small cardioactive peptide-like immunoreactivity and its colocalization with FMRFamide-like immunoreactivity in the central nervous system of the leech *Hirudo medicinalis. Cell Tissue Res.* **257,** 187–199.

Finney, M., and Ruvkun, G. (1990). The *unc-86* gene product couples cell lineage and cell identity in *C. elegans. Cell* **63,** 895–905.

Fuchs, P. A., Nicholls, J. G., and Ready, D. (1981). Membrane properties and selective connexions of identified leech neurones in culture. *J. Physiol.* **316,** 203–223.

Gao, W.-Q., and Macagno, E. R. (1987a). Extension and retraction of axonal projections by some developing neurons in the leech depends upon the existence of neighboring homologues. II. The AP and AE neurons. *J. Neurosci.* **18,** 295–313.

Gao, W.-Q., and Macagno, E. R. (1987b). Extension and retraction of axonal projections by some developing neurons in the leech depends upon the existence of neighboring homologues. I. The HA cells. *J. Neurobiol.* **18,** 43–59.

Gimlich, R. L., and Braun, J. (1985). Improved fluorescent compounds for tracing cell lineage. *Dev. Biol.* **109,** 509–514.

Gleizer, L., and Stent, G. S. (1990). Control of segment identity in the leech embryo. *Soc. Neurosci. Abstr.* **16,** 650.

Glover, J. C. (1987). Serotonin storage and uptake by identified neurons in the leech *Haementeria ghilianii. J. Comp. Neurol.* **256,** 117–127.

Glover, J. C., and Mason, A. D. (1986). Morphogenesis of an identified leech neuron: Segmental specification of axonal outgrowth. *Dev. Biol.* **115,** 256–260.

Gu, X., and Muller, K. J. (1990). Competitive interactions between neurons making axosomatic contacts in the leech. *J. Neurosci.* **10,** 3814–3822.

Ho, R. K., and Weisblat, D. A. (1987). A provisional epithelium in leech embryo: Cellular origins and influence on a developmental equivalence group. *Dev. Biol.* **120,** 520–534.

Huff, R., Furst, A., and Mahowald, A. P. (1989). *Drosophila* embryonic neuroblasts in culture: Autonomous differentiation of specific neurotransmitters. *Dev. Biol.* **134,** 146–157.

Kimble, J. (1981). Alterations in cell lineage following laser ablation of cells in the somatic gonad of *Caenorhabditis elegans. Dev. Biol.* **87,** 286–300.

Kimmel, C. B., and Warga, R. M. (1986). Tissue-specific cell lineages originate in the gastrula of the zebrafish. *Science* **231,** 365–368.

Kramer, A. P., and Weisblat, D. A. (1985). Developmental neural kinship groups in the leech. *J. Neurosci.* **5,** 388–407.

Kuhlman, J. R., Li, C., and Calabrese, R. L. (1985). FMRF-amide-like substances in the leech. I. Immunocytochemical localization. *J. Neurosci.* **5,** 2301–2309.

Kuwada, J. Y., and Goodman, C. S. (1985). Neuronal determination during embryonic development of the grasshopper nervous system. *Dev. Biol.* **110,** 114–126.

Li, C., and Calabrese, R. L. (1985). Evidence for proctolin-like substances in the central nervous system of the leech *Hirudo medicinalis. J. Comp. Neurol.* **232,** 414–424.

Loer, C. M., Schley, C., Zipser, B., and Kristan, W. B. (1986). Development of segmental differences in the pressure mechanosensory neurons of the leech *Haementeria ghilianii. J. Comp. Neurol.* **254,** 403–409.

Loer, C. M., Jellies, J., and Kristan, W. B. (1987). Segment-specific morphogenesis of leech Retzius neurons requires particular peripheral targets. *J. Neurosci.* **7,** 2630–2638.

Loer, C. M., and Kristan, W. B. (1989a). Central synaptic inputs to identified leech neurons are determined by peripheral targets. *Science* **244,** 64–66.

Loer, C. M., and Kristan, W. B. (1989b). Peripheral target choice by homologous neurons during embryogenesis of the medicinal leech. I. Segment-specific preferences of Retzius cells. *J. Neurosci.* **9,** 513–527.

Macagno, E. R. (1980). Number and distribution of neurons in the leech segmental ganglion. *J. Comp. Neurol.* **190,** 283–302.

Macagno, E. R., Peinado, A., and Stewart, R. R. (1986). Segmental differentiation in the leech nervous system: Specific phenotype changes associated with ectopic targets. *Proc. Natl. Acad. Sci. U.S.A.* **83,** 2746–2750.

Macagno, E. R., and Stewart, R. R. (1987). Cell death during gangliogenesis in the leech: Competition leading to the death of PMS neurons has both random and nonrandom components. *J. Neurosci.* **7,** 1911–1918.

Martindale, M. Q., and Shankland, M. (1988). Developmental origin of segmental differences in the leech ectoderm: Survival and differentiation of the distal tubule cell is determined by the host segment. *Dev. Biol.* **125,** 290–300.

Martindale, M. Q., and Shankland, M. (1990a). Segmental founder cells of the leech embryo have intrinsic segmental identity. *Nature (London)* **347,** 672–674.

Martindale, M. Q., and Shankland, M. (1990b). Neuronal competition determines the spatial pattern of neuropeptide expression by identified neurons of the leech. *Dev. Biol.* **139,** 210–226.

Morata, G., Macias, A., Urquia, N., and Gonzales-Reyes, A. (1990). Homoeotic genes. *Sem. Cell Biol.* **1,** 219–228.

Muller, K. J., Nicholls, J. G., and Stent, G. S. (1981). "Neurobiology of the Leech." Cold Spring Harbor, New York: Cold Spring Harbor Press.

Patterson, P. H. (1978). Environmental determination of autonomic neurotransmitter functions. *Ann. Rev. Neurosci.* **1,** 1–17.

Reh, T. A. (1987). Cell-specific regulation of neuronal production in the larval frog retina. *J. Neurosci.* **7,** 3317–3324.

Reh, T. A., and Tully, T. (1986). Regulation of tyrosine hydroxylase containing amacrine cell number in larval frog retina. *Dev. Biol.* **114,** 463–469.

Reinke, R., and Zipursky, S. L. (1988). Cell–cell interaction in the *Drosophila* retina: The *bride of sevenless* gene is required in photoreceptor cell R8 for R7 cell development. *Cell* **55**, 321–330.

Sandig, M., and Dohle, W. (1988). The cleavage pattern in the leech *Theromyzon tessulatum* (Hirudinea, Glossiphoniidae). *J. Morph.* **196**, 217–252.

Sawyer, R. T. (1986). "Leech Biology and Behaviour. Vol. I. Anatomy, Physiology, and Behaviour." Oxford: Clarendon Press.

Shafer, M. R., and Calabrese, R. L. (1981). Similarities and differences in the structure of segmentally homologous neurons that control the hearts in the leech, *Hirudo medicinalis. Cell Tissue Res.* **214**, 137–153.

Shankland, M. (1984). Positional determination of supernumerary blast cell death in the leech embryo. *Nature (London)* **307**, 541–543.

Shankland, M. (1987a). Differentiation of the O and P cell lines in the embryo of the leech. I. Sequential commitment of blast cell sublineages. *Dev. Biol.* **123**, 85–96.

Shankland, M. (1987b). Differentiation of the O and P cell lines in the embryo of the leech. II. Genealogical relationship of descendant pattern elements in alternative developmental pathways. *Dev. Biol.* **123**, 97–107.

Shankland, M. (1987c). Cell lineage in leech embryogenesis. *Trends Genet.* **3**, 314–319.

Shankland, M. (1991). Leech segmentation: Cell lineage and the formation of complex body patterns. *Dev. Biol.* **144**, 221–231.

Shankland, M., and Weisblat, D. A. (1984). Stepwise commitment of blast cell fates during the positional specification of the O and P cell lines in the leech embryo. *Dev. Biol.* **106**, 326–342.

Shankland, M., and Martindale, M. Q. (1989). Segmental specificity and lateral asymmetry in the differentiation of developmentally homologous neurons during leech embryogenesis. *Dev. Biol.* **135**, 431–448.

Shankland, M., Martindale, M. Q., Nardelli-Haefliger, D., Baxter, E. and Price, D. J. (1991). Origin of segmental identity in the development of the leech nervous system. *Devel. Suppl.* (in press).

Stent, G. S., Weisblat, D. A., Blair, S. S., and Zackson, S. L. (1982). Cell lineage in the development of the leech nervous system. *In* "Neuronal Development" (N. C. Spitzer, ed.), pp. 1–44. New York: Plenum Press.

Stewart, R. R., Spergel, D., and Macagno, E. R. (1986). Segmental differentiation in the leech nervous system: The genesis of cell number in the segmental ganglia of *Haemopis marmorata. J. Comp. Neurol.* **253**, 253–259.

Struhl, G. (1981). A gene product required for correct initiation of segmental determination in *Drosophila. Nature (London)* **293**, 36–41.

Stuart, D. K., Blair, S. S., and Weisblat, D. A. (1987). Cell lineage, cell death, and the developmental origin of identified serotonin- and dopamine-containing neurons in the leech. *J. Neurosci.* **7**, 1107–1122.

Sulston, J. E., and White, J. G. (1980). Regulation and cell autonomy during postembryonic development of *Caenorhabditis elegans. Dev. Biol.* **78**, 577–597.

Torrence, S. A., Law, M. I., and Stuart, D. K. (1989). Leech neurogenesis. II. Mesodermal control of neuronal patterns. *Dev. Biol.* **136**, 40–60.

Turner, D. L., and Cepko, C. L. (1988). A common progenitor for neurons and glia persists in rat retina late in development. *Nature (London)* **328**, 131–136.

Weeks, J. D. (1982). Segmental specialization of a leech swim-initiating interneuron (cell 205). *J. Neurosci.* **2**, 972–985.

Weisblat, D. A., Sawyer, R. T., and Stent, G. S. (1978). Cell lineage analysis by intracellular injection of a tracer enzyme. *Science* **202**, 1295–1298.

Weisblat, D. A., and Blair, S. S. (1984). Developmental indeterminacy in embryos of the leech *Helobdella triserialis. Dev. Biol.* **101**, 326–335.

Weisblat, D. A., Kim, S. Y., and Stent, G. S. (1984). Embryonic origins of cells in the leech *Helobdella triserialis. Dev. Biol.* **104,** 65–85.

Weisblat, D. A., and Shankland, M. (1985). Cell lineage and segmentation in the leech. *Phil. Trans. R. Soc. Lond. B* **312,** 39–56.

Wittenberg, G., Loer, C. M., Adamo, S. A., and Kristan, W. B. Jr. (1990). Segmental specialization of neuronal connectivity in the leech. *J. Comp. Physiol.* [A] **167,** 453–459.

Wysocka-Diller, J. W., Aisemberg, G. O., Baumgarten, M., Levine, M., and Macagno, E. R. (1989). Characterization of a homologue of bithorax-complex genes in the leech *Hirudo medicinalis. Nature (London)* **341,** 760–763.

Yau, K.-W. (1976). Physiological properties and receptive fields of mechanosensory neurones in the head ganglion of the leech: Comparison with homologous cells in segmental ganglia. *J. Physiol.* **263,** 489–512.

Zackson, S. L. (1984). Cell lineage, cell–cell interaction, and segment formation in the ectoderm of a glossiphoniid leech embryo. *Dev. Biol.* **104,** 43–60.

Zipser, B., and McKay, R. (1981). Monoclonal antibodies distinguish identifiable neurones in the leech. *Nature (London)* **289,** 549–554.

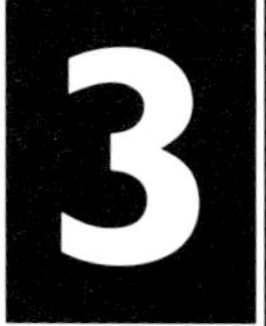

Control of Central Neurogenesis
in the Leech

Thomas Becker and Eduardo R. Macagno
Department of Biological Sciences
Columbia University
New York, New York

I. Introduction

Subdivision into segmental units, or neuromeres, is an important feature of the central nervous system (CNS) of animals with a segmented body plan, for example, annelids, arthropods, and vertebrates, although in the latter not all regions of the CNS may be truly segmented (Lumsden and Keynes, 1989). The individual neuromeres attain important differences in structure and size as they become specialized for distinct functions that correlate with their positions along the body axis. An intriguing problem, currently researched at many levels, is how these regional differences are generated in the developing animal from each set of segmental precursors. The specific aspect of this problem that we will consider in this chapter is the regulation of the number of neurons that constitute a neuromere. In particular, we will discuss recent work from our laboratory on the control of neurogenesis in the CNS of the medicinal leech *(Hirudo medicinalis)*. For other approaches to the problem of segmental differentiation in the leech, the reader is referred to Chapters 2 and 4.

In principle, the number of neurons in any particular region of the CNS may be determined by controlling the rate or amount of cell birth, the migration of cells into and out of the region, and the extent of cell death. Many of our current ideas about the mechanisms that regulate the size of central neuronal populations are derived from studies of vertebrate neurogenesis. A widely accepted view is that the number of central neurons in the adult vertebrate is attained, for the most part, through an initial overproduction of cells followed by the death of a significant fraction of them. Those that survive do so mainly because of extrinsic factors provided by interactions with their synaptic targets (Purves and Lichtman, 1985). Survival of spinal cord motor neurons, for example, has been shown to depend largely on their innervation of target muscles (reviewed in Williams and Herrup, 1988; Oppenheim, 1991). Likewise, sensory interneurons degenerate in the absence of contact with their presynaptic partners (e.g., Van der Loos and Woolsey, 1973; Woolsey *et al.,* 1981). In contrast to these observations, however, it appears that certain types of vertebrate neurons do not use such a strategy. For example, it has been reported recently that spinal cord interneurons do not undergo a significant level of regulatory cell death (McKay and Oppenheim, 1991).

In invertebrates, conversely, the sizes of neuronal populations have been thought to be achieved through a specified number of cell divisions and programmed cell death, with little or no effect from interactions with target cells (Purves and Lichtman, 1985). In insects, for instance, the ventral nerve cord is produced by segmentally repeated stereotyped sets of precursors, or neuroblasts (Bate, 1976; Hartenstein and Campos-Ortega, 1984), each of which divides a fixed number of times to produce an invariant subset of progeny (Taghert *et al.,* 1984, Doe and Goodman, 1985a,b; Hartenstein *et al.,* 1987). During embryogenesis of *Drosophila,* 40–50 neuroblasts per segment give rise to a ventral nervous system that contains comparable numbers of neurons in thoracic and abdominal segments (Hartenstein *et al.,* 1987). Subsequently, the larva undergoes a second phase of neurogenesis prior to metamorphosis, in which production of neurons in the thorax vastly exceeds neuronal birth in the abdomen (White and Kankel, 1978; Truman and Bate, 1988). The postembryonic precursors are unequally distributed: thoracic neuromeres contain about 47 neuroblasts and posterior abdominal neuromeres only 6 (Truman and Bate, 1988). Moreover, the thoracic neuroblasts undergo many more divisions than those in the abdomen. Since embryonic and postembryonic neuroblasts share a common origin (Prokop and Technau, 1991), segment-specific neurogenesis in the fruit fly appears to be a consequence of the selective survival of precursors.

Nonetheless, it is clear that cell death also contributes significantly to the regulation of cell number in the invertebrate CNS. In the locust *Schistocerca,* for example, the initial birth of ganglion cells is followed by extensive cell death in abdominal, but not in thoracic, segments. Although there is some differential generation of neurons (e.g., the medial neuroblast has about 100 progeny in the third thoracic segment but only about 90 in the first abdominal neuromere), most of the difference in neuron number among thoracic and abdominal neuromeres stems from the death of some 50% of the neurons in the latter (Goodman and Bate, 1981). This regulatory cell death is indepen-dent of the innervation of target muscles, since the removal of a limb bud has no effect on the differentiation of motor neurons that would normally in-nervate the missing muscles (Whitington *et al.,* 1982).

That fully differentiated motor neurons can survive in the absence of their target muscles has also been shown in beetles (Breidbach, 1987a) and in the leech (Baptista and Macagno, 1988b). Interestingly, during insect metamorph-osis, many motor neurons become disconnected from the periphery without dying, as they await remodeling of the CNS and peripheral tissues (e.g., Levine, 1986; Booker and Truman, 1987; Breidbach, 1987b; see also Chapter 9), although in the moth, up to 50% of the interneurons and motor neurons in the abdominal CNS degenerate after adult emergence (Truman and Schwartz, 1984). By comparison, a critical dependence on trophic factors for survival can be found in the arthropod visual system: the survival of cells in optic ganglia depends strongly on interactions with retinal axons in flies (Power, 1943; Meyerowitz and Kankel, 1978; Fischbach, 1983; Fischbach and Technau, 1984; Steller *et al.,* 1987) and in the small crustacean, *Daphnia magna* (LoPresti *et al.,* 1973; Macagno, 1979).

These examples, along with others, clearly demonstrate that differential distribution of precursors and cell death are important means for regula-ting the size of invertebrate and vertebrate neuronal populations. However, control over cell birth has also been proposed to have such a function (e.g., Kollros and Thiesse, 1988; reviewed in Williams and Herrup, 1988). Recently, two instances of innervation-dependent selective neurogenesis have been documented in invertebrates. One, the demonstration that innervation of a peripheral organ controls additional cell birth in two segmental ganglia of the ventral nerve cord of the leech, *Hirudo medicinalis* (Baptista and Macagno, 1988a; Baptista *et al.,* 1990), is the subject of this chapter. The second case is the demonstration that retinal innervation affects the genera-tion, as well as the survival, of neurons in the optic ganglia of *Drosophila* (Selleck and Steller, 1991). To what extent this mechanism will be found to contribute significantly to cell number regulation in other systems remains to be seen.

II. Early Neurogenesis in the Leech

The leech CNS comprises a chain of 21 midbody segmental ganglia, a head ganglion composed of a nonmetameric region (Weisblat *et al.*, 1984) and four fused neuromeres, and a tail ganglion derived from the fusion of seven neuromeres. Ganglia are connected to each other through paired connective nerves and innervate their own segments through bilateral anterior and posterior nerve roots (see Fig. 1A).

Early developmental events have been studied extensively in the glossiphoniid leech *Helobdella*. Glossiphoniid leeches have large eggs, in contrast to hirudinid leeches (the other extensively studied leech group); this has led to their extensive use in cell lineage studies by the injection of tracer dyes into individual precursors (Weisblat *et al.*, 1980; Stent and Weisblat, 1985). Early cleavage produces five bilateral pairs of stem cells, or teloblasts, designated M, N, O, P, and Q. Series of unequal divisions of each teloblast give rise to linear arrays, or bandlets, of primary blast cells. As they expand, the 10 bandlets merge to form a sheet of cells, the germinal plate. The earliest blast cells will eventually form the head, whereas later ones give rise to progressively more posterior segments, resulting in an anteroposterior order of development (Fernandez, 1980; Fernandez and Stent, 1982; Shankland, 1991; see also Chapter 2).

All five teloblasts contribute cells to the CNS (Weisblat *et al.*, 1984). Cell lineages, as far as is known, are invariant, since any particular identified neuron always stems from the same teloblast. Neurons of the same functional type do not, however, necessarily originate form the same precursor, nor do

Figure 1 A. Diagram showing a portion of the leech ventral nerve cord and the reproductive organs as seen in a young adult after partial dissection. The ganglia shown are those in midbody segments 4–7; ♂ penis and prostate; ♀ vagina; E, epididymides; o, ovaries; t, testisacs; *arrowheads,* vas deferens; *arrows,* branches of the root nerves innervating the genitalia. (Adapted from Baptista *et al.,* 1990.) B. The mean number of neurons in sex (M5 and M6; ---) and nonsex (M4 and M7; ---) ganglia in *Haemopis marmorata* plotted as a function of age. Since no significant difference was found between sex and nonsex ganglia at E20 or earlier stages, the means plotted at these early stages are for all ganglia. From E28 onwards, the difference is significant and the two types of ganglia are plotted separately. Emergence from the cocoon (the end of embryogenesis) occurs at about day 30 *(arrow).* Note the decrease in number up to E20, which is due to cell death. (Adapted from Stewart *et al.,* 1986.) C, D. Wholemounts of sex (M6) and nonsex (M7) adult ganglia, respectively, from the leech *Macrobdella decora.* The ganglia were stained with methylene blue to show the neuronal somata. Note the much greater number of small neurons in M6. In this figure, as well as those following, anterior is up and the dorsoventral axis is perpendicular to the page. Bar: 50 μm. (Adapted from Macagno, 1980.)

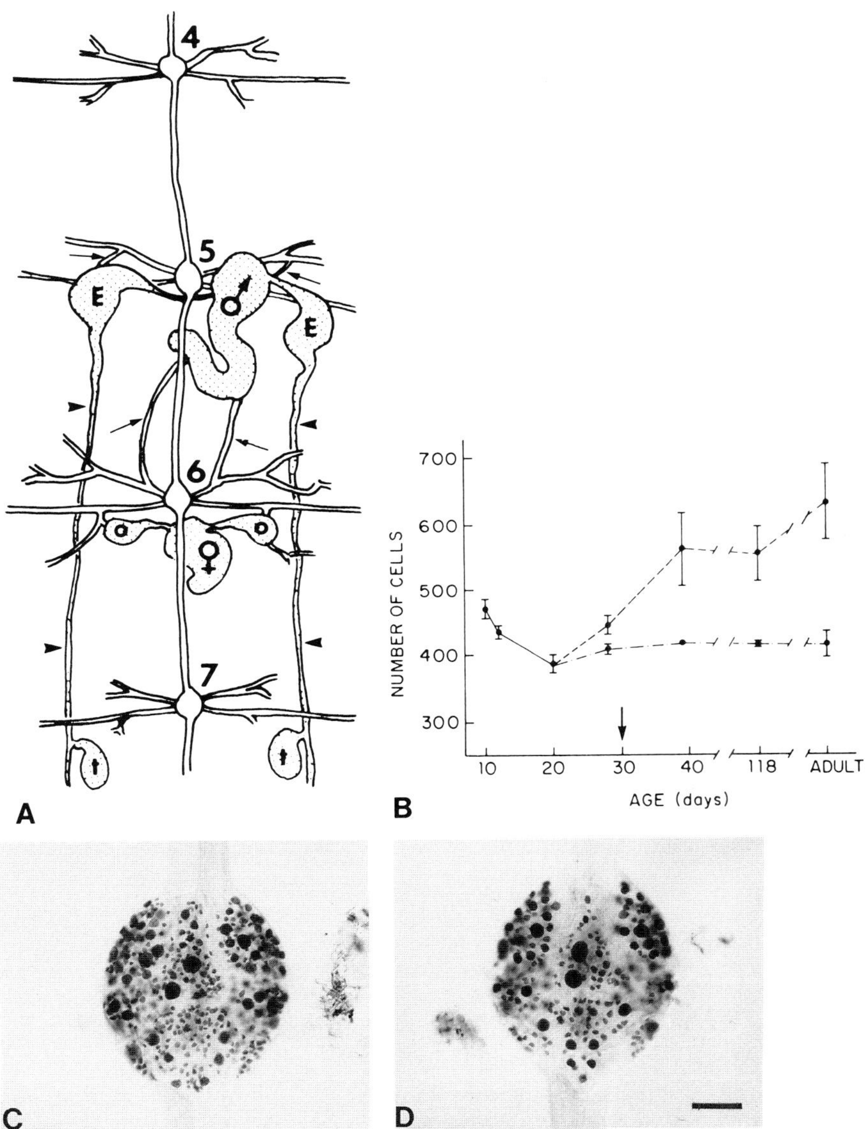

4
5
E
E
6
7
700
600
500
400
300
NUMBER OF CELLS
10   20   30   40   118   ADULT
AGE (days)
A
B
C
D

glia and neurons derive from separate lineages (Kramer and Weisblat, 1985). A significant amount of cell migration into the CNS does take place during gangliogenesis (Torrence and Stuart, 1986) and the clones of the different blast cell lineages intermingle as they coalesce into neuromeres (Weisblat *et al.*, 1984).

In hirudinid leeches, an initial overproduction of cells in segmental ganglia in the first third of embryogenesis (embryogenesis lasts 30 days at 22–23°C) is corrected during the second third by the degeneration of about 15% of the neurons (Stewart *et al.*, 1986; see Fig. 1B). This cell loss can be attributed in part to the death of homologous cells in all segments (e.g., Stewart *et al.*, 1987) and in part to the death of one of a bilateral pair of homologs in every segment (e.g., Macagno and Stewart, 1987). Segment-specific neuronal death, although suspected to occur, has yet to be convincingly documented in the generation of the leech ventral nerve cord.

III. Significant Segmental Differences in Cell Number in the Ventral Nerve Cord

In hirudinid leeches (e.g., *Hirudo medicinalis* and *Haemopis marmorata*), most of the midbody segmental ganglia (M1–M21) in the adult contain about 400 neurons, the main exceptions being the ganglia of the fifth and sixth midbody segments (M5 and M6), which innervate the male and female genitalia (see Fig. 1A). In these leeches, M5 and M6 (also termed the sex ganglia), contain additional complements of a few hundred small cells distributed throughout each ganglion (Macagno, 1980; see Fig. 1C,D). These cells, which are neurons by morphological and immunohistological criteria (Baptista and Macagno, 1988a), differentiate postembryonically and give the appearance of being added gradually to the neuron pool over several months (Stewart *et al.*, 1987; Baptista and Macagno, 1988a; see Fig. 1B). They are born only in the sex ganglia during the last third of embryogenesis (Baptista *et al.*, 1990). Using markers of mitotic activity (see subsequent text), we have determined that the early rounds of mitosis, common to all ganglia and ending at about embryonic day 10 (E10), are followed only in the sex ganglia by later rounds occurring between E20 and E30. These two distinct phases of neurogenesis, considered with the amenability of the leech embryo to microsurgical procedures, have made possible a detailed description of the early events leading to segment-specific neurogenesis.

IV. Birth of Extra Neurons in the Sex Ganglia Depends on Their Innervation of the Male Genitalia

The male genitalia are located in the fifth body segment and are innervated by branches of the anterior nerve roots of both M5 and M6; the female genitalia are found in the sixth body segment and are innervated only by branches of the posterior roots of M6 (Fig. 1A). If the male genitalia, which are innervated by the CNS no earlier than E12 (Jellies and Kristan, 1988), are ablated before E13, there is a complete absence of the extra neurons in the sex ganglia, as shown by cell counts in juveniles or adults (Baptista and Macagno, 1988a). Using the incorporation of 5-bromo-2'-deoxyuridine (BrdU) to detect mitotic cells (see Fig. 2), it was shown that the absence of the cells is due to their never being born rather than to their death following ablation of the male organ (Baptista *et al.,* 1990). Ablation of the female organ, in contrast, exerts no effect on the appearance of these neurons. If the sex ganglia are deprived of the nerve connection to the male organ, the extra neurons also fail to appear (Baptista and Macagno, 1988a; see Fig. 2B). These data are consistent with the hypothesis that the birth of the extra cells is induced by the male genitalia, and that the inductive signal is conveyed by the nerves connecting them to the CNS. These neurons, therefore, are called peripherally induced central (PIC) neurons.

Interestingly, although the PIC neurons are not born until after about E20, a signal from the peripheral target is not required after E16; animals whose male genitalia are ablated after E16 generate a full complement of PIC neurons (Baptista *et al.,* 1990). To further define the time of the interaction, we have recently begun a series of ablations and transplantations of the male organs. In one series of experiments, tissues were ablated at E10 and replaced at various later stages by a transplant of the same age; the number of PIC neurons was then counted. Our observations indicate that the critical period during which the sex ganglia must have access to the male genitalia is from E13 to E16 (unpublished results). However, these results did not tell us whether (1) the genitalia are only capable of sending the mitogenic signal at this time, (2) the CNS is only capable of receiving a signal at this time, or (3) both. We therefore began another series of experiments, in which we tested whether this critical period is defined by the CNS or the genitalia by transplanting older tissues into younger embryos. Our results show that male genitalia from animals as old as 40 days (10 days postembryonic) have the capacity to induce PIC neurons, provided the host is younger than E17 (see Fig. 2C; unpublished results). Thus, the existence of a critical period for the induction of the PIC neurons is a property of the CNS, not the periphery.

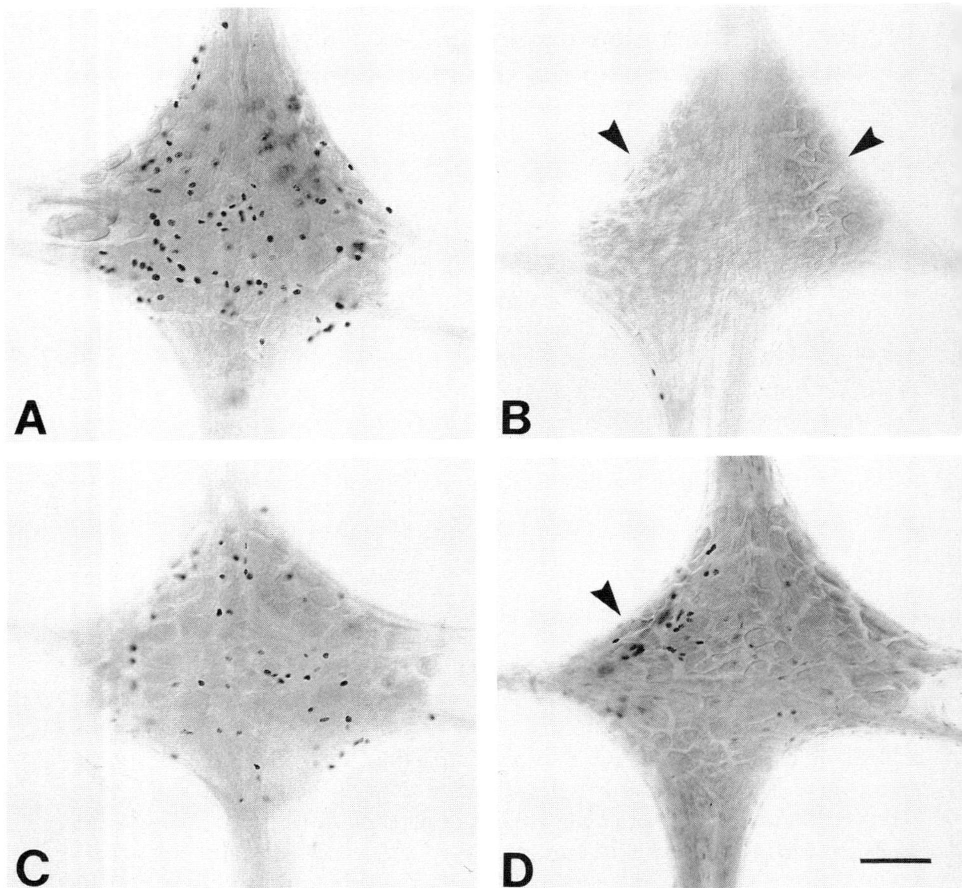

Figure 2 Wholemounts of sex ganglia from E24 embryos injected with BrdU and processed with anti-BrdU and horseradish peroxidase secondary antibodies to detect dividing cells that had incorporated the tracer in their nuclei (see Baptista *et al.*, 1990, for details of the technique). A. Normal sex ganglion showing labeled nuclei distributed widely. B. Ganglion that had the anterior root nerves cut *(arrowheads)* at E11. Note the almost complete lack of labeled nuclei. C. Sex ganglion from an animal that had its male genitalia removed at E11 and immediately replaced with the male genitalia of a 40-day-old donor. Labeled nuclei are present throughout the ganglion (compare with normal ganglion in A). D. Sex ganglion that had the anterior root on the left side *(arrowhead)* cut at E11. Note that the labeled nuclei are found mainly on the side of the root cut. Sex ganglia with unilateral root cuts show an asymmetric distribution of labeled cells, with most cells on the side of the cut root but a few cells on the opposite side. Bar: 20 μm.

Transplantation of the male genitalia, at E10 or later, to locations other than near M5 or M6 does not lead to the appearance of PIC neurons in those ganglia, despite their innervation of the ectopic male organ (Baptista and Macagno, 1988a; Passani *et al.,* 1991; but see Macagno *et al.,* 1986). Thus, the capacity to generate PIC neurons appears to be limited to the sex ganglia by this stage. Further, transplantation near M5 or M6 results in the birth of PIC neurons only if a nerve connection between the transplant and those ganglia is established. We therefore believe that the mitogenic signal is conveyed directly through these nerves, rather than diffusing from the male genitalia to the CNS through some other means.

Our data thus far show that (1) elements of the nerves linking the sex ganglia and the male genitalia are responsible for conveying a signal that triggers the birth of the PIC neurons, (2) the critical period for this mitogenic interaction is a property of the CNS and lies between E13 and E16; and (3) the interaction precedes the actual birth of the PIC neurons by several days, showing that their proliferation from their precursors, as well as their differentiation into mature neurons, is independent of the continued presence of the triggering signal. These conclusions raise several interesting questions, which we discuss in subsequent sections.

V. What Are the Precursors of the Peripherally Induced Central Neurons?

The distinct second wave of neurogenesis in the sex ganglia, separated from the more general early embryonic one by about 10 days, is somewhat reminiscent of the situation in holometabolous insects in which, prior to metamorphosis, the larval neuroblasts begin dividing and generate most of the imaginal nervous system. Segmental differences in cell numbers in the ventral CNS of the adult fly arise from segmental differences in the numbers of these neuroblasts (Truman and Bate, 1988). Although the embryonic thoracic and abdominal insect ganglia contain similar numbers of neurons, postembryonic addition of cells in the thoracic ganglia greatly exceeds the increase in cell number in the abdominal ganglia. The larval neuroblasts share a common lineage with, and are most likely to be identical to, their embryonic predecessors (Prokop and Technau, 1991).

In the leech, the neuroblasts that give rise to the PIC neurons could, in a similar fashion, be present only in the sex ganglia. An alternative possibility is that the precursors migrate into the sex ganglia from the male organ during the critical period. Several observations, however, argue against this possibility. First, as mentioned earlier, when the male organ of a 40-day-old animal (in which PIC neurons have already been generated) is transplanted back into an E10 animal that had its own genitalia ablated, PIC neurons are appropriately generated in the host (unpublished observations). It seems unlikely that a second population of precursors has migrated into the host CNS from this male organ. Second, male organs from E12–13 donors (in which the putative cell migration should just begin) never give rise to PIC neurons when transplanted into hosts older than E16. Third, ectopic male genitalia fail to elicit the generation of PIC neurons in ganglia other than M5 and M6, a result one would not expect if the male organ provided the precursors. We think, therefore, that it is likely that the precursors of the PIC neurons are present only in the sex ganglia, where they await the inductive signal from the male organ. An alternative explanation, also based on the sex ganglia being different from other ganglia, is that certain neurons that exist exclusively in the sex ganglia convey the mitogenic signal from the male genitalia to precursors that are present in all ganglia. Identification of the precursors will allow us to resolve this question in the future.

VI. What Is the Nature of the Mitogenic Signal?

When considering the possible nature of the inductive signal exchanged by the sex ganglia and the male genitalia, it is worth noting what we know at present about its attributes. First, the signal evidently originates in the male genitalia, and is conveyed by the nerve connection between these tissues and the CNS. The conveyor must be an element of the sex nerves, which includes afferent axons (Passani *et al.,* 1991), efferent axons from motor neurons in the sex ganglia [e.g., the RPE and LPE neurons (Zipser, 1979) or the Retzius cells (see Chapter 4)], and glial and epithelial cells. Second, the signal appears not to be highly diffusible, since disconnecting the male organs from the CNS prevents the birth of the PIC cells. Also, if only one sex ganglion is disconnected from the male genitalia by cutting both anterior nerve roots, the PIC cells are missing only from that ganglion and not from the other (Baptista and Macagno, 1988a; see Fig. 2B). This suggests that the signal cannot diffuse along the connective nerve between the sex ganglia, a relatively short distance. Furthermore, severing the connection on only one side often leads to the appearance of PIC neurons predominantly on one side of a sex ganglion (see Fig. 2D; unpublished data). Hence, the signal either must be released but have a very short range of action (e.g., it could turn over rapidly) or might be present on the surface of the cells that convey it and have its effects by direct cell-to-cell contact.

With respect to the possible involvement of cell-to-cell contact, it is interesting to note that the PIC neurons are born at or very close to the boundary between the neuropil and the surrounding glial packets, and then migrate to other locations (Fig. 3; unpublished observations). A hypothesis consistent with this and other observations is that the sex afferents project to the boundary of the neuropil and interact locally with PIC cell precursors, thereby conveying the mitogenic signal. Alternatively, a central neuron that projects to the male genitalia and has central neurites branching in the same region could play this role. The mitogenic signal could be a chemical factor transported by these cells from the periphery, or a particular pattern of electrical activity elicited by the target that triggers the expression or release of a mitogenic factor centrally. We are currently testing these hypotheses.

In the developing rat brain, and during metamorphosis in amphibians, neuronal proliferation appears to be strongly influenced by thyroid hormone (reviewed in Rohrer, 1990). Likewise, ecdysone triggers metamorphosis of the CNS in holometabolous insects (see, for example, Chapter 9). These hormones are small molecules that diffuse long distances to their site of action, however, and are therefore unlikely to mediate the described interactions in the leech. Unfortunately, little is known about leech hormones. The head ganglion of *Hirudo,* for example, is known to contain many neurosecretory cells (Sawyer, 1986), but its ablation has no effect on the appearance of the PIC cells (C. A. Baptista and E. R. Macagno, unpublished results). However, whether hormones do trigger the delayed differentiation of PIC neurons (FMRF-amide-like immunoreactivity of these neurons cannot be detected before animals are about 6 months old; Baptista and Macagno, 1988a), or play a role in determining the critical period during which the inductive interaction can have an effect, is not known at present.

In the chick embryo, it has been shown that embryonic gut and skeletal or cardiac muscle, when transplanted to a position in close proximity to the developing neural tube, causes a localized increase in the mitotic activity of nearby neuronal precursors (Rothman *et al.,* 1987; Fontaine-Perus *et al.,* 1990). A similar effect has been demonstrated for notochord implantations (Van Straaten *et al.,* 1985, 1990). This could mean that notochord and dermomyotome have mitogenic influences on developing neuroepithelia; indeed, there is evidence that mesodermal structures normally adjacent to the neural tube exert such influences on the developing CNS (Jessell *et al.,* 1989). Although it is not clear what the nature of these epigenetic interactions is,

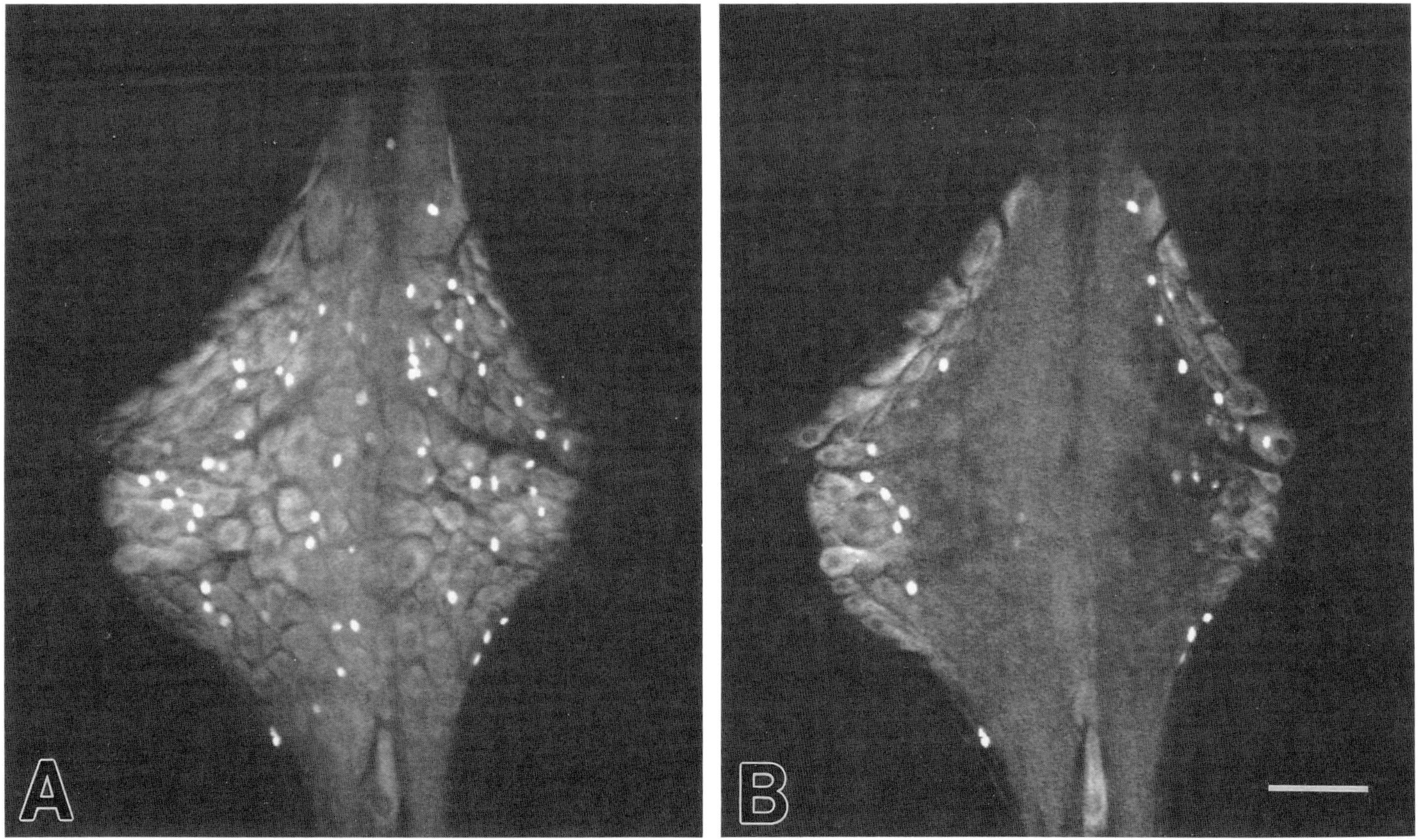

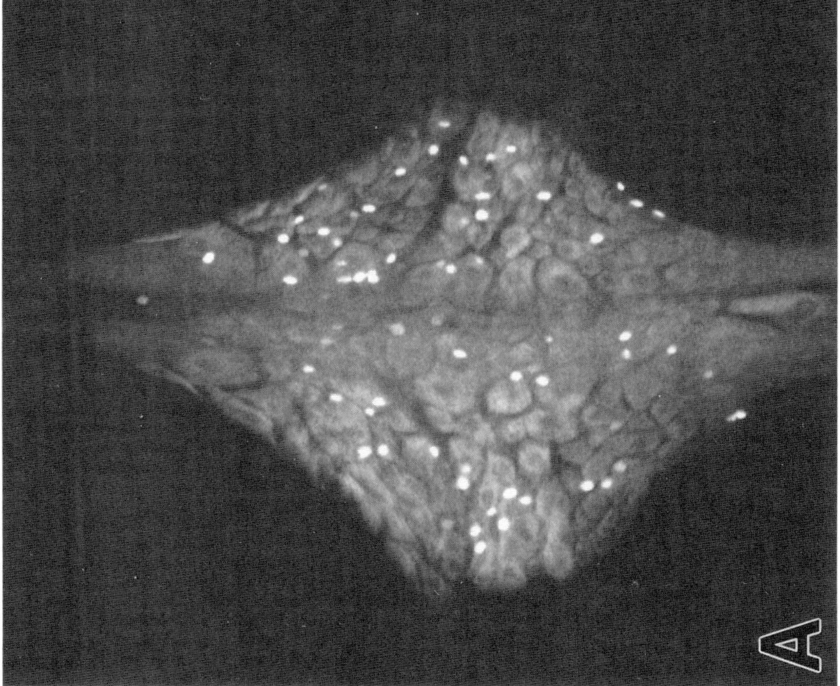

growth factors such as basic and acidic fibroblast growth factors (bFGF and aFGF), insulin, and insulin-like growth factor (IGF-1) have been found to have mitogenic effects on neuronal proliferation of embryonic cells from telencephalon of chick, mouse, and rat *in vitro* (reviewed in Rohrer, 1990). In contrast, nerve growth factor (NGF) has only been shown to prevent cell death (Levi-Montalcini, 1987; Barde, 1989; Thoenen and Barde, 1990). A possible role of any of these mitogenic substances *in vivo,* however, has not yet been assigned. One of the best examples of a localized mitogen, albeit acting on Schwann cells rather than neuronal precursors, is a heparin-binding protein expressed on the surface of peripheral embryonic neurons (Ratner *et al.,* 1988). It has been suggested that the cell surface, rather than a released factor, carries the signal. The PIC cells of the leech could be induced by a membrane-bound factor in a similar fashion, perhaps carried on the surfaces of the afferent fibers from the male organ, which enter the sex ganglia from both sides (Passani *et al.,* 1991). Induction could then take place by contact between the afferents and the precursors of the PIC cells.

In conclusion, knowledge of epigenetic influences on neuronal proliferation, whether signaled by diffusible substances or by direct cell-to-cell signaling, remains incomplete at best. The generation of the PIC neurons in the sex ganglia of the leech, which is triggered by a highly localized and apparently also specialized instructive signal, along with the dispensability of these cells under experimental conditions, provides an excellent model system for testing hypotheses experimentally and increasing our understanding of this phenomenon.

Acknowledgments

We thank Drs. Martin Shankland, Laura Wolszon, and Andreas Prokop for their critical comments on the manuscript. The work discussed here was supported in part by a grant from the National Institutes of Health.

Figure 3 Confocal images of a normal E23 sex ganglion showing anti-BrdU labeled nuclei. In this case, the primary antibody was visualized with biotinylated secondary antibodies and Texas Red–avidin. A series of 17 optical planes, 5 μm apart and perpendicular to the dorsoventral axis, was recorded. A. Projected image of all the planes showing the widely distributed labeled nuclei. B. Projected image of two of these planes in the center of the ganglion. The labeled nuclei are seen almost exclusively at the boundary of the neuropil (central uniform region) and interior to the cortical layer of the neuronal somata. Bar: 20 μm.

References

Baptista, C. A., and Macagno, E. R. (1988a). The role of the sexual organs in the generation of postembryonic neurons in the leech *Hirudo medicinalis. J. Neurobiol.* **19,** 707–726.

Baptista, C. A., and Macagno, E. R. (1988b). Modulation of the pattern of axonal projections of a leech motor neuron by ablation or transplantation of its target. *Neuron* **1,** 949–962.

Baptista, C. A., Gershon, T. R., and Macagno, E. R. (1990). Peripheral organs control central neurogenesis in the leech. *Nature (London)* **346,** 855–858.

Barde, Y. A. (1989). Trophic factors and neuronal survival. *Neuron* **2,** 1525–1534.

Bate, M. (1976). Embryogenesis of an insect nervous system. I. A map of the thoracic and abdominal neuroblasts in *Locusta migratoria. J. Embryol. Exp. Morph.* **35,** 107–123.

Booker, R., and Truman, J. W. (1987). Postembryonic neurogenesis in the CNS of the tobacco hornworm, *Manduca sexta.* I. Neuroblast arrays and the fate of their progeny during metamorphosis. *J. Comp. Neurol.* **255,** 548–559.

Breidbach, O. (1987a). Absence of sensory input does not affect persistent neurons in *Tenebrio molitor* metamorphosis (Insecta, Coleoptera). *Roux' Arch. Dev. Biol.* **196,** 486–491.

Breidbach, O. (1987b). The fate of persisting thoracic neurons during metamorphosis of the meal beetle, *Tenebrio molitor* (Insecta, Coleoptera). *Roux' Arch. Dev. Biol.* **196,** 93–100.

Doe, C. Q., and Goodman, C. S. (1985a). Early events in insect neurogenesis. I. Development and segmental differences in the pattern of neuronal precursor cells. *Dev. Biol.* **111,** 193–205.

Doe, C. Q., and Goodman, C. S. (1985b). Early events in insect neurogenesis. II. The role of cell interactions and cell lineage in the determination of neuronal precursor cells. *Dev. Biol.* **111,** 206–219.

Fernandez, J. (1980). Embryonic development of the glossiphoniid leech *Theromyzon rude:* Characterization of developmental stages. *Dev. Biol.* **76,** 245–262.

Fernandez, J., and Stent, G. S. (1982). Embryonic development of the hirudinid leech *Hirudo medicinalis:* Structure, development, and segmentation of the germinal plate. *J. Embryol. Exp. Morph.* **72,** 71–96.

Fischbach, K. F. (1983). Neural cell types surviving congenital sensory deprivation in the optic lobes of *Drosophila melanogaster. Dev. Biol.* **95,** 1–18.

Fischbach, K. F., and Technau, G. M. (1984). Cell degeneration in the developing optic lobes of the *sine oculis* and *small optic lobes* mutants of *Drosophila melanogaster. Dev. Biol.* **104,** 219–239.

Fontaine-Perus, J. C., Chanconie, M., LeDouarin, N. M., Gershon, M. D., and Rothman, T. P. (1990). Mitogenic effect of muscle on the neuroepithelium of the developing spinal cord. *Development* **107,** 413–422.

Goodman, C. S., and Bate, M. (1981). Neuronal development in the grasshopper. *Trends Neurosci.* **4,** 163–169.

Hartenstein, V., and Campos-Ortega, J. A. (1984). Early neurogenesis in wild type *Drosophila melanogaster. Roux's Arch. Dev. Biol.* **193,** 308–325.

Hartenstein, V., Rudloff, E., and Campos-Ortega, J. A. (1987). The pattern of proliferation of the neuroblasts in the wild-type embryo of *Drosophila melanogaster. Roux' Arch. Dev. Biol.* **196,** 473–485.

Jellies, J., and Kristan, W. B. (1988). An identified cell is required for the formation of a major nerve during embryogenesis of the leech. *J. Neurobiol.* **19,** 153–165.

Jessell, T. M., Bovolenta, P., Placzek, M., Tessier-Lavigne, M., and Dodd, J. (1989). Polarity and patterning in the neural tube: The origin and function of the floor plate. *Ciba Found. Symp.* **144,** 255–280.

Kollros, J. J., and Thiesse, M. L. (1988). Control of tectal cell number during larval development in *Rana pipiens. J. Comp. Neurol.* **278,** 430–445.

Kramer, A. P., and Weisblat, D. A. (1985). Developmental neural kinship groups in the leech. *J. Neurosci.* **5,** 388–407.

Levi-Montalcini, R. (1987). The nerve growth factor: Thirty-five years later. *EMBO J.* **6,** 1145–1154.

Levine, R. B. (1986). Reorganization of the insect nervous system during metamorphosis. *Trends Neurosci.* **6,** 315–319.

LoPresti, V. A., Macagno, E. R., and Levinthal, C. (1973). Structure and development of neuronal connections in isogenic organisms: Cellular interactions in the development of the optic lamina of *Daphnia. Proc. Natl. Acad. Sci. U.S.A.* **70,** 433–437.

Lumsden, A., and Keynes, R. (1989). Segmental patterns of neuronal development in the chick hindbrain. *Nature (London)* **337,** 424–428.

Macagno, E. R. (1979). Cellular interactions and pattern formation in the development of the visual system of *Daphnia magna* (Crustacea, Brachiopoda). I. Interactions between embryonic retinular fibers and laminar neurons *Dev. Biol.* **73,** 206–238.

Macagno, E. R. (1980). Number and distribution of neurons in leech segmental ganglia. *J. Comp. Neurol.* **190,** 283–302.

Macagno, E. R., Peinado, A., and Stewart, R. R. (1986). Segmental differentiation in the leech nervous system: Specific phenotypic changes associated with ectopic targets. *Proc. Natl. Acad. Sci. U.S.A.* **83,** 2746–2750.

Macagno, E. R., and Stewart, R. R. (1987). Cell death during gangliogenesis in the leech: Competition leading to the death of PMS neurons has both random and nonrandom components. *J. Neurosci.* **7,** 1911–1918.

McKay, S. E., and Oppenheim, R. W. (1991). Lack of evidence for cell death among avian spinal cord interneurons during normal development and following removal of targets and afferents. *J. Neurobiol.* (in press).

Meyerowitz, E., and Kankel, D. (1978). A genetic analysis of visual system development in *Drosophila melanogaster. Dev. Biol.* **62,** 112–162.

Oppenheim, R. W. (1991). Cell death during the development of the nervous system. *Ann. Rev. Neurosci.* **14,** 453–501.

Oppenheim, R. W., Prevette, D., Quin-Wei, Y., Collins, F., and MacDonald, J. (1989). Control of embryonic motoneuron survival *in vivo* by ciliary neurotrophic factor. *Science* **251,** 1616–1618.

Passani, M. B., Peinado, A., Engelman, H., Baptista, C. A., and Macagno, E. R. (1991). Normally unused positional cues guide ectopic afferents in the leech CNS. *J. Neurosci.* (in press).

Power, M. E. (1943). The effect of reduction in numbers of ommatidia upon the brain of *Drosophila melanogaster. J. Exp. Zool.* **94,** 33–71.

Prokop, A., and Technau, G. M. (1991). The origin of postembryonic neuroblasts in the ventral nerve cord of *Drosophila melanogaster. Development* **111,** 79–88.

Purves, D., and Lichtman, J. W. (1985). "Principles of Neural Development." Sunderland, Massachusetts: Sinauer.

Ratner, N., Hong, D., Lieberman, M. A., Bunge, R. P., and Glaser, L. (1988). The neuronal cell-surface molecule mitogenic for Schwann cells is a heparin binding protein. *Proc. Natl. Acad. Sci. U.S.A.* **85,** 6993–6996.

Rohrer, H. (1990). The role of growth factors in the control of neurogenesis. *Eur. J. Neurosci.* **2,** 1005–1015.

Rothman, T. P., Gershon, M. D., Fontaine-Perus, J. C., Chanconie, M., and LeDouarin, N. M. (1987). The effect of back-transplants of the embryonic gut wall on growth of the neural tube. *Dev. Biol.* **124,** 331–346.

Sawyer, R. T. (1986). "Leech Biology and Behaviour." Oxford: Oxford Science Publications.

Selleck, S. B., and Steller, H. (1991). The influence of retinal innervation on neurogenesis in the first optic ganglion of *Drosophila. Neuron* **6,** 83–99.

Shankland, M. (1991). Leech segmentation: Cell lineage and the formation of complex body patterns. *Dev. Biol.* **144,** 221–231.

Steller, H., Fischbach, K. F., and Rubin, G. M. (1987). *disconnected:* A locus required for neuronal pathway function in the visual system of *Drosophila. Cell* **50,** 1139–1153.

Stent, G. S., and Weisblat, D. A. (1985). Cell lineage in the development of invertebrate nervous systems. *Ann. Rev. Neurosci.* **8,** 45–70.

Stewart, R. R., Spergel, D., and Macagno, E. R. (1986). Segmental differentiation in the leech nervous system: The genesis of cell number in the segmental ganglia of *Haemopis marmorata. J. Comp. Neurol.* **253,** 253–259.

Stewart, R. R., Gao, W.-Q., Peinado, A., Zipser, B., and Macagno, E. R. (1987). Cell death during gangliogenesis in the leech: Bipolar cells appear and then degenerate in all ganglia. *J. Neurosci.* **7,** 1919–1927.

Taghert, P. H., Doe, C. Q., and Goodman, C. S. (1984). Cell determination and regulation during development of neuroblasts and neurones in grasshopper embryos. *Nature (London)* **307,** 163–165.

Thoenen, H., and Barde, Y. A. (1990). Physiology of nerve growth factor. *Physiol. Rev.* **60,** 1284–1335.

Torrence, S. A., and Stuart, D. K. (1986). Gangliogenesis in leech embryos: Migration of neural precursor cells. *J. Neurosci.* **6,** 2736–2746.

Truman, J. W., and Schwartz, L. M. (1984). Steroid regulation of neuronal death in the moth nervous system. *J. Neurosci.* **4,** 274–280.

Truman, J. W., and Bate, C. M. (1988). Spatial and temporal patterns of neurogenesis in the central nervous system of *Drosophila melanogaster. Dev. Biol.* **125,** 145–157.

Van der Loos, H., and Woolsey, T. A. (1973). Somatosensory cortex: Structural alterations following early injury to sense organs. *Science* **179,** 395–398.

Van Straaten, H. W. M., Thors, F., Wiertz-Hoessels, L., Hekking, J. W., and Drukker, J. (1985). Effect of a notochordal implant on the early morphogenesis of the neural tube and neuroblasts: Histometrical and histochemical results. *Dev. Biol.* **110,** 247–254.

Van Straaten, H. W. M., Hekking, J. W., Beursgens, J. P., Terwind-Rouwenhorst, E., and Drukker, J. (1990). Effect of the notochord on proliferation and differentiation in the neural tube of the chick embryo. *Development* **107,** 793–803.

Weisblat, D. A., Zackson, S. L., Blair, S. S., and Young, J. D. (1980). Cell lineage analysis by intracellular injection of fluorescent tracers. *Science* **209,** 1538–1541.

Weisblat, D. A., Kim, S. Y., and Stent, G. S. (1984). Embryonic origins of cells in the leech *Helobdella triserialis. Dev. Biol.* **104,** 65–85.

White, K., and Kankel, D. (1978). Patterns of cell division and cell movement in the formation of the imaginal nervous system in *Drosophila melanogaster. Dev. Biol.* **65,** 296–321.

Whitington, P. M., Bate, C. M., Seiffert, E., Ridge, K., and Goodman, C. S. (1982). Survival and differentiation of identified embryonic neurons in the absence of their target muscles. *Science* **215,** 973–975.

Williams, R. W., and Herrup, K. (1988). The control of neuron number. *Ann. Rev. Neurosci.* **11,** 423–453.

Woolsey, T. A., Durham, D., Harris, R. M., Simons, D. J., and Valentino, K. L. (1981). Somatosensory development. *In* "Development of perception" (Aslin, R. N., Alberts, J. R., and Petersen, M. R., eds.), Vol 1, pp. 259–292. New York: Academic Press.

Zipser, B. (1979). Identifiable neurons controlling penile eversion in the leech. *J. Neurophysiol* **42,** 255–464.

Intrinsic and Extrinsic Factors Influencing the Development of Retzius Neurons in the Leech Nervous System

Kathleen A. French and William B. Kristan, Jr.
Department of Biology
University of California, San Diego
La Jolla, California

I. Introduction
II. Adult Properties of Retzius Neurons
   A. Anatomical Features
   B. Physiology
III. Influences of Intrinsic Properties and Early Interactions
   A. Intrinsic Features
   B. Interactions with Ectodermal and Mesodermal Cells
IV. Later Peripheral Interactions
   A. Association with Reproductive Mesenchyme
   B. Results of Ablation and Transplantation of Reproductive Ducts
V. Summary
   References

I. Introduction

During the course of embryogenesis, neurons acquire their identities as the result of the interaction between two sets of influences: factors intrinsic to the cells themselves and factors in their surrounding environment. The transmission of intrinsic instructions depends largely on the mitotic lineage of each cell, whereas factors in the environment arise primarily from other cells in the neighborhood. Because the development of any cell depends on both classes of influence, it can be difficult to identify the unique contributions made by each of the factors and to distinguish their relative importance. In some cases, for example, in the nematode *C. elegans,* cell lineage probably plays a very significant role in determining cell fates (Stent and Weisblat, 1985), but even in *C. elegans* cellular interactions modulate developmental patterns in cellular equivalence groups (Sternberg, 1988). In other cases, cell–cell interactions are likely to play a major role in establishing neuronal identities; for example, in the development of the neural crest, events that take place during the migration of these cells probably strongly affect the final phenotype of the cell (LeDouarin, 1980a,b; Bronner-Fraser and Fraser, 1988). Intrinsic factors may contribute as well, because cell lineage can be determined for these cells, and lineage-based factors may limit the developmental potentialities of neural crest cells (Ziller *et al.,* 1987).

Cell–cell communication and factors originating in a cell's lineage may exert their influences at different stages of development. For example, early in insect development, cellular interactions among ventral ectodermal cells determine which cells will become neurons (Doe and Goodman, 1985b). The subsequent development of particular neurons proceeds through a predictable and regular pattern of cell division, making it possible to define the cell lineage of individual neurons (Doe and Goodman, 1985a). Such complex interactions between the two classes of controlling factors make it difficult to separate the influences of the factors.

One promising method for examining the relationship between intrinsic and extrinsic direction of neuronal development depends on following the development of individual identified neurons. Observing the development of particular neurons, rather than of entire populations in which it can be difficult to distinguish individuals, offers the hope that dynamic cellular responses to developmental signals can be identified and followed as they occur. When the cells being studied are readily identifiable throughout development, it is possible to manipulate the environment of each cell in a precise and understandable manner to further elucidate the contribution of individual developmental influences.

The Retzius (Rz) neurons in the central nervous system of the medicinal leech are ideal cells for this type of study. These neurons have been physiologically characterized and are known to contribute to identified behavior (Leake, 1986). For example, they modulate the function of muscles in a well-defined fashion (Mason and Kristan, 1982) and receive input from neuronal circuitry that generates the identifiable motor output driving swimming (Willard, 1981). Their development has received close attention from a number of different points of view, both descriptive and experimental. This work has shown that some aspects of Rz neuron development are likely to depend on information transmitted through their cell lineage, whereas other aspects of the development probably depend on interactions with cells in their environment. Thus, these cells provide a useful system in which to examine how the two classes of influences interact in shaping differentiation.

In leeches, neurons arise as the progeny of several ectodermal cell lineages (Weisblat and Shankland, 1985; see also Chapter 2). The fate of cells in each lineage is strongly determined, with only a limited ability for regulation among equivalence groups (Zackson, 1984; Kramer and Weisblat, 1985). Later in the development of particular leech neurons, however, cellular interactions assume more importance, as will be described for Rz neurons in this chapter (see also Chapter 3).

Rz neuron development has been studied in several leech species. These neurons appear to be remarkably alike from species to species; not only are they serotonergic, but the details of their central and peripheral structure seem to be strongly conserved among all species examined. This constancy of structure and biochemistry has been interpreted to imply that the details of Rz neuron development are probably very similar, or even identical, among the various species, and the choice of the species studied usually has depended on the general pattern of development of each species. Overall developmental strategy makes some species—the glossophoniid leeches, such as *Haementeria, Helobdella,* and *Theromyzon*—particularly well-suited for studying cell lineages and early development. In contrast, hirudinid leeches, such as *Hirudo,* are better suited for studying later development and the physiological properties of Rz neurons. As a result, we present in this chapter a summary of data from several species of leech, assuming that patterns observed in one species accurately represent events in all the species. As further data are accumulated, it should be possible to test directly the adequacy of this assumption.

II. Adult Properties of Retzius Neurons

A. Anatomical Features

Rz neurons can be recognized unambiguously in adult leeches based on their size and position in each midbody ganglion (Lent, 1981; Leake, 1986) and on their ability to take up and to synthesize the neurotransmitter serotonin (Glover, 1987). They are readily recognizable, as well, in developing leeches, based on the same properties (Blair, 1983; Glover and Mason, 1986; Glover *et al.,* 1987). In adult leeches, Rz neurons in the midbody ganglia assume one of two phenotypes (Glover and Mason, 1986; Jellies *et al.,* 1987). Most Rz neurons innervate the muscles and glands of the body wall and have 4 major

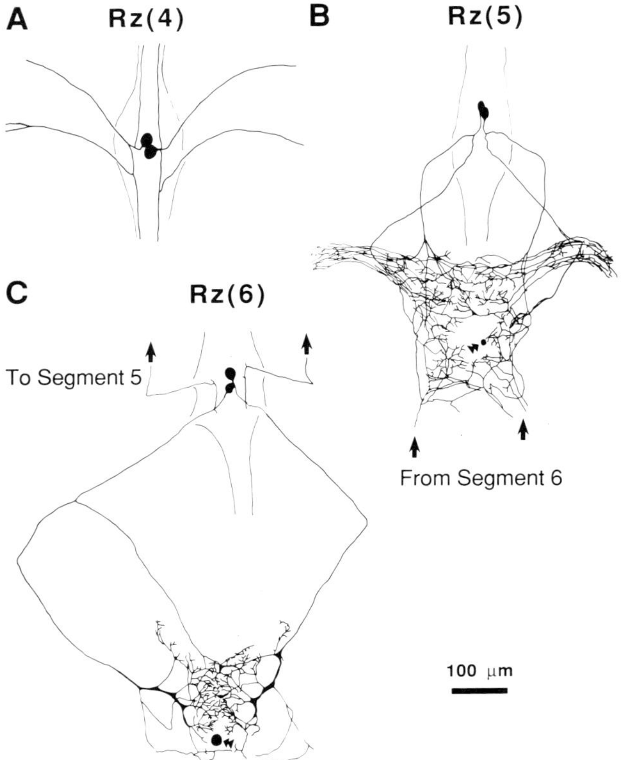

Figure 1 Peripheral anatomy of Retzius neurons. *Camera lucida* drawings of Rz neurons in *Hirudo*, labeled using an antibody to serotonin, in standard midbody segments and segments containing the male (midbody segment 5) and female (midbody segment 6) reproductive ducts. The soma and major central axons of each neuron have been drawn, but the central arborization in the neuropile has been eliminated. The outline of each ganglion is shown for orientation. A. Rz neurons in a representative standard midbody segment, segment 4. Peripheral axons extend into all four major peripheral nerves, only three of which can be seen this close to the ganglion, and each neuron sends a central axon to the next adjacent anterior and posterior ganglion. B. Rz neurons in the male segment. These cells do not send axons into the major peripheral nerves, but innervate the reproductive ducts near the ventral midline. The male reproductive ducts are innervated by both Rz(5) and Rz(6) (Glover and Mason, 1986; Jellies and Kristan, 1988); the major axons coming from Rz(6) are indicated by arrows. Rz neurons in segment 5 lack interganglionic axons, as do Rz neurons in segment 6. The male genital pore is indicated by double arrowheads. C. Rz neurons in the female segment. The anterior axon of each Rz neuron extends anteriorly and innervates the male reproductive ducts (*arrows*); the posterior peripheral axons innervate the female reproductive ducts. The female genital pore is indicated by double arrowheads.

axons, one in each ipsilateral interganglionic connective nerve and one in each ipsilateral root (Fig. 1A). In contrast, the Rz neurons of the two segments containing the male (midbody segment 5) and female (midbody segment 6) reproductive ducts innervate the reproductive ducts themselves, rather than the body wall, and lack axons in the interganglionic connectives (Fig. 1B,C). The morphological properties that distinguish the two phenotypes arise gradually (Glover and Mason, 1986; Jellies *et al.*, 1987) between day 10 of embryonic development (E10) in *Hirudo* and approximately day 20 of development (E20). These properties include length of interganglionic axons (Fig. 2A), lateral extent of peripheral axons (Fig. 2B), density of dendritic arborization in the neuropil of the ganglion (Fig. 2C), and size of the soma (Fig. 2D).

B. Physiology

In addition to these morphological features, the two phenotypes differ from one another physiologically (Loer and Kristan, 1989a; Wittenberg *et al.*, 1990). Rz neurons in all midbody segments except segments 5 and 6 [Rz(X)] are excited by pinching the tail, activating the neural circuit that drives swimming, or intracellularly stimulating pressure-sensitive mechanoreceptor neurons in the same ganglion (Fig. 2E). In contrast, the Rz neurons in the two reproductive segments [Rz(5,6)] receive none of this input and may even be inhibited when pressure-sensitive neurons are excited (Wittenberg *et al.*, 1990). Further, the two types of Rz neurons respond differently when acetylcholine (ACh) is ejected onto the soma; Rz(X) neurons rapidly depolarize and Rz(5,6) hyperpolarize or give a mixed response (Kristan and French, 1988). Pharmacological experiments have shown that the depolarizing and the hyperpolarizing responses are selectively blocked by different inhibitors, indicating that Rz(X) and Rz(5,6) express different types of acetylcholine receptors in their plasma membranes. Thus, the two Rz phenotypes differ morphologically and physiologically, and their distinctive properties characterize both peripheral and central portions of the neurons.

III. Influences of Intrinsic Properties and Early Interactions

A. Intrinsic Features

The early development of Rz neurons has been studied by injecting a long-lived tracer molecule into particular teloblasts and following the distribu-

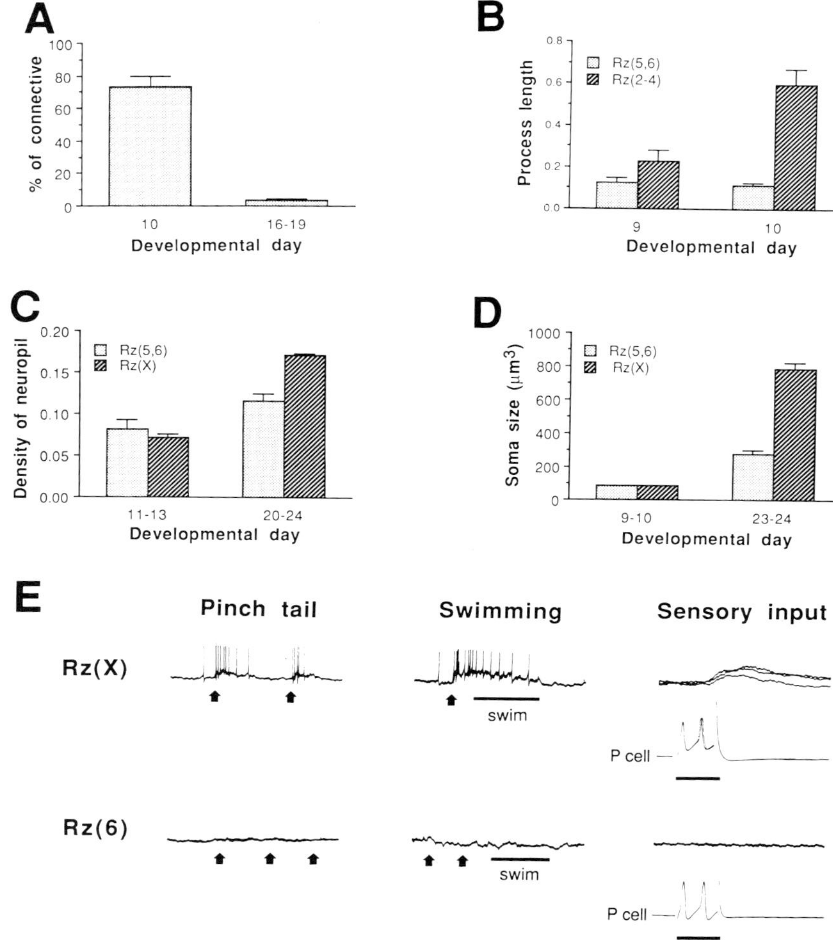

Figure 2 Features that distinguish Rz(X) and Rz(5,6) neurons in *Hirudo*. A. Length of central axons of Rz(5,6) expressed as a percentage of the distance between the ganglion containing the soma of the Rz neuron and the adjacent ganglia in the interganglionic connective nerves. On E10, Rz(X) central axons are indistinguishable from Rz(5,6) central axons. By E11, and through E19, the central axons of Rz(X) have invariably reached the adjacent ganglia, whereas the central axons of Rz(5,6) regress. (Data from Glover and Mason, 1986) B. The distance Rz peripheral axons extend from the ganglion into the periphery, expressed as a fraction of the distance to the edge of the embryo. C. Density of arborization in the central neuropil of the ganglion containing the soma of the Rz neuron. Neurons were labeled with an antibody to serotonin and drawn with *camera lucida*. The density of the arborization is expressed as the fraction of the ganglionic area that contained neurites of each Rz neuron. D. Size of soma. Antibody-labeled neurons were drawn with *camera lucida*, and the area of each soma was measured from the drawings. [Data (panels B–D) from Jellies *et al.*, 1987.] E. Synaptic inputs onto Rz neurons. Pinching the tail of a semi-intact leech, activating the central neuronal circuit that controls swimming, or exciting pressure-sensitive mechanoreceptor neurons (P cells) excites Rz(X) neurons but does not affect Rz(5,6) neurons. Adapted from Loer and Kristan, 1989a; copyright © 1989 by the AAAS.)

tion of the tracer during subsequent development. If an N teloblast contains tracer molecule, the ipsilataral Rz neuron also bears the tracer. Thus, Rz neurons develop from the N teloblast cell lineage (Blair, 1983; Stuart *et al.*, 1987); each of the paired Rz neurons arises from the ipsilateral n bandlet. (See Chapter 2 for a more thorough description of cell lineages in leech development.) Using a fluorescent tracer molecule also makes it possible to ablate particular labeled cells by illuminating them with intense light of an appropriate wavelength. Following such ablations, the development of particular cells can be studied in the absence of specific and defined cell–cell interactions. For example, if one N teloblast is ablated, each midbody ganglion contains only one Rz neuron, the Rz neuron that arose from the other N teloblast; hence, no other group of cells can regulate and generate Rz neurons. Further, only a specific subclass of cells in the n bandlet, namely the n_s cells, generate Rz neurons (Bissen and Weisblat, 1987).

Normally nascent Rz neurons are characterized by their production of serotonin and by the initial shape of their major axonal branches in the ganglion; during their early development, all midbody Rz neurons appear to be identical. The biochemical capacities to synthesize and to take up serotonin appear approximately simultaneously with the initiation of axonal outgrowth (Fig. 3). As Rz neurons extend processes into the central nervous system and then out into the peripheral body wall, the amount of serotonin that is measured in the nerve cord and then in the body wall increases steadily (Glover *et al.*, 1987). Even when the organization in the CNS has been seriously disrupted by ablating the progeny of teloblasts other than the ipsilateral N teloblast, Rz neurons can be recognized immunocytochemically because they contain serotonin (see subsequent text). Thus, Rz neurons or their lineal predecessors must not require interaction with cells from other teloblast lineages in order to synthesize the enzyme systems necessary for serotonergic neurotransmission.

Similarly, the earliest phase of process outgrowth from all Rz neurons appears to be invariant, even when organization in the developing CNS is extremely abnormal (Stuart *et al.*, 1989; Torrence *et al.*, 1989). In normal development, each Rz soma produces a single growth cone that grows away from the midline and then bifurcates. The two branches soon bifurcate once more in the ganglion to generate four major processes: two that will grow into the periphery by way of the ipsilateral roots and two that extend anteriorly and posteriorly into the interganglionic connectives of the CNS (Fig. 4A,B). At this stage, Rz neurons can be distinguished by two morphological properties, as well as by their serotonergic nature: their somata are larger than those of most other neurons in the CNS and the initial segment of the primary axon is unusually thick. These properties are maintained when many features have been disrupted by ablating other cell lineages (Fig. 4), and they allow Rz

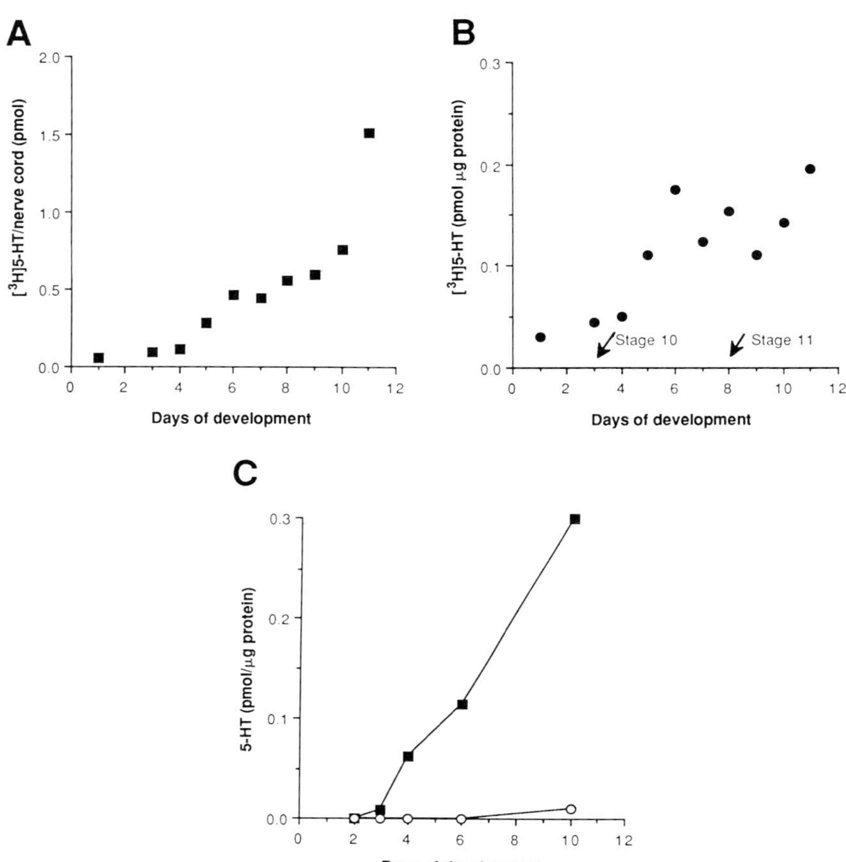

Figure 3 Development of synthesis and uptake of serotonin by neurons of *Haementeria*. Data for the first point on each of these graphs were taken two days prior to the onset of Stage 10, by which time the morphology of the ventral nerve cord and its ganglia are basically adult-like. By the end of Stage 11, which requires an additional 20 days at room temperature, the leech is ready for its first meal. Each ganglion contains serotonergic neurons other than Rz neurons, but the Rz neurons are larger than the others. A. Uptake of [³H]5-HT from the bathing solution, expressed as the amount taken up by each nerve cord. B. Specific uptake of [³H]5-HT by isolated nerve cords, normalized to the amount of protein, indicating an increase in the ability of neurons to sequester 5-HT. C. Amount of 5-HT measured in isolated nerve cords (■) and in body walls (○). (5-HT in body walls is presumably contained in peripheral axons of Rz neurons, because all other serotonergic neurons arborize entirely within the CNS.) (Data from Glover *et al.*, 1987.)

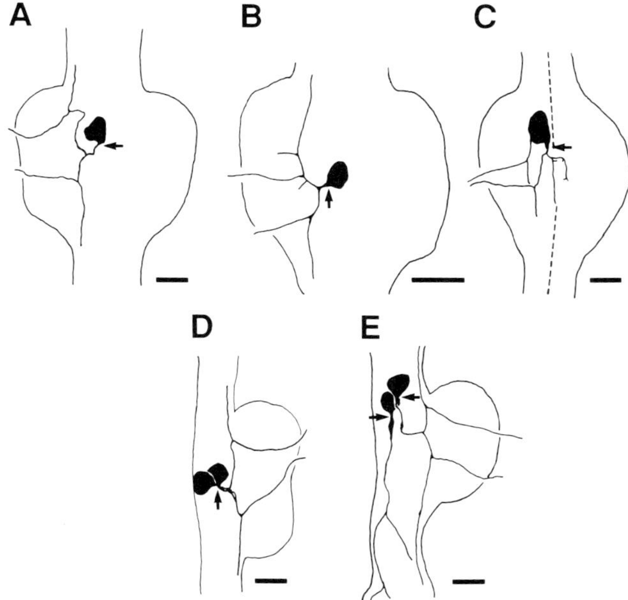

Figure 4 Somata and central branching of Rz neurons in *Theromyzon* and *Hirudo* embryos. Embryos were labeled by an antibody to serotonin, and cells were drawn with *camera lucida*. A. Normal soma and central branching pattern in a Stage 11 *Theromyzon*. Note the large soma and the thick initial segment of the single axon (*arrow*) that leaves the soma. (Data from Stuart *et al.*, 1989.) B. Normal soma and central branching pattern in a *Hirudo* embryo late on E10. The soma is large and the initial axonal segment is thick. The pattern of projection in the central nervous system is also very similar to the pattern in *Theromyzon*. (This pattern is found in all midbody segments at this stage of development). C. Rz neurons in a *Theromyzon* in which some ectodermal cell progeny were eliminated by ablating the parent teloblast cells. (See Fig. 5 for methods.) Although the central axons in this embryo do not follow the normal pathway, Rz neurons are recognizable based on their large somata and the thick initial segment of a single axon leaving the soma. (Data from Stuart *et al.*, 1989.) D,E. Retzius neurons in a *Theromyzon* in which mesodermal cells have been eliminated on one side of the embryo. (See Fig. 5 for methods.) In D, the Rz neurons lie close to one another, and their axons project together. In E, although the central projection of one of the Rz neurons is extremely abnormal, the neuron is still recognizable by its large soma and thick initial axonal segment. (Data from Torrence *et al.*, 1989.) Bar: 20 μm.

neurons to be identified even in embryos with very disorganized central nervous systems (Stuart *et al.*, 1989; Torrence *et al.*, 1989). It seems likely, therefore, that these morphological properties depend on information based in cell lineage or on early interactions among the progeny of the n bandlet ipsilateral to the Rz neuron, in a manner similar to the onset of serotonin synthesis and uptake.

B. Interactions with Ectodermal and Mesodermal Cells

Once Rz neurons have generated four processes, establishing the trajectory of each process depends, at least in part, on information gained from interactions with progeny of other teloblast lineages; Rz axonal projections in the CNS are disrupted by ablating cells derived from other teloblasts. For example, ablating the progeny of other ectodermal cells sometimes produces abnormal axonal projections in the CNS (Fig. 4C), as does ablating the mesodermal cell line ipsilateral to the Rz neuron (Fig. 4E). In fact, ablating the mesodermal cell line more dramatically disrupts Rz axonal projection (Torrence *et al.*, 1989) than does ablating ectodermal cell lines (Stuart *et al.*, 1989). When mesoderm is eliminated from one side of a developing leech, the Rz neuron from the side lacking mesoderm can be identified, but its axons establish a normal projection pattern only when the soma comes to lie on the side of the ganglion that is still in contact with mesoderm, that is, the side of the ganglion contralateral to the ablation. In those cases, both Rz neurons follow the same projection pathway: the pattern that would have been normal for the local Rz neuron (Fig. 4D).

The difference in severity of disruption that results from mesodermal and ectodermal ablation may imply that Rz somata must migrate in their ganglion to reach their final position and that the cues that direct this migration reside in, or on, the mesoderm (Torrence *et al.*, 1989). For example, when the mesodermal cell line is ablated, Rz somata often are seen to occupy an abnormal position in their ganglion (Fig. 5A,C). By contrast, ablating the contralateral n bandlet, or other ectodermal cell lines, does not disrupt the distribution of Rz somata (Fig. 5A,B; Stuart *et al.*, 1989), but ablating ectodermal cell lines does disrupt the pattern of Rz axonal projection.

IV. Later Peripheral Interactions

A. Association with Reproductive Mesenchyme

The differences between Rz(X) and Rz(5,6) begin to appear in *Hirudo* embryos during E10, the period when Rz axons grow into the periphery far enough for Rz(5) and Rz(6) axons to approach the developing reproductive ducts. At this time, the posterior processes of Rz(5,6) first come in contact with the embryonic reproductive ducts (Jellies *et al.*, 1987), particularly the

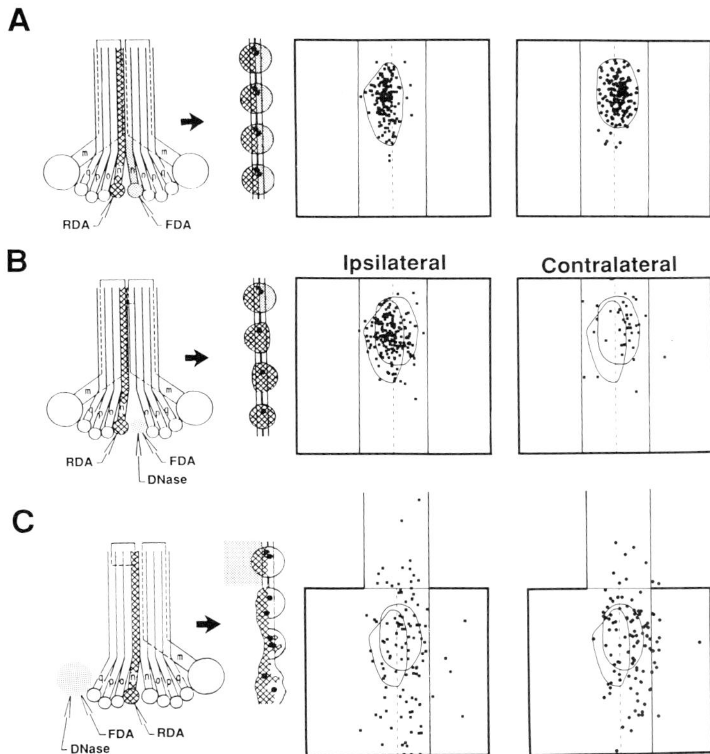

Figure 5 Effect on the position of Rz somata of ablating embryonic cell lines in *Theromyzon*. A. Fluorescent markers were injected into the left and right N teloblasts of an embryo, and the position of each Rz neuron (descended from the N lineage) was plotted. The ganglion is diagramatically represented as a rectangle, the dotted line shows the ventral midline, and the fine vertical lines indicate the lateral edges of the axon bundles running in the interganglionic connective nerves. The oval lines enclose the smallest area containing 95% of the somata plotted. (Data from Stuart *et al.,* 1989.) B. Positions of Rz somata in embryos in which the N teloblast lineage (one of four ectodermal lineages) was ablated on one side and label was injected into the N teloblast lineage on the other side. Some Rz neurons were located on the N-ablated side, indicating that they had migrated into that side. Most somata were, nonetheless, located in the region expected from measurements done on normal embryos; these are indicated on each diagram. "Ipsilateral" and "contralateral" refer to the side injected with the marker molecule. (Data from Stuart *et al.,* 1989.) C. Positions of Rz somata in embryos in which the M teloblast lineage (mesodermal) was ablated on one side and the N teloblast lineage was labeled on the side ipsilateral to the ablation. Conventions in the diagrams are as stated; vertical lines extending above the heavy rectangle indicate the lateral boundaries of the interganglionic connective nerves. (Data from Torrence *et al.,* 1989.)

mesenchymal cells of the ducts (French *et al.,* 1992). Once Rz(5,6) axons have reached the reproductive ducts, the trajectory and properties of their growth cones change dramatically (Fig. 6). As all Rz axons leave the ganglion and grow into the periphery, they fasciculate with and follow axons in peripheral nerves that were established at least a day earlier. [Among the first axons in the peripheral nerves are those of pressure-sensitive mechanosensory neurons, whose somata lie in the midbody ganglia (Kuwada, 1985).] Although Rz(X) axons continue to follow this established path, Rz(5,6) axons leave the path when they pass the embryonic reproductive ducts. Within a few hours their growth cones enlarge and turn back toward the ventral midline (Fig. 6A,B). Over the next several days, the axons of Rz(5,6) arborize around the male and female genital pores, which lie on the ventral midline, and all vestiges of other peripheral axons and the central axons are lost (Fig. 6C,D). Rz(5) innervates

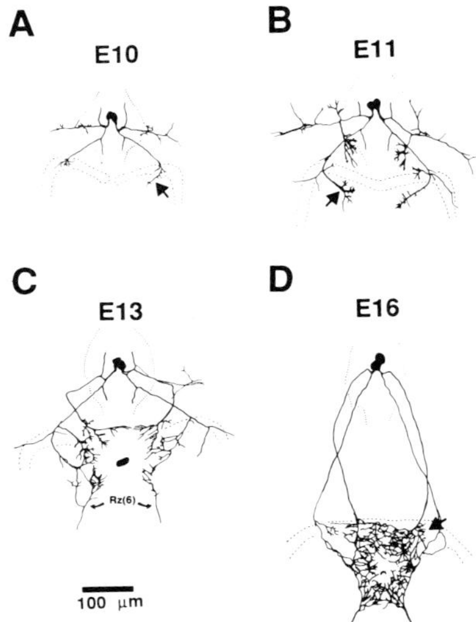

Figure 6 Development of the peripheral innervation of the male reproductive ducts in midbody segment 5 of *Hirudo.* Embryos were labeled with an antibody to serotonin and were drawn with *camera lucida.* The boundary of the ganglion is shown by dotted lines, and the outline of the reproductive duct epithelium is indicated by dashed lines. A. Initial peripheral branching pattern late on E10. A branch extends toward the ventral midline and posterior to the ganglion (*arrow*). B. More complex branching and enlarged growth cones on the anterior and posterior (*arrow*) peripheral axons on E11. C. On E13, innervation of the male ducts by both Rz(5) and Rz(6) (*arrows*) initially centers on the male genital pore. Arrows indicate axons from the anterior branch of Rz(6). D. On E16, small sprouts extend laterally along the horns of the male ducts, away from the ventral midline (*arrow*). Eventually, the entire duct is heavily innervated (Fig. 1). (Data from French *et al.,* 1992.)

the male genital pore and reproductive ducts; Rz(6) innervates both the male and the female reproductive structures.

B. Results of Ablation and Transplantation of Reproductive Ducts

Two observations imply that the enlargement and elaboration of growth cones that are seen on the axons of Rz(5,6) late in E10 and into E11 (Fig. 7A), and the subsequent modification of the Rz developmental program, depend on contact with reproductive mesenchyme and not on some intrinsic property of the Rz neurons in segments 5 and 6. First, when reproductive duct tissue is transplanted into a more posterior nonreproductive segment, a branch of the local Rz neuron produces enlarged and elaborate growth cones (Fig. 7B) and heavily innervates the tissue (Loer and Kristan, 1989b; French *et al.*, 1992). In these experiments, segments of the body wall containing embryonic reproductive ducts are surgically removed from embryos and transplanted into an incision along the ventral midline of more posterior standard segments in sibling embryos. The transplanted pieces of body wall include both the male and the female reproductive ducts or, in some cases, only the male reproductive ducts. Such transplants are most likely to induce enlarged Rz growth cones and to become heavily innervated if the surgery is performed on E10. Earlier transplants prove to be technically impossible; later transplants are usually ignored by the local Rz neuron. When pieces of body wall lacking reproductive ducts are removed from midbody segments 5 and 6 and transplanted into standard segments, the resident Rz neurons do not enlarge their growth cones or arborize extensively within the tissue.

In a second type of experiment, ablating the reproductive ducts during E10 prevents the development of the distinctive morphological (Fig. 8A,B) features of normal Rz(5,6); instead, the Rz neurons in midbody segments 5 and 6 develop morphological features that are much more typical of Rz(X), including an orthogonal branching pattern among the muscles of the body wall, anterior- and posterior-going central axons, an enlarged soma, and dense arborization in the ipsilateral neuropile (Loer *et al.*, 1987). Surgery that removes part of the body wall but leaves the reproductive ducts intact has no influence on Rz(5,6) development. If the reproductive ducts are removed from only one side of the embryo, one Rz neuron in midbody segment 5 or 6 contacts a residual reproductive duct and the other one is deprived of such contact. When this occurs, the Rz neuron innervating the duct takes on the Rz(5,6) morphology, while the Rz neuron lacking contact with the duct differentiates more similarly to Rz(X), suggesting that contact between the Rz neuron and the cells in the duct is crucial to generating the Rz(5,6) morphol-

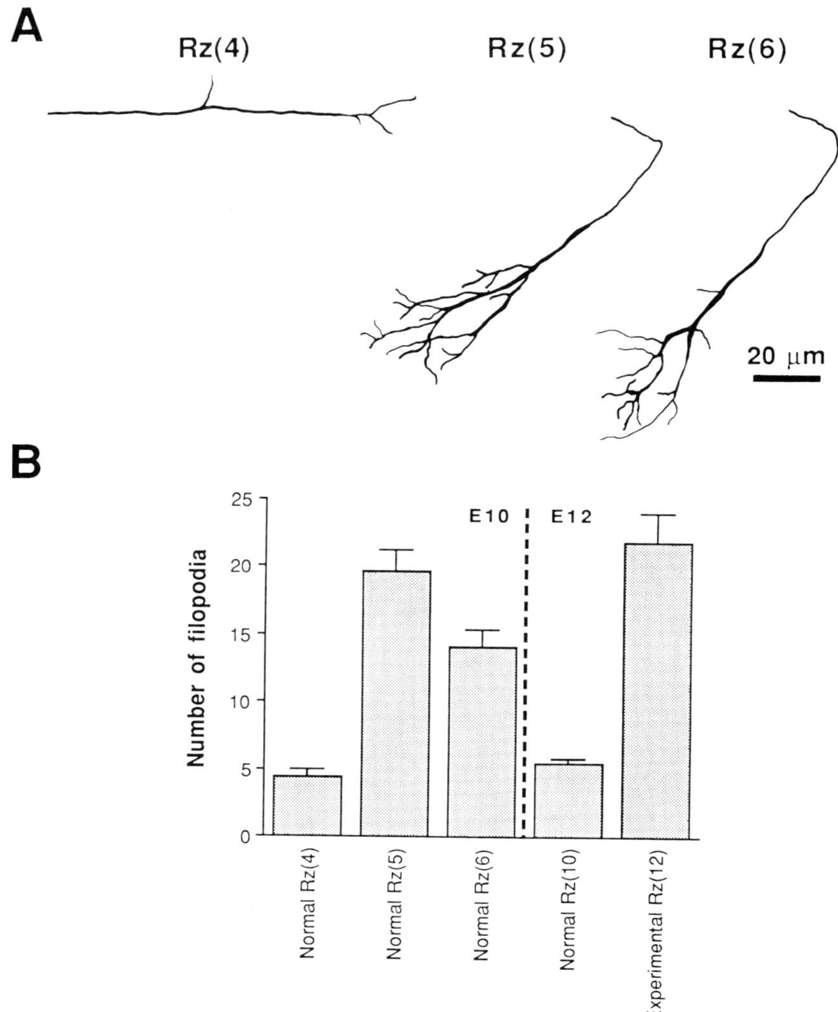

Figure 7 Complexity of growth cones in Rz neurons that make or lack contact with reproductive duct tissue. A. *Camera lucida* drawings of the ends of Rz peripheral axons in midbody segments 4, 5, and 6 in one typical normal embryo. B. Number of Rz axonal branches counted in midbody segments 4, 5, and 6 of 10 normal embryos (20 hemi-embryos) and midbody segments 10 (standard) and 12 (experimental) of embryos in which ectopic reproductive ducts were transplanted into segment 12. Error bars show the standard error of the mean.

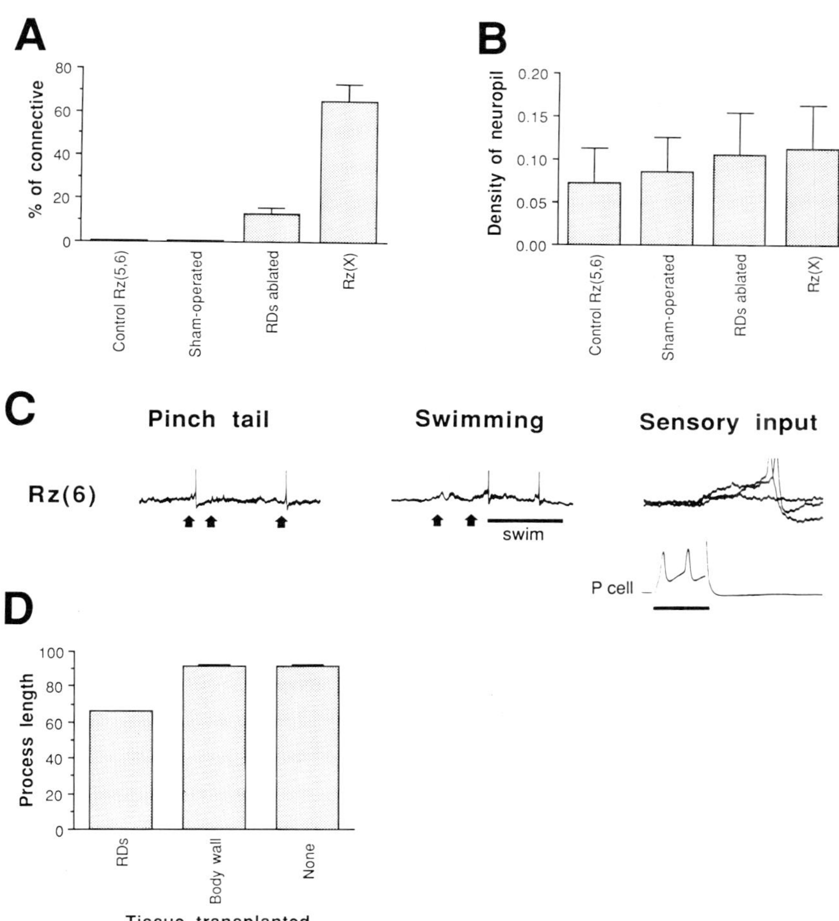

Figure 8 Effect of ablation and transplantation of embryonic reproductive duct tissue on the development of Rz neurons in *Hirudo*. A. Length of Rz(5,6) axons and of Rz(X) axons, expressed as a percentage of the distance between the ganglion housing the Rz soma and the adjacent ganglion. Cells were visualized by filling them with horseradish peroxidase. Lengths of Rz(5,6) axons are shown for normal control embryos, for embryos in which the reproductive duct tissue was ablated during E10, and for embryos in which body wall, but not reproductive duct tissue, was ablated in segments midbody 5 and 6 (sham-operated). The lengths of Rz(X) axons in these embryos are shown for comparison. Error bars show the standard error of the mean. (Data from Loer *et al.*, 1987.) B. Density of neuropile, as measured for Fig. 2C, in embryos under the same conditions as described in A. (Data from Loer *et al.*, 1987.) C. Synaptic inputs onto Rz(6) neurons in a juvenile leech following the ablation of reproductive duct tissue during E10. (Data from Loer and Kristan, 1989a.) D. Peripheral process length on E20, as measured in Fig. 2B, in segment 12, after reproductive duct (RD) tissue or some other part of the body wall had been transplanted into the segment on E10. "None" shows data for normal embryos with no surgical manipulation. (Data from Loer and Kristan, 1989b.)

ogy. As in the transplant experiments, ablations generate the most striking results if the surgical manipulations are performed on E10.

Morphology is not the only property of Rz(5,6) that is sensitive to the presence of the embryonic reproductive ducts. Ablating the reproductive tissue on E10 changes the physiological properties of Rz(5,6) as well (Fig. 8C; Loer and Kristan, 1989a).

Other observations are consistent with the results of these surgical manipulations. For example, in adult leeches that were found to have an abnormal segmental distribution of reproductive ducts, the morphology of the Rz neurons was also abnormal; Rz neurons innervating the reproductive ducts lacked central axons, regardless of the segment in which they lay (Macagno *et al.,* 1986). Early manipulations of segmental relationships between cells in the N teloblast and cells from mesodermal cell lineages have also indicated that contact with reproductive ducts modifies the developmental program of Rz neurons. When reproductive tissue was moved into novel segments by causing mesodermal bandlet cells on one side of the embryo to slip along the embryonic axis (for more details, see Chapter 2), Rz neurons in the segments containing the "ectopic" reproductive tissue acquire at least some of the properties of normal Rz(5,6) neurons (Gleizer and Stent, 1990). In normal development, these Rz neurons would have differentiated into Rz(X). In similar experiments, when an n bandlet is made to slip, placing Rz neurons that would normally have grown up to be Rz(X) in segments containing the embryonic reproductive ducts, Rz neurons contacting reproductive ducts take on at least some aspects of the Rz(5,6) phenotype. In these experiments, the Rz neurons that would normally have become Rz(5,6) are moved into standard midbody segments, and they fail to acquire the Rz(5,6) phenotype (Chapter 2). However, following surgical transplantation of reproductive tissue into nonreproductive segments, when the local Rz neuron innervates the ectopic tissue, its growth is disrupted (Fig. 8D), but it is not transformed into the Rz(5,6) phenotype (Loer and Kristan, 1989b). Clearly the interaction between Rz neurons and their reproductive duct targets is complex, and timing may play a crucial and as yet unexplored role.

V. Summary

The development of Rz neurons in leeches depends on the actions of a hierarchy of controlling factors, which appear to operate approximately sequentially to modulate the development of these neurons (Fig. 9). Cell lineage relationships play a dominant role early in development and cell–cell inter-

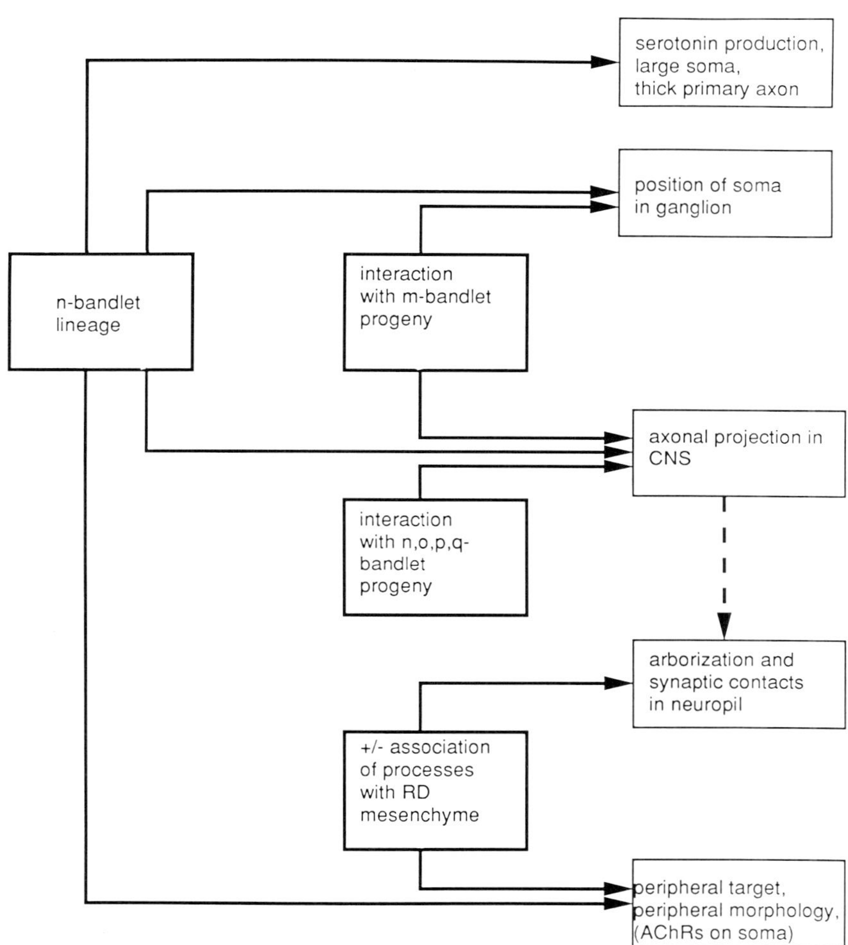

Figure 9 Summary of influences molding the differentiation of Rz neurons. Features of Rz neurons are listed on the right; mechanisms that influence Rz cell differentiation are listed on the left. The arrows indicate which developmental mechanisms contribute to the various features of differentiated Rz neurons. The dotted vertical line in the right column indicates that the axonal projection in a ganglion probably must be correct, or very nearly so, in order for synaptic contacts made onto and by the Rz neuron to be normal but, as yet, no experimental evidence supports this statement.

actions modulate later development. Rz neurons invariably arise from a particular subset of cells derived from the N teloblast, and each segment-equivalent of N teloblast progeny can generate only one Rz neuron (Blair, 1983; Bissen and Weisblat, 1987). Serotonergic neurotransmitter chemistry, a large soma, and a thick initial axonal segment appear to be determined by lineage, rather than by interactions with progeny of other ectodermal teloblasts. (Interactions among the progeny of the same N teloblast cannot be ruled out based on current experimental results.) Early interactions with the progeny of other ectodermal cell lines and with the mesoderm affect the position taken by Rz somata and regulate the pathways followed as their axonal growth cones move through their own ganglion. Once the growth cones have entered nerves—the interganglionic connectives and the roots leading to the periphery—they fasciculate with other axons already following these paths. Still later, if processes of Rz neurons encounter the embryonic reproductive duct cells, they arborize in and innervate this tissue; this interaction again modulates their differentiation, generating the Rz(5,6) phenotype. Each interaction appears to be necessary for the normal development of Rz neurons. If interaction between Rz(5,6) and reproductive duct cells does not occur, the Rz neurons take on the morphological and physiological properties of the Rz(X) phenotype. If the interaction with mesoderm or other ectodermal cells is disrupted, Rz neurons fail to find appropriate pathways through the CNS or into the periphery. Finally, if the N teloblast lineage is destroyed, no Rz neurons differentiate at all.

The development of Rz neurons differs from other well-studied systems in some ways, and shares important features with other systems. For example, the basic plan of Rz neuron development, in which cell lineage plays an important role early and cell interactions are more important later, contrasts with insect neuronal development. In insects, interactions among ectodermal cells are important early, determining which cells will become neuroblasts (Doe and Goodman, 1985a,b), and lineage is important later. On the other hand, the fine tuning of Rz neuronal identity in the reproductive segments, based on contact with target organs, is reminiscent of the development of the sympathetic innervation of mammalian sweat glands (Landis *et al.,* 1988; Schotzinger and Landis, 1988, 1990; Stevens and Landis, 1990). In these developing sympathetic neurons, the basic structure and identity of the neurons remains specified—they are sympathetic neurons—and it is their neurotransmitter that is modified following contact with their targets.

Three features have contributed to our current understanding of how intrinsic and extrinsic factors interact to mold the differentiation of Rz neurons. (1) The neurons can be identified very early in development. (2) Their developmental progress can be followed essentially continuously from early cleavage to adulthood. (3) They and their neighboring cells can be manipulated experimentally. In the future, these features should allow us to understand the physiological and molecular aspects of Rz neuron differentiation at the same level of detail with which we now understand their morphological development. It then seems likely that this information will contribute to understanding other, similar neuronal development in the same detail.

Acknowledgments

This work was supported by research grants from the March of Dimes and the National Institutes of Health (NS 25916).

References

Bissen, S. T., and Weisblat, D. A. (1987). Early differences between alternate n blast cells in leech embryo. *J. Neurobiol.* **18,** 251–269.

Blair, S. S. (1983). Blastomere ablation and the developmental origins of identified monoamine-containing neurons in the leech. *Dev. Biol.* **95,** 65–72.

Bronner-Fraser, M., and Fraser, S. E. (1988). Cell lineage analysis reveals multipotency of some avian neural crest cells. *Nature (London)* **335,** 161–164.

Doe, C. Q., and Goodman, C. S. (1985a). Early events in insect neurogenesis I. Development and segmental differences in the pattern of neuronal precursor cells. *Dev. Biol.* **111,** 193–205.

Doe, C. Q., and Goodman, C. S. (1985b). Early events in insect neurogenesis II. The role of cell interactions and cell lineage in the determination of neuronal precursor cells. *Dev. Biol.* **111,** 206–219.

French, K. A., Jordan, S. M., Loer, C. M., and Kristan, W. B., Jr. (1992). Mesenchyme of reproductive ducts guides growth cones and modifies the developmental program of Retzius neurons in the medicinal leech. *Dev. Biol.* (in press).

Gleizer, L., and Stent, G. S. (1990). Control of segment identity in the leech embryo. *Soc. Neurosci. Abstr.* **16,** 650.

Glover, J. C. (1987). Serotonin storage and uptake by identified neurons in the leech, *Haementeria ghilianii. J. Comp. Neurol.* **256,** 117–127.

Glover, J. C., and Mason, A. (1986). Morphogenesis of an identified leech neuron: Segmental specification of axonal outgrowth. *Dev. Biol.* **115,** 256–260.

Glover, J. C., Stuart, D. K., Cline, H. T., McCaman, R. E., and Stent, G. (1987). Development of neurotransmitter metabolism in embryos of the leech *Haementeria ghilianii. J. Neurosci.* **7,** 581–594.

Jellies, J., Loer, C. M., and Kristan, W. B., Jr. (1987). Morphological changes in leech Retzius neurons after target contact during embryogenesis. *J. Neurosci.* **7,** 2618–2629.

Jellies, J., and Kristan, W. B., Jr. (1988). An identified cell is required for the formation of a major nerve during embryogenesis in the leech. *J. Neurobiol.* **19,** 153–165.

Kramer, A. P., and Weisblat, D. A. (1985). Developmental neural kinship groups in the leech. *J. Neurosci.* **5**, 388–407.

Kristan, W. B., Jr., and French, K. A. (1988). Segment-specific differences in ACh receptors on leech Retzius neurons. *Soc. Neurosci. Abstr.* **14**, 164.

Kuwada, J. Y. (1985). Pioneering and pathfinding by an identified neuron in the embryonic leech. *J. Embryol. Exp. Morph.* **86**, 155–167.

Landis, S. C., Siegel, R. E., and Schwab, M. (1988). Evidence of neurotransmitter plasticity *in vivo*. II. Immunocytochemical studies of rat sweat gland innervation during development. *Dev. Biol.* **126**, 129–140.

Leake, L. D. (1986). Leech Retzius cells and 5-hydroxytryptamine. *Comp. Biochem. Physiol.* **83C**, 229–239.

LeDouarin, N. (1980a). Migration and differentiation of neural crest cells. *Curr. Topics Dev. Biol.* **16**, 32–85.

LeDouarin, N. M. (1980b). The ontogeny of the neural crest in avian embryo chimeras. *Nature (London)* **286**, 663–669.

Lent, C. M. (1981). Morphology of neurons containing monoamines within leech segmental ganglia. *J. Exp. Zool.* **216**, 311–316.

Loer, C. M., Jellies, J., and Kristan, W. B., Jr. (1987). Segment-specific morphogenesis of leech Retzius neurons requires particular peripheral targets. *J. Neurosci.* **7**, 2630–2638.

Loer, C. M., and Kristan, W. B., Jr. (1989a). Central synaptic inputs to identified leech neurons determined by peripheral targets. *Science* **244**, 64–66.

Loer, C. M., and Kristan, W. B., Jr. (1989b). Peripheral target choice by homologous neurons during embryogenesis of the medicinal leech. II. Innervation of ectopic reproductive tissue by nonreproductive Retzius cells. *J. Neurosci.* **9**, 528–538.

Macagno, E. R., Peinado, A., and Stewart, R. R. (1986). Segmental differentiation in the leech nervous system: Specific phenotypic changes associated with ectopic targets. *Proc. Nat. Acad. Sci. U.S.A.* **83**, 2746–2750.

Mason, A., and Kristan, W. B., Jr. (1982). Neuronal excitation, inhibition and modulation of leech longitudinal muscle. *J. Comp. Physiol.* **146**, 527–536.

Schotzinger, R. J., and Landis, S. C. (1988). Cholinergic phenotype developed by noradrenergic sympathetic neurons after innervation of a novel cholinergic target *in vivo*. *Nature (London)* **335**, 637–639.

Schotzinger, R. J., and Landis, S. C. (1990). Acquisition of cholinergic and peptidergic properties by sympathetic innervation of rat sweat glands requires interaction with normal target. *Neuron* **5**, 91–100.

Stent, G. S., and Weisblat, D. A. (1985). Cell lineage in the development of invertebrate nervous systems. *Ann. Rev. Neurosci.* **8**, 45–70.

Sternberg, P. W. (1988). Control of cell fates within equivalence groups in *C. elegans*. *Trends Neurosci.* **11**, 259–264.

Stevens, L. M., and Landis, S. C. (1990). Target influences on transmitter choice by sympathetic neurons developing in the anterior of the eye. *Dev. Biol.* **137**, 109–124.

Stuart, D. K., Blair, S. S., and Weisblat, D. A. (1987). Cell lineage, cell death and the developmental origin of identified serotonin- and dopamine-containing neurons in the leech. *J. Neurosci.* **7**, 1107–1122.

Stuart, D. K., Torrence, S. A., and Law, M. I. (1989). Leech neurogenesis. I. Positional commitment of neural precursor cells. *Dev. Biol.* **136**, 17–39.

Torrence, S. A., Law, M. I., and Stuart, D. K. (1989). Leech neurogenesis. II. Mesodermal control of neuronal patterns. *Dev. Biol.* **136**, 40–60.

Weisblat, D. A., and Shankland, M. (1985). Cell lineage and segmentation in the leech. *Phil. Trans. R. Soc. Lond. B* **312**, 39–56.

Willard, A. L. (1981). Effects of serotonin on the generation of the motor program for swimming in the medicinal leech. *J. Neurosci.* **1**, 936–944.

Wittenberg, G., Loer, C. M., Adamo, S. A., and Kristan, W.B., Jr. (1990). Segmental specialization of neuronal connectivity in the leech. *J. Comp. Physiol. A* **167**, 453–459.

Zackson, S. L. (1984). Cell lineage, cell interactions and segment formation in the embryo of a glossiphoniid leech. *Dev. Biol.* **104**, 143–160.

Ziller, C., Fauquet, M., Kalcheim, C., Smith, J., and LeDouarin, N. M. (1987). Cell lineages in peripheral nervous system ontogeny: Medium-induced modulation of neuronal phenotypic expression in neural crest cell cultures. *Dev. Biol.* **120**, 101–111.

The Generation of Neuronal Diversity
in the *Drosophila* Embryonic
Central Nervous System

Chris Q. Doe
Department of Cell and Structural Biology
University of Illinois
Urbana, Illinois

Both simple and complex behaviors, from the crawling of a *Drosophila* larva to Vladmir Horowitz playing the piano, are controlled by the integrated function of a diverse array of neurons. We know little about how neuronal diversity is generated, despite its importance for understanding the development and function of the central nervous system (CNS). In most organisms the number, complexity, and inaccessibility of most neurons, as well as the difficulty of genetic analysis, are major obstacles in understanding the generation of neuronal diversity.

There are several reasons for using *Drosophila* to study the cellular and molecular mechanisms controlling the generation of neuronal diversity. The CNS is relatively small, with only 250 neurons per hemisegment. Each neuron has a stereotyped cell lineage from a unique precursor cell, and individual neuronal precursors and their progeny can often be identified by their size, position, or pattern of gene expression. The combination of invariant lineages and probes for individual neurons is extremely valuable: experimental or genetic manipulations can be used to define the time of neuronal determination and the genes involved. Few other systems offer the combination of identified precursor cells, invariant cell lineages, molecular probes for specific neurons, and facile molecular genetic analysis. In this chapter I will describe experiments using both grasshopper and *Drosophila* embryos. Moving back and forth between these organisms is justified by the known similarities in cellular and molecular mechanisms of neurogenesis. For example, many criteria can be used to identify homologous precursor cells and neurons in both organisms (Taghert and Goodman, 1984; Thomas *et al.*, 1984; Doe *et al.*, 1988a,b; Valles and White, 1988; Patel *et al.*, 1989a).

I will begin by briefly describing early *Drosophila* development and the morphological events of neurogenesis (Fig. 1). Three hours after fertilization (embryonic development takes 22 hr at 25°C), the *Drosophila* embryo is a football-shaped blastoderm of about 5000 cells arranged in a single layer surrounding the central yolk (Campos-Ortega and Hartenstein, 1985). The ventral-most cells will invaginate to form the mesoderm, whereas the dorsal-most cells produce the peripheral nervous system (PNS) and dorsal epidermis. The lateral cells will form the "neurogenic region," which generates the CNS and ventral epidermis (Fig. 1). The two halves of the neurogenic region are brought together at the ventral midline after gastrulation.

During the 4 hr following gastrulation, the neurogenic region goes through three phases of neuroblast formation, as well as two rounds of mitosis (Campos-Ortega and Hartenstein, 1985). Neuroblast formation involves the enlargement of single ectodermal cells and their delamination into the embryo, forming a subectodermal layer of neuroblasts. The first two phases of neuroblast formation generate three columns of neuroblasts along the dorsal–ventral (DV) axis: medial (next to the ventral midline), intermediate, and lateral (adjacent to the dorsal ectoderm). In each hemisegment (one half of the bilaterally symmetric neurogenic region), the first 10 neuroblasts (SI class) form in all columns: 4 medial neuroblasts, 2 intermediate neuroblasts, and 4 lateral neuroblasts (Fig. 2) (Jimenez and Campos-Ortega, 1990). The next set of neuroblasts (SII class) results in the addition of 2 neuroblasts to the medial column and 4–6 neuroblasts to the intermediate column (Hartenstein and Campos-Ortega, 1984; C. Q. Doe, unpublished results). The last phase of neuroblast formation (SIII class) adds neuroblasts throughout the neurogenic region, giving a total of ~25 neuroblasts, roughly arranged in four columns and six rows (Doe *et al.*, 1988a; Jimenez and Campos-Ortega, 1990). In larger arthropod embryos (e.g., grasshopper, *Manduca*, and crayfish), the neuroblast pattern is arranged in 7 distinct rows and 4 columns (Patel *et al.*, 1989a).

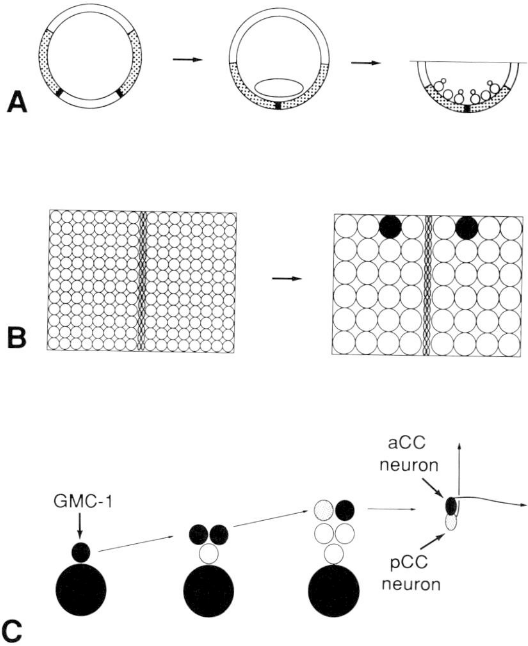

Figure 1. Formation of the embryonic *Drosophila* CNS. A. Cross-sectional view through blastoderm *(left)*, postgastrula *(center)*, and germ band extended stages *(right;* only half the embryo is shown). At the blastoderm stage *(left)*, all cells look identical but each region has different developmental fates: the dorsal ectoderm *(top)* give rise to dorsal epidermis and peripheral nervous system; the neurogenic region *(stippled)* give rise to ventral epidermis and the CNS; the prospective mesectodermal cells *(black)* produce neurons and nonneuronal cells along the ventral midline; the prospective mesoderm *(bottom)* invaginates to form the somatic and visceral musculature. At gastrulation *(center)*, the mesoderm has invaginated and the mesectodermal cells come together at the ventral midline. Soon after gastrulation *(right)*, neuroblasts *(large circles)* delaminate from the neurogenic region and begin to produce progeny *(small circles)*. For clarity, the mesoderm is not shown. B. Ventral view of neuroblast formation in one segment. Initially there are 60–70 ectodermal cells per hemisegment *(left)*; at specific times during the next 4 hr of development, individual ectodermal cells enlarge and delaminate into the embryo to form a stereotyped array of neuroblasts *(right)*. Neuroblast 1-1 is shown in black and its lineage is represented in C. The smaller ovals show the position (but not the actual number) of mesectodermal cells on the ventral midline. C. Cross-sectional view of the neuroblast 1-1 lineage shown at approximately 45-min intervals; the ventral surface of the embryo is toward the bottom of the figure. Each neuroblast divides asymmetrically to generate a chain of ganglion mother cells (GMCs) that divide once symmetrically to produce a pair of postmitotic neurons. For neuroblast 1-1, the first daughter cell (GMC-1) expresses the *ftz* and *eve* genes immediately after birth, and always gives rise to the aCC and pCC neurons (dark and light stipple, respectively).

In the *Drosophila* embryo, the neuroblasts are smaller and the pattern is less ordered. Nevertheless, a growing number of neuroblasts in this stereotyped array can be uniquely identified due to their position, time of formation, or pattern of gene expression (Doe *et al.*, 1988a; Jimenez and Campos-Ortega, 1990) (Fig. 2).

Soon after formation, each neuroblast begins a stereotyped cell lineage, which transforms the two-dimensional neuroblast pattern into a three-dimensional CNS. Neuroblasts are stem cells, dividing asymmetrically to generate an average of 5 smaller ganglion mother cells (GMCs) during embryogenesis. Each GMC divides to produce a pair of postmitotic neurons (Fig. 1c). Studies in a variety of insects, including *Drosophila*, show that an identified neuroblast always contributes a characteristic group of neurons to the CNS (Raper *et al.*, 1984; Taghert and Goodman, 1984; Thomas *et al.*, 1984; Doe *et al.*, 1988a;

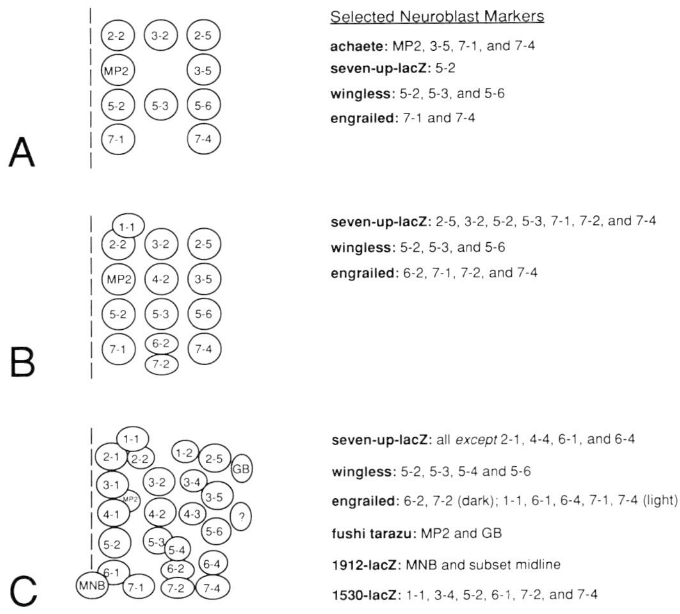

Figure 2. Maps and markers for embryonic *Drosophila* neuroblasts. A: all SI neuroblasts. B: SI and some SII neuroblasts. C: SI, SII, and some SIII neuroblasts. Stages are from Campos-Ortega and Hartenstein (1985); hours are from time of egg deposition; germ band refers to percent extension from posterior tip of egg.

C. Q. Doe, unpublished results). Some GMCs can be unambiguously identified at the time they are born by their birth order from an identified neuroblast or by their position and pattern of gene expression. In addition, neurons can often be identified by their characteristic axon morphology.

In this chapter I will briefly discuss the process of neuroblast formation (see Chapter 6 for more details). Neuroblast formation refers to the process by which individual cells of the neurogenic region enlarge and delaminate to form neuroblasts; the remaining superficial cells develop into the ventral epidermis. In the following section I will discuss the mechanisms controlling the fate of individual neuroblasts, GMCs, and neurons.

I. Neuroblast Formation

Two classes of genes are involved in neuroblast formation, the proneural and the neurogenic genes (Fig. 3). Although they have similar names, the genes perform opposite functions. Proneural genes (Chapter 8) are named after their function: to promote neural development. Thus, loss-of-function mutations in proneural genes result in a *decrease* in the number of neuroblasts formed (Jimenez and Campos-Ortega, 1990). In contrast, the neurogenic genes are named after their mutant phenotype: loss of neurogenic gene function results in an *increase* in the number of neuroblasts formed (Lehmann *et al.*, 1983). Both classes of genes have been recently and extensively reviewed (see Chapter 6 and references therein), and will be described briefly here.

A. Proneural Gene Function

The proneural genes include the regionally expressed *achaete* (*ac;* T5 transcript), *scute* (*sc;* T4 transcript), *lethal of scute* (*l'sc;* T3 transcript), and *asense* (*ase;* T1 transcript) genes. The ubiquitously expressed *daughterless* gene is also usually considered a proneural gene (see Chapter 8). Loss of proneural gene function results in the formation of fewer neuroblasts (Fig. 3); as more proneural genes are removed, more neuroblasts are missing (Cabrera *et al.*, 1987; Jimenez and Campos-Ortega, 1990; Martin-Bermundo *et al.*, 1991). Conversely, increasing the amount of proneural gene function (by adding extra copies of the wild-type genes) results in excessive neuroblast formation (Brand and Campos-Ortega, 1988). The loss-of-function and gain-

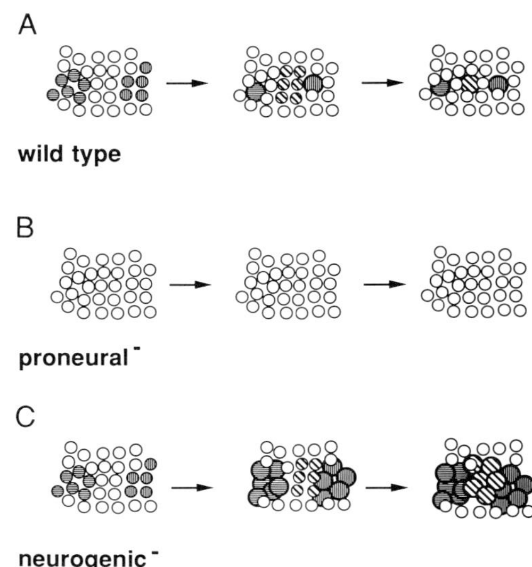

Figure 3. Expression and function of the proneural genes in wild-type and mutant embryos. A. Wild type. Only a subset of the ectoderm of the neurogenic region is shown. The regionally expressed proneural genes are first detected in clusters of 4–6 cells. Not all clusters express a particular gene at the same time; here two clusters are shown developing first, followed by a third cluster later in development (small patterned circles). One cell in each cluster will form a neuroblast and maintain expression (large patterned circles). B. Proneural‾. Loss of proneural gene expression (open circles) results in a decrease in neuroblast formation. C. Neurogenic‾. Loss of neurogenic gene function results in all cells of the proneural expressing cluster (small patterned circles) developing into neuroblasts (large patterned circles). Ultimately, most (probably all) cells of the neurogenic region develop as neuroblasts, and there is a corresponding loss of ventral epidermis.

of-function phenotypes of proneural mutations suggest that the role of the proneural genes is to repress epidermal development and promote neural development. This is supported by double mutant experiments described in section I.C.

The RNA and protein expression patterns for several proneural genes has been described (Cabrera *et al.,* 1987; Romani *et al.,* 1987; Cabrera, 1990; J. Skeath and S. Carroll, personal communication). The *ac* protein is first detected in four clusters of 4–6 ectodermal cells in stereotyped positions in each hemisegment of the neurogenic region (Fig. 4). One neuroblast will develop from each cluster; soon after neuroblast formation, the ectodermal cells of the cluster lose *ac* expression. The neuroblast maintains expression briefly, but *ac* protein is not detectable by the time the neuroblast produces its first progeny. *ac* expression reappears in a more complex pattern of ectodermal clusters slightly later, preceding formation of several SII neuroblasts; presumably these clusters also give rise to a single *ac*-positive neuroblast. Similarly, a polyclonal antibody detects *l'sc* protein in clusters of 4–6 ectodermal cells, with each cluster producing a *l'sc*-positive neuroblast (Martin-Bermundo *et al.,* 1991). Interestingly, a second polyclonal antibody (made to a short *l'sc* peptide) reveals only the neuroblast expression of *l'sc* (Cabrera, 1990). This suggests that there are posttranslational differences between ecto-

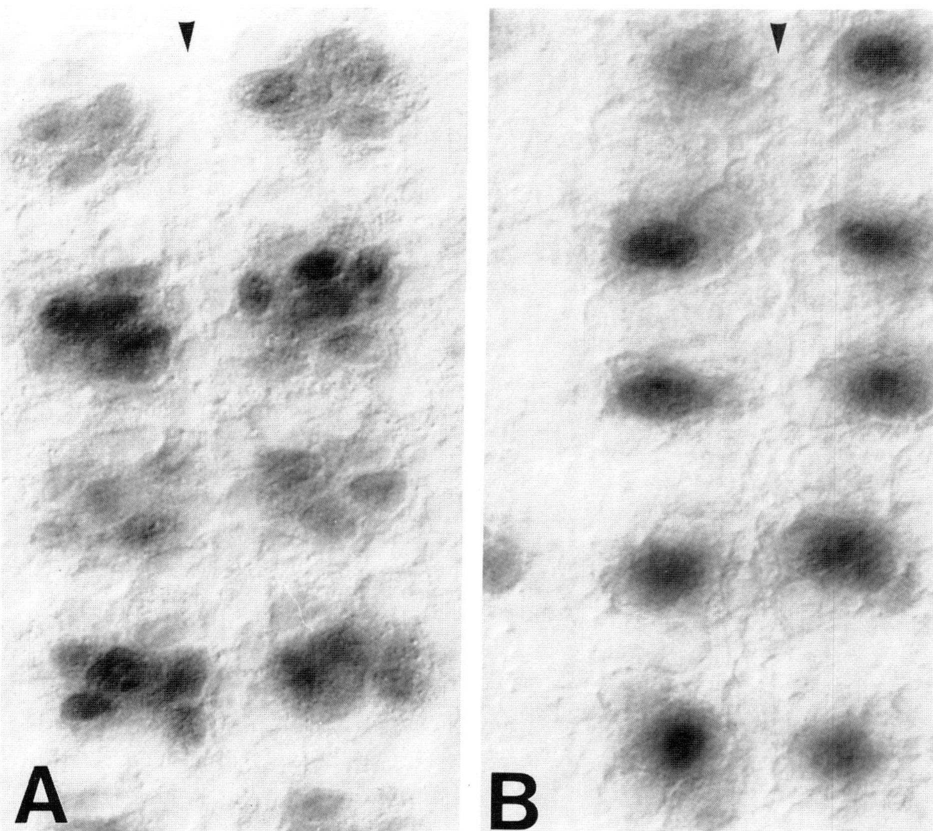

Figure 4. Expression of a proneural gene product (the *ac* protein) in clusters of ectodermal cells and neuroblasts. A. Cluster of ectodermal cells in the neurogenic region that express the *ac* protein. B. One neuroblast developing from each cluster retains *ac* protein expression, whereas the remaining cells of the cluster lose expression. The ventral midline is indicated *(arrowhead)*. Figure kindly provided by J. Skeath and S. Carroll.

dermal and neuroblast *l'sc* proteins. Not surprisingly, the peptide used to generate Cabrera's antibody contains both a serine and a tyrosine that may be phosphorylated. Thus the *l'sc* protein may be phosphorylated in the ecto-dermal cell clusters, but dephosphorylated in the enlarging neuroblast. All known proneural genes encode basic helix-loop-helix proteins, similar to *myc* and Myo-D gene products. It will be interesting to explore the molecular parallels between the triggering of neurogenesis by AS-C proteins and the promotion of myogenesis by the Myo-D class of proteins.

The pattern of AS-C expression has led to the speculation that these genes may be involved in neuroblast specification (Cabrera *et al.*, 1987; Cabrera, 1990). However, the evidence is not conclusive. Embryos lacking AS-C function were probed with antibodies against proteins expressed in subsets of neuroblasts and GMCs (Jimenez and Campos-Ortega, 1990). None of the proteins were found to be overexpressed or ectopically expressed. Rather, each was expresses in a subset of its normal pattern. These results are consistent with AS-C⁻ embryos having a reduction in neuroblast number but no change in neuroblast identity (Jimenez and Campos-Ortega, 1990). Evidence consistent with this interpretation can be found by examining the role of the AS-C in adult neurogenesis (see Chapter 8). Many neurons of the adult sensory nervous system are identified cells, derived from a unique precursor similar to a neuroblast. Loss of *ac* or *sc* expression results in the absence of some, but not all, sensory precursors and their neuronal progeny; the identity of the remaining sensory neurons is unaltered, although they developed without *ac* or *sc* expression (A. Ghysen, personal communication). Similarly, misexpression of either *ac* or *sc* in sensory precursors where they are not usually expressed does not alter precursor specification (Rodriguez *et al.*, 1990). Combined, these data support a role for proneural genes in the for-mation, but not the specification, of neuroblasts or sensory precursors.

B. Neurogenic Gene Function

Well-studied neurogenic genes are *Notch, Delta, big brain, mastermind, neuralized,* the *Enhancer-of-split* Complex [E(spl)-C], and *shaggy* (Lehmann *et al.*, 1983; Bourouis *et al.*, 1989). Loss-of-function mutations in any neu-rogenic gene results in all cells of the neurogenic region developing into neuroblasts (Fig. 3), whereas an increase in neurogenic gene function results in the development of fewer neuroblasts (Brand and Campos-Ortega, 1988; Lehmann *et al.*, 1983). Embryos lacking neurogenic gene function have an initially normal pattern of *l'sc* and *ac* gene expression, but expression is never restricted to a single neuroblast; instead, all cells of the cluster apparently differentiate into neuroblasts (Cabrera, 1990; J. Skeath and S. Carroll, personal communication). This shows that neurogenic gene function is required to restrict AS-C gene expression to a single cell of the cluster. When AS-C gene expression is maintained in all cells of the cluster, all differentiate into neuroblasts (Fig. 3).

How might the neurogenic genes limit AS-C gene expression to a single cell per cluster? Cell interactions are clearly involved in the process. In grasshopper embryos, when a neuroblast is ablated, one of the adjacent cells will enlarge to replace it; this implies that when a neuroblast is present, it inhibits the adjacent cells from developing into neuroblasts (Doe and Goodman, 1985b). Intercellular signaling of this kind has been termed lateral inhibition (Wigglesworth, 1940). In *Drosophila,* one direct consequence of the lateral inhibition signal may be the loss of AS-C gene expression in cells adjacent to the developing neuroblast. The lateral inhibition signal and its reception may be mediated by the products of the neurogenic genes *Notch* and *Delta,* which are membrane proteins with extracellular EGF-like repeats (Wharton *et al.,* 1985; Kopczynski *et al.,* 1989). In particular, the *Notch* protein is quite similar to proteins encoded by the genes *lin-12* and *glp-1,* which mediate cell interactions in the nematode (Greenwald, 1989). The lateral inhibition signal ultimately leads to a loss of AS-C gene expression in the cells adjacent to the developing neuroblast; these cells generate ventral epidermis.

C. The "Default" Pathway of the Neurogenic Region Is Epidermal Development

What triggers the genes of the epidermal differentiation pathway: activation by the neurogenic genes or the absence of repression by proneural gene products? This question can be answered by looking at embryos mutant for both AS-C and neurogenic gene function. If neurogenic gene activity is required for epidermal development, the double mutants should be missing ventral epidermis due to a lack of neurogenic gene function. In fact, the double mutants produce some ventral epidermis, indicating that the neurogenic genes are not necessary for ventral epidermal development. This should not be surprising, because the neurogenic genes are not required for the development of the dorsal-most epidermis (Lehmann *et al.,* 1983). Apparently it is the lack of proneural gene expression that allows epidermal development (Brand and Campos-Ortega, 1988). This shows that the default state of the neurogenic region, lacking both AS-C and neurogenic gene function, is differentiation into epidermis. It also suggests that proneural genes act to modify this default state by triggering neural development.

D. Homeotic Genes Control Segment-Specific Neuroblast Formation

The neuroblast pattern in the embryonic thoracic and abdominal segments of several insects is different, with more neuroblasts present in the thorax (Bate, 1976; Campos-Ortega and Hartenstein, 1985; Doe and Goodman, 1985a; Booker and Truman, 1987). This difference is even more striking in the late larval and adult CNS (Truman and Bate, 1989). Because segmental identity of the epidermis and some larval CNS structures) is controlled by the homeotic genes (reviewed in Doe and Scott, 1988), it is likely that they also control the formation of segment-specific embryonic neuroblasts. Homeotic genes are expressed in the neurogenic region during the period of embryonic neuroblast formation (Carroll *et al.*, 1988). Furthermore, evidence that a homeotic gene can control segment-specific neuroblast formation has been observed in the moth *Manduca.* The *Octopod* gene is required for suppressing the formation of thorax-specific neuroblasts in the first abdominal segment (Booker and Truman, 1989). How might homeotic genes control the segment-specific spatial array of neuroblasts? A clear prediction is that homeotic gene products regulate the spatial expression of the proneural genes, thereby producing different neuroblast patterns in the thoracic and abdominal segments.

II. Generation of Neuronal Diversity

Our working model is that there are three classes of genes controlling cell fate in the developing CNS (Fig. 5). First, genes expressed regionally in the neurogenic region provide positional cues. Second, in response to these positional cues, "neuroblast identity" genes are expressed in overlapping subsets of neuroblasts and their progeny. Each neuroblast identity gene is expressed in a subset of GMCs produced from each neuroblast; the pattern of GMC expression can be in lineal homologs (e.g., only first-born GMCs) or positional homologs (e.g., transiently in every newly born GMC) or can be lineage-specific (e.g., all GMCs from one neuroblast) (Fig. 6). The function of the neuroblast identity genes is to translate positional cues into specific neuroblast lineages. Third, "GMC and neuronal identity" genes are expressed in subsets of GMCs in response to the neuroblast identity genes; these genes control the identity of individual GMCs and the subsequent pair of neurons. Examples of each class of genes are known: certain segmentation genes

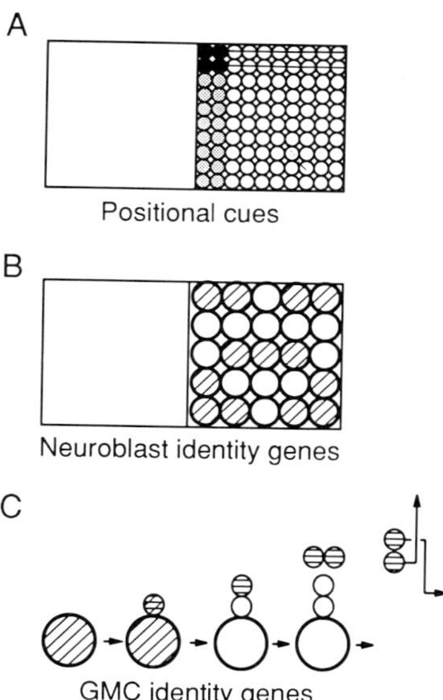

Figure 5. A model for a gene regulatory hierarchy controlling the specification of cell fate in the embryonic CNS. A. Regionally expressed genes (⊘ and ⊖) are expressed in overlapping patterns in the ectoderm of the neurogenic region, so clusters of 4–6 cells express a unique combination or concentration of gene products (●). B. Neuroblast identity genes are expressed in subsets of neuroblasts in response to the positional cues (diagonal stripes). Each neuroblast identity gene may be expressed in a subset of GMCs produced from a neuroblast; the pattern of GMC expression can be in lineally related GMCs, positionally related GMCs, or lineage-specific GMCs (see Fig. 6). The function of the neuroblast identity genes is to translate positional cues into a specific neuroblast lineage, that is, the number of cell cycles and the fate of the GMCs produced. C. GMC and neuronal identity genes (horizontal stripes) are expressed in subsets of GMCs and neurons, but not neuroblasts, in response to the particular combination of neuroblast identity genes present in a GMC. These genes are required for the establishment of unique GMC and neuronal fates.

provide positional cues in the neuroectoderm (Patel *et al.*, 1989b; J. Skeath and S. Carroll, personal communication), *prospero (pros)* is a neuroblast identity gene (Doe *et al*, 1991), and the homeobox genes *fushi tarazu (ftz)* and *even-skipped (eve)* are expressed in specific GMCs and control GMC and neuronal fates (Doe *et al.*, 1988a,b).

A. Positional Cues

In this section I will first summarize the evidence that positional cues control neuroblast identity, and describe genes that may encode these cues.

Then I will discuss the timing of neuroblast specification, and whether positional cues establish equivalence groups in the neurogenic region.

1. NEUROBLAST IDENTITY IS SPECIFIED BY POSITIONAL CUES IN THE NEUROGENIC REGION

There are three reasons to believe that positional cues specify neuroblast identity. First, a strong correlation exists between the position and the identity of a neuroblast, but there is no known relationship between cell lineage and the identity of a neuroblast. In grasshopper embryos it is possible to predict the identity of individual neuroblasts with 100% certainty based solely on the position of the neuroblast in the neurogenic region (Raper *et al.*, 1984; Taghert and Goodman, 1984; Doe and Goodman, 1985a). Although the *Drosophila* neuroblast pattern is compressed and slightly more variable, it is still obvious that specific neuroblasts always develop in stereotyped locations (Doe *et al.*, 1988a; Jimenez and Campos-Ortega, 1990; C. Q. Doe, unpublished data). In contrast, cell lineage plays no obvious role in specifying neuroblast

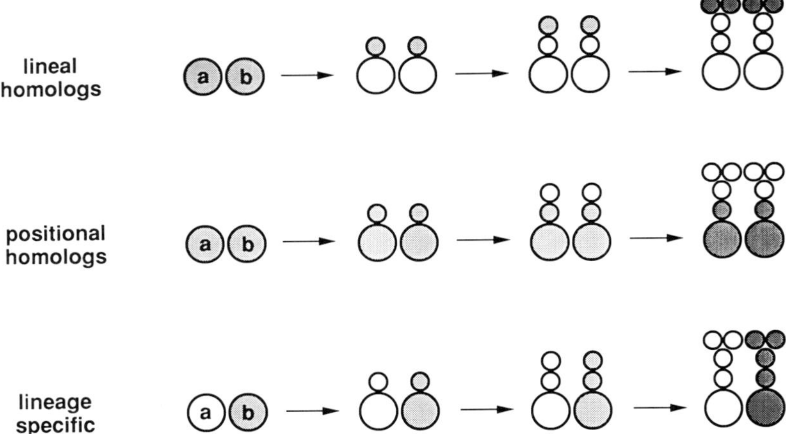

Figure 6. Schematic of three possible patterns of neuroblast identity gene expression. Two neuroblast lineages are shown in each example. Lineal homologs. Expression is restricted to lineally related cells: newly formed neuroblasts (large shaded circles), GMC-1s (small shaded circles), and their neuronal descendants. The *hunchback* gene is expressed in a pattern similar to this one. Positional homologs. Expression is restricted to positionally related cells; in this example only neuroblasts (large shaded circles) and the adjacent newly formed GMCs (small shaded circles) express the gene. This expression pattern occurs when newly born GMCs express the gene transiently. The *pros* gene is expressed in a pattern similar to this one. Lineage specific. Expression is restricted to a subset of neuroblasts and their progeny (shaded circles). The *en* gene is expressed in a pattern similar to this one.

fate. The SI neuroblasts develop directly (no intervening mitoses) from blastoderm cells that have completed cell cycle 14, and there is no correlation between the lineage and position of blastoderm cells (Minden *et al.*, 1989).

The phenotype of *Drosophila* neurogenic mutations also provides clues toward the mechanism of neuroblast specification. Neurogenic mutations result in all cells of the neurogenic region developing as neuroblasts (Lehmann *et al.*, 1983). The neuronal precursor MP2 can be identified by its position in the neurogenic region and its expression of the *ftz* gene (Doe *et al.*, 1988a). MP2 initially develops like a neuroblast—it enlarges, delaminates, and assumes a position in the neuroblast array. In embryos mutant for the neurogenic gene *Delta*, a cluster of 4–6 adjacent ectodermal cells differentiates as MP2 (C. Q. Doe, unpublished results). It is improbable that these MP2s are lineally related; their common fate is likely to be due to a common position in the neurogenic region.

Finally, evidence for position-specific neuroblast determination comes from neuroblast ablation experiments in the grasshopper embryo. When a laser microbeam is used to ablate a single neuroblast, an adjacent ectodermal cell will often enlarge and assume the fate of the killed neuroblast. Any of the surrounding ectodermal cells can replace the ablated neuroblast, thus ruling out cell lineage as a factor in neuroblast specification. The position of enlargement is the best and only predictor of neuroblast identity (Doe and Goodman, 1985b).

2. WHAT ARE THE POSITIONAL CUES CONTROLLING NEUROBLAST SPECIFICATION?

Positional cues must be molecules with restricted or graded distribution in the neurogenic region; presumably a unique combination of these cues specifies individual neuroblast identity, but the mechanisms used could vary. First, there might be positionally restricted expression of genes that may act as cell autonomous cues present in ectodermal cells of the neurogenic region; each neuroblast would be specified by the inheritance of a unique combination of molecules. Second, diffusible molecules may be released from stereotyped positions along the anterior–posterior (AP) or (DV) axis; a concentration gradient of the factor(s) may contribute to neuroblast specification. Third, interactions between cells of the neurogenic region, or between ectoderm and the underlying mesoderm, may lead to positional specification of individual neuroblasts. In the following sections I will discuss the asymmetric distribution of gene products in the AP and DV axes, and consider whether they could mediate neuroblast specification by one of the three mechanisms just mentioned.

a. Positional Cues along the Anterior/Posterior Axis

The best candidates for positional cues along the AP axis are the pair rule and segment polarity genes (Nüsslein-Volhard and Weischaus, 1980). Pair rule genes are expressed at cellular blastoderm in a bisegmental or "pair rule" periodicity, whereas segment polarity genes are expressed slightly later, usually in a stripe in every segment (see chapter by Howard).

At least two pair rule genes are expressed in the neurogenic region during SI neuroblast formation (*eve* and *ftz*; C. Q. Doe, N. Patel, and C. S. Goodman, unpublished results). Pair rule genes have been proposed to subdivide each segment into four molecularly distinct ectodermal regions (Ingham *et al.*, 1988); it is likely that each of these domains generates a single row of SI neuroblasts. Recently several probes have become available that distinguish between different SI neuroblasts (Figs. 2 and 4); using these markers it should be possible to determine whether pair rule genes directly contribute to SI neuroblast specification. Interestingly, all pair rule mutations alter the pattern of *ac* in the SI neuroblasts (where it is expressed in the MP2, 3-5, 7-1, and 7-4 neuroblasts; Fig. 2), whereas segment polarity mutations show little or no alterations (J. Skeath and S. Carroll, personal communication). These data suggest that the AP position at which the first four *ac*-positive SI neuroblast form is controlled by pair rule gene activity. Given that neuroblast formation and neuroblast specification are closely linked (see Section II.A.4), it is likely that pair rule genes contribute to SI neuroblast specification as well. The SII and SIII neuroblasts develop after pair rule gene expression disappears from the ectoderm; good candidates for positional cues controlling the fate of these neuroblasts are the segment polarity genes.

Each segment polarity gene is expressed in one or two stripes per segment in a different register along the AP axis (reviewed in DiNardo and Heemskerk, 1990). Patel *et al.* (1989b) used a number of neuron-specific markers to assay development of embryos lacking various segment polarity genes. Although a neuroblast can be identified by the family of neurons it produces, it is risky to use neurons as an assay for the identity of a neuroblast in mutant embryos. The mutation may alter GMC or neuron fate, rather than neuroblast identity. This caveat is especially relevant for the segment polarity genes known to be expressed in GMCs and neurons (see Table 1). Nevertheless, embryos with mutations in *patched* or a deficiency removing the tandem *gooseberry* genes have phenotypes consistent with a role in neuroblast specification. Each mutant shows alterations in the CNS that mimics those observed in the epidermis, suggesting that *patched* and *gooseberry* gene products give positional cues to ectodermal cells of the neurogenic region prior to neuroblast formation. These cues may be used to specify the identity of both epidermal precursors and neuroblasts. Mutations in *Cell, hedgehog, wingless (wg)* or the deficiency removing both *gooseberry* genes produce complex alterations in GMC and neuronal fates that are not consistent with a simple change of neuroblast identity (Patel *et al.*, 1989b). These genes presumably have multiple functions during neurogenesis.

It is important to note that many segment polarity genes (and pair rule genes) are expressed in ectodermal stripes as well as subsequently in neuroblasts, GMCs and neurons (Carroll and Scott, 1986; DiNardo *et al.*, 1986; Frasch *et al.*, 1987; Martinez-Arias *et al.*, 1988; van den Heuvel *et al.*, 1989; T. Gutjahr, N. Patel, C. S. Goodman, and M. Noll, personal communication). Expression in each cell or tissue type (ectoderm, neuroblast, GMC or neuron) is likely to be independently regulated, as shown by several examples. First, the pattern of expression in each tissue is often strikingly different: the pair rule genes *ftz* and *eve* are expressed in the ectoderm with bisegmental periodicity, and in segmental repeats in the CNS (Carroll and Scott, 1986; Frasch *et al*, 1987), whereas the segment polarity gene *en* is expressed in a neuroblast and several GMCs in regions where the ectoderm does not express *en* (C. Q. Doe, unpublished results). Second, gene regulatory interactions are usually different in each tissue (Table 2). The pair rule genes *ftz* and *eve* are clearly regulated differently in the CNS vs. ectoderm (Doe *et al*, 1988a,b). The segment polarity genes *en* and *wg* also illustrate this difference: in the ectoderm, *en* and *wg* are required to maintain high levels of expression of each other, whereas in the CNS, expression of *en* or *wg* is independent of each other (Martinez-Arias *et al.*, 1988; Patel *et al.*, 1989b). Thus it is likely that segmentation genes, and other genes, function at multiple levels during neurogenesis: in ectodermal cells, neuroblasts, GMCs or neurons (or all of the above). In each cell type the gene might participate in a unique gene regulatory hierarchy.

Genes of the segment polarity class encode nuclear proteins [e.g., *engrailed (en)*], predicted cell-surface proteins (e.g., *patched*), and secreted proteins (e.g., *wingless*). Each gene may control neuroblast specification by one of the three possibilities mentioned earlier: cell autonomous inheritance by a group of ectodermal cells or a neuroblast, cell interactions within the neurogenic region, or diffusion of a secreted protein across the neurogenic region. Future experiments should include assaying the pattern of neuroblast-specific genes (see Table 1) in embryos mutant for each segment polarity gene.

b. Genes Subdividing the Neurogenic Region along the Dorsal–Ventral Axis

If pair-rule or segment polarity genes specify differences between each of the six rows of neuroblasts, what distinguishes the four neuroblasts in a particular row? The initial embryonic DV polarity is controlled by a group of maternal effect genes whose action results in a ventral-to-dorsal nuclear localization gradient of the *dorsal* protein (Rushlow *et al.*, 1989). However, the

TABLE I
Known and Candidate Neuroblast Identity Genes

Gene	Expression in each hemisegment			Protein motifs	Controls GMC identity?	References
	Neuroectoderm	NBs[a]	GMCs + neurons			
prospero	none	most	subset GMCs no neurons	divergent homeodomain	yes	Doe *et al.*, 1991; Chu-LaGraff *et al.*, 1991.
runt	none	subset	subset	novel nuclear	yes	Kania *et al.*, 1990; J. Duffy, M. Kania, P. Gergen, personal communication.
polyhomeotic	none	subset	subset	Zn finger	yes	Smouse *et al.*, 1988; Dura *et al.*, 1988; H. Brock, personal communication
seven-up	subset (clusters)	subset	subset	Zn finger; steroid receptor	yes	Mlodzik *et al.*, 1990; Y. Hiromi, personal communication
wingless	subset (stripes)	4	few or none	secreted protein	yes	van den Huevel *et al.*, 1989; Patel *et al.*, 1989b; Q. Chu-LaGraff and C. Q. Doe, unpublished results.
83C	none	subset	few or none	Zn finger	yes	X. Cui and C. Q. Doe, unpublished results.
hunchback	?	all	subset	Zn finger	?	Tautz *et al.*, 1987. C. Q. Doe, unpublished results.
64A	none	subset	?	Zn finger	?	E. Bier and Y. Jan, personal communication.
cut	none	subset	subset	homeodomain	?	C. Q. Doe, K. Blochlinger, and Y. Jan, unpublished results.

gooseberry-neuro	none	subset	subset	homeodomain	?	Baumgarten *et al.,* 1987; N. Patel, T. Gutjahr, M. Noll, and C. S. Goodman, personal communication.
gooseberry	subset (stripes)	subset	subset	homeodomain	?	Baumgarten *et al.,* 1987; N. Patel, T. Gutjahr, M. Noll, and C. S. Goodman, personal communication.
engrailed	subset (stripes)	8	subset	homeodomain	?	Patel *et al.,* 1989a.
pox neuro	none	2	subset	paired-box	?	Bopp *et al.,* 1989; M. Noll, personal communication.
44C	subset (stripes)	all	?	helix-loop-helix	?	E. Bier and Y. Jan, personal communication.
lethal of scute	subset (clusters)	most	none	helix-loop-helix	?	Cabrera *et al.,* 1987; Romani *et al.,* 1987.
scute	subset (clusters)	subset	none	helix-loop-helix	?	Cabrera *et al.,* 1987; Romani *et al.,* 1987.
achaete	subset (clusters)	subset	none	helix-loop-helix	?	Cabrera *et al.,* 1987; Romani *et al.,* 1987.
asense	none	subset	none	helix-loop-helix	?	Alonso and Cabrera, 1988.

[a]The number of neuroblasts expressing the gene in every thoracic hemisegment (about 25 neuroblasts are in each thoracic hemisegment).

dorsal protein does not directly influence neuroblast identity, because the protein is undetectable by the time of neurogenesis (Rushlow *et al.*, 1989). Presumably the *dorsal* protein regulates zygotic genes whose products play a role in neuroblast specification.

Only a few genes are known to be regionally expressed along the DV axis during neurogenesis, and most of these are localized in cells adjacent to the neurogenic region. The midline genes are expressed in the specialized ventral midline cells between the two halves of the neurogenic region; this group includes *orthodenticle, single-minded, slit, Star,* and *rhomboid* (Mayer and Nüsslein-Volhard, 1988; Rothberg *et al.,* 1988; Thomas *et al.,* 1988; Bier *et al.,* 1990; Finkelstein *et al.,* 1990; Klambt *et al.,* 1991). At least two of these genes, *rhomboid* and *slit,* encode putative membrane proteins (Rothberg *et al.,* 1988; Bier *et al.,* 1990), which could affect the specification of neuroblasts adjacent to the ventral midline through cell–cell interactions. The *deca-pentaplegic* gene is expressed in a stripe along the dorsal ectoderm (St. Johnston and Gelbart, 1987), well outside the neurogenic region, but it en-codes a protein with homology to transforming growth factor β (Padgett *et al.,* 1987), and could affect neuroblast specification if neuroblasts at different DV positions are exposed to different levels of the potentially diffusible *deca-pentaplegic* protein.

A final possibility is that there may be no cues expressed along the DV axis. Differences in neuroblast specification along this axis may be due to the

---

TABLE 2
Selected Tissue-Specific Gene Regulatory Differences[a]

CNS	References	Blastoderm or epidermis	References
ftz | *en*	C. Q. Doe (unpublished results)	*ftz* + *en*	Howard and Ingham (1986); DiNardo and O'Farrell (1987)
ftz + *Ubx* in RP1, 2, 3	Doe *et al.* (1988a)	*ftz* + *Ubx*	Duncan (1986); Ingham and Martinez-Arias (1986)
ftz + *eve* in RP2	Doe *et al.* (1988a)	*ftz* | *eve*	Harding *et al.* (1986); Ingham *et al.* (1988)
ftz | *Ubx* in aCC, pCC	Doe *et al.* (1988a)		
ftz | *eve* in aCC, pCC	Doe *et al.* (1988a)		
ftz | *ftz*	Doe *et al.* (1988a)	*ftz* + *ftz*	Hiromi *et al.* (1987)
eve | *ftz*	Doe *et al.* (1988b)	*eve* − *ftz*	Carroll and Scott (1986)
wg | *en*	Patel *et al.* (1989b)	*wg* + *en*	Martinez-Arias *et al.* (1988)

[a]\|, has no effect on; +, activates or maintains; −, represses.

different times of neuroblast formation. Neuroblast formation is not a synchronous event; with a few exceptions, the neuroblasts of each row form at different times (Campos-Ortega and Hartenstein, 1985). Segment polarity gene expression is continually modified during neurogenesis; thus, early- and late-forming neuroblasts of the same row may assume different fates due to changes in segment polarity gene expression.

We have only begun to identify genes regionally expressed in the neurogenic region. The mutant phenotype of genes encoding positional cues in the neuroectoderm may well be subtle, especially for genes expressed along the DV axis. There are few ventral cuticular markers distributed asymmetrically, so these genes may have been missed in previous saturation mutageneses (Nüsslein-Volhard and Weischaus, 1980). Screens looking for defects in the CNS have been done with a few probes, but certainly not to saturation. Analysis of candidate genes will be facilitated by new markers for individual neuroblasts (e.g., enhancer trap lines). These probes can be used to assay the fate of identified neuroblasts at the time they form in embryos mutant for the genes just described.

3. TIMING OF NEUROBLAST SPECIFICATION

Initial neuroblast specification probably occurs by the time a neuroblast has produced its first GMC, since each neuroblast generates a characteristic set of progeny. It can begin in ectodermal cells either prior to neuroblast formation or in the period after neuroblast formation but before cell division begins (Fig. 7). Several *Drosophila* genes are expressed in clusters of 4–6 ectodermal cells in the neurogenic region; one cell in each cluster maintains expression and differentiates as a neuroblast. This suggests that positional specification can occur in groups of neuroectodermal cells, prior to neuroblast formation (Fig. 7A). One gene with this type of expression is *seven-up (svp),* which controls cell fate in the eye disc (Mlodzik *et al.,* 1990) and is a candidate neuroblast identity gene. The AS-C genes are also initially expressed in clusters of 4–6 ectodermal cells in the neurogenic region. The cells of the cluster that do not form the neuroblast rapidly lose AS-C expression, while the developing neuroblast maintains expression. Although the functions of the AS-C genes and *svp* have not been conclusively determined, it is likely that the former genes control neuroblast formation, whereas the latter gene controls neuroblast identity. Thus, the same set of positional cues may regulate both neuroblast formation and neuroblast specification. It would be interesting to know whether the *svp* and AS-C clusters are congruent; a cell-for-cell match would provide additional evidence for a common mechanism coordinating the timing and position of neuroblast formation with the fate of the neuroblast.

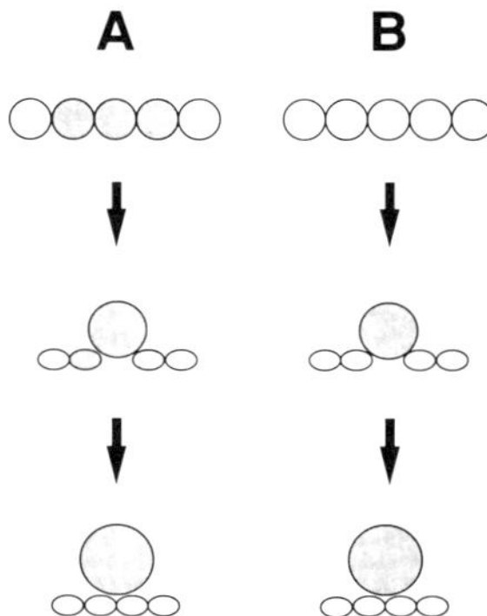

Figure 7. Timing of neuroblast specification. A. Positional specification may occur in clusters of 4–6 ectodermal cells (shaded) in the neurogenic region; only one of these cells will ultimately form a neuroblast. This model is supported by expression of the *svp* gene and several enhancer trap lines in clusters of 4–6 ectodermal cells prior to their expression in the neuroblast derived from the cluster. B. Neuroblast specification may occur after the neuroblast has formed. Expression of *pros* occurs only in newly formed neuroblasts.

4. DO NEUROBLAST EQUIVALENCE GROUPS EXIST?

As mentioned in section II.A.3, gene expression patterns in the *Drosophila* neuroectoderm are often in clusters of 4–6 cells, from which one cell will form a neuroblast (e.g., *sc, ac, l'sc, svp,* and several enhancer trap lines). In grasshopper embryos, clusters of 4–6 neuroectodermal cells differentiate concurrently into one neuroblast and associated nonneuronal cells (Doe and Goodman, 1985a), with all cells of the cluster capable of forming the neuroblast (Doe and Goodman, 1985b). These data raise the possibility that the insect neuroectoderm contains "equivalence groups" (Kimble, 1981) committed to forming a specific neuroblast and its support cells. If so, these equivalence groups should have a restricted developmental potential: to produce a single, unique neuroblast. However, ablation experiments in grasshopper embryos suggest that ectodermal cells have the ability to form two or three different neuroblasts, indicating that ectodermal cells are not clustered into equivalence groups committed to produce specific neuroblasts.

First, all cells of a putative neuroblast equivalence group appear to differentiate concurrently. An ablated neuroblast is not replaced if it is surrounded by previously differentiated neuroblasts (for example, if the late-forming neuroblast 7-3 is ablated; Doe and Goodman, 1985b). This suggests that no individual cell in the putative equivalence group remains capable of replacing the neuroblast once it has differentiated; all cells of the equivalence group appear to differentiate into nonneuronal cells in parallel with neuroblast formation. Second, when an ablated neuroblast is adjacent to ectodermal cells that have not yet differentiated (for example, if the early-forming neuroblast 1-1 is ablated), regulation can still occur to produce a new neuroblast. Presumably all of the cells in the putative "neuroblast 1-1 equivalence group" have differentiated into either neuroblast 1-1, nonneuronal cells, or died; the only nearby cells with the potential to replace the neuroblast are at the adjacent future neuroblast 1-2 position, suggesting that one of these ectodermal cells switches from a neuroblast 1-2 fate to that of neuroblast 1-1. Similarly, when neuroblast 7-4 is ablated, the only remaining ectodermal cells are at the adjacent future neuroblast 7-3 position. Neuroblast 7-3 gives rise to a pair of serotonergic neurons. When one of the ectodermal cells at position 7-3 replaces the ablated neuroblast 7-4, duplicated serotonergic neurons are never observed, suggesting that the ectodermal cells at position 7-3 are not committed to the neuroblast 7-3 fate.

Positional cues certainly exist within the neurogenic region, and apparently define groups of 4–6 cells with a similar developmental fate, but these cues do not *irreversibly* determine ectodermal cell fate. Cells finding themselves in a new position—e.g. following a neuroblast ablation—can regulate and switch their fate to correctly replace the ablated neuroblast. Ultimately, transplantations of neuroectodermal cells from one position (e.g., the 7-3 position) to a new location (e.g., the 1-1 position) will clarify whether equivalence groups exist in the insect neuroectoderm.

B. Neuroblast Identity Genes

As described earlier, positional cues exist in the neuroectoderm from which neuroblasts delaminate. Our model is that positional cues control expression of neuroblast identity genes in subsets of neuroblasts or in clusters of ectodermal cells preceding the formation of a single neuroblast. The role of neuroblast identity genes is to trigger a unique neuroblast cell lineage by regulating two processes: the neuroblast cell cycle and the identity of each GMC. Each neuroblast divides a characteristic number of times; how neuroblast identity genes control the number of divisions a neuroblast makes is unknown. A testable hypothesis for how neuroblast identity genes control GMC fate is that each GMC inherits a unique combination of neuroblast identity gene products. Neuroblast identity genes could be expressed in a lineage-specific pattern, in the lineal homologs of each neuroblast, or in a specific position in neuroblast lineages (Fig. 6). Genes with expression patterns similar to each of these classes have been described: *en* (subset of neuroblast lineages), *hunchback* (neuroblasts followed by most GMC-1s and their neuronal progeny), and *prospero* (neuroblasts and newly born GMCs but not neurons). Many genes are expressed in neuroblasts and GMCs, but have yet to be carefully analyzed for either expression pattern or mutant phenotype. I will begin by examining the evidence that several neuroblast cell lineages are autonomous (at least for the early progeny); these data provide much of the impetus for proposing the neuroblast identity gene model. I will next describe the phenotype and expression of *prospero (pros),* a neuroblast identity gene. Other candidate neuroblast identity genes will be discussed at the end of this section.

I. INVARIANT NEUROBLAST CELL LINEAGES

A number of different mechanisms can be imagined for the specification of neuroblast progeny: environmental influences, neuroblast–GMC cell interactions, neuroblast–neuroblast interactions, and quantitatively or qualitatively different factors passed from the neuroblast to each GMC in the lineage. Two lines of evidence show that for several neuroblast lineages, specification of the early GMCs is controlled by the parental neuroblast, rather than by environmental influences. First, when a grasshopper neuroblast is killed after it has generated two or three GMCs, it can be replaced by an adjacent ectodermal cell. The new neuroblast begins its cell lineage with the first GMC, not the third or fourth GMC. The development of these "heterochronic" neuroblasts suggests that the identity of a GMC is due to its birth order, or cell lineage, rather than to environmental cues (Doe and Goodman, 1985b).

A second type of experiment is the *in vitro* culture of isolated *Drosophila* neuroblasts. Isolated neuroblasts will divide in culture to generate GMCs and neurons. The neuroblast lineage results in a group of cells around the isolated neuroblast. When these *in vitro* neuroblast lineages are assayed for serotonergic or dopaminergic neurons, in each case about 1 in 25 shows immunoreactive neurons (Huff *et al.,* 1989). Interestingly, in the embryo about 1 in 25 neuroblast lineages generates serotonergic neurons and 1 in 25 lineages generates dopaminergic neurons. Both in embryos and *in vitro,* the first born GMCs generate the neurotransmitter-expressing neurons (Huff *et al.,* 1989). Apparently specification of neurotransmitter type occurs normally *in vitro,* which strongly suggests that GMC specification is due to factors inherited from the neuroblast or interactions between GMC and neuroblast. Neurotransmitter expression *in vitro* requires one cycle of DNA synthesis in the neuroblast (Huff *et al.,* 1989), suggesting that GMC specification occurs during the interval between S phase and mitosis. Interestingly, this is the exact stage in the cell cycle during which ferret cortical neurons acquire their laminar fates (McConnell, 1988; see also Chapter 12). We expect that each *Drosophila* neuroblast expresses a unique combination of neuroblast identity genes at the time each GMC is born. The progression of a neuroblast through

S phase might switch, or "reset," gene expression so the next GMC inherits a different set of neuroblast identity gene products.

2. *PROSPERO* IS A NEUROBLAST IDENTITY GENE

To identify neuroblast identity genes that control GMC fate, we isolated embryonic lethal mutations that met the following criteria: (1) early development (prior to neurogenesis) occurs normally, (2) the normal number of neuroblasts is formed, (3) the neuroblasts divide to produce GMCs, and most importantly, (4) there is altered expression of *eve, ftz,* and *en* genes in newly born GMCs. A change in gene expression in newborn GMCs would be the earliest sign of a defective neuroblast cell lineage. The *prospero (pros)* gene was discovered in this screen as well as in an enhancer trap screen, by virtue of expression in a subset of neuroblasts and GMCs (Doe *et al.,* 1991). The earliest detectable defect in *pros* embryos is a change in GMC gene expression (Fig. 8). In wild-type embryos, *eve* is first expressed in five GMCs in each hemisegment; these GMCs are produced by at least three neuroblasts and give rise to the aCC and pCC neurons, six CQ neurons, and the RP2 neuron (Doe *et al.,* 1988a,b; Patel *et al.,* 1989b). In *pros* embryos, these GMCs and neurons do not express *eve.* These GMCs and neurons also lack *ftz* expression (Doe *et al.,* 1991). However, other GMCs and neurons in *pros* embryos show normal *eve* expression: the five *eve*-positive GMCs at the lateral side of the CNS develop normally into the 10 "*eve*-lateral" (EL) neurons (Fig. 8).

Loss of *pros* function does not result only in the absence of gene expression from GMCs and neurons, as is seen for *ftz* and *eve. en* is expressed in more neurons in *pros* embryos that in wild-type embryos. *en* is normally expressed in four clusters of cells in the posterior half of each neuromere: six large ventral midline (VM) neurons, six to eight smaller dorsal midline (DM) cells (probably neurons), bilateral clusters of about eight mediolateral (ML) neurons, and bilateral clusters of about six lateral (L) neurons at the edge of the CNS. In *pros* embryos, the neurons between the ML and L neurons express *en;* normally they do not. In addition, the number of small *en*-positive DM cells is increased four- to fivefold, to 20–30 *en*-positive cells (Fig. 8). There is also a complete absence of the large *en*-positive VM cells (Doe *et al.,* 1991).

It is important to determine whether the GMCs that normally express *eve* and *ftz* actually survive and differentiate in *pros* embryos. In wild-type embryos, one *ftz*- and *eve*-positive GMC produces the identifiable aCC and pCC neurons, which are born at the anterior edge of each segment and then migrate anteriorly, stopping just posterior to the future location of the posterior commissure (Thomas *et al.,* 1984). The mature aCC and pCC neurons have a characteristic size, position in the CNS, and axon morphology. In *pros* embryos the GMC that normally would produce the aCC and pCC neurons

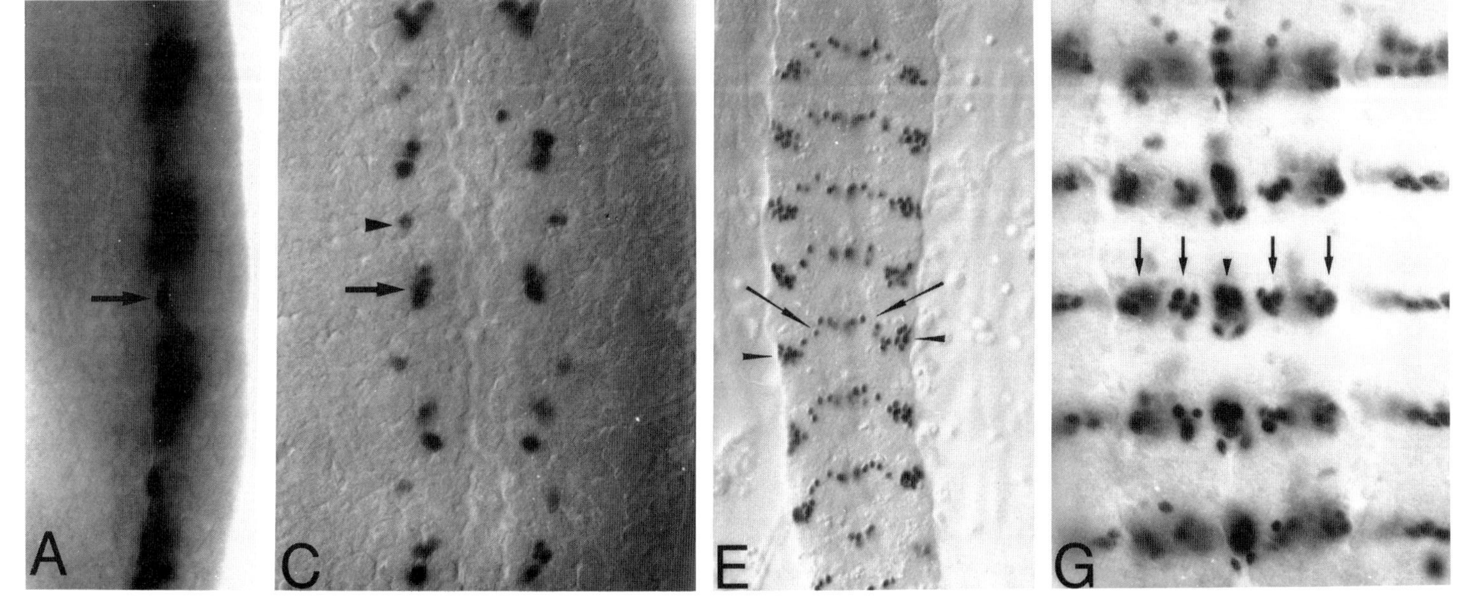

Figure 8. *prospero* is required for correct gene expression in GMCs and neurons. A, B. *ftz* expression at 7.5 hr of development; lateral view, anterior up. A. Wild-type embryo showing the aCC and pCC neurons *(arrow)*. B. *pros* embryos do not express *ftz* in the aCC and pCC neurons *(arrow)*. C, D. *eve* expression at 7 hr of development; ventral view, anterior up. C. Wild-type embryo showing aCC and pCC neurons together with two CQ neurons *(arrow)* and the single GMC that will give rise to the RP2 neuron *(arrowhead)*. D. *pros* embryos do not express *eve* in these cells. The approximate positions of the unstained cells are indicated: aCC, pCC, and CQ neurons *(arrow)*; GMC precursor of RP2 *(arrowhead)*. At this stage other cells near the telson continue to express *eve (bottom)*, as do the cells of the amnioserosa (out of the plane of focus). E, F. *eve* expression in the 13-hr CNS; dorsal view, anterior up. E. Wild-type embryo showing the cluster of ten EL neurons *(arrowhead)* and the more medial CQ neurons *(arrow)*; the aCC, pCC, and RP2 neurons are out of the plane of focus. F. *pros* embryo showing normal *eve* expression in the EL neurons *(arrowhead)*, but no expression in the CQ neurons *(arrow)*. Occasionally one or several CQ neurons express *eve (asterisk-arrow)*. The aCC, pCC, and RP2 neurons do not express *eve* and are out of the plane of focus. G, H. *en* expression in the 13-hr CNS; dorsal view, anterior up. G. Wild-type embryo showing *en*-positive L neurons *(outer arrow)*, ML neurons *(inner arrows)* and DM cells *(arrowhead)*. Six larger *en*-positive VM neurons are out of the plane of focus. H. A higher magnification view of the CNS of a *pros* embryo showing *en*-positive neurons in the location of the L and ML clusters *(arrows)*, with additional *en*-positive neurons in between. There is an increase in the number of *en*-positive DM cells *(arrowhead)* and a total absence of large VM *en*-positive neurons (out of the plane of focus).

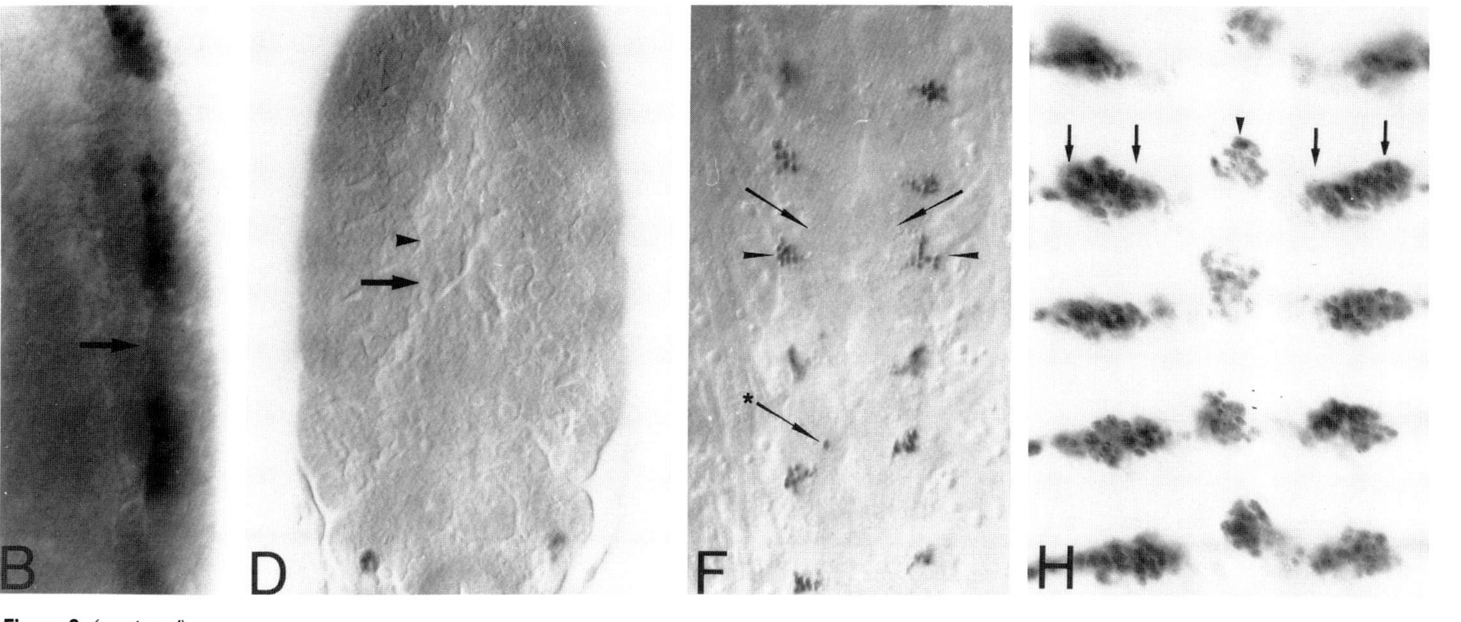

Figure 8 *(continued)*

does not express *ftz,* or *eve,* yet the neuronal progeny of this GMC ("aCC" and "pCC") migrate to the appropriate position and can be unambiguously identified due to their size, position, and aspects of their axon morphology. Not surprisingly, the "aCC" and "pCC" neurons in *pros* embryos show striking defects in axon morphology; it is not known whether these pathfinding errors are due to altered neuron identities or incorrect cues required for normal pathfinding. Combined, these results suggest that in *pros* embryos a subset of neuroblasts generates aberrant cell lineages, as detected by the loss or gain of gene expression in identified GMCs; these GMCs divide to produce several identifiable neurons (Doe *et al.,* 1991).

Due to the nature of *pros* mutations—aberrant neuroblast cell lineages and incorrect GMC specification—*pros* expression is expected in a subset of neuroblasts and GMCs. Indeed, *pros* transcripts are observed in all but two of the neuroblasts in each hemisegment (Fig. 9). The two *pros*-negative cells are considered neuroblasts based on size, morphology, and position in the neuroblast array. During neuroblast formation, the transcript is clearly restricted to neuroblasts; no signal is seen in the ventral neuroectoderm from which neuroblasts delaminate (Fig. 9). In addition, the transcript is observed in many of the GMCs born early in neurogenesis. In general, the *pros* transcript is not detectable in neurons, although it may be expressed in a small number of neurons or transiently in young neurons (Fig. 9).

The *pros* gene encodes two classes of transcripts, one 6.4 kb and one 6.5 kb; the shorter transcript lacks an 87-base pair exon in the protein coding region (Chu-LaGraff *et al.,* 1991). A nearly full-length cDNA has been sequenced, and the predicted protein has a highly divergent homeodomain. Interestingly, the alternatively spliced exon lies in the homeobox; thus, each transcript may produce a homeodomain that differs at the five N-terminal amino acids. Crystal structure of the *en* homeodomain shows that the N-terminal "arm" of the homeodomain makes contacts with nucleotides in the minor groove (Kissinger *et al.,* 1990); perhaps the two predicted homeodomains produced from the *pros* gene have different DNA binding specificities. The phenotype of embryos lacking *pros* function includes changes in *eve,* *ftz,* and *en* gene expression in specific GMCs; it will be interesting to determine whether the *pros* protein interacts directly with the promoters of these genes. How *pros* expression is limited to specific GMCs, and how it regulates gene expression in some, but not all, of these GMCs, is currently unknown.

3. CANDIDATE NEUROBLAST IDENTITY GENES

In addition to *pros,* four other genes have phenotypes suggesting a role in GMC specification: *runt, svp, polyhomeotic (ph),* and *wg.* The *runt* gene is expressed in a subset of neuroblasts and encodes a novel nuclear protein

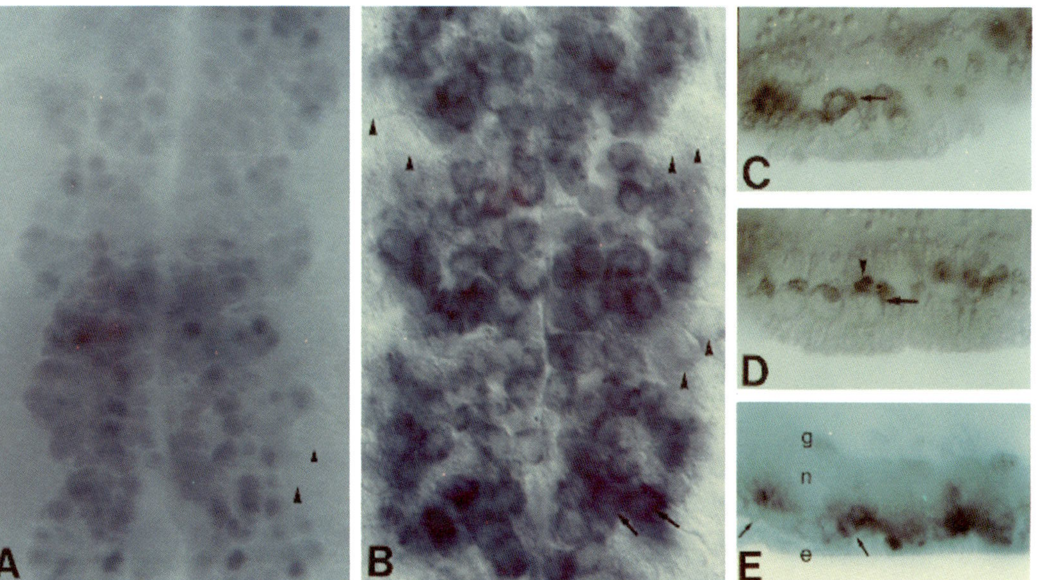

FIGURE 9. *prospero* is expressed in neuroblasts and early-born GMCs but not in neurons. A. Enhancer trap detection showing *lac Z* expression in a pattern matching that of the *pros* gene in a 6-hr embryo (ventral view of about 2.5 segments; compare with B). Arrowheads indicate neuroblasts that do not express *lacZ* B. Expression of the *pros* transcript in most neuroblasts (in an embryo similar in age to that in A). The majority of neuroblasts expresses *pros* *(arrows)*, but two per hemisegment do not *(arrowheads)*. Based on size, morphology, and position in the neuroblast array, these two *pros*-negative cells are neuroblasts; neither is the glioblast. C,D,E. Neuroblast, GMC, and neuronal expression shown in optical cross section, detected with HRP reaction product. The ventral surface of the embryos is toward the bottom of the photographs. C. *pros* expression in a newly formed neuroblast *(arrow)*; GMCs have not yet been born. D. *pros* expression in newly born GMCs *(arrowhead)* is often stronger than neuroblast expression *(arrow)*. This photograph also illustrates the lack of *pros* expression in the ventral ectoderm from which the neuroblasts develop *(below arrow)*. E. Neuroblast expression continues in 7.5-hr embryos *(arrows)*, but no neuronal expression (n) is detected; the cell on the dorsal surface expressing *pros* is one of the longitudinal glia (g). *pros* is not expressed in the epidermis (e).

(Kania *et al.*, 1990). Temperature shift experiments can be used to inactivate *runt* protein during neurogenesis. Loss of *runt* function during the time of neuroblast expression results in absence of the *eve*-positive EL neurons, suggesting that *runt* function is required in neuroblasts to control GMC identity and consequently EL neuron fate (J. Duffy, M. Kania, and P. Gergen, personal communication). However, it is not yet known whether the missing *eve*-positive neurons are never born, die, or assume an abnormal (*eve*-negative) fate.

The *svp* gene is expressed in a subset of neuroblasts and GMCs, and encodes a protein with both a steroid ligand binding domain and a Zn-finger domain (Mlodzik *et al.*, 1990). Embryos lacking *svp* function have abnormal *eve* expression in a subset of neurons (Y. Hiromi, personal communication). The *ph* gene also encodes a putative Zn-finger protein that is expressed in many neuroblasts (F. Maschat and H. Brock, personal communication). Mutations in *ph* affect the expression of *eve, en,* and other homeobox genes in the CNS (Dura and Ingham, 1988; Smouse *et al.*, 1988), suggesting that *ph* may control the lineage of many neuroblasts.

The segment polarity gene *wg* encodes a secreted protein that is expressed in three SI neuroblasts (Fig. 2; van den Huevel *et al.*, 1990; Q. Chu-LaGraff and C. Q. Doe, unpublished results). Loss of *wg* function results in the loss of *eve* expression in the RP2 neuron and its GMC precursor (Patel *et al.*, 1989a), which is born from an SII neuroblast (neuroblast 4-2) that does not express *wg* (Q. Chu-LaGraff and C. Q. Doe, unpublished results). Temperature shift experiments using a *wg*^{ts} allele can be used to allow some *wg* function during segmentation while still observing the CNS defect. Thus *eve* expression in the neuroblast 4-2 lineage could be due, in part, to *wg* function in an adjacent SI neuroblast. This indicates that neuroblast identity genes can act autonomously, as presumed for the nuclear *runt* and *svp* proteins, or via interactions between neuroblasts as presumed for the secreted *wg* protein (Q. Chu-LaGraff and C. Q. Doe, unpublished results).

It is interesting that the overwhelming majority of genes expressed in neuroblasts are putative transcription factors (Table 1). This supports the hypothesis that the overlapping expression of neuroblast identity genes may control GMC specification. Because GMC identity seems to be determined between S phase of the neuroblast and its subsequent mitosis (Huff *et al.*, 1989), we expect that the expression of neuroblast identity genes is modified after S phase of each neuroblast cell cycle. In this manner, each GMC could inherit a unique combination of gene products. The subsequent step in GMC specification may involve the expression of a characteristic set of genes in each GMC; this class of genes, expressed in a subset of GMCs (but not neuroblasts) in response to neuroblast identity gene function, can be termed GMC and neuronal identity genes.

C. GMC and Neuronal Identity Genes

Two genes, *ftz* and *eve,* have been tested for their role in GMC and neuron specification (Doe *et al.,* 1988a,b). These genes are expressed in a number of GMCs soon after their birth; I will focus on the GMCs derived from neuroblast 4-2 (NB 4-2). GMC-1 expresses both *ftz* and *eve,* one daughter cell differentiates into the RP2 neuron and the other assumes an unknown fate (possibly undergoing programmed cell death; C. Q. Doe, unpublished results). GMC-2 expresses *ftz,* but not *eve,* and probably generates the RP1 and RP3 neurons (Fig. 9). The role of *ftz* in GMC specification was tested by using a *ftz* gene construct with the CNS enhancer deleted; this allows normal blastoderm stripe expression but removes detectable CNS expression (Doe *et al.,* 1988a). Only one defect is observed in the CNS of these embryos: *eve* is not expressed in GMC-1 of NB 4-2, and the resulting "RP2" neuron shows abnormal axon morphology, mimicking the RP1 and RP3 axons. Thus, loss of *ftz* (and *eve*) alters the specification of GMC-1 towards that of GMC-2 (Fig. 10).

To determine if the defect in GMC-1 specification is due to the loss of *ftz* or the loss of *eve,* embryos lacking only *eve* CNS expression were examined. A temperature-sensitive mutation was used to inactivate the *eve* protein during neurogenesis, while allowing earlier segmentation to occur normally (Doe *et al.,* 1988b). Interestingly, the loss of *eve* alone produces the same phenotype as the loss of both *ftz* and *eve* (Fig. 10).This result suggests that the transformation of GMC-1 to GMC-2 identity is solely due to the loss of *eve* function. It is not known when the *eve* protein is required for RP2 development: the shift to nonpermissive temperature included stages during which *eve* is expressed in GMC-1 as well as in the neurons. More precise temperature shifts will be required to determine the time at which the *eve* protein acts to control GMC or neuronal fate.

The NB 4-2 lineage provides an opportunity to assign a few genes to the steps of GMC specification. Factors in GMCs result in the expression of *ftz* in GMC-1 and GMC-2. One of these GMC factors is the *pros* gene product, since embryos mutant for *pros* do not express *ftz* in these GMCs. *pros* transcript is detected in NB 4-2 and its first progeny (GMC-1). Expression of *ftz* in GMC-1 is necessary but not sufficient for the activation of *eve* expression. The activity of the *eve* protein in GMC-1 or its daughter RP2 neuron is required for correct RP2 pathfinding. The *eve* protein has a homeodomain, and its function presumably involves the regulation of gene expression in GMC-1 or the RP2 neuron. Discovering the genes controlled by *eve* will be an important step in bridging the gap between gene regulation and the morphological differentiation of a neuron. Obvious candidates include the fasciclin genes, which are expressed in several *eve*-positive neurons (Hortsch and Goodman, 1990, and

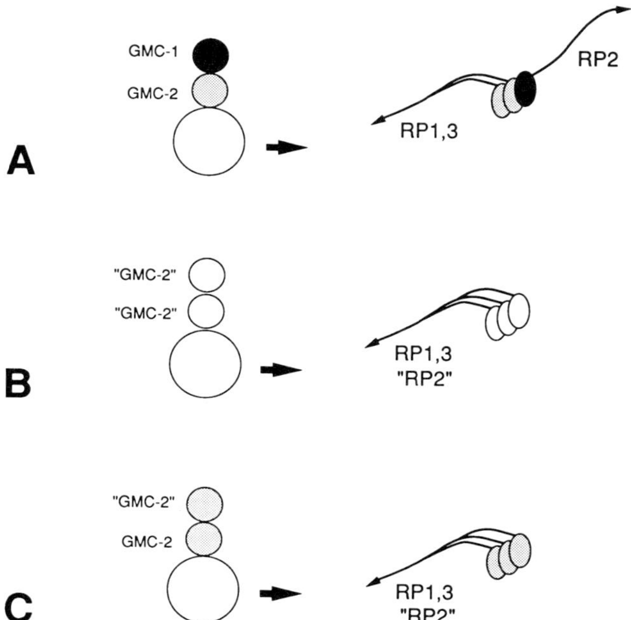

Figure 10. GMC and neuronal fate is controlled by *ftz* and *eve*. A. In wild-type embryos, *ftz* and *eve* are both expressed in GMC-1 from neuroblast 4-2, which develops into the RP2 neuron and a neuron of unknown fate. GMC-2 expresses only *ftz*, and develops into the RP1 and RP3 neurons. B. Loss of *ftz* prevents expression of *eve* in GMC-1; GMC-1 produces a neuron resembling RP1 and RP3 ("RP2"). This indicates an alteration of cell fate from GMC-1 towards GMC-2. C. Loss of *eve* has no effect on *ftz* expression in GMC-1 or GMC-2; again GMC-1 produces a neuron resembling RP1 and RP3, showing that loss of *eve* alone is sufficient to transform GMC-1 towards GMC-2.

references therein), and the I-POU gene, which is expressed in the same neurons as *eve*, but slightly later in development (Treacy *et al.*, 1991).

What controls the fate of sibling neurons? Cell lineage plays a key role: the type of neurons that develop depends on their parental GMC. However, sibling neurons often assume different fates, for example, RP2 and its sibling or the aCC and pCC neurons. Experiments in grasshopper indicate that sibling neurons are born with equivalent fates, but cell interactions between the pair can assign each a particular identity (Kuwada and Goodman, 1985). When one neuron is killed immediately after birth the surviving neuron always differentiates into one type of neuron (the 1° fate). If one neuron is killed slightly later, several hours after its birth, its sibling takes the 1° and 2° fate with equal probability, showing that the neuron has already been specified. Ablation of many of the nearby cells has no effect on the fate of the sibling neurons. Thus cell interactions between sibling neurons seem to be required to specify neuronal fate. This can be considered an example of a two-cell neural equivalence group (Kuwada and Goodman, 1985).

III. Gene Regulatory Hierarchies in the Central Nervous System

It has become increasingly clear that epidermis, endoderm, mesoderm, and CNS show distinctive hierarchies of gene expression; a few examples of tissue-specific gene regulation are shown in Table 2. For example, *eve* is required for the correct expression of *ftz* in the cellular blastoderm; the converse can be observed in the CNS, where *ftz* is required to activate *eve* in the RP2 neuron. Not only are there obvious differences in gene regulation between tissues, but even in the CNS there are neuron-specific gene regulatory interactions. *ftz* and *eve* are expressed in the RP2, aCC, and pCC neurons, but *eve* requires *ftz* only in the RP2 neuron. A sobering thought (especially for those who want to study neuronal gene regulation *in vitro*) is the possibility of unique gene regulatory hierarchies in individual neurons.

IV. Perspectives

We currently have a sketchy understanding of how neuronal diversity is generated in the *Drosophila* CNS. We know that positional cues specify neuroblast identity, but we know very little about the molecules or mechanisms used. We know that the proneural genes are expressed in clusters of 4–6 cells, and that they trigger neural development. Proneural gene expression is negatively regulated by the neurogenic genes, perhaps directly by the genes of the E(spl)-C or posttranslationally by the *shaggy* kinase. Recently progress has been made in characterizing the molecular mechanisms controlling neuroblast cell lineages. In some neuroblast lineages GMC fate is specified autonomously by birth order, or cell lineage, from a particular neuroblast. Determination of GMC identity seems to occur just prior to neuroblast mitosis; it is proposed that specific combinations of neuroblast identity gene products mediate GMC cell fates. Of the five neuroblast identity genes implicated in controlling neuroblast lineages, four encode putative transcription factors *(pros, svp, runt* and *pb)*.

To fully understand the mechanisms of GMC specification, new genes will have to be identified, and genes currently known to be expressed in neuroblasts will have to be carefully analyzed to determine their loss-of-function phenotypes. The arrival of enhancer trap screens will lead to a rapid increase in the number of genes known to be expressed at the right time and place for both neuroblast and GMC specification, as well as provide useful markers for specific cells. In addition, genes isolated by DNA homology (e.g., homeobox genes) and previously identified genes (e.g., segmentation genes) are often discovered to be expressed in neuroblasts. Identifying new genes will be relatively easy; the challenge will be to determine how each gene contributes to neuroblast or GMC specification.

Two areas need to be actively pursued. First, it will be vital to characterize individual neuroblast lineages in more detail: we know only a few neurons derived from GMCs born early in some lineages, and we do not know the complete lineage of any neuroblast. In particular, it is critical to determine the entire lineage of specific neuroblasts, for example, neuroblast 1-1, which produces the aCC and pCC neurons, or neuroblast 4-2, which generates the RP neurons. Second, the relationship between neuroblast identity gene expression and the neuroblast cell cycle needs to be investigated: does S phase (or G_2) trigger a change in gene expression and, if so, how is the new pattern of gene expression regulated?

Early CNS development is virtually identical among arthropods (Patel *et al.*, 1989a; Thomas *et al.*, 1984). Might fundamental similarities extend to more distantly related organisms, such as vertebrates? Genes known to play a role in CNS development are also conserved between *Drosophila* and vertebrates. Recently, two AS-C homologs have been identified in rats; as expected, they are expressed in a subset of CNS precursor cells during early neurogenesis (Johnson *et al.*, 1990; Lo *et al.*, 1991). Vertebrate homologs to the *Drosophila* pair-rule gene *eve* and the segment polarity genes *wg* and *en* have been identified. Each of these genes is expressed in the developing CNS (Wilkinson *et al.*, 1987; Davis *et al.*, 1988; Bastian and Gruss, 1990) and the mouse *wg* and *en* homologs are necessary for the correct development of specific regions of the mouse brain (McMahon and Bradley, 1990; Joyner *et al.*, 1991). In addition, homeotic genes specify segment-specific differences in the CNS of both *Drosophila* and vertebrates (reviewed in Doe and Scott, 1988). These results suggest that characterization of *Drosophila* CNS development will provide insight into the mechanisms controling neuronal diversity in both flies and vertebrates.

Acknowledgments

I would like to thank J. Skeath, S. Carroll, J. Duffy, M. Kania, J. P. Gergen, N. H. Patel, T. Gutjahr, M. Noll, C. S. Goodman, E. Bier, Y. Jan, J. Campos-Ortega, E. Knust, A. Ghysen, H. Brock, Y. Hiromi, and S. McConnell for providing data prior to publication; J. Skeath and S. Carroll for Figure 4; and D. Smouse for commenting on an early version of this chapter. The research described here has been supported by the Searle Scholars Program, an NSF Presidential Young Investigator Award, and NIH RO1-27056.

References

Alonso and Cabrera (1988). The achaete-scute complex of Drosophila melanogaster comprises four homologous genes. *EMBO J.* **7**, 2585–2591.

Bastian, H., and Gruss, P. (1990). A murine *even-skipped* homologue, *Evx 1,* is expressed during early embryogenesis and neurogenesis in a biphasic manner. *EMBO J.* **9**, 1839–1852.

Bate, C. M. (1976). Embryogenesis of an insect nervous system. I. A map of the thoracic and abdominal neuroblasts in *Locusta migratoria. Embryol. Exp. Morph.* **35**, 107–123.

Baumgartner, S., Bopp, D., Burri, M., and Noll, M. (1987). Structure of two genes at the *gooseberry* locus related to the *paired* gene and their spatial expression during *Drosophila* embryogenesis. *Genes Devel.* **1**, 1247–1267.

Bier, E., Jan, L. Y., and Jan, Y. N. (1990). *rhomboid,* a gene required for dorsoventral axis establishment and peripheral nervous system development in *Drosophila melanogaster. Genes Devel.* **4**, 190–203.

Booker, R., and Truman, J. W. (1987). Postembryonic neurogenesis in the CNS of the tobacco hornworm *Manduca sexta.* I. Neuroblast arrays and the fate of their progeny during metamorphosis. *J. Comp. Neurol.* **255**, 548–559.

Booker, R., and Truman, J. W. (1989). *Octopod,* a homeotic mutation of the moth *Manduca sexta,* influences the fate of identifiable pattern elements within the CNS. *Development* **105**, 621–628.

Bopp, D., Jamet, E., Baumgartner, S., Burri, M., and Noll, M. (1989). Isolation of two tissue-specific *Drosophila* paired-box genes, Pox meso and Pox neuro. *EMBO J.* **8**, 3447–3457.

Bourouis, M., Heitzler, P., El Messal, M., and Simpson, P. (1989). Mutant *Drosophila* embryos in which all cells adopt a neural fate. *Nature (London)* **341**, 442–444.

Brand, M., and Campos-Ortega, J. A. (1988). Two groups of interrelated genes regulate early neurogenesis in *Drosophila melanogaster. Roux's Arch. Dev. Biol.* **197**, 457–470.

Cabrera, C. V. (1990). Lateral inhibition and cell fate during neurogenesis in *Drosophila:* The interactions between *scute, Notch* and *Delta. Development* **109**, 733–742.

Cabrera, C. V., Martinez-Arias, A., and Bate, M. (1987). The expression of three members of the *achaete-scute* gene complex correlates with neuroblast segregation in *Drosophila. Cell* **50**, 425–533.

Campos-Ortega, J. A., and Hartenstein, V. (1985). "The embryonic development of *Drosophila melanogaster.*" New York: Springer-Verlag.

Carroll, S. B., and Scott, M. P. (1985). Localization of the *fushi tarazu* protein during *Drosophila* embryogenesis. *Cell* **43**, 47–57.

Carroll, S. B., and Scott, M. P. (1986). Zygotically active genes that affect the spatial expression of the *fushi tarazu* segmentation gene during early *Drosophila* embryogenesis. *Cell* **45**, 113–126.

Carroll, S. B., DiNardo, S., O'Farrell, P. H., White, R. A. H., and Scott, M. P. (1988). Temporal and spatial relationships between segmentation and homeotic gene expression in *Drosophila* embryos: Distributions of the *fushi tarazu, engrailed, Sex combs reduced, Antennapedia,* and *Ultrabithorax* proteins. *Genes Devel.* **2**, 350–360.

Davis, C. A., Noble-Topham, S. E., Rossant, J., and Joyner, A. L. (1988). Expression patterns of the homeobox-containing gene *En-2* delineates a specific region of the developing mouse brain. *Genes Devel.* **2**, 361–371.

DiNardo, S., Kuner, J. M., Theis, J., and O'Farrell, P. H. (1985). Development of embryonic pattern in *D. melanogaster* as revealed by accumulation of the nuclear *engrailed* protein. *Cell* **43**, 59–69.

DiNardo, S., and O'Farrell, P. H. (1987). Establishment and refinement of segmental pattern in the *Drosophila* embryo: Spatial control of *engrailed* expression by pair-rule genes. *Genes Devel.* **1**, 1212–1225.

DiNardo, S., and Heemskerk, J. (1990). Molecular and cellular interactions responsible for intrasegmental patterning during *Drosophila* embryogenesis. *Sem. Cell Biol.* **1**, 173–183.

Doe, C. Q., and Goodman, C. S. (1985a). Early events in insect neurogenesis. I. Development and segmental differences in the pattern of neuronal precursor cells. *Dev. Biol.* **111**, 193–205.

Doe, C. Q., and Goodman, C. S. (1985b). Early events in insect neurogenesis. II. The role of cell interactions and cell lineages in the determination of neuronal precursor cell. *Dev. Biol.* **111**, 206–219.

Doe, C. Q., Hiromi, Y., Gehring, W. J., and Goodman, C. S. (1988a). Expression and function of the segmentation gene *fushi tarazu* during *Drosophila* neurogenesis. *Science* **239**, 170–175.

Doe, C. Q., Smouse, D., and Goodman, C. S. (1988b). Control of neuronal fate by the *Drosophila* segmentation gene *even-skipped. Nature (London)* **333**, 376–378.

Doe, C. Q., and Scott, M. P. (1988). Segmentation and homeotic gene function in the developing nervous system of *Drosophila. Trends Neurosci.* **11**, 101–106.

Doe, C. Q., Chu-LaGraff, Q., Wright, D. M., and Scott, M. P. (1991). The *prospero* gene specifies cell fates in the *Drosophila* central nervous system. *Cell* **65**, 451–464.

Duncan, I. M. (1986). Control of *bithorax* complex functions by the segmentation gene *fushi tarazu* of Drosophila melanogaster. *Cell* **47**, 297–309.

Dura, J., and Ingham, P. (1988). Tissue- and stage-specific control of homeotic and segmentation gene expression in *Drosophila* embryos by the *polyhomeotic* gene. *Development* **103**, 733–741.

Finkelstein, R., Smouse, D., Capaci, T. M., Spradling, A. C., and Perrimon, N. (1990). The *orthodenticle* gene encodes a novel homeo domain protein involved in the development of the *Drosophila* nervous system and cellar visual structures. *Genes Devel.* **4**, 1516–1527.

Frasch, M., Hoey, T., Rushlow, C., Doyle, H., and Levine, M. (1987). Characterization and localization of the *even-skipped* protein in *Drosophila. EMBO J.* **6**, 749–759.

Greenwald, I. (1989). Cell–cell interactions that specify certain cell fates in *C. elegans* development. *Trends Genet.* **5**, 237–241.

Harding, K., Rushlow, C., Doyle, J. H., Hoey, T., and Levine, M. (1986). Cross-regulatory interactions among pair-rule genes in *Drosophila. Science* **233**, 953–959.

Hartenstein, V., and Campos-Ortega, J. A. (1984). Early neurogenesis in wild-type *Drosophila melanogaster. Roux's Arch. Dev. Biol.* **193**, 308–325.

Hortsch, M., and Goodman, C. S. (1990). *Drosophila* fasciclin I, a neural cell adhesion molecule, has a phosphatidylinositol lipid membrane anchor that is developmentally regulated. *J. Biol. Chem.* **265,** 15104–15109.

Hiromi, Y., and Gehring, W. J. (1987). Regulation and function of the *Drosophila* segmentation gene *fushi tarazu. Cell* **50,** 963–974.

Howard, K., and Ingham, P. W. (1986). Regulatory interactions between the segmentation genes *fushi tarazu, hairy,* and *engrailed* in the *Drosophila* blastoderm. *Cell* **44,** 949–957.

Huff, R., Furst, A., and Mahowald, A. P. (1989). *Drosophila* embryonic neuroblasts in culture: Autonomous differentiation of specific neurotransmitters. *Dev. Biol.* **134,** 146–157.

Ingham, P. W., and Martinez-Arias, A. (1986). The correct activation of *Antennapedia* and *bithorax* complex genes requires the *fushi tarazu* gene. *Nature (London)* **324,** 592–597.

Ingham, P. W., Baker, N. E., and Martinez-Arias, A. (1988). Regulation of segment polarity genes in the *Drosophila* blastoderm by *fushi tarazu* and *even-skipped. Nature (London)* **331,** 73–75.

Jimenez, F., and Campos-Ortega, J. A. (1990). Defective neuroblast commitment in mutants of the *achaete-scute* complex and adjacent genes of *D. melanogaster. Neuron* **5,** 81–89.

Johnson, J. E., Birren, S. J., and Anderson, D. J. (1990). Two rat homologues of *Drosophila achaete-scute* specifically expressed in neuronal precursors. *Nature (London)* **346,** 858–861.

Joyner, A. L., Herrup, K., Auerbach, B. A., Davis, C. A., and Rossant, J. (1991). Subtle cerebellar phenotype in mice homozygous for a targeted deletion of the *En-2* homeobox. *Science* **251,** 1239–1243.

Kania, M. A., Bonner, A. S., Duffy, J. B., and Gergen, J. P. (1990). The *Drosophila* segmentation gene *runt* encodes a novel nuclear regulatory protein that is also expressed in the developing nervous system. *Genes Devel.* **4,** 1701–1713.

Kimble, J. (1981). Alterations in cell lineage following laser ablation of cells in the somatic gonad of *Caenorhabditis elegans. Develop. Biol.* **87,** 286–300.

Kissinger, C. R., Liu, B., Martin, B. E., Kornberg, T. B., and Pabo, C. O. (1990). Crystal structure of an engrailed homeodomain–DNA complex at 2.8 Å resolution: A framework for understanding homeodomain–DNA interactions. *Cell* **63,** 579–590.

Klambt, C., Jacobs, J. R., and Goodman, C. S. (1991). The midline of the *Drosophila* central nervous system: A model for the genetic analysis of cell fate, cell migration, and growth cone guidance. *Cell* **64,** 801–815

Kopczynski, C. C., Alton, A. D., Fechtel, K., Kooh, P. I., and Muskavitch, M. A. T. (1989). Complex spatio-temporal accumulation of alternative transcripts from the neurogenic gene *Delta* during *Drosophila* embryogenesis. *Development* **107,** 623–636.

Kuwada, J. Y., and Goodman, C. S. (1985). Neuronal determination during embryonic development of the grasshopper nervous system. *Dev. Biol.* **110,** 114–126.

Lehmann, R., Jimenez, F., Dietrich, U., and Campos-Ortega, J. A. (1983). On the phenotype and development of mutants of early neurogenesis in *Drosophila melanogaster. Roux's Arch. Dev. Biol.* **192,** 62–72.

Lo, L.-C., Johnson, J. E., Wuenscell, C. W., Saito, T., and Anderson, D. J. (1991). Mammalian *achaete-scute* homolog 1 is transiently expressed by spatially restricted subsets of early neuroepithelial and neural crest cells. *Genes and Develop.* **5,** 1524–1537.

McConnell, S. K. (1988). Fates of visual cortical neurons in the ferret after isochronic and heterochronic transplantation. *J. Neurosci.* **8,** 945–974.

McMahon, A. P., and Bradley, A. (1990). The *Wnt-1 (int-1)* proto-oncogene is required for development of a large region of the mouse brain. *Cell* **62,** 1073–1085.

Martin-Bermundo, M. D., Martinez, C., Rodriguez, A., and Jimenez, F. (1991). Distribution and function of the *lethal of scute* gene product during early neurogenesis in *Drosophila Development* **113,** 445–454.

Martinez-Arias, A., Baker, N. E., and Ingham, P. W. (1988). Role of segment polarity genes in the definition and maintenance of cell states in the *Drosophila* embryo. *Development* **103,** 157–170.

Mayer, U., and Nüsslein-Volhard, C. (1988). A group of genes required for pattern formation in the ventral ectoderm of the *Drosophila* embryo. *Genes Devel.* **2,** 1496–1511.

Minden, J., Aagard, D., Sedat, J., and Alberts, B. (1989). Direct cell lineage analysis in *Drosophila melanogaster* by time lapse three-dimensional microscopy in living embryos. *J. Cell Biol.* **109,** 505–520.

Mlodzik, M., Hiromi, Y., Weber, U., Goodman, C. S., and Rubin, G. M. (1990). The *Drosophila seven-up* gene, a member of the steroid receptor gene superfamily, controls photoreceptor cell fates. *Cell* **60,** 211–224.

Nüsslein-Volhard, C., and Wieschaus, E. (1980). Mutations affecting segment number and polarity in *Drosophila. Nature (London)* **287,** 795–801.

Padgett, R. W., St. Johnson, R. D., and Gelbart, W. M. (1987). A transcript from a *Drosophila* pattern gene predicts a protein homologous to the transforming growth factor-β family. *Nature (London)* **325,** 81–84.

Patel, N. H., Martin-Blanco, E., Coleman, K. G., Poole, S. I., Ellis, M. C., Kornberg, T. B., and Goodman, C. S. (1989a). Expression of *engrailed* proteins in arthropods, annelids, and chordates. *Cell* **58,** 955–968.

Patel, N. H., Schafer, B., Goodman, C. S., and Holmgren, R. (1989b). The role of segment polarity genes during *Drosophila* neurogenesis. *Genes Devel.* **3,** 890–904.

Raper, J. A., Bastiani, M. J., and Goodman, C. S. (1984). Pathfinding by neuronal growth cones in grasshopper embryos. I. Divergent choices made by growth cones of sibling neurons. *J. Neurosci.* **3,** 20–30.

Ready, D. F. (1989). A multifaceted approach to neural development. *Trends Neurosci.* **12,** 102–110.

Rodriguez, I., Hernandez, R., Modolell, I., and Ruiz-Gomez, M. (1990). Competence to develop sensory organs is temporally and spatially regulated in *Drosophila* epidermal primordia. *EMBO J.* **9,** 3583–3592.

Romani, S., Campuzano, S., and Modolell, J. (1987). The *achaete-scute* complex is expressed in neurogenic regions of *Drosophila* embryos. *EMBO J.* **6,** 2085–2092.

Rothberg, J. M., Hartley, D. A., Walther, Z., and Artavanis-Tsakonas, S. (1988). *slit:* An EGF-homologous locus of *D. melanogaster* involved in the development of the embryonic central nervous system. *Cell* **55,** 1047–1059.

Rushlow, C. A., Han, K., Manley, J. L., and Levine, M. (1989). The graded distribution of the *dorsal* morphogen is initiated by selective nuclear transport in *Drosophila. Cell* **59,** 1165–1177.

Smouse, D., Goodman, C. S., Mahowald, A. P., and Perrimon, N. (1988). *polyhomeotic:* A gene required for the embryonic development of axon pathways in the central nervous system of *Drosophila. Genes Devel.* **2,** 830–842.

St. Johnston, R. D., and Gelbart, W. M. (1987). *Decapentaplegic* transcripts are localized along the dorsal–ventral axis of the *Drosophila* embryo. *EMBO J.* **6,** 2785–2791.

Taghert, P. H., and Goodman, C. S. (1984). Cell determination and differentiation of identified serotonin-immunoreactive neurons in the grasshopper embryo. *J. Neurosci.* **4,** 989–1000.

Tautz *et al.* (1987). Finger protein of novel structure encoded by *hunchback,* a second member of the gap class of *Drosophila* segmentation genes. *Nature (London)* **327,** 383–389.

Thomas, J. B., Bastiani, M. J., Bate, M., and Goodman, C. S. (1984). From grasshopper to *Drosophila:* A common plan for neuronal development. *Nature (London)* **310,** 203–207.

Thomas, J. B., Crews, S. T., and Goodman, C. S. (1988). Molecular genetics of the *single-minded* locus: A gene involved in the development of the *Drosophila* nervous system. *Cell* **52,** 143–151.

Treacy, M. N., He, X., and Rosenfeld, M. G. (1991). I-POU: A POU-domain protein that inhibits neuron-specific gene activation. *Nature (London)* **350,** 577–584.

Truman, J. W., and Bate, M. (1989). Spatial and temporal pattern of neurogenesis in the central nervous system of *Drosophila melanogaster. Dev. Biol.* **125,** 145–157.

Valles, A., and White, E. (1988). Serotonin-containing neurons in *Drosophila melanogaster:* Development and distribution. *J. Comp. Neurol.* **268,** 414–428.

van den Heuvel, M., Nusse, R., Johnston, P., and Lawrence, P. A. (1989). Distribution of the *wingless* gene product in *Drosophila* embryos: A protein involved in cell–cell communication. *Cell* **59,** 739–749.

Wharton, K. A., Johansen, K. M., Xu, T., and Artavanis-Tsakonas, S. (1985). Nucleotide sequence from the neurogenic locus *Notch* implies a gene product that shares homology with proteins containing EGF-like repeats. *Cell* **43,** 567–581.

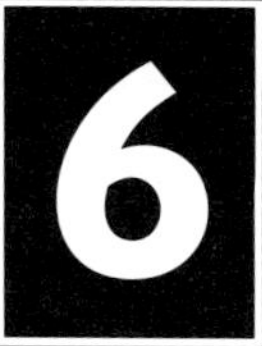

Initial Determination of the Neurectoderm in *Drosophila*

Ralph J. Greenspan
Department of Neurosciences
Roche Institute of Molecular Biology
Nutley, New Jersey

I. Introduction

In all organisms that have nervous systems, the cells that become neurons start out with the capacity to become either neural or epidermal. The first step in the determination of neuronal identity is thus a decision taken by cells of the embryonic ectoderm about which pathway of development to follow. The cellular arrangements and dynamics of this decision are not necessarily alike in all organisms, nor do they necessarily use the same genes and macromolecules. It seems likely, however, that in all cases the cells must interact with each other in some fashion to bring about the choice of cell fate.

The genetic foundations of the neural–epidermal decision have been best studied in the fruit fly, *Drosophila melanogaster.* Genes required in the process were discovered initially because of mutant phenotypes, and their products have subsequently been identified by means of molecular techniques. Although the process is still poorly understood, the studies in the fruit fly, in conjunction with relevant work on other organisms, have been informative about the nature of the macromolecules involved and suggestive of their actual roles.

The subject matter of this field has been extensively reviewed in recent years (Campos-Ortega, 1985; Artavanis-Tsakonas, 1988; Campos-Ortega, 1988; Knust and Campos-Ortega, 1989; Campos-Ortega and Knust, 1990a,b; Hartley, 1990; Campos-Ortega and Jan, 1991; see also relevant discussions in Way, 1990; Simpson, 1990). The rationale, therefore, for writing another chapter on the subject is to offer a fresh perspective.

A great many findings, both genetic and molecular, have been made in this area, and a great deal of phenomenology has thus been generated. Much of this information has yet to be incorporated into a detailed model. The following pages constitute an attempt to make sense of the findings on the embryonic neural–epidermal decision in *Drosophila,* to the extent that they lend themselves to the task. I have not tried to be exhaustive or comprehensive (e.g., regarding all of the genetic information pertaining to later times in development), since this has been amply seen to by others. Instead, I have tried to construct a framework, sometimes hypothetical, for thinking about the genetic foundations of this choice of cell fate.

II. The Neural–Epidermal Decision

A. Where Do Neurons and Epidermal Cells Come From?

The nervous system of *Drosophila* is derived from the ventro-lateral portion of the blastoderm (Fig. 1), called the "neurogenic region" (Hartenstein and Campos-Ortega, 1984). This was first observed in histological preparations of early embryos made by Poulson (1950), in which neuroblasts were

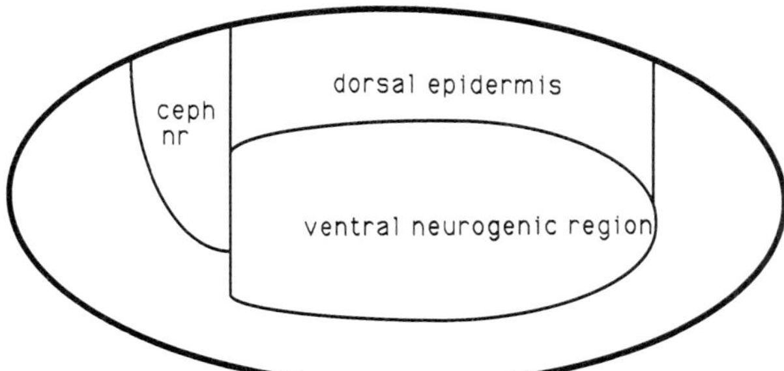

Figure 1. Diagram representing a side view of the blastoderm stage of a *Drosophila* embryo, showing the cephalic (ceph nr) and ventral neurogenic regions, as well as the portion giving rise to the dorsal epidermis.

observed to delaminate inward from the single layer of cells extending around the periphery of the egg. Those cells remaining on the periphery in this region become the ventro-lateral epidermis; those delaminating gave rise to the nervous system. Closer scrutiny revealed that the presumptive neuroblasts were actually interspersed among the presumptive epidermal cells; only 1 in 4 became a neuroblast (Fig. 2; Poulson, 1950; Hartenstein and Campos-Ortega, 1984). Moreover, the pattern and number of neuroblasts produced in each hemisegment of the embryo is characteristic (Hartenstein and Campos-Ortega, 1984). The dorsal epidermis is derived from the dorso-lateral region of the blastoderm, a region that does not give rise to neuroblasts (Poulson, 1950).

Poulson's histological observations on the site of origin of neuroblasts and epidermis were subsequently confirmed by two kinds of fate map. One utilized genetic mosaics to measure the "embryological distance" between structures (Kankel and Hall, 1976) and the other relied on the transplantation of marked cells from one embryo to another (Technau and Campos-Ortega, 1986). These studies have shown that both the central nervous system and portions of the epidermis map to this ventro-lateral region of the embryo. They have likewise shown that dorsal epidermis is derived from more dorsal regions of the blastoderm.

B. Why Invoke a Decision Process?

The fact that both neural and epidermal precursors are derived from the same region of the embryo does not, in itself, require that cells undergo a decision process. One might imagine that the same factors providing posi-

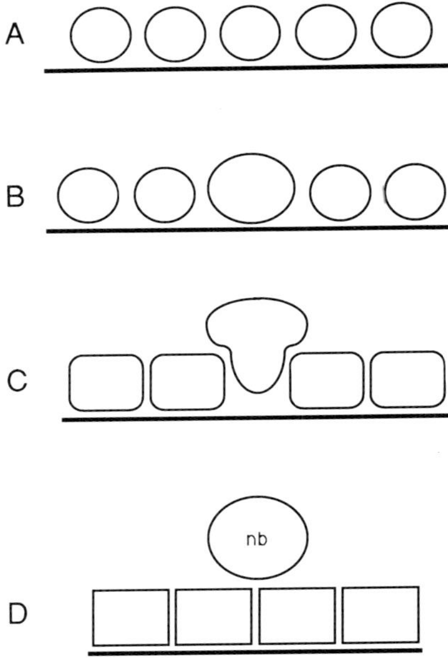

Figure 2. Neuroblast delamination in *Drosophila* embryo. A. All cells start out equivalent. B. Presumptive neuroblast becomes enlarged. C. Assumptive neuroblast slips out of the layer of cells around the periphery of the embryo. D. Presumptive neuroblast comes to lie internally. Cells remaining on the periphery become an epithelium of epidermal precursors.

tional coordinates to the embryo as a whole (Hedgecock and Hall, 1990) could also specify neural and epidermal cell fates.

The inference that there is a neural–epidermal decision comes from the phenotypes of a set of mutations that subvert the decision-making process. The mutations are termed "neurogenic" because they produce too many neurons and misappropriate cells into the neural pathway at the expense of the epidermal pathway (see Section III,B,C). First observed by Poulson (1937,1940) for deletions and mutations at the *Notch* locus (Fig. 3), this neuralizing phenotype has subsequently been found for mutations of *Delta, mastermind, big brain, neuralized,* and the *Enhancer-of-split* complex [*E(spl)-C*; Lehmann *et al.,* 1981,1983].

Figure 3. Phenotypes of wild-type and *Notch⁻* embryos of *Drosophila.* External cuticle, secreted by epidermis, of mature wild-type embryo (a) and *Notch⁻* embryo (b). Only a small patch of dorsal cuticle is present in *Notch⁻* embryos. Central and peripheral nervous system of wild-type (c) and *Notch⁻* (d) embryos, midway through embryogenesis. Bar: 40μm.

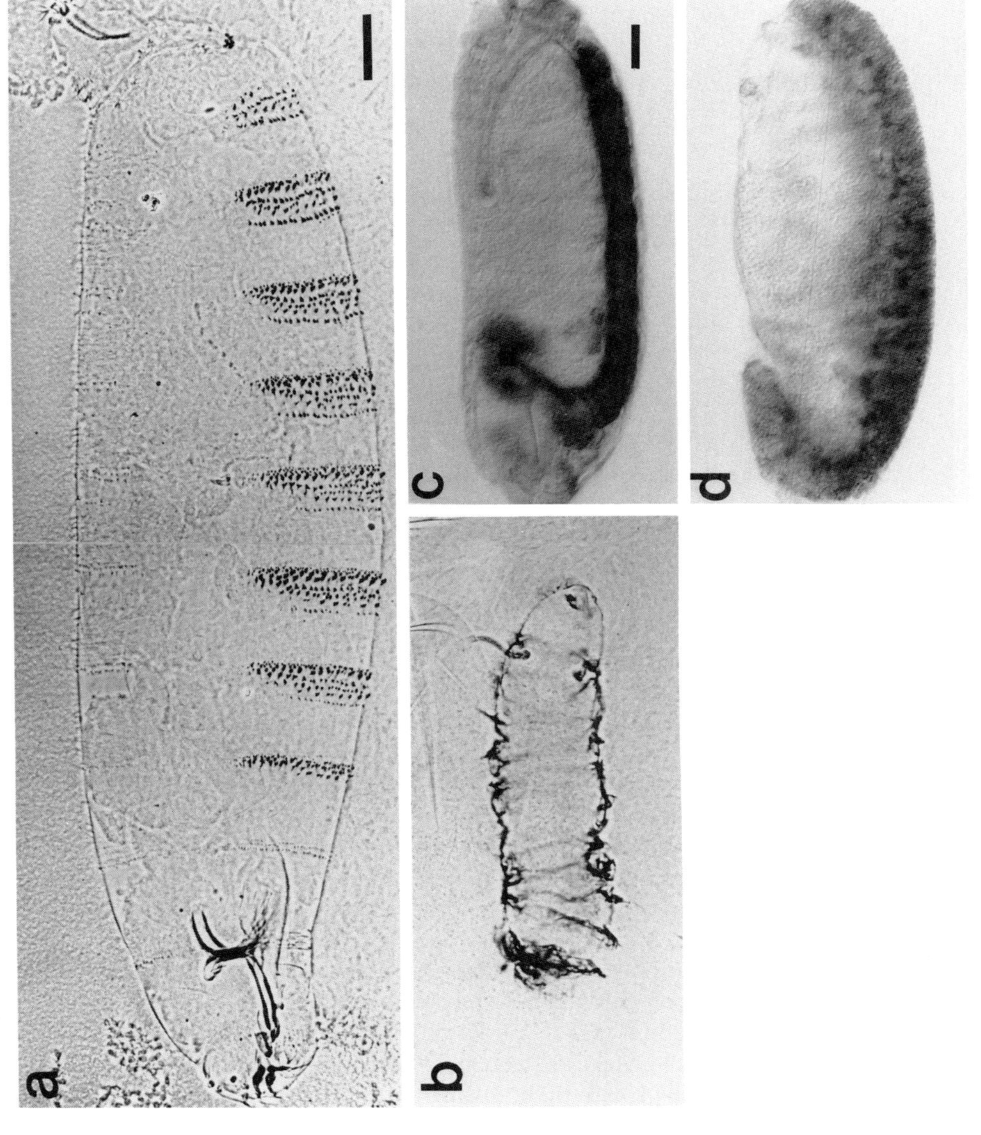

Absence of any of these genes apparently causes all of the cells in the neurogenic region to choose the neural pathway and none to become epidermal. The association of these genes with a neural–epidermal decision, rather than simply with the formation of epidermis *per se,* derives from the fact that all of the mutants produce epidermis normally in the dorsal region of the embryo. Thus, the neurogenic mutations only exhibit defective embryonic development in the neurogenic region, where the cells must make the neural–epidermal decision.

C. A Decision Implies an Interaction between Cells

If cells have a choice of fate, then some external agent must prompt them to choose one rather than the other, if the decision is to be regulated. A decision could conceivably be wholly an internal event for each cell, but this would preclude any control over the final proportion and distribution of cells choosing each alternative fate. In this instance, the external agents appear to be a cell's immediate neighbors. There is little direct evidence for interactions between presumptive neural and epidermal cells in *Drosophila,* but there are suggestions of it, as well as close analogies with other invertebrates in which such interactions have been demonstrated. Moreover, there are indications that interactions may occur not only between neural and epidermal precursors, but also between presumptive epidermal cells

1. HINTS FROM *DROSOPHILA*

The presence of cell interactions is suggested, as implied earlier, by the fact that the ratio of neuroblasts to epidermal precursors is constant (1:3), that the neuroblasts are initially interspersed among the cells of the region, and that they arise in a reproducible pattern in each segment (Hartenstein and Campos-Ortega, 1984). It is difficult to imagine a nonlineage system of positional specification so exact that each neuroblast could be distinguished from its nonneural neighbors so accurately without some communication between them.

Further indications come from experiments in which cells were transplanted from the dorsal region of the embryo, which makes epidermis but no neuroblasts, to the ventral region. Under these conditions, transplanted dorsal cells are capable of giving rise to neuroblasts, suggesting that they do so as a result of interactions with their new neighbors in the neurogenic region (Technau and Campos-Ortega, 1986).

Additional suggestions come from the structure and location of products from two of the neurogenic genes, *Notch* and *Delta.* These genes, whose normal products are required for proper proportioning of neural and epidermal precursors (see Section IV,B), code for transmembrane proteins with considerable extracellular domains (Wharton *et al.*, 1985; Kidd *et al.*, 1986; Vassin *et al.*, 1987; Kopczynski *et al.*, 1988). They are thus likely candidates for mediating interactions between cells.

2. ANALOGIES FROM GRASSHOPPER EMBRYOS

Neuroblasts arise from the grasshopper neurectoderm in a process resembling that of *Drosophila* in several respects. (1) The cells appear to be uniform initially. (2) Neuroblasts arise interspersed among their neighbors and are never immediately adjacent to each other. (3) The number and pattern of neuroblasts is regulated (Doe and Goodman, 1985a). (They differ inasmuch as the neighboring cells do not become epidermis, but nonneural accessory cells.) These cells thus appear to be communicating with each other. Moreover, direct evidence for communication between these cells has been provided by laser ablation experiments.

When a presumptive neuroblast is killed selectively, one of its immediate neighbors, which would otherwise have never done so, takes on the neuroblast fate (Doe and Goodman, 1985b). The reversibility of the neighboring cell's fate lasts for a finite period, after which no replacement can occur. These findings have been interpreted to mean that a presumptive neuroblast inhibits its immediate neighbors from adopting the neuroblast fate (Fig. 4). The neurogenic genes of *Drosophila* have been nominated as the agents that carry out an analogous set of events in that organism's neurectoderm (Doe and Goodman, 1985b).

3. HOMOLOGIES FROM *CAENORHABDITIS ELEGANS*

Two genes have been identified in the nematode, *C. elegans,* that govern decisions of cell fate and also bear a strong structural resemblance to the *Notch* gene of *Drosophila.* These genes, *lin-12* and *glp-1,* encode transmembrane proteins with significant sequence homology to *Notch* (see IV,B,1 Yochem *et al.*, 1988; Austin and Kimble, 1989; Yochem and Greenwald, 1989). As for the neurogenic genes of *Drosophila,* when either of these nematode genes is mutant, there is a defect in cell fate decision-making and, as in the grasshopper embryo, these decisions require cell interactions.

When worms are mutant for *lin-12,* cell fate decisions in particular lineages are affected so too many of one type are produced at the expense of another, just as when *Drosophila* embryos are mutant for *Notch* (Greenwald *et al.*, 1983; Seydoux *et al.*, 1990). The cell fate decisions mediated by *lin-12* have been shown to require interactions between the relevant cells.

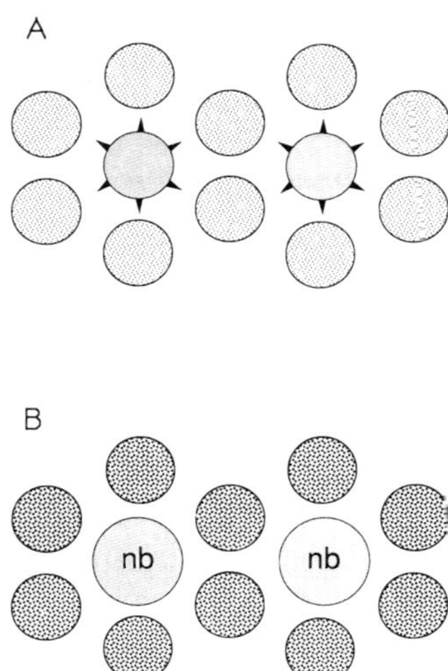

Figure 4. Model of Doe and Goodman (1985b), in which presumptive neuroblasts in the grasshopper neurepithelium inhibit their neighbors from adopting the neuroblast fate. Neuroblasts (nb) are surrounded by cells that will become epidermal precursors.

In the formation of the vulva, for example, two cells will make the choice between becoming an anchor cell or a ventral uterine precursor cell (Fig. 5). When either one of the cells is killed by laser ablation, the remaining one becomes an anchor cell (Kimble, 1981; Seydoux and Greenwald, 1989), indicating that both must be present in order for one to become a ventral uterine precursor cell. No other neighboring cells are required. Similarly, when *lin-12* function is lacking, both will become anchor cells. This finding, in conjunction with the fact that the gene codes for a transmembrane protein, suggests that the gene is somehow involved in the interaction (Greenwald *et al.*, 1983; Seydoux *et al.*, 1990).

Similar arguments apply to the *glp-1* gene in *C. elegans*. It resembles both *lin-12* and *Notch* in sequence (Yochem and Greenwald, 1989; Austin and Kimble, 1989) and it is required in a developmental decision that involves cell interactions (Kimble and White, 1981). The decision in this case involves whether cells of the germ line will proliferate or enter meiosis. When the key regulatory cell, the "distal tip" cell, is ablated, the germ cells do not proliferate and go directly into meiosis. The same result is seen when the *glp-1* gene is mutant (Kimble, 1981).

The strong evidence favoring the involvement of *lin-12* and *glp-1* in cell interactions, in conjunction with their structural and functional similarities to *Notch,* bolster the argument that the neural–epidermal decision in *Droso-*

phila that requires *Notch* is a cell fate decision involving cell interactions (Fig. 5). Although it has generally been assumed that this interaction must be between neuroblasts and epidermal precursors, there are indications from developmental genetic studies that it may also occur between epidermal precursors (see Section IV,B).

D. Default States in Cell Fate Decisions

In each of the demonstrations of cell interactions cited, the choice that the cells take in the absence of an interaction may be defined as a default state.

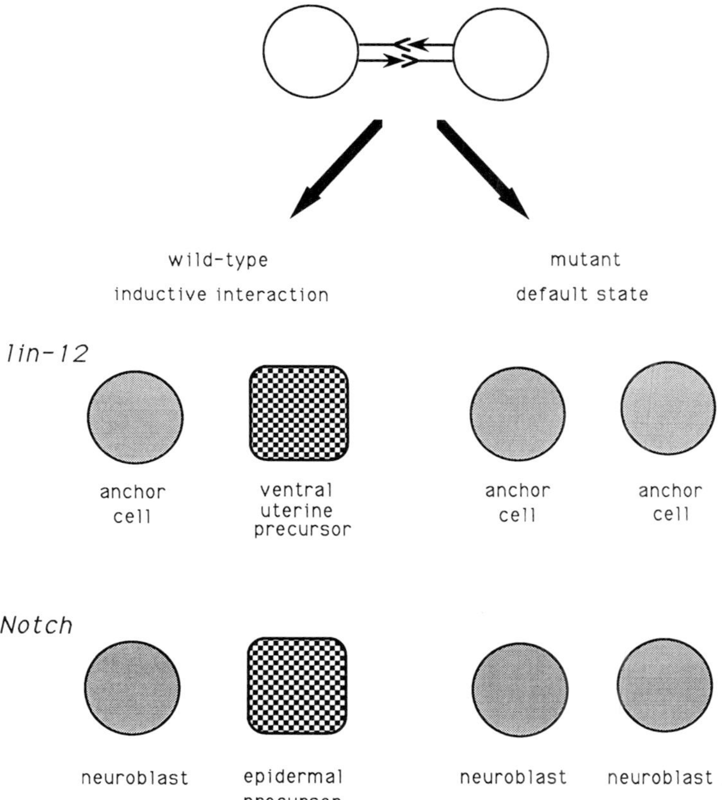

Figure 5. Analogous functions of *lin-12* and *Notch* in enabling cells to depart from their default state following interactions between neighbors.

Thus, in the grasshopper neurepithelium the default state is the neuroblast pathway, in the nematode vulva it is the anchor cell, and in the germ line it is meiosis. This means that the *lin-12* and *glp-1* genes function to enable cells to leave the default state.

The concept of a default state has traditionally been applied to induction in vertebrate embryos, as a description of the developmental outcome of tissues that fail to receive inductive signals. The classical case is primary embryonic induction, in which ectoderm can be induced to become neural, but will become epidermis otherwise (Slack, 1983). Induction implies that one tissue signals another so it may advance to the next developmental stage. This, too, may be applied to the cases just cited. In the grasshopper, the presumptive neuroblast signals to its immediate neighbors not to become neuroblasts. In the nematode, the presumptive anchor cell signals to the presumptive ventral uterine precursor and, similarly, the distal tip cell signals the germ cells to undergo mitosis.

The neural–epidermal decision in *Drosophila* resembles these events in the grasshopper and nematode in many respects, as discussed earlier. By analogy, the default state in the neurogenic region of the *Drosophila* embryo is the neuroblast state. Cells are able to leave this state when the neurogenic genes *Notch, Delta, mastermind, big brain, neuralized,* and the E(spl)-C are functioning properly.

III. Genetic Mechanisms in the Neural–Epidermal Decision: Controlling Gene Expression

Any developmental decision must, at some stage, affect transcription in the cells taking part. In the neural–epidermal decision, this must encompass gene expression that distinguishes cells of the neurogenic region as a whole, as well as control mechanisms that enact the choice of cell fate.

Genes putatively involved in the neural–epidermal decision in *Drosophila* have been identified based on the phenotypes of mutations. For the majority of these, the neurogenic genes, that phenotype consists of the misrouting of cells so too many of them follow the neuroblast pathway. Another smaller group of genes has also begun to be identified in which neuroblasts are missing. Molecular characterization of genes from both sets has provided information about the kinds of proteins they make, as well as where and when they are expressed. These findings, in conjunction with experiments establishing relationships between genes and testing their site of action, make it possible to begin drawing the outlines of how the decision occurs.

A. Becoming a Neuroblast

1. THE *ACHAETE–SCUTE* COMPLEX

A gene complex near the tip of the *X* chromosome appears to be involved in delineating the neurogenic region. Genes of the *achaete–scute* complex (AS-C) were originally identified because of their effects on bristle development (i.e., peripheral nervous system development; see Chapter 8). They were subsequently shown to be necessary for embryonic neural development (Jimenez and Campos-Ortega, 1979, 1987; White, 1980). A chromosomal deletion of the entire complex produces a severe reduction in the embryonic CNS. Subdivision of the complex, by means of smaller deletions, reveals a graded effect; the more genes that are deleted, the more severe the deficits in neural tissue.

The earliest phenotype associated with a deletion of the complex is the failure of a subset of neuroblasts (~25%) to form during the stage at which neuroblasts delaminate from the ectodermal epithelium (Fig. 6; Jimenez and Campos-Ortega, 1990). In later stages of embryogenesis, a considerable number of the remaining neurons die as well, resulting in a significantly reduced central nervous system (Jimenez and Campos-Ortega, 1979,1987,1990; White, 1980).

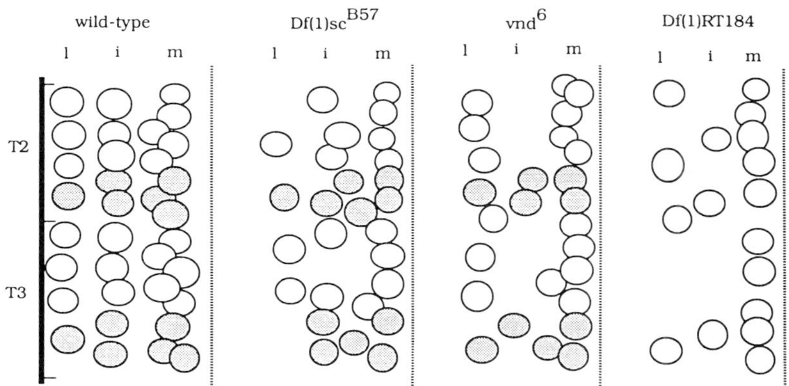

Figure 6. Map of neuroblasts from two thoracic hemisegments (T2 and T3) of the ventral nervous system in embryos that are wild type, deleted of the AS-C [Df(l)sc^{B57}] mutant for *vnd* (*vnd^6*), and deleted of both the AS-C and *vnd* [Df(l)RT184] Circles represent neuroblasts arranged in lateral (l), intermediate (i), and medial (m) rows. Shaded circles indicate neuroblasts lying at segmental boundaries. [Reproduced with permission from Cell Press and the authors, Jimenez and Campos-Ortega (1990).]

a. Defining the Neurogenic Region: Expression of AS-C in Embryos

Three transcripts (T3, T4, and T5) have been identified in the confines of the complex whose temporal and spatial distribution correlate almost completely with the neurogenic region during the time of the neural–epidermal decision (Campuzano *et al.*, 1985; Cabrera *et al.*, 1987; Romani *et al.*, 1987; Brand and Campos-Ortega, 1988; Cabrera, 1990). The deficit of neuroblasts in embryos deleted of *AS-C*, in conjunction with the expression patterns of T3, T4, and T5, strongly implicates these transcripts in the determination process.

The protein product of T3 appears to undergo a change in antigenicity that suggests even more strongly that it is a determinant of neuroblast fate. Whereas the T3 RNA is expressed widely in the neurogenic region (though not in every cell), an antibody to the C-terminus of the T3 protein detects in only a subset of these cells, the delaminating neuroblasts (Cabrera, 1990). This result indicates that the T3 protein becomes modified so that its original epitope continues to appear only in those cells committed to being neuroblasts. The antibodies may recognize a dephosphorylated phosphopeptide. The important point is that this particular T3 epitope marks cells that have made the decision to become neuroblasts. Analogous information does not yet exist for T4 or T5.

b. AS-C Expression and the Default State

If T3 marks commitment to the neuroblast fate, then its pattern suggests that all (or at least most) cells of the neurogenic region are initially specified as neuroblasts but only a subset of them ultimately follow that pathway. This is reminiscent of the discussion of neuroblast as default state (see Section II), in which cells of the neurogenic region are determined so they will adopt the default state if deprived of the action of the neurogenic genes (*Notch*, etc.). In fact, when all these cells remain in the default state in embryos mutant for *Notch* or *Delta*, the T3 epitope is detectable in the full complement of cells that have transcribed it (Cabrera, 1990). This result supports the idea that transcription of *AS-C* parallels the readiness of the cells to become neuroblasts, whereas persistence of the T3 epitope indicates that they have committed to it. Normally, the decision takes most of them out of the neuroblast pathway (~75%). However, in neurogenic mutants in which no decision is made, they all become neuroblasts.

c. AS-C Products Resemble Transcription Factors

The sequences of these three transcripts show considerable similarity to each other and their products share a common domain, the so-called helix-loop-helix (HLH) motif (Villares and Cabrera, 1987; Alonso and Cabrera,

1988). They share this motif with a variety of other proteins known to bind DNA that have been implicated in the regulation of gene expression (Murre *et al.,* 1989a,b). Moreover, the T3 protein has been shown to form heterodimers *in vitro* with another putative transcription factor, the product of the *daughterless* locus (Cronmiller, 1988; Caudy *et al.,* 1988), the heterodimers of which are transcriptionally active (Murre *et al.,* 1989b).

Sequence homologies are most useful in suggesting where a gene might act. In this case, they suggest that T3, T4, and T5 act in the nucleus. Given the phenotype in their absence and their pattern of expression, it is plausible that their role is to control the expression of genes that commit cells to the neuroblast fate.

2. THE *ventral nervous system condensation defective* GENE

Although the evidence points to a role of the *AS-C* in defining the neurogenic region and committing cells to the neuroblast fate, it must be borne in mind that absence of *AS-C* activity does not eliminate all neuroblasts, only 25% of them (Jimenez and Campos-Ortega, 1990). Another gene in the same region of the *X* chromosome, *ventral nervous system condensation defective (vnd),* produces a failure in neural development analogous in many respects to deletions of the *AS-C* (White, 1980; White *et al.,* 1983). At the time of neuroblast delamination, approximately 25% of the neuroblasts fail to appear in *vnd* embryos (Jimenez and Campos-Ortega, 1990). Neither the product of the *vnd* locus nor its expression pattern at the time of neuroblast commitment and delamination are known.

Absence of *AS-C* and *vnd* activity eliminate nonoverlapping sets of neuroblasts (Jimenez and Campos-Ortega, 1990). Thus, embryos that are mutant for both genes are depleted of approximately 50% of their neuroblasts. This result suggests that other genes are yet to be identified in whose absence the remaining neuroblasts will be eliminated.

3. COMBINATORIALS IN NEUROBLAST DETERMINATION

The expression pattern of the *AS-C* transcripts appears to be more widespread in the neurogenic region than the neuroblast deficit in embryos deleted of the locus (discussed earlier). This discrepancy may be explained in the context of the potential for *AS-C* products to complex with other putative transcription factors. These factors, and others yet to be identified, may participate in a combinatorial system to generate positional identity among presumptive neuroblasts. Thus, they may be functioning throughout the neurogenic region as part of such complexes, but only be rate-limiting with respect to the generation of specificity in some portions of the region. Other factors, in turn, would fulfill this rate-limiting role in other places. The *vnd* product, should it turn out to be a transcription factor, is a good candidate for another combinatorial player, one that is rate-limiting in a different set of presumptive neuroblasts (see previous text).

B. Becoming an Epidermal Precursor

If the genes of the *AS-C* and *vnd* make cells neuroblasts, then one might expect that there is an analogous set of genes that commits cells to the epidermal fate. Genes of the *E(spl)* complex, one of the neurogenic genes, may fill this role.

1. THE *ENHANCER-OF-SPLIT* COMPLEX

E(spl) is a complex of genes on the third chromosome, at least some of whose members are required for cells to choose the epidermal pathway in the neural--epidermal decision. The locus was originally identified by a spontaneous mutation [*E(spl)*^{D}] that enhanced the severity of mutations in the *split (spl)* gene (Welshons, 1956; Lindsley and Grell, 1968). *spl* is an allele of the *Notch* locus that is viable and mild in its phenotype, with no effects on embryonic development, but with abnormalities in compound eye development (see Chapter 7). Although this might have led some to speculate about the possible involvement of *E(spl)* in the embryonic neural–epidermal decision, no one did so until the discovery of lethal mutations at the locus that produced the characteristic neurogenic phenotype of appropriating all cells of the neurogenic region into the neuroblast pathway (Lehmann *et al.*, 1981, 1983).

Genetic analysis of *E(spl)* has yielded many mutations and deletions that show a wide spectrum of phenotypic severity (Lehmann *et al.*, 1981,1983; Knust *et al.*, 1987a; Preiss *et al.*, 1988; Ziemer *et al.*, 1988). Severity refers both to the consistency of lethality and to the extent of neuralization of the neurogenic region. Many of these variants produce neurogenic phenotypes and their severity correlates with the amount of DNA that is deleted (Knust *et al.*, 1987b; Preiss *et al.*, 1988; Ziemer *et al.*, 1988). No single point mutation produces as severe a neurogenic phenotype as a deletion of at least 30 kb of DNA from the region; larger deletions produce still more severe neuralization (Knust *et al.*, 1987b; Preiss *et al.*, 1988). This is reminiscent of the graded effect of various sized deletions of the *AS-C* (discussed earlier). In fact, there are many respects in which the genetic and molecular properties of the *E(spl)* complex mirror those of the *AS-C.*

a. Defining the Epidermogenic Region: Expression of the E(spl) Complex in Embryos

The first respect in which *E(spl)* resembles *AS-C* is in the initial expression pattern of its transcripts. Fifteen transcripts have been identified so far, of which six are expressed in virtually identical patterns, m4, m5, m7, m8, mβ, and mδ are all expressed throughout the neurogenic region just prior to neuroblast delamination (Knust *et al.*, 1987b; Knust and Campos-Ortega, 1989; E. Knust, H. Schrons, F. Grawe, and J.A. Campos-Ortega, unpublished observations). Since the neurogenic region also gives rise to the ventro-lateral epidermis, this pattern of expression correlates with the fact that these cells have the capacity to make the epidermal choice in the neural–epidermal decision.

The expression of these transcripts is reciprocal in some respects to that of the *AS-C* T3 protein (discussed earlier). Many of the *E(spl)* transcripts (m4, m5, m7, mβ, and mδ) disappear from the cells that delaminate and become neuroblasts, but continue to be expressed in the epidermal precursors that were the immediate neighbors of neuroblasts just before delamination (Knust and Campos-Ortega, 1989; E. Knust, H. Schrons, F. Grawe, and J.A. Campos-Ortega, unpublished observations). They differ from the *AS-C* transcripts, however, because their segregation into the epidermal precursors is regulated transcriptionally.

Nonetheless, they share with T3 the important similarity of marking one subset of the cells making the neural–epidermal decision, in this case the epidermal precursors. Their expression in the cells lying immediately adjacent to the delaminating neuroblasts, in conjunction with their turning off in the neuroblasts, implies that they are intimately involved in the commitment to the epidermal pathway.

b. Several E(spl) Products Resemble Transcription Factors

Many of the transcripts from the *E(spl)* complex show sequence similarity to the family of DNA-binding proteins containing the HLH motif, including five of those whose patterns of expression were just described m5, m7, m8, mβ, and mδ (E. Knust, H. Schrons, F. Grawe and J.A. Campos-Ortega, unpublished observations). This represents another aspect of similarity to the *AS-C,* suggesting a role for these products in the regulation of gene expression. In this case, the genes regulated are likely to be in the epidermal precursors.

One of these products appears to be the principal site of the lesion in the original *E(spl)*[D] mutation, indicating its potential for interacting with the product of *Notch* (see previous text). This allele exhibits several molecular lesions mapping to m8 as well as to m9/m10, a transcription unit with two overlapping products (Preiss *et al.*, 1988; Klambt *et al.*, 1989). Functional evidence favors m8 as the site of the crucial *E(spl)*[D] lesion, based on transformation experiments. Introduction of a DNA fragment containing the m8 unit cloned from *E(spl)*[D] DNA into wild-type flies reproduces the dominant mutant phenotype (Klambt *et al.*, 1989). The implications of an interaction between m8 and the *spl* allele of *Notch* are not immediately obvious since one is a putative transcription factor and the other is a cell surface protein (see subsequent text).

c. Other Products of the Complex

The m9/m10 overlapping transcription unit shows sequence similarity to a G-protein (Hartley *et al.*, 1988). This is intriguing with respect to its possible involvement in intracellular communication in the neural–epidermal decision. The expression pattern of m9/m10 differs, however, from that of m4, m5, m7, m8, mβ, and mδ inasmuch as it persists in the neuroblasts after delamination rather than in the epidermal precursors (Hartley *et al.*, 1988; see previous text). Nonetheless, transformation with wild-type sequences containing m9/m10 can partially rescue the neuralization produced by a deletion of the *E(spl)* complex. Moreover, the *E(spl)*[E73] mutation, which is exclusive to the m9/m10 transcription unit, shows a weak neurogenic phenotype (Preiss *et al.*, 1988). Thus, m9/m10 appears to have a role in the developmental decision, but not necessarily in the same cells or at the same stage in the process.

As mentioned previously, the molecular alterations associated with *E(spl)*[D] map to both m8 and the m9/m10 unit. Although the m8 lesion is sufficient to reproduce the dominant phenotype (Klambt *et al.*, 1989), and therefore is capable of interacting with the *spl* allele of *Notch,* there is evidence that a mutation in the m9/m10 unit can also interact with some alleles of *Notch.* The *E(spl)*[E73] mutation, even when heterozygous, exacerbates the effects of *notchoid* alleles (*nd* and *nd*[2]), which are mild viable alleles of the *Notch* locus that affect wing morphology (Xu *et al.*, 1990).

This implies an interaction between the genes. In this case, the protein encoded by m9/m10 may associate with the cytoplasmic tail of the *Notch* protein; the *notchoid* mutations map to the cytoplasmic tail portion of the gene (Xu *et al.*, 1990; see subsequent text).

d. The E(spl) Complex and Epidermal Commitment

The evidence points to a central role for members of the *E(spl)* complex in the epidermal option of the neural–epidermal decision. Deletions of the complex result in failure of cells in the neurogenic region to become epidermal; expression of several of its transcripts correlates exactly with epidermal commitment, and reciprocally with neuroblast commitment.

Moreover, there are indications that the *E(spl)* complex lies at the end of the neural–epidermal decision-making process. One indication comes from studies of the relationship between the various neurogenic genes. Such relationships can be discerned by varying the number of wild-type (normal) copies of one locus in the presence of a mutant genotype at another locus. When experiments of this sort were carried out with the various neurogenic genes, extra copies of the *E(spl)* complex were found in most cases to influence the extent of neuralization in embryos mutant for another neurogenic gene (de la Concha *et al.*, 1988). In most instances, the effect was an ameliorization of the mutant phenotype. Conversely, extra copies of any other neurogenic gene had no effect on the neuralization present in embryos deleted for the *E(spl)* complex.

If there is sequential order to the action of these genes, then a mutation should act as a dam blocking any further effects downstream. Thus, extra copies should only be effective if they are downstream from the block. It is this lack of reciprocity that suggests that *E(spl)* acts later than the other genes. Given all of these findings, along with the likelihood that several of its products are transcription factors, it seems reasonable to suggest that members of the *E(spl)* complex carry out the final stage of commitment to the epidermal fate.

C. Implementing the Decision

In the framework presented here, genes of the *AS-C* and *E(spl)* complexes (and perhaps *vnd*) carry out the final steps in the neural–epidermal decision at the level of gene regulation. This concept is based primarily on the phenotypes of embryos deleted for either complex, the patterns of expression of their transcripts, and the sequence homology to transcription factors.

A key point in the argument is the selective turning on of the *AS-C* T3 protein in neuroblasts and of the *E(spl)* transcripts m4, m5, m7, m8, mβ, and mδ in epidermal precursors. Tracing the process back a step, there must be other genes whose products regulate those of *AS-C* and *E(spl)*. Although there is no direct evidence for this, there are two possible candidates for this kind of function among the other neurogenic genes, by virtue of their resemblance to proteins that regulate gene expression.

1. *mastermind*

The *mastermind (mam)* locus encodes a protein that does not closely resemble any other known protein, but that contains unusual homopolymeric sequences, alternating runs of amino acids, and tightly clustered acidic or basic sequences (Smoller *et al.*, 1990). Although these characteristics are not exclusively associated with any single kind of function, they are all features shared by a variety of transcription factors and gene regulatory proteins.

Moreover, the *mam* protein is found in cell nuclei, supportive of a possible role in gene regulation (Smoller *et al.,* 1990).

The locus produces at least five transcripts, apparently by alternative splicing (Smoller *et al.,* 1990). Two of these transcripts are expressed during the time of neuroblast segregation, with little apparent selectivity with respect to cell type. Initially, expression appears along a narrow band encompassing mesoderm, and endoderm, gradually expanding to include ventral ectoderm (Bettler *et al.,* 1991).

There is evidence for genetic interactions between *mam* and *Notch,* based on the finding that specific mutations of *mam* can ameliorate the effects of specific *Notch* mutations (Xu *et al.,* 1990).

2. neuralized

The sequence of the product of the *neuralized (neu)* locus (G.L. Bouliane and Y-N. Jan, personal communication) contains two distinct regions with strong resemblance to transcription factors: a HLH motif (Murre *et al.,* 1989a,b) and a homeodomain (Gehring and Hiromi, 1986). From this information, it seems feasible to suggest that *neu* acts to regulate gene expression.

As in the case of *mam,* the *neu* gene appears to be expressed in both neuroblasts and epidermal precursors at the time of neuroblast segregation (G.L. Bouliane and Y-N. Jan, personal communication). Should this be true of both protein products as well, it would distinguish them from the *AS-C* and *E(spl)* products. This would be intriguing with regard to the possibility that both of these components might exert opposite regulatory effects on two different cell types.

IV. Genetic Mechanisms in the Neural–Epidermal Decision: Genes Taking Part in Interactions between Cells

Proteins on the cell surface are obvious candidates for involvement in cell interactions. Three of the neurogenic genes fall into this category: *big brain, Delta,* and *Notch.*

A. *big brain*

The *big brain (bib)* gene stands apart from the rest of the neurogenic genes, as well as from most other developmental genes, in several respects.

Its predicted amino acid sequence resembles membrane channel proteins, such as the major intrinsic protein (MIP) of mammalian lens fiber cells (Rao *et al.,* 1990). This is a class of genes that hitherto has not been implicated in developmental events such as the determination of cell fate, and it is not obvious how it would take part in such a process.

Furthermore, it is the only one of the neurogenic mutations that shows no genetic interactions with the rest. Extra copies of the normal *bib* locus have no effect on the phenotype of other neurogenic mutations and extra copies of other neurogenic loci have no effect on the phenotype of *bib⁻* embryos (de la Concha *et al.,* 1988). This suggests that it functions independently of the other genes.

The pattern of expression of *bib* is also somewhat different from the other genes. It is expressed throughout the cells of the neurogenic region at the time neuroblast segregation begins. Subsequently, it is lost from the neuroblasts soon after they delaminate, but persists in the epidermal precursors until just after the end of neuroblast segregation (Rao *et al.,* 1990).

Since it codes for a channel-like protein, *bib* may be involved in allowing communication between cells undergoing the decision-making process. This reasoning, and *bib*'s expression pattern, would suggest that it is initially required for signaling from neuroblasts to epidermal precursors (discussed in Section II,C), since it is present on both at first. Its persistence in the presumptive epidermis suggests that it may subsequently be involved in an interaction between those cells as well. Such a hypothesis is not out of line with conclusions drawn from developmental genetic findings about the time and place of *Notch* gene action, and its putative role in stabilizing the choice of cell fate (see subsequent text).

B. *Delta* and *Notch*

The genes *Delta (Dl)* and *Notch (N)* are the best candidates for mediators of cell interactions of all the neurogenic genes. Both genes encode transmembrane proteins with large extracellular domains; these domains have significant sequence homology to each other. There are also several independent lines of evidence indicating that the products of *Delta* and *Notch* interact with each other.

1. IMPLICATIONS FROM SEQUENCE COMPARISONS

The first indications the *Delta* and *Notch* might be directly involved in cell interactions came from their sequences (Fig. 7). The predicted amino acid sequences for each, based on the DNA, contained a putative signal sequence and a transmembrane domain, indicative of a transmembrane protein (Wharton *et al.*, 1985; Kidd *et al.*, 1986; Vassin *et al.*, 1987; Kopczynski *et al.*, 1988). Antibodies raised against portions of the *Notch* protein and against synthetic peptides have confirmed that it is indeed a transmembrane protein with a large extracellular domain (Johansen *et al.*, 1989; Kidd *et al.*, 1989).

Both gene products also contain a large region in the putative extracellular domain with numerous repeats of a specific EGF-like arrangement of cysteines. This cysteine motif is also found in a variety of proteins involved in adhesion and extracellular binding, such as laminin (Montell and Goodman,

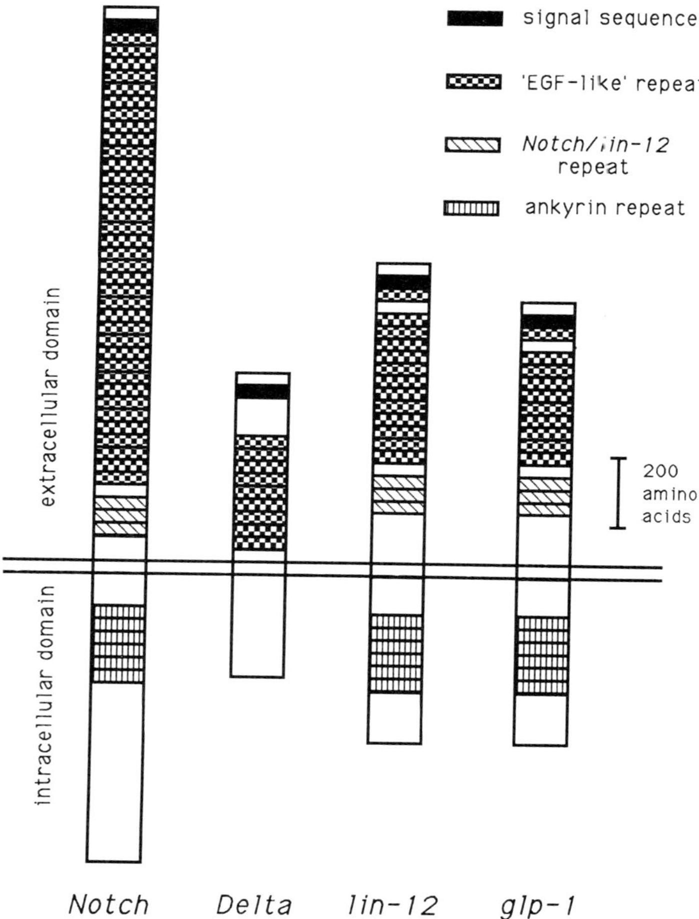

Figure 7. Structural homologies in *Notch*, *Delta*, *lin-12*, and *glp-1*.

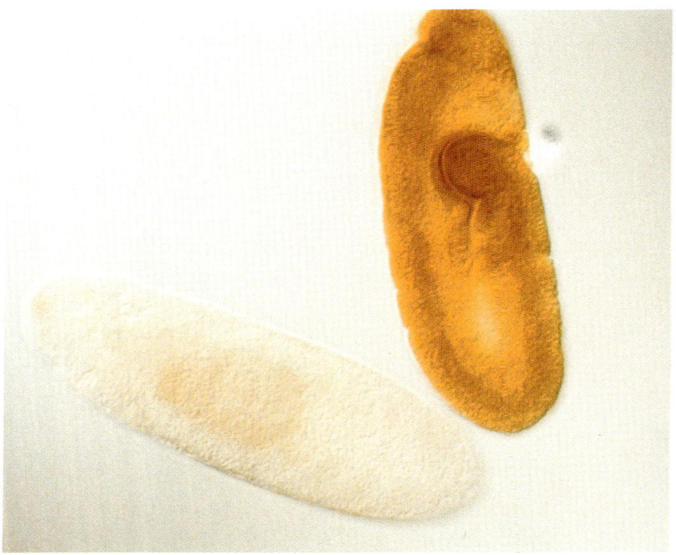

FIGURE 8. Wild-type and *Notch⁻* embryos of *Drosophila,* from the stage just after neuroblast delamination, stained with antibody to the *Notch* protein.

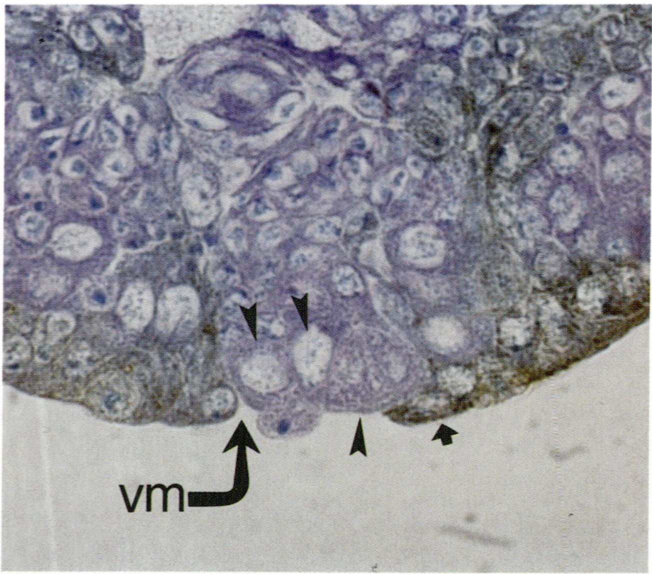

FIGURE 9. Embryo mosaic for a *Notch* mutation stained with an antibody to the *Notch* protein, showing the ventral midline (vm). To the left of the ventral midline are wild-type cells, to the right a mosaic patch. The darkly staining *Notch*⁺ cells juxtapose to nonstaining *Notch⁻* cells. The *Notch*⁺ cells around the periphery of the embryo *(small arrow)* are wild-type epidermal cells, whereas the *Notch⁻* cells are neuroblasts *(arrowheads).*

1988), epidermal growth factor, and various clotting factors (Wharton *et al.*, 1985; Kidd *et al.*, 1986). In fact, the cysteine repeats and the overall structure—large extracellular domain, single membrane spanning domain—give these proteins a strong resemblance to adhesion molecules (Davis, 1990; Greenspan, 1990).

In addition to their resemblance to each other, *Delta* and *Notch* also share homology with two genes in the nematode *C. elegans* that are involved in developmental decisions, *lin-12* and *glp-1* (see Section II,C,3; Yochem *et al.*, 1988; Yochem and Greenwald, 1989; Austin and Kimble, 1989). All these genes have in common the overall resemblance to transmembrane proteins as well as the repeated cysteine motifs in the putative extracellular domain.

Notch shares additional homologies with *lin-12* and *glp-1* in the proximal portion of the extracellular domain, where a different cysteine motif appears, and in the cytoplasmic domain, where a motif found in the cytoskeletal anchoring protein ankyrin is found (Lux *et al.*, 1990). The extensive similarities suggest that the genes may carry out analogous functions, an idea supported by experiment (see subsequent text).

In addition to its similarity to ankyrin, the cytoplasmic tail also contains a motif present in the cytoplasmic tail of the neural cell adhesion molecule NCAM (Barbas *et al.*, 1988). This fact, along with the ankyrin homology, may offer a clue that the vehicle of its function is the cytoskeleton, as would be expected for an adhesion-like molecule (Greenspan, 1990).

2. EXPRESSION OF *DELTA* AND *NOTCH*

Delta and *Notch* are both expressed throughout the neurogenic region during the time of neuroblast segregation (Hartley *et al.*, 1987; Kopczynski and Muskavitch, 1989; Haenlin *et al.*, 1990). They are also expressed in many other places at many other times (Fig. 8). Immunocytochemical staining for *Notch* protein in whole mounts of embryos has confirmed the finding that it is expressed on the surface of all cells in the neurogenic region during the time of neuroblast segregation (Johansen *et al.*, 1989; Kidd *et al.*, 1989; Fehon *et al.*, 1991).

Staining of sections from embryos at a slightly later stage, however, indicates the *Notch* immunoreactivity is lost from neuroblasts but retained by epidermal precursors (Hoppe and Greenspan, 1990; Fehon *et al.*, 1991). This suggests that the distribution of the protein is uniform at first, as would be expected for cells that are equivalent until they make a developmental choice, but that it is lost from neuroblasts concomitant with their taking on that fate. A similar time and pattern of disappearance for *Delta* RNA from neuroblasts has also been described (Haenlin *et al.*, 1990).

These findings have a bearing on the possible role of these molecules in mediating interactions between epidermal precursors (Greenspan, 1990; Hoppe and Greenspan, 1990; see subsequent text).

3. WHERE *NOTCH* ACTS

A gene's pattern of expression is often a poor predictor of what the phenotype of a mutation in that gene will be. Most genes are expressed over a much wider area than is affected when they are mutant. *Notch* is a good example of this, given its ubiquity of expression in the embryo (Fig. 8; see Johansen *et al.,*1989; Kidd *et al.,* 1989; Fehon *et al.,* 1991) relative to the domain of its phenotype in mutant embryos (Fig. 3). Thus, identifying which cells express *Notch* is not the same as identifying which cells require *Notch* for proper development. Genetic mosaics, individuals in which some cells are mutant and others are normal, are needed to accomplish this task.

The results of genetic mosaic studies of embryos have identified the epidermal precursor as the cell that must express a normal *Notch* product in order to make the correct choice of cell fate (Hoppe and Greenspan, 1986;1990). That is, when mutant and normal cells are juxtaposed, those cells that choose the epidermal pathway are always *Notch*$^+$ (Fig. 9). Stated another way, *Notch* must be expressed by those cells leaving the default state (cf., Greenspan, 1990). The same is true for mosaic studies of *Notch* action at later times in development (Cagan and Ready, 1989; Heitzler and Simpson, 1991).

[A different result was obtained in mosaics produced by cell transplantation (Technau and Campos-Ortega, 1987). This appears to be dependent on the technique employed, since these cell transplants are the only case in which nonautonomy was obtained. It may be that singly dissociated cells sometimes take on different properties when transplanted, or that the technique has special problems associated with these mutations.]

A role for *Notch* in cells departing from the default state lends further strength to the analogies between it and the genes *lin-12* and *glp-1* (see Section II,C,3). Mosaic studies for these mutations in *C. elegans* have revealed a similar functional role for them: they are required in the cells that will leave the default state (Austin and Kimble, 1987; Seydoux and Greenwald, 1989; Seydoux *et al.,* 1990).

A clue about where *Delta* is required has been revealed by studies of cells transfected with *Delta* and *Notch.* Such cells become capable of adhering to each other, suggesting that *Delta* and *Notch* may interact with each other physically (Fehon *et al.,* 1990; Lieber *et al.,* 1990). This extends previous findings that mutations at the two loci can interact (Brand and Campos-Ortega, 1990; Xu *et al.,* 1990), and suggests that *Delta* may be used by cells adjacent to those expressing, and perhaps requiring, *Notch.* Mosaic studies of adult sensory neuron development point to the neuroblast as the site of *Delta* action (Hehzler and Simpson, 1991). Preliminary embryonic studies gave an opposite result, suggesting that, like *Notch, Delta* is required in epidermal cells (R. Greenspan, unpublished observations).

4. WHEN *NOTCH* ACTS

The time during which *Notch* acts has also been defined to some extent. Results have been obtained from mitotic recombination experiments (Hoppe and Greenspan, 1990), in which the time of induction of mutant clones in a mosaic can be controlled, and by temperature shifts of a temperature-sensitive mutant combination (R.J. Greenspan, unpublished observations). These techniques reveal that *Notch* is required from the onset of neuroblast segregation, as expected, until some time after it is complete, a result that was not expected.

In particular, mutant clones induced by mitotic recombination show that the action of the *Notch* gene continues to be required for cells to become epidermal precursors, even after the majority of neuroblasts have segregated (Hoppe and Greenspan, 1990). These results have been interpreted to indicate that *Notch* plays a role in the maintenance and stabilization of the neural–epidermal decision (Greenspan, 1990; Hoppe and Greenspan, 1990).

Additional evidence favoring a period of stabilization for the neural–epidermal choice comes from two independent sources. Poodry has shown that a temperature-sensitive mutation affecting membrane cycling, *shibire*[ts], will produce a neurogenic phenotype if placed at its restrictive temperature during the time that the neural–epidermal decision is taking place (Poodry, 1990). The time during which embryos are susceptible to this manipulation is longer than simply the time of neuroblast delamination, as is the case for the temperature-sensitive *Notch* genotype referred to earlier (R.J. Greenspan, unpublished observations).

In a different kind of experiment, Technau *et al.* (1988) removed presumptive epidermal cells from the neurogenic region after neuroblast delamination and found that these cells can switch their fate if placed back into a younger embryo. Both of these results support the idea that determination to become epidermal requires a period of maintenance and stabilization (Greenspan, 1990), a concept that is well established in studies of the determined state.

5. ADHESION AND THE ROLE OF *NOTCH*

Differential adhesion is necessarily an important condition for the morphogenetic movement associated with neuroblast delamination and epithelium formation by the epidermal precursors. The neuroblasts distinguish themselves by their failure to adhere to their neighbors, resulting in their slipping out of the peripheral epithelium. The resemblance of *Notch* to an adhesion molecule has already been pointed out (see Greenspan, 1990), as has its capability of mediating cellular adhesion *in vitro* (Fehon *et al.*, 1990). If one also considers its persistent requirement by epidermal cells and its disappearance from neuroblasts and concomitant retention by epidermal cells (Hoppe and Greenspan, 1990), *Notch* begins to look like an agent of differential adhesiveness. That is, if *Notch* makes epidermal precursors stick to each other preferentially, then neuroblasts would slip out of the epithelium and the remaining cells would adhere to each other to maintain and stabilize themselves as an epithelium. This postulates a role for *Notch* in interactions between epidermal precursor cells that is consistent with its place and time of action.

C. Genetic Balance

The genetic basis for developmental decisions appears increasingly to involve a balance of gene expression, in which quantitative differences can effect qualitative changes. The neural–epidermal decision supplies many such examples, not surprisingly, given the necessity of subdividing homogeneous cells of equivalent potential.

The idea that a balance is important comes from studies in which changes in the amount or activity of a particular gene product counteract the effects of mutations in other genes or produce opposing phenotypes for opposite changes in gene activity. These phenomena have been demonstrated for the *AS-C, vnd,* and the *E(spl)* complex, the genes provisionally designated as committing cells to the neural or epidermal pathways, respectively.

Absence of the *AS-C* and *vnd* results in a failure of neuroblast development, whereas absence of any of the neurogenic genes results in misappropriation of cells into the neuroblast pathway (discussed earlier). When an embryo mutant for a neurogenic mutation is also deficient for *AS-C* and *vnd* (or *AS-C* alone), the neurogenic phenotype is not as severe (Brand and Campos-Ortega, 1988). That is, fewer cells are misappropriated into the neuroblast pathway. Conversely, when an otherwise wild-type embryo carries extra copies of the normal *AS-C* and *vnd* loci, a partial neurogenic phenotype is produced (Jimenez and Campos-Ortega, 1990). Thus, it appears that the amount of *AS-C* and *vnd* activity relative to that of the neurogenic genes is crucial to the cells' choice of pathway. The more the genes are active, the more likely they are to tip the balance toward the neural pathway.

The *E(spl)* complex mirrors *AS-C* in this respect, as in so many others (see previous text). In addition to the possibility of testing extra copies of the wild-type complex, there is a dominant allele, $E(spl)^D$, that behaves as if the gene product is overactive or overproduced. When embryos carry extra copies of the wild-type locus, or multiple copies of $E(spl)^D$, they develop with a deficit of neural tissue, apparently stemming from a reduced complement of neuroblasts (Knust *et al.*, 1987a). This suggests that the amount of *E(spl)* activity relative to that of some other genes (e.g., *AS-C* and *vnd*) determines pathway choice, and more activity biases the cells more toward the epidermal pathway.

There are indications that increased levels of *Notch* activity can give rise to an antineurogenic phenotype, based on studies of adult sensory neuron development (Palka *et al.*, 1990). However, a counterpart of this effect in the embryonic neural–epidermal decision has not been seen yet.

The *AS-C* (including *vnd*) and the *E(spl)* complex have been considered in this chapter as the two genetic poles of the neural–epidermal decision. It seems fitting, therefore, that their levels of expression relative to each other should be so effective in tipping the balance toward either neural or epidermal development.

D. Maternal Contributions

The neural–epidermal decision is one of the first determinative events following gastrulation in *Drosophila* (Poulson, 1950; Campos-Ortega and Hartenstein, 1985). As such, it is principally dependent on zygotic gene expression, that is, transcription occurring after fertilization. There are, however, several genes whose expression during oogenesis is required for normal accomplishment of the neural–epidermal decision.

The maternal requirement for expression of the neurogenic loci has been revealed by eliminating the function of these genes during oogenesis (Jimenez and Campos-Ortega, 1982). The results indicate that elimination of the maternal as well as the zyogtic contribution of most of these genes can exacerbate somewhat the neurogenic phenotype, without qualitatively altering it (Jimenez and Campos-Ortega, 1982). This affects how far dorsally the neuralization extends. Elimination of the maternal component alone is insufficient to produce neurogenic phenotypes, in contrast to the fact, previously denoted, that elimination of the zygotic component alone is sufficient to produce such a phenotype. Thus, the significance of maternal expression for the neurogenic genes does not appear to be great.

Several other loci have been identified which, when the maternal component is eliminated, affect the neural–epidermal decision. For four of these, *almondex, pecanex, l(1)EA24,* and *l(1)3PP4,* both maternal and zygotic expression must be eliminated to produce the neurogenic phenotype (Jimenez and Campos-Ortega, 1982; Perrimon *et al.,* 1984, 1989). For two other loci, *l(1)1PP22* and *l(1)5PP1,* elimination of the maternal component alone is sufficient to affect the embryo (Perrimon *et al.,* 1989). Most of these mutations (except *almondex* and *pecanex)* are recessive lethal mutations with lethal phases in the larval or pupal periods.

The finding of five maternal effect loci affecting the neural–epidermal decision on the *X* chromosome alone (Perrimon *et al.,* 1989) suggests that there are likely to be more (as many as 20–30) elsewhere in the genome. This fact has been disturbing to some, since it suggests that a neurogenic phenotype can be produced rather nonspecifically.

Alternatively, it may be germane to the involement of many cellular components in developmental events, components involved in many different aspects of development that are prepackaged into the egg because they will be required early on in large amounts. The mutant phenotypes for such genes will thus depend on the stage at which gene activity is eliminated. This has already been seen for the zygotically acting *shibire*[ts] mutant (see Section IV,B,4), which affects membrane cycling in general, but produces a neurogenic phenotype if its activity is interrupted at the appropriate time in embryogenesis. Thus, these maternal-effect neurogenic loci are candidates for functions involving ubiquitous machinery that might be involved in the control of cell shape, movement, or communication. Given the hints of cytoskeletal involvement from sequence motifs in *Notch* (see Section IV,B,1), some of these genes may turn out to encode such components.

V. The Neural–Epidermal Decision: Tilting the Balance and Keeping It Tilted

The picture that emerges from an examination of the genes involved in the neural–epidermal decision is, unfortunately, incomplete. Not all the genes have been characterized to the same extent and, undoubtedly, not all the genes are known yet. In spite of these deficiencies, it is possible to draw the outlines of the process and make some suggestions about how it might work.

There appear to be genes whose role is to define the cells that may take part in the decision and to set these cells in the default (neuroblast) state. *AS-C* and *vnd* are the best candidates for constituting at least some of these genes.

Likewise, there appear to be genes whose role is to commit cells irreversibly to the epidermal pathway. The *E(spl)* complex is the best candidate for playing this part. The rest of the genes are presumably required to tilt the balance in the neurogenic region and to bring those cells that will leave the default state to the final stage of committing to the epidermal pathway.

The symmetry-breaking event is still a mystery. There is some indication that the cells destined to become neuroblasts are not always the same cells. That is, one cell in a cluster will become a neuroblast (Cabrera, 1990; Heitzler and Simpson, 1991), but the choice of cell may well be random. Thus, just as *AS-C* seems to define the domain of the neurogenic region in a global sense, its interaction with positional cues in the embryo may also define the narrow domain in which a neuroblast of one particular identity will arise. In this narrow domain of roughly 4–6 cells (Cabrera, 1990), it may then be a stochastic process to choose which one will delaminate.

A stochastic process of the same sort is known to be involved in the designation of which amoebae will become aggregation centers during development of the cellular slime mold, *Dictyostelium discoideum* (Bonner, 1971). The slime mold presents an analogous situation because all cells start out equally capable of becoming aggregation centers. As soon as one does so, its immediate neighbors are inhibited from adopting the same fate. The process of choosing an aggregation center cell is known to be stochastic and depend on where in the cell cycle an amoeba is at the time the trigger for development—starvation—occurs (McDonald, 1986). All that is required for such a mechanism is asynchrony of cell divisions and a mechanism for the designated cell to communicate with its neighbors.

Asynchrony of cell division is a characteristic of cells in the neurogenic region of the fly embryo (Foe, 1989). Although it is not yet clear which genes constitute the signaling machinery, it is easy to imagine that, once the balance is tilted, a cascade of gene expression ensues, distinguishing those cells starting to be neuroblasts from those starting to be epidermal. Such a picture predicts that there is a sensitive means of detecting slight differences between initially identical cells, as well as a strong feedback mechanism to reinforce that difference once it is detected.

One finding that supports the idea of a cascade involves the *Notch* locus. There is reason to believe, as described in Section IV,B,2, that once symmetry is broken, the level of expression of *Notch* starts to change (and perhaps of other genes not yet documented fully). It is known that in the development of adult sensory neurons, the neural–epidermal decision can be biased by manipulating the number of copies of the *Notch* locus (Heitzler and Simpson, 1991). This suggests that an imbalance in *Notch* expression is necessary for the choice of cell fate. There are several candidates among the neurogenic genes for possible regulators of *Notch,* including the nuclear gene *mam* and putative transcription factor *neu*. Perhaps one of these will turn out to constitute part of the predicted feedback loop.

Because of the reciprocal nature of this developmental choice, there must be reciprocal effects on gene expression in the two populations of cells. The evidence suggests that *AS-C* and *vnd* must be repressed in epidermal precursors, whereas *E(spl)* must be repressed in neuroblasts, as *Notch* apparently is. Given the suggestion that these gene complexes represent commitment to one pathway or the other, it may be useful to think of their regulation as endpoints in the process.

This begs the question of how an endpoint is achieved. The resemblances of *Notch* to an adhesion molecule have already been discussed, as has the role of adhesion in establishing the difference between delaminating neuroblasts and the epithelium of epidermal precursors (see Section IV,B,5). Aside from establishing an epithelium and, by default, bringing about delamination, is there any reason to believe that an adhesion-like molecule could also be receptorlike and influence gene expression? If so, then the morphogenetic event would be inextricably bound up with the choosing of cell fate as reflected in altered gene expression.

There are indications that cell shape and tissue architecture *per se* can affect gene expression, presumably mediated through the cytoskeleton (Ben-Ze'ev *et al.*, 1980; Clayton *et al.*, 1985). The homologies of *Notch*'s cytoplasmic tail to proteins that interact with the cytoskeleton (see Section IV,B,1) suggest that it has the requisite properties for fulfilling such a function. In this scheme, *Notch*'s role in stabilizing and maintaining the determined state (see Section IV,B,4) would involve a stabilization of the epidermal epithelium which, in turn, would lead to the correct constellation of gene expression in those cells. Some other neurogenic gene, such as *mam* with its unusual structure and nuclear localization, may convey signals from the cytoskeleton to the nucleus. Alternatively, or perhaps as part of the same process, *Notch* may communicate with the nucleus by way of the G-protein-like product of the m9/10 transcripts of *E(spl)*.

In the absence of further functional studies on the other relevant genes, it is difficult to sketch in the rest of the picture. *Delta* appears to be capable of interacting with *Notch,* as adduced from *in vitro* cell adhesion assays; the evidence from mutant interactions suggests that it actually does so *in vivo*. Where or when it acts is less clear, though evidence from adult sensory neuron development suggests the neuroblast as its site of action (Heitzler and Simpson, 1991). Embryonic mosaic studies have yet to be carried out for *Delta* and the other neurogenic genes. Such functional studies are crucial in drawing conclusions about a gene's action, given the observation that many genes are expressed more widely than their mutant phenotype would have implied.

VI. Conclusion

The neural–epidermal decision in the *Drosophila* embryo is paradigmatic for determination in the earliest stages of nervous system development. While exemplifying a process known to all organisms with nervous systems, it provides a unique glimpse into the genetic components of the decision. The picture is not yet complete, but it clearly includes some features already familiar from developmental genetics and other features that are new and strange.

Familiar are the transcription factors [*AS-C* and *E(spl)*] whose relatives have appeared in many other developmental contexts. They have the capability of interacting with other such factors to produce specificity by virtue of their ability to form combinations with each other. Less familiar, but recognizable, are gene products resembling other nuclear proteins (*mam* and *neu*) and a G-protein [m9/10 of *E(spl)*]. Their familiarity, however, extends only as far as the sequence resemblance. They could still harbor functional surprises. Least familiar are the membrane proteins (*bib*, *N*, and *Dl*) with possible involvement in communication, adhesion, and stabilization. It is among these genes that new mechanisms of development are most likely to be discovered.

References

Alonso, M. C., and Cabrera, C. V. (1988). The *achaete–scute* complex of *Drosophila melanogaster* comprises four homologous genes. *EMBO J.* **7**, 2585–2591.

Artavanis-Tsakonas, S. (1988). The molecular biology of the *Notch* locus and the fine tuning of the differentiation in *Drosophila*. *Trends Genet.* **4**, 95–100.

Austin, J., and Kimble, J. (1987). *glp-1* is required in the germ line for regulation of the decision between mitosis and meiosis in *C. elegans*. *Cell* **51**, 589–599.

Austin, J., and Kimble, J. (1989). Transcript analysis of *glp-1* and *lin-12*, homologous genes required for cell interactions during development of *C. elegans*. *Cell* **58**, 565–571.

Barbas, J. A., Chaix, J-C., Steinmetz, M., and Goridis, C. (1988). Differential splicing and alternative polyadenylation generates distinct NCAM transcripts and proteins in the mouse. *EMBO J.* **7**, 625–632.

Ben-Ze'ev, A., Farmer, S. R., and Penman, S. (1980). Protein synthesis requires cell-surface contact while nuclear events respond to cell shape in anchorage-dependent fibroblasts. *Cell* **21**, 365–372.

Bettler, D., Schmid, A., and Yedvobnick, B. (1991). Early ventral expression of the *Drosophila* neurogenic locus *mastermind*. *Devel. Biol.* **144**, 436–439.

Bonner, J. T. (1971). Aggregation and differentiation in the cellular slime molds. *Ann. Rev. Microbiol.* **25**, 75–92.

Brand, M., and Campos-Ortega, J. A. (1988). Two groups of interrelated genes regulate early neurogenesis in *Drosophila melanogaster. Roux' Arch. Dev. Biol.* **197,** 457–470.

Brand, M., and Campos-Ortega, J. A. (1990). Second-site modifiers of the *split* mutation of *Notch* define genes involved in neurogenesis in *Drosophila melanogaster. Roux' Arch. Dev. Biol.* **198,** 275–285.

Cabrera, C. V. (1990). Lateral inhibition and cell fate during neurogenesis in *Drosophila:* The interactions between *scute, Notch,* and *Delta. Development* **109,** 733–742.

Cabrera, C. V., Martinez-Arias, A., and Bate, M. (1987). The expression of three members of the *achaete–scute* gene complex correlates with neuroblast segregation in *Drosophila. Cell* **50,** 425–433.

Cagan, R. L., and Ready, D. F. (1989). *Notch* is required for successive cell decisions in the developing *Drosophila* retina. *Genes Devel.* **3,** 1099–1112.

Campos-Ortega, J. A. (1985). Genetics of early neurogenesis of *Drosophila melanogaster. Trends Neurosci.* **8,** 245–250.

Campos-Ortega, J. A. (1988). Cellular interactions during early neurogenesis of *Drosophila melanogaster. Trends Neurosci.* **11,** 400–405.

Campos-Ortega, J. A. (1990). Mechanisms of a cellular decision during embryonic development of *Drosophila melanogaster. In* "Genetic Regulatory Hierarchies in Development" (T. R. F. Wright, ed.), pp. 403–453. New York: Academic Press.

Campos-Ortega, J. A., and Hartenstein, V. (1985). "The Embryonic Development of *Drosophila melanogaster.*" Berlin: Springer-Verlag.

Campos-Ortega, J. A., and Knust, E. (1990a). Genetic and molecular mechanisms of neurogenesis in *Drosophila melanogaster. J. Physiol.* **84,** 1–10.

Campos-Ortega, J. A., and Knust, E. (1990b). Molecular analysis of a cellular decision during embryonic development of *Drosophila melanogaster:* Epidermogenesis or neurogenesis. *Eur. J. Biochem.* **190,** 1–10.

Campos-Ortega, J. A., and Jan, Y. N. (1991). Genetic and molecular basis of neurogenesis in *Drosophila melanogaster. Ann. Rev. Neurosci.* **14,** 399–420.

Campuzano, S., Carramolino, L., Cabrera, C. V., Ruiz-Gomez, M., Villares, R., Boronat, A., and Modelell, J. (1985). Molecular genetics of the *achaete–scute* gene complex of *Drosophila melanogaster. Cell* **40,** 327–338.

Caudy, M., Vassin, H., Brand, M., Tuma, R., Jan, L. Y., and Jan Y. N. (1988). *daughterless,* a gene essential for both neurogenesis and sex determination in *Drosophila,* has sequence similarities to *myc* and the *achaete–scute* complex. *Cell* **55,** 1061–1067.

Clayton, D. F., Harrelson, A., and Darnell, J. E., Jr. (1985). Dependence of liver-specific transcription on tissue organization. *Mol. Cell. Biol.* **5,** 2623–2632.

Cronmiller, C., Schedl, P., and Cline, T. W. (1988). Molecular characterization of *daughterless,* a *Drosophila* sex determination gene with multiple roles in development. *Genes Devel.* **2,** 1666–1676.

Davis, C. G. (1990). The many faces of epidermal growth factor repeats. *New Biol.* **2,** 410–419.

de la Concha, A., Dietrich, U., Weigel, D., and Campos-Ortega, J. A. (1988). Functional interactions of neurogenic genes of *Drosophila melanogaster. Genetics* **118,** 499–508.

Dietrich, U., and Campos-Ortega, J. A. (1984). The expression of neurogenic loci in imaginal epidermal cells of *Drosophila melanogaster. J. Neurogenet.* **1,** 315–332.

Doe, C. Q., and Goodman, C. S. (1985a). Early events in insect neurogenesis. I. Development and segmental differences in the pattern of neuronal precursor cells. *Dev. Biol.* **111,** 193–205.

Doe, C. Q., and Goodman, C. S. (1985b). Early events in insect neurogenesis. II. The role of cell interactions and cell lineage in the determination of neuronal precursor cells. *Dev. Biol.* **111,** 206–219.

Fehon, R. G., Kooh, P. J., Rebay, I., Regan, C. L., Xu, T., Muskavitch, M. A. T., and Artavanis-Tsakonas, S. (1990). Molecular interactions between the protein products of the neurogenic loci *Notch* and *Delta,* two EGF-homologous genes in *Drosophila. Cell* **61,** 523–534.

Fehon, R. G., Johansen, K., Rebay, I., and Artavanis-Tsakonas, S. (1991). Complex cellular and subcellular regulation of *Notch* expression during embryonic and imaginal development of *Drosophila:* Implications for *Notch* function. *J. Cell Biol.* **113** 657–669.

Foe, V. (1989). Mitotic patterns reveal early commitment in the *Drosophila* embryo. *Development* **107,** 1–22.

Friedlander, D. R., Mege, R-M., Cunningham, B. A., and Edelman, G. M. (1989). Cell sorting-out is modulated by both the specificty and amount of different cell adhesion molecules (CAMs) expressed on cell surfaces. *Proc. Natl. Acad. Sci. U.S.A.* **86,** 7043–7047.

Gehring, W. J., and Hiromi, Y. (1986). Homeotic genes and the homeobox. *Ann. Rev. Genet.* **20,** 147–173.

Greenspan, R. J. (1990). The *Notch* gene, adhesion and developmental fate in the *Drosophila* embryo. *New Biol.* **2,** 595–600.

Greenwald, I. S., Sternberg, P. W., and Horvitz, H. R. (1983). The *lin-12* locus specifies cell fates in *Caenorhabditis elegans. Cell* **34,** 435–444.

Haenlin, M., Kramatschek, B., and Campos-Ortega, J. A. (1990). The pattern of transcription of the neurogenic gene *Delta* of *Drosophila melanogaster. Development* **110,** 905–914.

Hartenstein, V., and Campos-Ortega, J. A. (1984). Early neurogenesis in wild-type *Drosophila melanogaster. Roux' Arch. Dev. Biol.* **193,** 308–325.

Hartley, D. A. (1990). Early neurogenesis. *Sem. Cell Biol.* **1,** 185–196.

Hartley, D. A., Xu, T., and Artavanis-Tsakonas, S. (1987). The embryonic expression of the *Notch* locus of *Drosophila melanogaster* and the implications of point mutations in the extracellular EGF-like domain of the predicted protein. *EMBO J.* **6,** 3407–3417.

Hartley, D. A., Preiss, A., and Artavanis-Tsakonas, S. (1988). A deduced gene product from the *Drosophila* neurogenic locus. *Enhancer of split,* shows homology to mammlain G-protein β subunit. *Cell* **55,** 785–795.

Hedgecock, E. M., and Hall, D. H. (1990). Homologies in the neurogenesis of nematodes, arthropods, and chordates. *Sem. Neurosci.* **2,** 159–172.

Heitzler, P., and Simpson, P. (1991). The choice of cell fate in the epidermis of *Drosophila. Cell* **64,** 1083–1092.

Hoppe, P. E., and Greenspan, R. J. (1986). Local function of the *Notch* gene for embryonic ectodermal pathway choice in *Drosophila. Cell* **46,** 773–783.

Hoppe, P. E., and Greenspan, R. J. (1990). The *Notch* locus of *Drosophila* is required in epidermal cells for epidermal development. *Development* **109,** 875–885.

Jimenez, F., and Campos-Ortega, J. A. (1979). A region of the *Drosophila* genome necessary for CNS development. *Nature (London)* **282,** 310–312.

Jimenez, F., and Campos-Ortega, J. A. (1987). Genes in subdivision 1B of the *Drosophila melanogaster* X-chromosome and their influence on neural development. *J. Neurogenet.* **4,** 179–200.

Jimenez, F., and Campos-Ortega, J. A. (1990). Defective neuroblast commitment in mutants of the *achaete–scute* complex and adjacent genes of *Drosophila melanogaster. Neuron* **5,** 81–89.

Johansen, K. M., Fehon, R. G., and Artavanis-Tsakonas, S. (1989). The *Notch* gene product is a glycoprotein expressed on the cell surface of both epidermal and neuronal precursor cells during *Drosophila* development. *J. Cell Biol.* **10,** 2427–2440.

Kankel, D. R., and Hall, J. C. (1976). Fate mapping of the nervous system and other internal tissues in genetic mosaics of *Drosophila melanogaster Dev. Biol.* **48,** 1–24.

Kidd, S., Kelley, M. R., and Young, M. W. (1986). Sequence of the *Notch* locus of *Drosophila:* Relationship of the encoded protein to mammalian clotting and growth factors. *Mol. Cell. Biol.* **6,** 3094–3108.

Kidd, S., Baylies, M. K., Gasic, G. P., and Young, M. W. (1989). Structure and distribution of the *Notch* protein in developing *Drosophila. Genes Devel.* **3,** 1113–1129.

Kimble, J. (1981). Alterations in cell lineage following laser ablation of cells in the somatic gonad of *Caenorhabditis elegans. Dev. Biol.* **87,** 286–300.

Kimble, J., and White, J. G. (1981). On the control of germ cell development in *Caenorhabditis elegans. Dev. Biol.* **81,** 208–221.

Klambt, C., Knust, E., Tietze, K., and Campos-Ortega, J. A (1989). Closely related transcripts encoded by the neurogenic gene complex *Enhancer of split* of *Drosophila melanogaster. EMBO J.* **8,** 203–210.

Knust, E., Bremer, K. A., Vassin, H., Ziemer, A., Tepass, U., and Campos-Ortega, J. A. (1987a). The *Enhancer of split* locus and neurogenesis in *Drosophila melanogaster. Dev. Biol.* **122,** 262–273.

Knust, E., Tietze, K., and Campos-Ortega, J. A. (1987b). Molecular analysis of the neurogenic locus *Enhancer of split* of *Drosophila melanogaster. EMBO J.* **6,** 4113–4123.

Knust, E., and Campos-Ortega, J. A. (1989). The molecular genetics of early neurogenesis in *Drosophila melanogaster. BioEssays* **11,** 95–100.

Kopczynski, C. C., Alton, A. K., Fetchel, K., Kooh, P. J., and Muskavitch, M. A. T. (1988). *Delta,* a *Drosophila* neurogenic gene, is transcriptionally complex and encodes a protein related to blood coagulation factors and epidermal growth factor of vertebrates. *Genes Devel.* **2,** 1723–1735.

Kopczynski, C. C., and Muskavitch, M. A. T. (1989). Complex spatio-temporal accumulation of alternative transcripts from the neurogenic gene *Delta* during *Drosophila* embryogenesis. *Development* **107,** 623–636.

Lehmann, R., Dietrich, U., Jiminez, F., and Campos-Ortega, J. A. (1981). Mutations of early neurogenesis in *Drosophila. Roux' Arch. Dev. Biol.* **190,** 226–229.

Lehmann, R., Jimenez, F., Dietrich, U., and Campos-Ortega, J. A. (1983). On the phenotype and development of mutants of early neurogenesis in *Drosophila melanogaster. Roux' Arch. Dev. Biol.* **192,** 62–74.

Lieber, T., Krane, J. F., Hassel, B., Campos-Ortega, J. A., and Young, M. W. (1990). Cellular and genetic interactions between the *Drosophila Notch* and *Delta* proteins. (in press).

Lindsley, D. L., and Grell, E. H. (1968). "Genetic Variations of *Drosophila melanogaster.*" Carnegie Inst. Wash., Publ. 627.

Lux, S. E., John, K. M., and Bennett, V. (1990). Analysis of cDNA for human erythrocyte ankyrin indicates a repeated structure with homology to tissue-differentiation and cell-cycle control proteins. *Nature (London)* **344,** 36–42.

McDonald, S. A. (1986). Cell cycle regulation of center initiation in *Dictyostelium discoideum. Dev. Biol.* **117,** 546–549.

Montell, D. J., and Goodman, C. S. (1988). *Drosophila* substrate adhesion molecule: Sequence of laminin B1 chain reveals domains of homology with mouse. *Cell* **53,** 463–473.

Murre, C., Schoenleber-McCaw, P., and Baltimore, D. (1989a). The amphipathic helix-loop-helix: A new DNA-binding and dimerization motif in immunoglobulin enhancer binding, *daughterless, MyoD,* and *myc* proteins. *Cell* **56,** 777–783.

Murre, C., Schoenleber-McCaw, P., Vassin, H., Caudy, M., Jan, L. Y., Jan, Y. N., Cabrera, C. V., Buskin, J. N., Hauschka, S. D., Lassar, A. B., Weintraub, H., and Baltimore, D. (1989b). Interactions between heterologous helix-loop-helix proteins generate complexes that bind specifically to a common DNA sequence. *Cell* **58,** 537–544.

Palka, J., Schubiger, M., and Schwaninger, H. (1990). Neurogenic and antineurogenic effects from modifications at the *Notch* locus. *Development* **109,** 167–175.

Perrimon, N., Engstrom, L., and Mahowald, A. P. (1984). Developmental genetics of the 2E-F region of the *Drosophila* X chromosome: A region rich in "developmentally important" genes. *Genetics* **108,** 559–572.

Perrimon, N., Engstrom, L., and Mahowald, A. P. (1989). Zygotic lethals with specific maternal effect phenotypes in *Drosophila melanogaster*. I. Loci on the *X* chromosome. *Genetics* **121**, 333–352.

Poodry, C. (1990). *shibire,* a neurogenic mutant of *Drosophila*. *Dev. Biol.* **138**, 464–472.

Poulson, D. F. (1937). Chromosomal deficiencies and the embryonic development of *Drosophila melanogaster*. *Proc. Natl. Acad. Sci. U.S.A.* **23**, 133–137.

Poulson, D. F. (1940). The effects of certain X-chromosome deficiencies on the embryonic development of *Drosophila melanogaster*. *J. Exp. Zool.* **83**, 271–325.

Poulson, D. F. (1950). Histogenesis, organogenesis, and differentiation in the embryo of *Drosophila melanogaster. In* "Biology of Drosophila" (M. Demerec, ed.), pp. 168–274. New York: Wiley.

Preiss, A., Hartley, D. A., and Artavanis-Tsakonas, S. (1988). The molecular genetics of *Enhancer of split,* a gene required for embryonic neural development in *Drosophila melanogaster*. *EMBO J.* **6**, 2085–2092.

Rao, Y., Jan, L. Y., and Jan, Y. N. (1990). Similarity of the product of the *Drosophila* neurogenic gene *big brain* to transmembrane channel proteins. *Nature (London)* **345**, 163–167.

Romani, S., Campuzano, S., and Modelell, J. (1987). The *achaete–scute* complex is expressed in neurogenic regions of *Drosophila* embryos. *EMBO J.* **6**, 2085–2092.

Seydoux, G., and Greenwald, I. (1989). Cell autonomy of *lin-12* function in a cell fate decision in *C. elegans*. *Cell* **57**, 1237–1245.

Seydoux, G., Schedl, T., and Greenwald, I. (1990). Cell–cell interactions prevent a potential inductive interaction between soma and germline in *C. elegans*. *Cell* **61**, 939–951.

Simpson, P. (1990). Lateral inhibition and the development of the sensory bristles of the adult peripheral nervous system in *Drosophila*. *Development* **109**, 509–520.

Slack, J. M. W. (1983). "From Egg to Embryo." Cambridge: Cambridge University Press.

Smoller, D., Friedel, C., Schmid, A., Bettler, D., Lam, L., and Yedvobnick, B. (1990). The *Drosophila* neurogenic locus *mastermind* encodes a nuclear protein unusually rich in amino acid homopolymers. *Genes Devel.* **4**, 1688–1700.

Steinberg, M. S., and Poole, T. J. (1981). Strategies for specifying form and pattern: Adhesion-guided multicellular assembly. *Phil. Trans. R. Soc. Lond. B* **295**, 451–460.

Technau, G. M., and Campos-Ortega, J. A. (1986). Lineage analysis of transplanted individual cells in embryos of *Drosophila melanogaster*. II. Commitment and proliferative capabilities of neural and epidermal cell progenitors. *Roux' Arch. Dev. Biol.* **195**, 445–454.

Technau, G. M., and Campos-Ortega, J. A. (1987). Cell autonomy of expression of neurogenic genes of *Drosophila melanogaster*. *Proc. Natl. Acad. Sci. U.S.A.* **84**, 4500–4505.

Technau, G. M., Becker, T., and Campos-Ortega, J. A. (1988). Reversible commitment of neural and epidermal progenitor cells during embryogenesis of *Drosophila melanogaster*. *Roux' Arch. Dev. Biol.* **197**, 413–418.

Vassin, H., Bremer, K. A., Knust, E., and Campos-Ortega, J. A. (1987). The neurogenic gene *Delta* of *Drosophila melanogaster* is expressed in neurogenic territories and encodes a putative transmembrane protein with EGF-like repeats. *EMBO J.* **6**, 3431–3440.

Villares, R., and Cabrera, C. (1987). The *achaete–scute* gene complex of *D. melanogaster:* Conserved domains in a subset of genes required for neurogenesis and their homology to *myc*. *Cell* **50**, 415–424.

Way, J. C. (1990). Determination of cell type in the nervous system. *Sem. Neurosci.* **2**, 173–184.

Welshons, W. J. (1956). *Dros. Inf. Serv.* **30**, 157–158.

Wharton, K. A., Johansen, K. M., Xu, T., and Artavanis-Tsakonas, S. (1985). Nucleotide sequence from the neurogenic locus *Notch* implies a gene product which shares homology with proteins containing EGF-like repeats. *Cell* **43**, 567–581.

White, K. (1980). Defective neural development in *Drosophila melanogaster* embryos deficient for the tip of the X-chromosome. *Dev. Biol.* **80**, 322–344.

White, K., DeCelles, N. L., and Enlow, T. C. (1983). Genetic and developmental analysis of the locus *vnd* in *Drosophila melanogaster*. *Genetics* **118**, 483–497.

Wiseman, L. L., Steinberg, M. S., and Phillips, H. M. (1972). Experimental modulation of intercellular cohesiveness: Reversal of tissue assembly patterns. *Dev. Biol.* **28**, 498–517.

Xu, T., Rebay, I., Fleming, R. J., Scottgale, T. N., and Artavanis-Tsakonas, S. (1990). The *Notch* locus and the genetic circuitry involved in early *Drosophila* neurogenesis. *Genes Devel.* **4**, 464–475.

Yochem, J., Weston, K., and Greenwald, I. (1988). The *Caenorhabditis elegans lin-12* gene encodes a transmembrane protein with overall similarity to *Drosophila Notch*. *Nature (London)* **335**, 547–550.

Yochem, J., and Greenwald, I. (1989). *glp-1* and *lin-12*, genes implicated in cell–cell interactions in *C. elegans*, encode similar transmembrane proteins. *Cell* **58**, 553–563.

Ziemer, A., Tietze, K., Knust, E., and Campos-Ortega, J. A. (1988). Genetic analysis of *Enhancer of split*, a locus involved in neurogenesis in *Drosophila melanogaster*. *Genetics* **119**, 63–74.

Cell Choice and Patterning in the *Drosophila* Retina

Ross Leigh Cagan and S. Lawrence Zipursky
Department of Biological Chemistry
Howard Hughes Medical Institute
School of Medicine
University of California at Los Angeles
Los Angeles, California

DETERMINANTS OF NEURONAL IDENTITY

189

I. Introduction

The importance of interactions between cells during development has been known for at least a century. For example, when Roux (1888) simply pierced one cell of a two-cell embryo, the remaining cell produced half an embryo. However when Spemann (1928) separated the two cells using a fine hair, both cells produced fully formed embryos. The simplest interpretation is that the two cells are totipotent and interact to regulate their development. However, the mechanisms through which such interactions occur remain a mystery. Could such a fundamental mechanism generate the enormous cellular diversity seen in the nervous system? Recent work suggests that interactions between cells do indeed play an important role in regulating the number, position, and fate of cells. In the developing vertebrate eye, such interactions have been inferred from lineage studies using viral markers (Turner and Cepko, 1987). More direct evidence has come from studies with invertebrates, where interactions can be examined between individual identified cells. Ablation studies in the grasshopper and nematode have shown a requirement for particular cells in the specification of their neighbor(s) (e.g., Doe and Goodman, 1985; Sulston *et al.*, 1983). Furthermore, genetic mosaic studies in the fruitfly have identified genes in which expression is required in an identified cell for the proper specification of its neighbor (Reinke and Zipursky, 1988; Tomlinson *et al.*, 1988; Karpilow *et al.*, 1989). These developmental systems, which have provided strong evidence for the importance of cell–cell interaction in the specification of cell fate, are also beginning to yield insights into its mechanisms.

Current work on the role of cell–cell interactions in regulating cell fate have focused on several key issues: (1) characterizing the cues, both molecular and cellular, that regulate cell fate determination; (2) identifying the cells producing these cues as well as those that receive them; and (3) understanding how other cells are prevented from responding to these cues. The structural simplicity of the fly's retina provides several advantages for studying these questions. Its development has been examined morphologically in careful detail, and it is one of the few developmental systems that have been described at the level of individual identifiable cells In addition, it allows us to make use of the powerful genetic techniques available in *Drosophila.* These techniques, some of which are discussed in this chapter, have led to the isolation of several genes important for cell fate decisions.

II. Structure of the Compound Eye

Perhaps the most striking feature of the fly eye is its regularity. It is composed of a reiterated pattern of hexagonally arranged unit eyes called ommatidia punctuated by precisely spaced sensory bristles. Each ommatidium is identical to the next, containing a core of 14 cells and surrounded by an interweaving hexagonal lattice. The structure of a single adult ommatidium is shown in Figs. 1 and 2. At the center of the ommatidium are 8 photoreceptor cells (R cells). These cells fall into three classes based on their spectral sensitivity and synaptic connectivity: R1–R6, R7, and R8. The R cells contain specialized light-gathering rods known as rhabdomeres. The rhabdomeres of R1–R6 have a large cross-sectional profile and extend the length of the ommatidia, whereas those of R7 and R8 are thinner and found solely in the apical and basal regions, respectively. Light passing into these rods activates a photosensitive rhodopsin, resulting in a signal carried through the axon to the underlying optic lobe. The cytoplasm contains small brown ommachrome pigment granules that play a role in the R cell's adaptation to light; these granules have proven useful for genetic mosaic studies.

Between the R cells are 4 cone cells that secrete the central part of the overlying optical lens and also the pseudocone. The cone cells extend the length of the ommatidium from just under the pseudocone to the floor of the retina. In this basal region the cones are filled with large brown ommachrome pigment granules. Surrounding the apical reach of the cone cells are two primary pigment cells. These cells also secrete the central portion of the lens and in addition help optically insulate the apical portion of the cluster. Between ommatidia is an interweaving hexagonal lattice composed of secondary and tertiary pigment cells. These cells, which contain the red pigment that gives the fly eye its striking red color, optically insulate the cluster and also contribute to lens formation. The secondaries and tertiaries produce an actin-rich matrix, the fenestrated membrane, which acts as the floor of the eye. Evenly spaced in this lattice are the sensory bristles, originally formed by four cells of which two—the neuron and glial cell—remain in the adult.

III. Description of Eye Development

The *Drosophila* life cycle lasts about 9 days at 25°C. It includes a day of embryogenesis, 4 days of larval development, and 4 days of pupation.[1] As the

---

[1]For convenience, we include the first 10 hr after larval development—sometimes referred to as pupariation—as part of pupation.

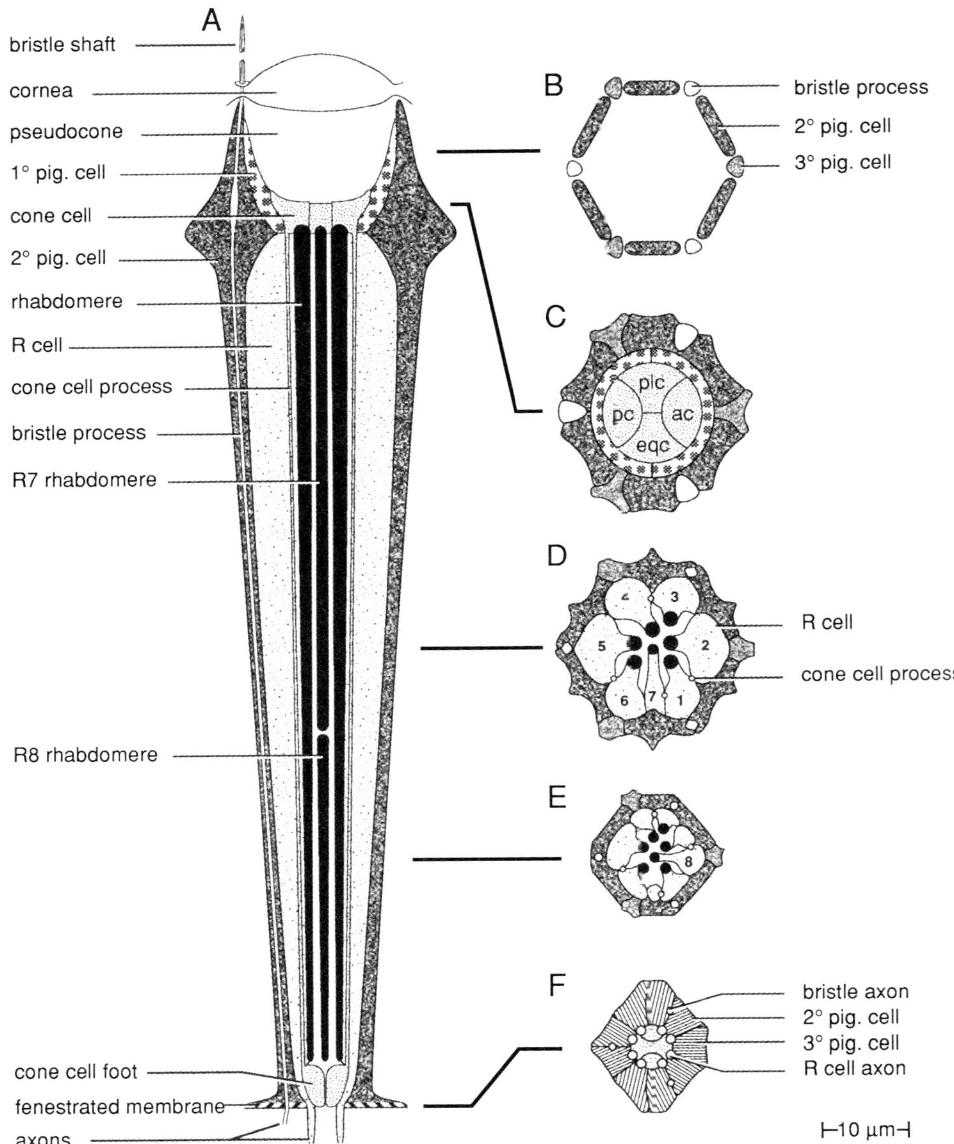
bristle shaft
cornea
pseudocone
1° pig. cell
cone cell
2° pig. cell
rhabdomere
R cell
cone cell process
bristle process
R7 rhabdomere
R8 rhabdomere
cone cell foot
fenestrated membrane
axons
A
B
bristle process
2° pig. cell
3° pig. cell
C
plc
pc
ac
eqc
D
R cell
cone cell process
E
F
bristle axon
2° pig. cell
3° pig. cell
R cell axon
10 μm

embryo develops, it sets aside small islands of epithelia, referred to as imaginal discs, to form most of the adult cuticular structures. Estimates of the number of cells initially set aside to form the eye vary between 6 and 20 cells. (Garcia-Bellido and Merriam, 1969; Wieschaus and Gehring, 1976). These cells divide during embryogenesis and the subsequent three larval stages to form a columnar epithelium, which in the mature larva is composed of about 2000 cells (Becker, 1957). Until the final larval stage, the cells in the eye disc appear to be identical and undifferentiated.

A. The Morphogenetic Furrow

Ommatidial assembly begins midway through the last larval stage. Cells at the posterior edge of the eye disc stop dividing and displace their nuclei downward, causing a groove in the epithelial sheet. This groove, referred to as the morphogenetic furrow, runs in a dorsal–ventral line across the disc. As developmental time continues, the nuclei of more anterior cells move downward, causing the morphogenetic furrow to move anteriorly. Posterior to the furrow, the nuclei of some of these cells move back up toward the apical surface; these cells have begun differentiating into identifiable neuronal cell types. the remaining cells re-enter the cell cycle. The furrow's anterior progression results in a smooth gradient of developmental maturity: the most posterior cells are the most mature and cells near the morphogenetic furrow are developmentally younger (Figs. 3,4). A new row of ommatidial clusters

---

Figure 1. The adult retina. A. A schematic longitudinal view of a single ommatidium, drawn to scale. B. A cross-sectional view 5 μm below the lens. The secondary and tertiary pigment cells and bristles, which form the hexagonal lattice, are the most apical cells. At this level, the lattice surrounds the pseudocone. C. A cross-sectional view 12 μm below the lens. The anterior and posterior cone cells are separated by the equatorial and polar cones. They are enwrapped by two primary pigment cells and the surrounding hexagonal lattice. D. A cross-sectional view 20–80 μm below the lens. Seven R cells can be seen. The dark circles extending from each R cell are photosensitive structures called rhabdomeres. The R cells are surrounded by the hexagonal lattice. The cone cells are thin threads, and the primary pigment cells do not extend to this depth. E. A cross-sectional view 80–115 μm below the lens. R8 is visible at this depth; its rhabdomere replaces that of R7 in the center. F. A cross-sectional view 120 μm below the lens. The feet of the secondary and tertiary pigment cells widen into the filamentous fenestrated membrane. At the center, the cone cells have enlarged into pigment-containing sacs; the anterior and posterior cone cells contact each other (compare with C). Abbreviations: 1° pig. cell, primary pigment cell; 2° pig. cell, secondary pigment cell; 3° pig. cell, tertiary pigment cell; ac, anterior cone cell; eqc, equatorial cone cell; pc, posterior cone cell; plc, polar cone cell. Anterior is to the right; bar 10 μm (From Cagan and Ready, 1989b; reprinted by permission of the publisher.)

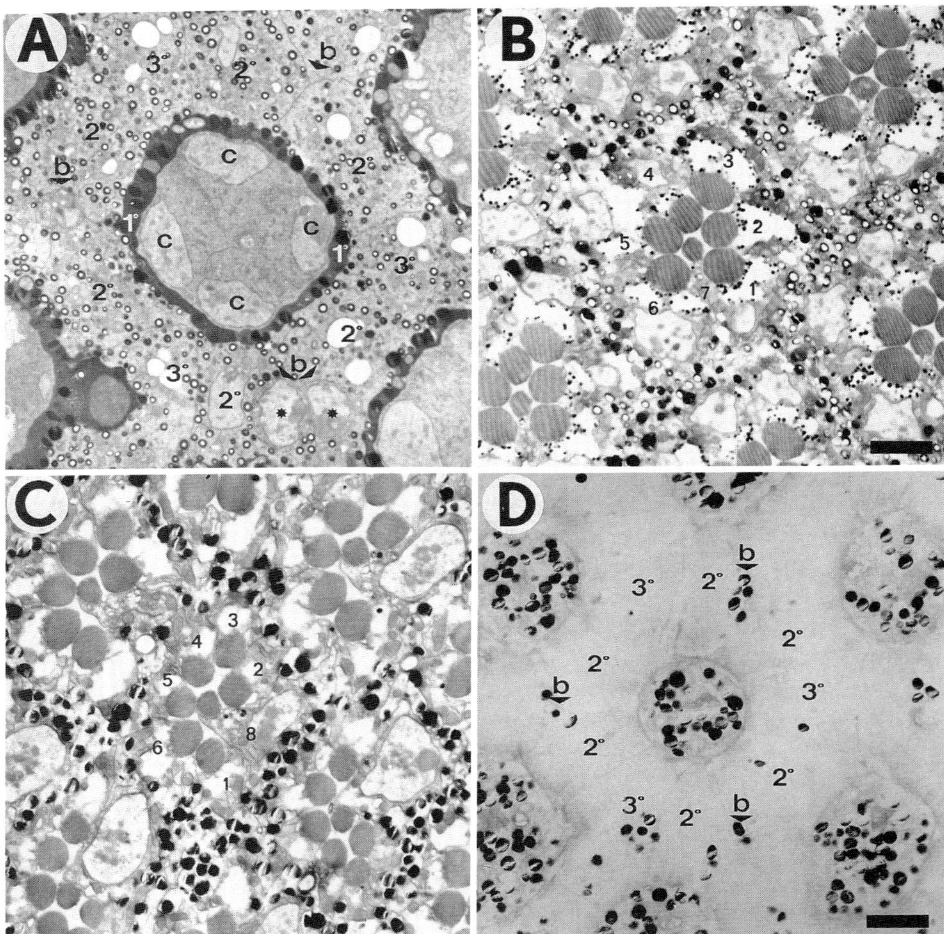

Figure 2. Electron micrographs showing four descending cross-sectional views of an adult ommatidium. For comparison, see schematic view in Fig. 1. A. A section 10 μm below the lens. The four cone cells are enwrapped by two primary pigment cells. The primaries contain large ommachrome pigment granules. The surrounding secondary and tertiary pigment cells contain smaller pteridine pigment granules. Arrowheads and asterisks indicate the nuclei of the neuron and thecogen that compose the adult bristle group. B. A section 30 μm below the lens. R1–R7 can be seen with their darkly stained rhabdomeres. Surrounding the R cells are the secondary and tertiary pigment cells. Their pigment granules stain more darkly than in A. C. A section 100 μm below the lens. Again seven rhabdomeres can be seen, but the R7 rhabdomere is replaced in the center by that of R8. D. A section at the base of the retina. The base of the secondary and tertiary pigment cells forms the fibrous fenestrated membrane; the outline of their feet can still be seen. Abbreviations: 1–8, R1–R8; 1°, primary pigment cell; 2°, secondary pigment cell; 3°, tertiary pigment cell; b, bristle process; c, cone cell. Anterior is to the right. Bar: 2 μm (A,B) bar: 3 μm (C,D). (From Cagan and Ready, 1989b; reprinted by permission of the publisher.)

arises every 2 hr (Campos-Ortega, 1980). Since each eye contains nearly 30 rows, the morphogenetic furrow requires 2 days of larval life plus 10 hr of pupation to complete its anterior progression.

How can discrete, evenly spaced ommatidial units arise from an apparently homogeneous epithelial sheet? In grasshoppers, elegant ablation experiments have provided one possible answer (Doe and Goodman, 1985). Neuroblasts in the grasshopper CNS arise among a small population of cells in the neural epithelium. If a cell that appeared to be initiating the process of neuroblast formation is ablated at an early stage, a neighboring cell takes its place. This switch has to be made in a certain developmental period: later ablations have no effect. Drawing on this work and past models, Doe and Goodman proposed that neuroblasts prevent neighboring cells from assuming the same cell fate by presenting an inhibitory substance to their neighbors. In this manner, founder cells can be spaced at regular intervals (Fig. 5). Ablating the neuroblast removes the inhibition, freeing other cells to take its place.

Could spacing of ommatidia in the fly eye take place in a similar manner? Perhaps a founder cell arises via a stochastic process at the morphogenetic furrow. It inhibits formation of a founder by surrounding cells; cells outside its inhibitory influence are free to start new ommatidial clusters. This founder then initiates recruitment of other cells to begin an ommatidial cluster (as discussed subsequently). Through this process, a regular array of ommatidial clusters could emerge. Since early clusters are separated by several cells, this model requires that either the founder cells are initially near each other and later move apart or the inhibitory factor diffuses across several cell diameters.

B. Development of the R Cell Cluster

Ommatidial assembly begins near the morphogenetic furrow. Figure 3B shows a tracing of the disc's surface near the furrow as visualized with cobalt sulfide. These cells have aggregated into small, evenly spaced clusters that are the precursors to the ommatidia. The row of cell clusters just posterior to the furrow usually consists of 6–8 cells, including one central cell contacted by 5–7 cells around its posterior face (Fig. 3). By the third row posterior to the furrow, each cluster has 5 cells: the fate of the cells eliminated from the cluster is not clear (Tomlinson and Ready, 1987a; Cagan and Ready, 1989b). The remaining 5 cells in each group express neural- and R-cell-specific antigens and extend axons in a defined sequence: first R8, followed by R2 and R5, and then R3 and R4. Following a round of cell divisions in the surrounding undifferentiated pool of cells, R1 and R6 are added to the cluster, followed by R7. The addition of R7 by row 8 gives the ommatidial cluster its full complement of eight R cells, with R8 surrounded by the remaining seven R cells.

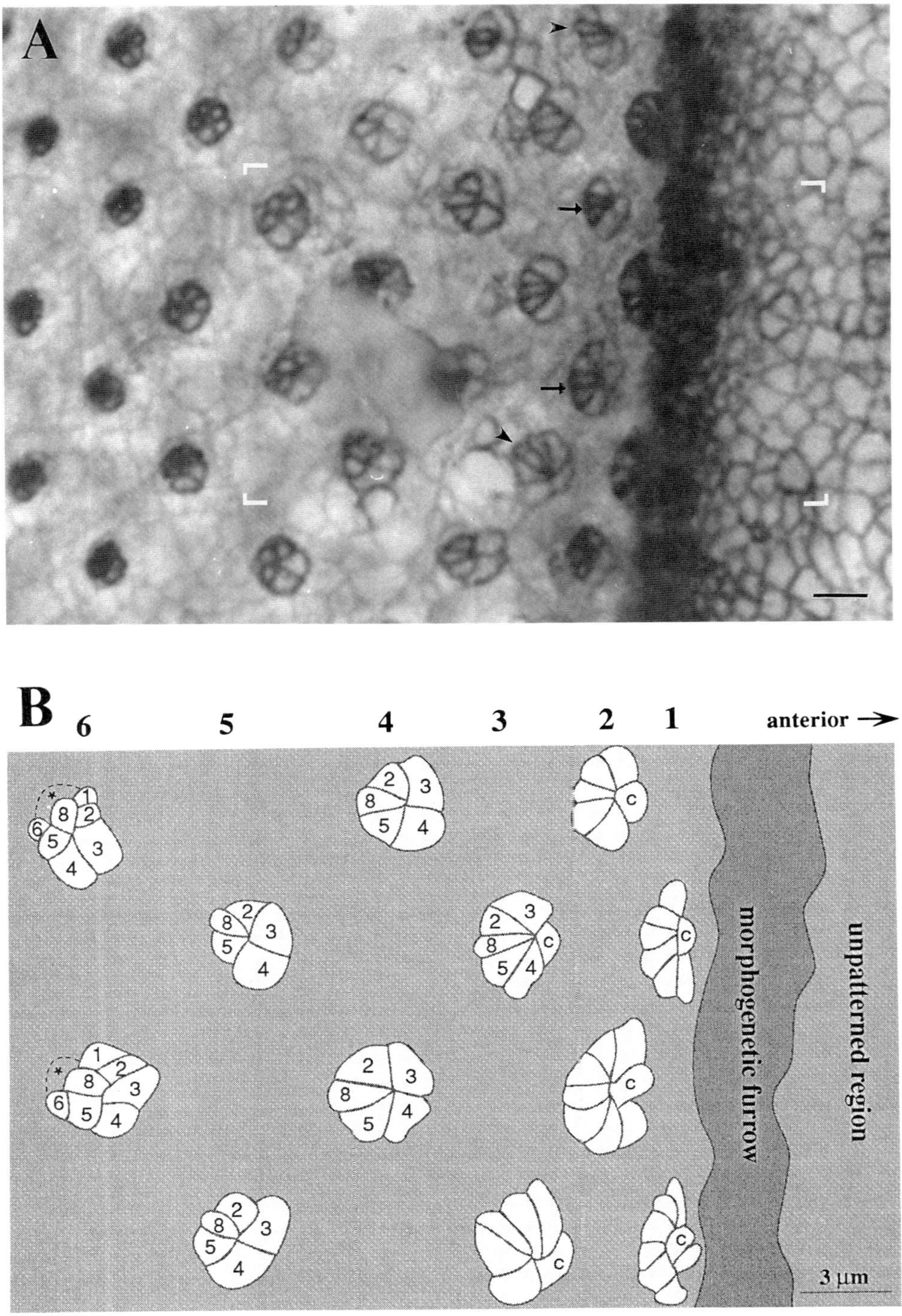

A
B
6
5
4
3
2
1
anterior →
1
2
8
2
3
5
4
6
8
2
3
5
4
c
8
2
3
5
4
8
2
3
5
4
c
2
3
8
c
5
4
c
1
2
8
3
6
5
4
2
3
8
5
4
c
2
3
8
5
4
c
morphogenetic furrow
unpatterned region
3 μm

I. Larval development

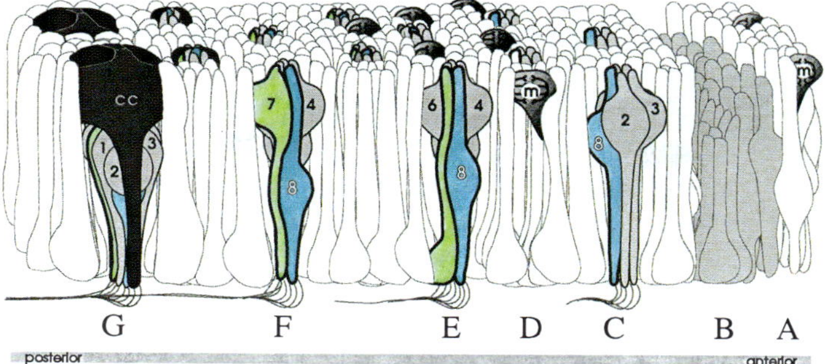

II. Pupal development

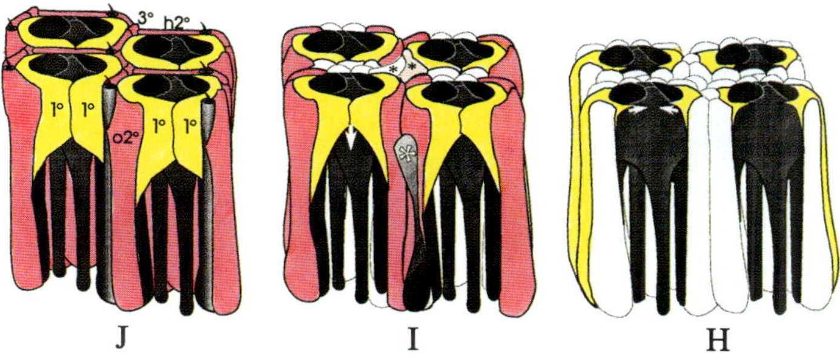

FIGURE 4. A schematic view of ommatidial development. For clarity, only a few stages of development are shown. The upper panel shows stages during late larval development; the lower panel shows early pupal stages. A. Ahead of the morphogenetic furrow, cells are proliferating and unpatterned, with nuclei distributed throughout the depth of the eye field. B. The cells' nuclei descend basally, resulting in the groove referred to as the morphogenetic furrow. C. Behind the furrow, cells cluster into evenly spaced ommatidial primordia. The first cells in the group are R2, R3, R4, R5, and R8. D. Subsequent ommatidial cells are derived from a second round of cell divisions. E. The first cells added from this second round of cell divisions are R1 and R6 (for clarity, R1, R2, and R3 are not shown). Between them is another cell that is destined to differentiate as R7. F. The first indication of R7's development is the apical movement of its nucleus. At this point, all eight R cells have been added to the cluster. G. The last cells to be added to the cluster are the four cone cells, whose nuclei rise over the periphery of the R cell cluster. As a result, the R cells will soon no longer project to the apical surface. Three stages of pupal development are shown in H, I, and J. The R cells are deleted for clarity. H. Beginning some 20 hr after pupariation, two cells, contacting the anterior and posterior cone cells, begin to enwrap the cluster at the apical surface *(arrows)*. These will become the anterior and posterior primary pigment cells, respectively. I. Having contacted each other at the apical surface, the two primaries extend this contact basally *(arrow)*. Concurrently, the hexagonal lattice begins to take shape. Cells stretch between ommatidia to become the secondary and tertiary pigment cells *(black asterisks)*, while other cells undergo programmed cell death *(white asterisk)*. J. By 60 hr, cell death has removed unneeded cells, moving each ommatidium into register with its neighbor. Each cell has taken its characteristic place in the eye field. The bristles, now shown in the diagram, arise between ommatidia shortly after pupariation. Abbreviations: 2–8, R cells R2–R8; cc, cone cell; 1°, primary pigment cell; h2°, horizontal secondary pigment cell; o2°, oblique secondary pigment cell; 3°, tertiary pigment cell; b, bristle; m, mitotic cell.

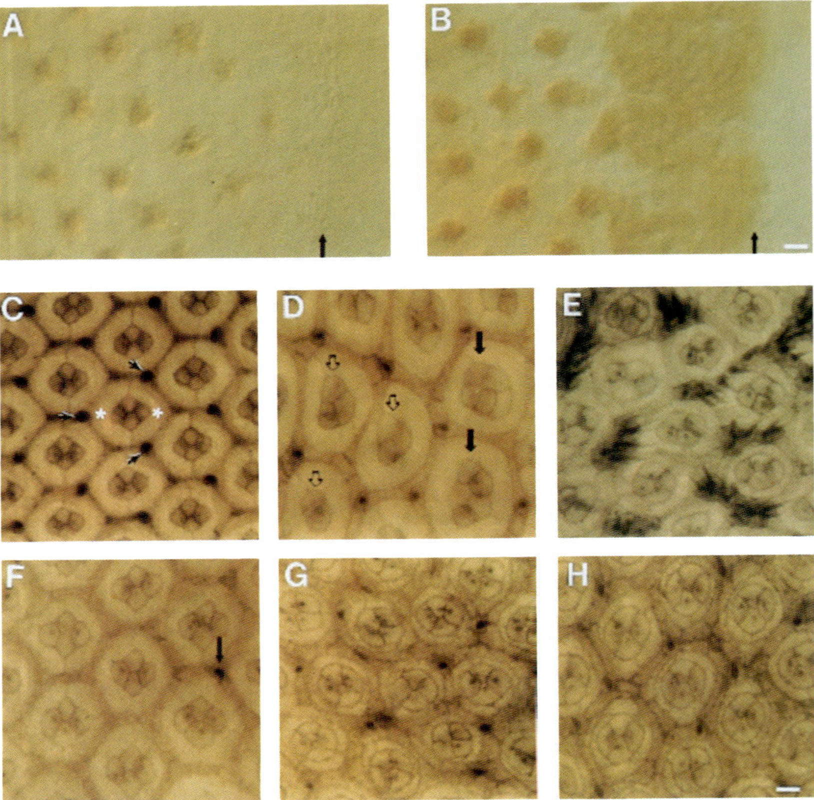

FIGURE 5. *Notch* activity is required for the development of each cell type in the developing eye. The temperature-sensitive *Notch* allele, N^{ts1}, was used to reduce *Notch* activity at successive stages of ommatidial development. A, B. Anti-HRP antibody staining of wild-type and N^{ts1} late larval eye disks. The morphogenetic furrow is near the right edge of each panel *(arrow)*. A. Wild-type disk. Behind the furrow, the cells that group together into developing ommatidia can be recognized with anti-HRP antibody. The ommatidial clusters are evenly spaced; the unstained region between them contains undifferentiated cells. B. N^{ts1} disk shifted to 32°C for 16 hr. Nearly all the cells just posterior to the furrow stained with anti-HRP antibody, revealing their neural identity. More posteriorly, ommatidial clusters are abnormally large. C–H. Apical surface of five N^{ts1} disks that received 8-hr temperature shifts at successive developmental stages. Disks were then returned to the permissive temperature, dissected 65 hr after pupariation, and stained with cobalt sulfide to highlight the surface. Time refers to the hours after pupariation during which the developing pupa received a heat shock. C. No heat shock treatment. In each ommatidium, the central four cone cells are surrounded by two primary pigment cells (*) and a hexagonal lattice of secondary and tertiary pigment cells and three bristles *(arrows)* (see also Figs. 1D, 8G to identify cells). By this stage, the R cells are no longer at the surface. D. 0–8 hr: solid arrows indicate ommatidia with too many cone cells. Open arrows indicate ommatidia with too few. E. 8–16 hr: the lattice is dominated by bristles. F. 16–24 hr: the surrounding hexagonal lattice lacks bristles (arrow indicates a lone exception). G. 28–36 hr.: the cone cells are surrounded by cells with thin apical profiles. All these outer cells will become secondary-like pigment cells; few primary pigment cells will develop. This is a phenocopy of *facet–glossy* (H). Anterior is to the right. Bar: 5 μm (A,B); 3 μm (C–H).

C. Addition of the Cone Cells

During the next stage of ommatidial assembly, the four cone cells are added along the periphery of each cluster. Beginning at about row 10 the anterior and posterior cone cells are added, followed some two rows later by the equatorial and polar cone cells. This is the "four-cone-cell stage" (Tomlinson, 1985) and marks the end of ommatidial assembly in the larva. The nuclei of the cone cells move over the top of the R cells, allowing first the anterior and posterior cone cells, then the equatorial and polar cone cells, to establish contact across the top of the cluster (Fig. 4G). As a result the R cells are excluded from the surface, and will remain beneath the cone cell nuclei into adulthood.

D. Addition of the Pigment Cells

Ten hours after puparium formation and some 15–20 hr after formation of the cone cells, pigment cells are first added at the posterior edge of the disc. Two precursor cells, one contacting the anterior cone cell and the other contacting the posterior cone cell, begin to enwrap the inner cluster. These cells will differentiate into the two primary pigment cells. Shortly after appearance of the primary pigment cells, cells in the undifferentiated pool sort themselves into the hexagonal lattice. Some cells stretch between primary pigment cells from two adjoining clusters, whereas others contact primaries from three clusters. These cells will become the oblique secondary pigment cells and tertiary pigment cells, respectively. The last cells to differentiate are the horizontal secondary pigment cells. They also arise between two adjoining ommatidia, but contact two pairs of primary pigment cells (Fig. 4I,J). As the

---

Figure 3. The surface of a late larval disk as visualized with cobalt sulfide. A. Near the morphogenetic furrow, cells arise in well-spaced clusters. Two ommatidia near the furrow, indicated with solid arrows, contain two strongly stained cells at their posterior face. Two other ommatidial clusters, indicated with arrowheads, contain one strongly stained cell; based on its position, we believe this strongly stained cell will differentiate as R8. The bracketed region is traced in B. B. Tracing of a portion of A to highlight the developing ommatidial clusters. The numbers above the image refer to row numbers posterior to the morphogenetic furrow. In Row 1, clusters of 6–8 cells are already strongly stained with cobalt sulfide. The other cells in the cluster are grouped around the central mystery cell. By Row 4 the 5-cell precluster is evident, containing R2, R3, R4, R5, and R8. In the upper cluster in Row 3, R3 and R4 are pinching together. After a wave of cell divisions (not shown), R1 and R6 stain strongly (Row 6). At this stage, a single cell resides between R1 and R6. This cell will become R7. Abbreviations: c, central mystery cell; 1–8, R1–R8. Anterior is to the right; bar 5 μm (A); bar: 3 μm (B).

cells of the hexagonal lattice stretch between primary pigment cells, many of
their neighbors in the undifferentiated pool die. These cells undergo morphological changes that are characteristic of programmed cell death (see
subsequent text).

E. Tightening the Ommatidial Pattern: Programmed Cell Death

The eye may provide an excellent model system for studying the role of
cell–cell interaction in regulating cell death. Most of the deaths occur during
a discrete period of ommatidial development; as with other cell decisions, cell
death appears to require cell–cell communication. Cell death is important for
proper eye development: producing an excess of cells early in development
ensures that the retina will contain a sufficient number of cells to create all the
cell types it will need later. When the last cell types are produced, unneeded
cells are then eliminated to refine the ommatidial pattern.

Cells that are removed in the retina undergo classical programmed cell
death or "apoptosis", a process distinct from death due to simple trauma
(Wyllie *et al.*, 1980). Apoptotic cells undergo a stereotyped series of morphological changes that appear to be the same from nematodes to humans.

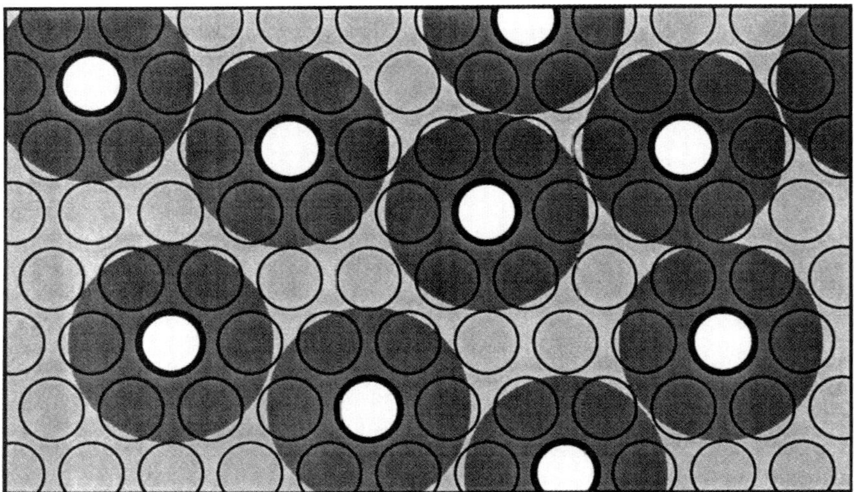

Figure 6. A model for spacing of neurons. A central founding cell (white) arises in a stochastic manner.
This central cell then inhibits other nearby cells from also becoming founders. The surrounding dark
circle represents the zone of inhibition produced by the central cell.

This includes detachment from the apical surface, a refractile appearance of the cytoplasm, condensation of the chromatin, and eventual phagocytosis by a neighboring cell. In *C. elegans,* in which control of cell death has been studied extensively, it has been shown that apoptosis is under strict genetic control (e.g., Hedgecock *et al.,* 1983).

In the retina, several mutations (e.g., *facet-glossy*) block primary pigment cell development and cell death, suggesting that primaries select, directly or indirectly, which cells will die. Moreover, cells in the retina appear not to be selected for death simply by their failure to respond to directive cues. Rather, preventing primary pigment cell development prevents cell death, suggesting that cells must be actively directed to die. Interestingly, when cells are prevented from dying, as in *facet-glossy* eyes, they invariably differentiate instead into cells that resemble secondary pigment cells. As with their neighbors, these cells will differentiate into secondary pigment cells unless specifically directed away from that fate into programmed cell death.

A similar situation was seen for development of the linker cell in nematodes (Sulston *et al.,* 1980). Although most cell deaths in the nematode are cell autonomous, the programmed death of the linker cell can be rescued by ablating the neighboring P12.pa cell. This suggests that contact with its neighbor directs the linker cell to die. The P12.pa cell has been dubbed the "killer cell" for its role in the linker cell's death. Similarly in the retina, when the primary pigment cell is removed by mutation, no cell death is observed.

F. Development of the Bristle

In several respects, formation of the bristle complex seems to stand apart from ommatidial development. Remarkably, the first bristles arise, not at the posterior edge of the eye disc, but at its center. Addition of later bristles occurs progressively more peripherally, radiating out toward the disc's edge. This radiating pattern is superimposed on the posterior-to-anterior progression of ommatidial development. Furthermore, the cells that give rise to each bristle rarely make contact with already differentiated cells in the surrounding ommatidia. Instead, they arise in the pool of undifferentiated cells found between ommatidia.

The first bristles begin differentiating early in pupation, somewhat before the primary pigment cells appear. The first sign of bristle development is the appearance of bristle mother cells; these cells stain strongly with cobalt sulfide and are found between ommatidia in the pool of undifferentiated cells. The bristle mother cell undergoes two rounds of cell division to produce the four cells that compose the bristle. The trichogen and tormogen are created first and will later secrete the bristle and bristle shaft, respectively. The sensory neuron and its support cell, the thecogen, are the last cells to arise. These four cells align themselves in a row. The neuron then moves under the thecogen, the trichogen enwraps the neuron and thecogen, and finally the tormogen enwraps the inner three. The result is a sensory structure whose cross-sectional profile resembles a bull's eye, with the neuron at the center (Fig. 7).

G. Production of Secondary Structures

The addition and sorting of cells is mostly completed within 60 hr of pupation. By this stage, the eye is a striking crystalline lattice with each cell in its proper position. Each cell must next produce its characteristic secondary structures. The cone cells and primary pigment cells secrete the high central portion of the corneal lens. The secondary and tertiary pigment cells secrete the low portion of the lens. R cells stack fingers of microvilli to form rhabdomeres, which are specialized light-gathering rods. Meanwhile, the cells in the

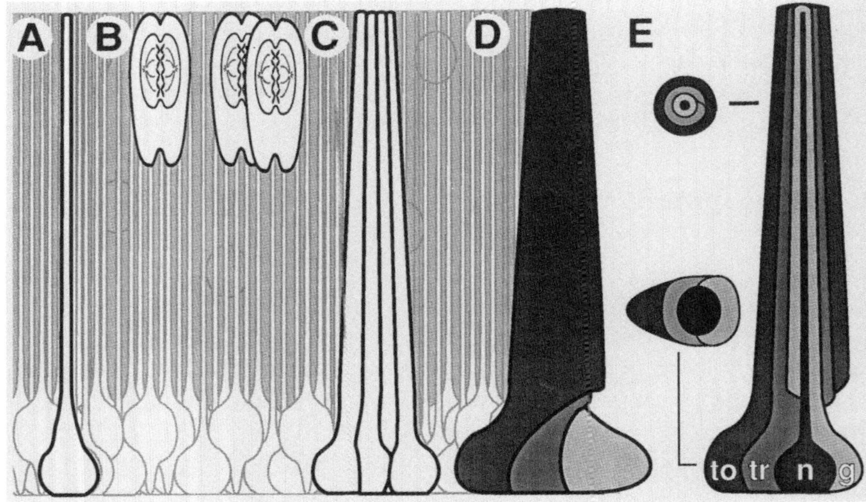

Figure 7. Schematic of bristle development. For clarity, the cells are not drawn to scale. A. The bristle group is derived from a single mother cell. B. Two rounds of cell division result in four cells. C. First to appear are the trichogen and tormogen, then the neuron and thecogen. The four cells are aligned in a row: tormogen–trichogen–neuron–thecogen. D. The thecogen slides over the neuron, then the trichogen and tormogen enwrap the inner two. E. A cut-away view of the bristle group of a 60-hr pupa, showing the neuron (n), the thecogen or glial cell (g), the trichogen (tr), and the tormogen (to). The neuron is occluded from the top by the thecogen. Anterior is approximately to the right. (From Cagan and Ready, 1989b; reprinted by permission of the publisher.)

eye elongate, increasing the distance from the lens to the floor fourfold. The result of this developmental process is the beautifully structured optical unit portrayed schematically in Fig. 1.

IV. Developmental Analysis of the Retina

A. Cell Lineage Relationships as Assessed by Genetic Mosaic Analysis

Until the mid-1970s, most researchers assumed that arthropod ommatidia developed from a single cell in a lineage-dependent manner. This view was not surprising since each ommatidium contained eight R cells: three rounds of cell divisions would yield eight cells from a single precursor. Indeed, Bernard (1937) inferred just such a lineage relationship between members of an ommatidium in the ant. How could such an idea be tested? In many systems lineage can be tested using genetic mosaics. In the fly such mosaics can be generated with mitotic recombination. Mitotic recominbation in the eye commonly exploits the *white* gene as a cell marker. When flies heterozygous for *white* are irradiated, recombination commonly occurs between a cell's sister chromatids to produce a daughter homozygous for *white*. If this daughter then undergoes many rounds of cell divisions, it will produce a readily visible patch of unpigmented *white*[−] cells surrounded by pigmented *white*[+] cells (Fig. 8). All the cells in the mutant patch are derived from a single progenitor.

Ready, Hansen, and Benzer (1976) showed that ommatidia at the clone boundaries frequently contained cells of both genotypes. Furthermore, they showed that the various R cells in an ommatidium could be genetically different, ruling out a strict cell lineage mechanism for generating them. They also found that an unpigmented clone derived from a single precursor cell early in development could give rise to both R cells and pigment cells, an observation that argued against specific stem cell populations that generate these different cell types. Lawrence and Green (1979) extended these observations by analyzing mosaic patches generated at late stages of development. They could find no strict lineage relationships between any of the R cells or between R cells and pigment cells. Hence, in the absence of any data supporting cell lineage relationships between cells, it was concluded that cell fate determination during ommatidial assembly is a consequence of cell–cell interactions.

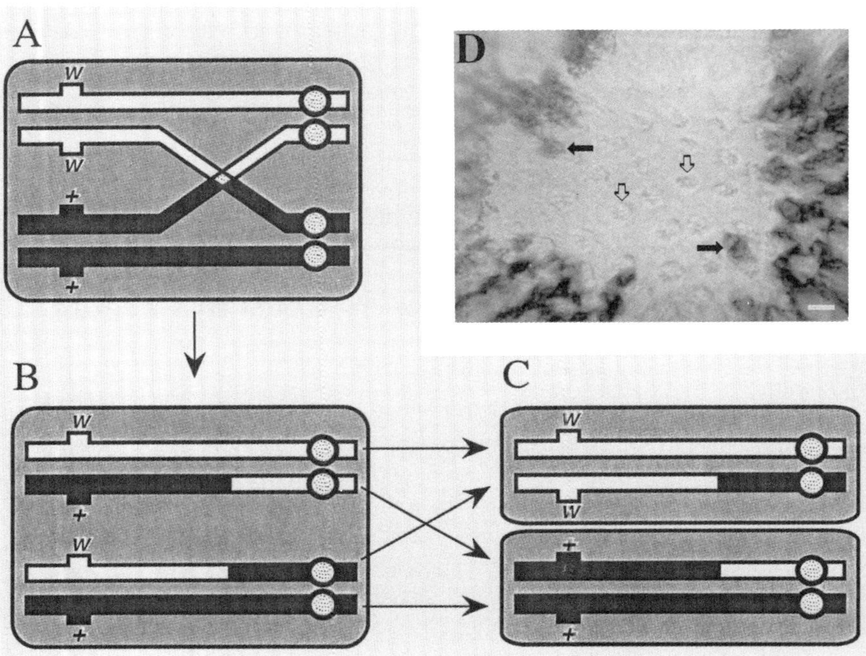

Figure 8. Producing genetic mosaics by irradiation. If mitotically active cells heterozygous for a mutation are irradiated, a patch of homozygous tissue can sometimes be produced. A. In this example, the cell is heterozygous for the visible marker *white (w): w/+*. The *w* chromosome is represented as white and the + chromosome as black. Before the late larval stage, cells in the eye disc are mitotically active. Irradiation, subsequent to chromosomal duplication but before chromosomal segregation, can cause breakage of the DNA strands. B. A chimeric chromosome can result by homologous recombination. C. If the chromosomes then segregate as shown, the daughter cells will give rise to a red pigmented (+/+) clone and a white unpigmented clone. D. An example of a mosaic patch induced by irradiation. In this example, *w* has been linked to the *Notch* allele *facet–glossy (fa^g)* to assess *fa^g*'s autonomy (see text). The open arrows indicate two unpigmented ommatidia in the patch. The solid arrows indicate two pigmented cells that, due to the mixing of cells during proliferation, are in the *w* patch. Mixed areas such as these are especially useful for demonstrating that *fa^g* is required autonomously for primary pigment cell development (see text). Bar: 8 μm.

B. Sequential Differentiation of R Cells

Since each cell's lineage does not lead it to its appropriate fate, the information needed to make a proper choice must come from its environment. The model currently favored is that cells direct the fate of their neighbors by direct cell–cell contact. The best method of testing this model is direct ablation of neighboring cells or removing identified cells and studying them *in vitro*. However, cells in the fly retina are generally too small to manipulate or easily ablate. Nevertheless, three lines of evidence led to the proposal that direct cell–cell contact specify cell fate. First, Lebovitz and Ready (1986) cut away large portions of the eye disc early in development, removing areas that contained differentiated cells. When the remaining small pieces were cultured, ommatidia developed normally in a posterior-to-anterior gradient. They concluded that the information required to direct cell fate was present locally.

Morphological studies provided a second piece of evidence in support of this view. Waddington (1962), Ready *et al.* (1976), and Campos-Ortega (1980) showed that cells achieve stereotyped positions in the retina, both in the adult and in the eye disc. Using electron microscopy, Tomlinson (1985) provided a detailed description of ommatidial development near the morphogenetic furrow. He found that contacts made between cells are highly stereotyped, even during the earliest stages of their development. By the third row posterior to the morphogenetic furrow, each R cell in the initial five-cell cluster is precisely positioned. Later when R1, R6, and R7 arise, they consistently contact R2/R8, R5/R8, and R1/R6/R8, respectively. A similar precision of contacts is seen during differentiation of the cone cells. The extreme invariance of these contacts led to the view that unique contacts directed a cell to assume a specific cell fate.

Antibodies provided the third evidence supporting this view. Using neuron- and R-cell-specific antibodies 22C10 and anti-HRP, Tomlinson and Ready (1987a) showed that R cells differentiated in a specific and invariant order. Neuronal antigens appeared first in R8, then R2 and R5, then R3 and R4, then R1 and R6, and finally in R7. They surmised that this sequence of antigen expression reflected the sequence of R cell determination, and it led them to a model based on the sequential induction of cell identities.

C. Sequential Induction Model

Based on the morphology and order of R cell differentiation, Tomlinson and Ready proposed a combinatorial model, in which contacts with previously differentiated cells direct cells to new fates. In other words, the position of each cell decides its fate. More specifically, they proposed that two cells that by chance contact R8 early in ommatidial development become R2 or R5. Next, cells contacting R8 and R2 or R5 become R3, R4, R1, or R6. An undifferentiated cell in contact with R8 and R1/R6 becomes R7. Cells contacting the R cells would become cone cells. Subsequent work by Cagan and Ready (1989b) extended this model to later development. Primary pigment cells could arise from contacts with the anterior and posterior cone cells. In turn, contact with the primaries could direct development of the secondary and tertiary pigment cells (Fig. 9).

At each step, cells are recruited from the surrounding undifferentiated pool of cells. In this manner, a cell's position decides its developmental fate. Implicit in this model is the concept that communication between cells occurs by the binding of specific receptors and ligands between neighboring cells. Consistent with this idea, at least three transmembrane proteins have been found that are involved in specifying cell fate. These three proteins, products of *sevenless, bride of sevenless,* and *Notch,* will be discussed in Section V.

D. Evidence That Specific Cellular Interactions Regulate Development

Genetic mosaics provide a means for determining the site of action of a particular gene. When a mutation in a gene affects the development of a particular cell type, it is important to determine whether the normal gene

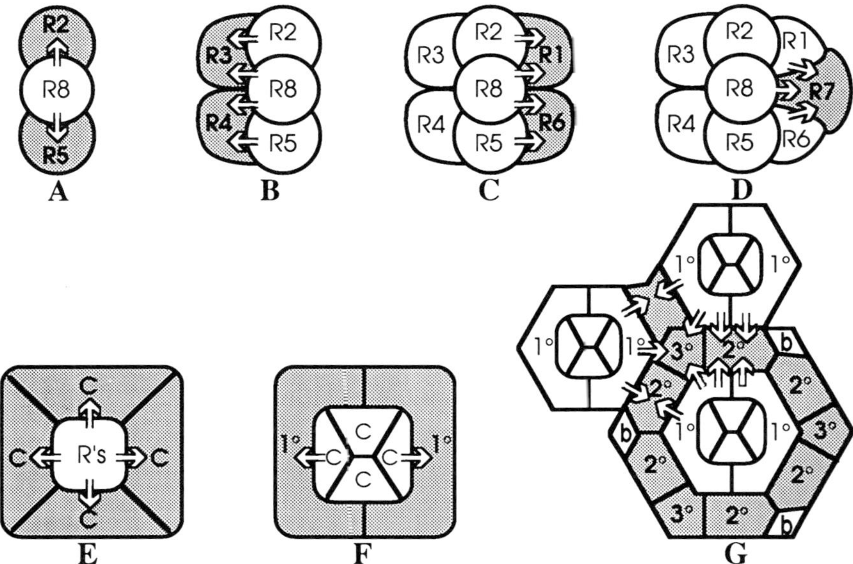

Figure 9. The sequential induction model. As proposed by Tomlinson and Ready (1987a) and Cagan and Ready (1989b), cell fate is determined by the sequential accumulation of determinative events; this information is transmitted via interactions between neighboring cells. As a result, each cell's position within the cluster decides its fate. For example, R8 directs two neighboring cells to differentiate as R2 and R5 (A); R8, R2, and R5 specify R3 and R4 (B), and so on (C–G). The flow of determinative information is indicated by arrows. Abbreviations: R, R cell; c, cone cell; 1°, primary pigment cell; 2°, secondary pigment cell; 3°, tertiary pigment cell; b, bristle.

product is required in the cells affected (i.e., autonomously) or elsewhere (i.e., nonautonomously). The strategy is similar to that outlined previously: use mitotic recombination to generate patches of marked (e.g., *white)* mutant tissue and examine the genetically mixed ommatidia found at the clonal boundaries. Indeed, genetic mosaics have not only proven useful for examining the requirement of various genes during development, they have also provided the best evidence that cells control the development of their neighbors.

The first genetic evidence for the induction of cell fate by a neighboring cell came from studies of the *bride of sevenless (boss)* gene. In *boss* mutants, R7 is missing (Reinke and Zipursky, 1988). The defect occurs early in development, when a cell positioned to become R7 fails to express neural- or R-cell-specific markers (Hart *et al.,* 1990). Genetic mosaics using the visible markers *white* or *chaoptic* were produced to decide which cell required normal *boss* function. These analyses demonstrated that the *boss* genotype of R8 alone determined whether R7 will develop; an R7 cell can form if, and only if, R8 is *boss$^+$*. If R8 is *boss$^-$*, the R7 cell invariably fails to form. Since the *boss* defect is seen early, this mosaic study provides strong evidence that differentiating cells in the retina do indeed play a role in directing other cell fates. The fact that R7's development requires *boss* in an adjoining cell is compatible with the idea that this interaction is mediated through direct cell–cell contact.

Mosaic analysis of another gene, *retina aberrant in pattern* or *rap,* has also shown the importance of R8 in ommatidial assembly. *rap* flies have severely roughened eyes, a result of scattered ommatidia that contain varying numbers of R cells (Karpilow *et al.,* 1989). These defects occur very early in ommatidial development: aberrations can be seen in ommatidial clustering near the morphogenetic furrow. Using genetic mosaic analysis, *white rap* cells were generated in a wild-type background. Normal ommatidia that contained R cells of mixed genotype were examined; abnormal ommatidia could not be examined, since the identity of R cells is difficult to determine if they are out of position. Whenever genotypically mixed but developmentally normal ommatidia were examined, R8 was always *rap$^+$*, regardless of the *rap* genotype of the other ommatidial cells. Again, the proper assembly of the ommatidium is affected by a mutant allele in R8. The *rap* gene is a good candidate for helping direct either the fate of R8 or its ability to recruit cells correctly into an ommatidial cluster.

Finally, work on another gene has shown that R cells other than R8 are responsible for proper recruitment of cells. *rough* flies gain their name from the roughened appearance of the adult eye, the result of ommatidia containing varying numbers of R cells. A mosaic analysis of genotypically mixed ommatidia of normal cellular composition revealed that *rough* was required only in R2 and R5 for normal development: whenever these two cells were genotypically wild type at the *rough* locus, the ommatidium was normal (Tomlinson *et al.,* 1988). As in the case of *rap,* the genotype of R2 and R5 in mutant ommatidia could not be assessed. These data indicate that *rough* is required in R2 and R5 for the normal development of R3 and R4. Whether this effect is direct or indirect will be discussed in Section V.E.

V. The Role of Specific Genes in Regulating Eye Development

Several different approaches have been used in an effort to understand the molecular basis of the developmental decisions that regulate eye development. The first, and certainly the most powerful, approach has been the use of classical genetics to identify mutations that disrupt specific stages of ommatidial assembly. These genes have then been characterized using standard genetic and molecular techniques. The ability to compare development in mutant and wild-type eyes at the level of individual identifiable cells has proven a powerful way to assign potential roles to these genes. Some, such as *boss, rough,* and *sev,* are involved in specific steps along the developmental pathway, whereas others, such as *Notch,* affect a wide variety of cell decisions.

Since the eye develops in the mature larva, mutations in genes essential not only for eye development but for embryogenesis as well are often lethal to the embryo. Mutations in these genes can be difficult to isolate if flies do not survive long enough to develop eyes. The role of these essential genes can be determined through genetic mosaic analysis, creating patches of mutant tissue specifically in the eye. Alternatively, conditionally lethal mutations, such as the temperature-sensitive *Notch* allele N^{ts1}, can also be used to reduce a gene's activity at selected developmental stages.

Recently a powerful new method, the enhancer trap technique (O'Kane and Gehring, 1987; Bier *et al.,* 1989), has provided an opportunity for broad screening of essential genes expressed in the eye (e.g., Mlodzik *et al.,* 1990; see below). The enhancer trap screens involve mobilizing a transposable element containing the *Escherichia coli lacZ* gene into sites throughout the genome. Individual lines can be established that contain an insertion into a single site. The mobile element itself contains only a weak promoter to drive expression of the *lacZ* gene. If the construct transposes to a site near an enhancer that is controlling expression of a closely linked gene, the construct can come under the regulation of the enhancer. The result is the expression of the *lacZ* gene in a pattern similar to that of the endogenous gene. Its pattern of expression can be visualized immunologically or by using a chromogenic substrate. If the construct has inserted into the coding sequence of the gene, a mutation results. If not, mutations can often be created by re-mobilizing the element: excision is occasionally imprecise, removing DNA adjacent to the insert. Another important feature of screening with these enhancer traps is that they provide a molecular tag for cloning the gene.

A. *Notch* Plays a Permissive Role in Eye Development

Notch is a member of the neurogenic class of loci that are required in the embryo to limit the number of cells in the ventral ectoderm that assume a neuroblast cell fate (Poulson, 1937; Lehmann *et al.,* 1983; see Chapter 6). Interestingly, *Notch* is also required for proper eye development (Welshons, 1965; Dietrich and Campos-Ortega, 1984; Cagan and Ready, 1989a; Marko-poulou *et al.,* 1989). Using the *Notch* temperature-sensitive allele N^{ts1}, Cagan and Ready (1989a) found that *Notch* played a surprisingly general role in eye development. N^{ts1} flies placed at 32°C suffer a loss of *Notch* function. Shifting N^{ts1} flies to 32°C for brief periods during various stages of ommatidial assembly allowed the effects of reducing *Notch* activity on each developmental decision to be examined.

Larval temperature shifts resulted in recruitment of too many R cells in ommatidia near the morphogenetic furrow (see Fig. 5B). By contrast, these shifts blocked addition of R cells to more mature ommatidia (i.e., further posterior from the furrow). For example R7 was lost, resulting in an ommatidium with only seven R cells. When flies received successively later temperature pulses, the fates of potential cone cells, then bristles, and finally pigment cells were changed in much the same manner. Each cell type was affected if the temperature shift occurred at the stage during which that cell normally began its differentiation.

In addition to affecting cell decisions directly, these temperature shifts showed how early defects can cascade into later ones. For example, an early reduction in *Notch* activity resulted in ommatidia with too many R cells; even after returning the flies to the permissive temperature, these clusters subsequently recruited too many cone cells into the cluster (Fig. 9D). An especially striking example was seen for development of the primary pigment cells. Brief temperature shifts in the mature larva affected cone cells; in this region development of the primary pigment cells was abnormal as well. This effect on primaries occurred even if the larva was returned to the permissive temperature a full day before primaries were added to the cluster. The simplest interpretation is that normal primary pigment cell development requires normal cone cell development. This provides strong evidence that cells do indeed play an important role in recruiting later cell types into the cluster.

Since local cell communication plays an important role in eye development, it is important to determine which of two interacting cells requires *Notch* activity. The question of *Notch*'s autonomy can be answered in the eye by making use of an unusual allele of *Notch, facet-glossy (fa^g). facet-glossy* flies have a retrotransposon insertion in the second intron of *Notch* (Kidd and Young, 1986; Markopoulcu *et al.*, 1989). The result of this insertion is the selective loss of primary pigment cells and the absence of cell death during development (Cagan and Ready, 1989a). This phenotype can be phenocopied by temperature shifts of N^{ts1} and N^{ts1}/fa^g in young pupae (Shellenbarger and Mohler, 1975), indicating that the loss of primary pigment cells in *facet-glossy* flies is due to a stage-specific reduction of *Notch* activity. The specificity of *facet-glossy*'s defects allowed an examination of the autonomy of *Notch. white fa^g* patches were produced in a wild type background by mitotic recombination, and genetically mixed ommatidia were examined. In the 115 mosaic ommatidia examined, all but one primary pigment cell were *white$^+$* (R. Cagan and D. Ready, unpublished observations). Thus the primary pigment cells required normal *Notch* activity autonomously to develop properly.[2] For a discussion of *Notch*'s autonomy in the embryo, see Chapter 6.

The broad range of decisions that require normal *Notch* activity in both neural and nonneural precursors suggests *Notch* does not directly specify particular cell fates. Rather, *Notch* appears to act permissively to allow other more specific interactions to occur. When *Notch* activity is reduced (e.g., by temperature shifts), cells appear to be unable to receive and act on information available from their neighbors. For example, near the morphogenetic furrow this communication restricts the number of cells that assume an R cell fate, whereas at later stages it appears to be required for the inductive interactions needed for the addition of other R cells. Based on the phenotype of *Notch* embryos, Hartenstein and Campos-Ortega (1984) have proposed that *Notch* plays a similarly important role in communication among neighbors in the ventral ectoderm (see Chapter 6).

B. A *Drosophila* Homolog of the EGF Receptor Controls the Number of R Cell Clusters

Recent studies have shown that the *DER* locus, which encodes a homolog of the epidermal growth factor receptor, plays an important role at several

---

[2]This single exception was expected, since *facet–glossy* eyes have a few primary pigment cells, indicating that penetrance is not 100%.

stages of fly development. An analysis of some of these alleles indicates that *DER* plays a key role in determining the number of ommatidial clusters arising at the furrow. Baker and Rubin (1989) found that flies containing a dominant *DER* allele, *Ellipse,* had small eyes with only a few ommatidia, although these ommatidia were normally structured (Fig. 10A). An examination of the morphogenetic furrow in *Ellipse* flies revealed the origin of the defect: newly forming ommatidia are spaced much farther apart than normal. Baker and Rubin suggest that the activity of *DER* could act to help regulate the number of clusters forming at the morphogenetic furrow, with high activity inhibiting cluster formation. Consistent with this view are preliminary results that suggest that the density of clusters may be increased in mitotically induced patches in the eyes of the partial-loss-of-function *DER* allele *torpedo* (R. Clifford, R. Cagan, and T. Schupbach, unpublished results).

C. The *sevenless* Gene Encodes a Receptor That Regulates R7 Development

Whereas *Notch* seems to be used by all cells in the eye to mediate cellular interactions, other genes play a more specific role. Two of these, *sevenless* and *bride-of-sevenless,* are involved in the specification of a single fate: that of R7. Tomlinson and Ready (1986) used their detailed knowledge of early ommatidial development to take a closer look at development of R7 in *sevenless* eyes. They were surprised to find that a cell did indeed appear to join the ommatidial cluster between R1 and R6 in the developing eye disc. However, this cell failed to differentiate into a neuron. Using electron micrographs, they serially reconstructed developing *sevenless* ommatidia and concluded that the cell in the place of R7 developed instead as an equatorial cone cell. Examining genetic mosaics generated by mitotic recombination, Campos-Ortega *et al.* (1979) and Tomlinson and Ready (1986) concluded that *sevenless* was required autonomously by the cell destined to become R7. They suggested that *sevenless* might be required in a pathway of cell–cell communication, and that a potential R7 cell required *sevenless* protein to receive or interpret proper instructions from its neighbor(s).

The structure of *sevenless* is consistent with this model. The *sevenless* gene encodes a transmembrane protein with a large extracellular domain, a proposed uncleaved signal sequence and a stretch of 22 amino acids proposed to span the membrane (Hafen *et al.,* 1987). Within the proposed intracellular carboxy terminus is a region with high homology to tyrosine kinases (Hafen *et al.,* 1987; Basler and Hafen, 1988; Bowtell *et al.,* 1988; Simon *et al.,* 1989). Similar sequences are found in membrane-bound receptors, such as those for epidermal growth factor and platelet-derived growth factor. In these proteins,

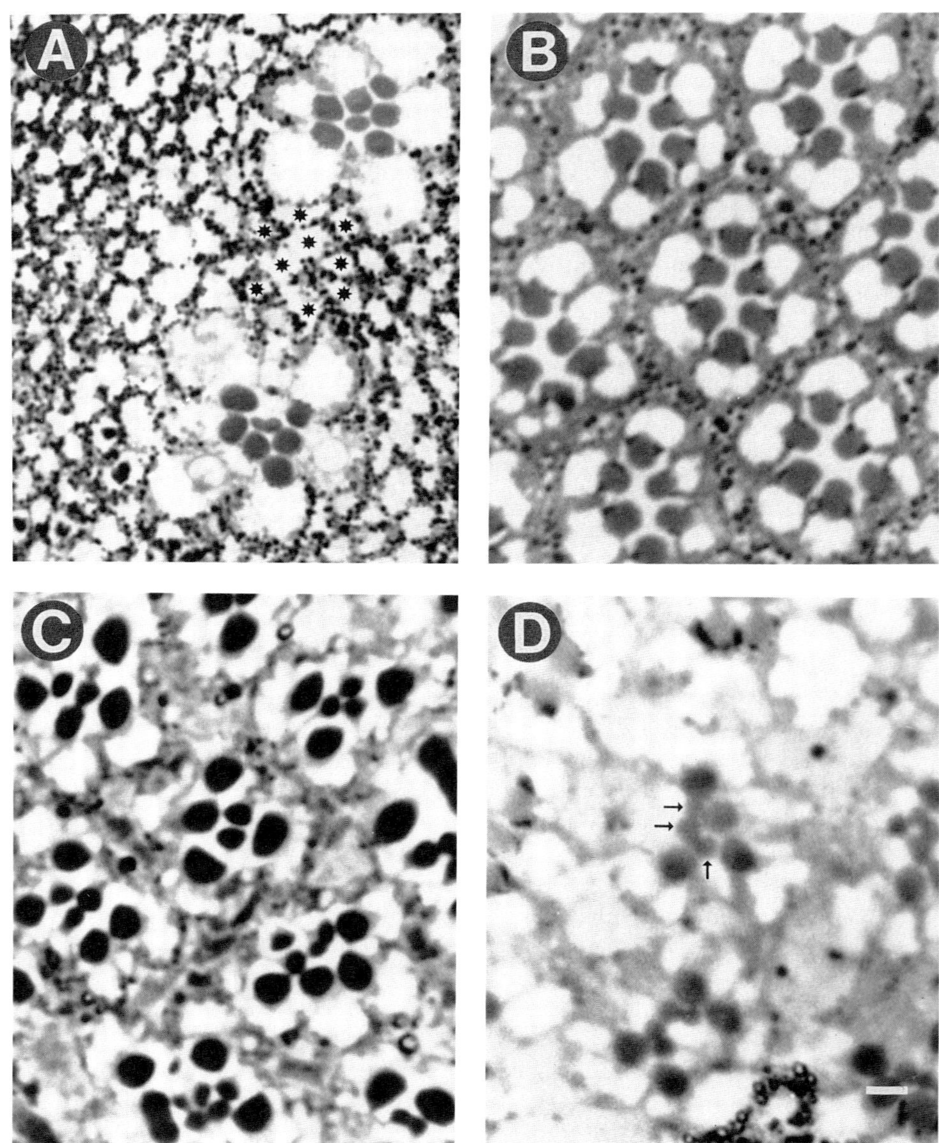

tyrosine kinase activity appears to transduce a signal when the extracellular portion binds an appropriate ligand (Hunter and Cooper, 1986). The membrane localization of *sevenless* has been confirmed biochemically and by visualization with antibodies directed to the sevenless protein (Banerjee *et al.,* 1987; Tomlinson *et al.,* 1987; Simon *et al.,* 1989). Thus, the structure and cell-surface localization of *sevenless* suggest it may directly bind a ligand from a neighboring cell. This direct interaction may then lead the receiving cell into the R7 developmental pathway. Consistent with this idea, when a truncated form of *sevenless* was expressed at high levels in cells that normally express *sevenless,* these cells were misrouted into the R7 pathway of development (Basler *et al.,* 1991).

Is expression of *sevenless* sufficient to direct a cell to become R7? Apparently not. Banerjee *et al.* (1987) and Tomlinson *et al.* (1987) found *sevenless* to be expressed on other R cells before appearing on R7. Banerjee *et al.* describe antisevenless staining in the apical microvilli of all R cells and cone cells. Tomlinson *et al.* find similar results, although their antibodies did not detect staining in R8, R2, and R5. Instead they describe a complex pattern of expression in the other R cells and cone cells. Thus, *sevenless* is necessary to direct a cell into the R7 pathway, but expression in a given cell is not sufficient.

To decide if the timing of *sevenless* expression is important, Basler and Hafen (1989) and Bowtell *et al.* (1989) fused the *sevenless* structural gene to the heat-inducible promoter hsp-70. By putting this construct into *sevenless* flies, *sevenless* expression could be turned on or off simply by changing the flies' ambient temperature. When a mature *sevenless* larva was heat pulsed, all cells in the developing eye expressed high levels of *sevenless* transcript. Ommatidia near the morphogenetic furrow at the time of the heat pulse recruited a single normal R7 cell. No other cells were obviously affected. Thus, *sevenless* appears to be required only at the time when an R7 cell is developing, and expression of *sevenless* in other cells will not redirect them into the R7 pathway. Thus, although the *sevenless* protein may indeed receive a signal

Figure 10 The adult ommatidial structure of four eyes containing mutations in genes required for normal eye development. A. Mutations in the *DER* allele *Ellipse* affect the spacing of ommatidial clusters. Instead of a single secondary and tertiary pigment cell between ommatidia, *Ellipse* eyes often have several intervening cells. In the example shown there are nine intervening cells (asterisks). B. Mutations in the *boss* gene specifically remove R7. As a result, the ommatidia's apical profiles contain six R cells with large rhabdomeres, but none with a small rhabdomere. C. Mutations in the *rough* gene affect early R cell identity. Ommatidia contain aberrant numbers of R cells. D. *svp* ommatidia are characterized by an excess of R7-like cells. The small rhabdomeres of three of these cells are indicated with arrows. Sections near the surface of the mutant eyes as visualized with light microscopy; compare with Figs. 1D,2A. Anterior is to the right; bar: 5 μm.

directing a cell to become R7, regulation of the *sevenless* pathway must lie elsewhere.

D. The *boss* Gene Encodes a Membrane-Bound Ligand of *sevenless*

Mutations in the *bride-of-sevenless (boss)* gene give a phenotype similar to *sevenless:* loss of R7 (Fig. 10B). However, as we have discussed in the previous section, this phenotype is strictly correlated with loss of *boss* activity in R8. Is *boss* the ligand that binds to the putative receptor encoded by *sevenless?* Its sequence appears to encode a 912-amino acid transmembrane protein with a large N-terminal extracellular domain (501 a.a.), a smaller intracellular C-terminal domain (120 a.a.), and seven transmembrane domains (Hart *et al.,* 1990). Although *boss* does not appear to contain any obviously conserved sequences, the seven transmembrane domains would give the *boss* protein a structure similar to a family of receptors involved in translating binding of an extracellular signal into intracellular information (e.g., LH receptor, β-adrenergic receptor, and the rhodopsins). However, since no specific sequences are conserved, the significance of *boss'* structural similarity to this family of receptors remains unclear.

The sevenless protein was localized with antibodies ot the region of R7 that juxtaposes R8, leading Tomlinson *et al.* (1987) to propose that the ligand activating *sevenless* is produced in R8. Consistent with this model, the boss protein is made exclusively in R8: antibodies directed to the boss protein recognized it in the endoplasmic reticulum of R8 only (Krämer *et al.,* 1991). Interestingly, boss is concentrated mainly in the apical microvilli of R8, much as the sevenless protein is found mainly in the microvilli of the surrounding cells. Perhaps the strongest morphological evidence that boss is a ligand of sevenless is that it is found in a multivesicular body (MVB) in R7. Localization to similar MVBs has been seen for other receptor/ligand complexes such as those for EGF, LDL, insulin, and asialoglycoprotein (e.g., Felder *et al.,* 1990; Ullrich and Schlessinger, 1990). The localization of boss in R7 is lost in a *sevenless*-null mutant, and remains in a *sevenless*-defective (but protein-positive) mutant, suggesting that boss requires only the presence of sevenless protein and not *sevenless* activity for uptake.

Perhaps the strongest evidence that the proteins encoded by *boss* and *sevenless* interact directly was found by expressing each in *Drosophila* Schneider (S2) cells (Krämer *et al.,* 1991). S2 cells expressing either *boss* or *sevenless* remain as a single cell suspension. When the two cell populations were mixed, large aggregates formed consisting of both cell types. This aggregation was blocked with antibodies directed to either the boss or sevenless proteins, indicating that boss and sevenless are interacting directly to bind the cells together. Interestingly, the boss protein is internalized into vesicles in the sevenless-expressing cells, reminiscent of the MVBs seen *in vivo*. Whether the interaction with boss is sufficient for activation of the sevenless tyrosine kinase is currently under study.

E. The *rough* Gene Encodes a Homeobox Protein That Specifies Cell Fate

As discussed earlier, the *rough* gene is required in R2 and R5 for the proper development of R3 and R4. Unfortunately, whether *rough* affects R cells added after R3 and R4 is unknown, since poor ommatidial packing makes it difficult to assess cell identities (Fig. 10C). The *rough* gene has been cloned and sequenced. The predicted rough protein contains 350 amino acids, including a 61-amino acid domain similar to sequences shown to bind DNA in other proteins (Saint *et al.,* 1988; Tomlinson *et al.,* 1988). This region, termed the homeobox, is a transcriptional regulator which is also found in other developmentally important genes throughout the animal kingdom (for a review, see De Robertis *et al.,* 1990). Antibodies generated against the *rough* protein stain first in nearly all cells in the morphogenetic furrow, quickly resolving specifically to R2, R3, R4, and R5 (Kimmel *et al.,* 1990).

The presence of a homeobox motif in *rough* suggests that it is involved directly in regulating genes. But for what purpose? Perhaps *rough* is part of a pathway used by R2 and R5 to control the development of R3 and R4. This would explain its nonautonomous requirement. Alternatively, R2 and R5 could use *rough* directly for proper differentiation; when they develop abnormally, R3 and R4 are affected as a secondary consequence.

To better decide *rough*'s role in development, Kimmel *et al.* (1990) and Basler *et al.* (1990) attached the *rough* coding region to the promoter of *sevenless,* a gene expressed in R7 as well as in other ommatidial cells. R7 can be identified by its short thin rhabdomere and by expression of the R7-specific rhodopsins, Rh3 and Rh4. Expressing *rough* ectopically in R7 produced a cell in the position of R7 that contained a long thick rhabdomere and expressed the R1–R6 specific rhodopsin, Rh1. Genetic mosaics indicated that this transformation was cell autonomous, suggesting that expression of *rough* is sufficient to direct a cell into an R1–R6 fate. Given the requirement of the *rough* gene in R2 and R5 for normal ommatidial assembly, it is tempting to speculate that expression of *rough* in R7 has transformed it into an R2/R5 identity.

This result suggests that *rough*'s effects on R3 and R4 development are indirect. Development in R3 and R4 is abnormal, presumably because they require normal R2/R5 development. A closer look at early development of *rough* eyes appears to confirm this: R2 and R5 show aberrations in their position and expression of neural markers. In addition, cells in the position of R2 and R5 often express boss protein, indicating an early misrouting into the R8 pathway (Van Vactor *et al.,* 1991). These studies highlight an important distinction when considering the nature of autonomy and nonautonomy, especially in developmental systems that rely on complex interactions to specify a phenotype. Distinguishing between direct and indirect requirements for a gene is easier when cell-specific markers exist that can unambiguously identify individual cell types early in eye development.

F. The *seven-up* Gene Specifies R1, R3, R4, and R6 Cell Fates

seven-up was one of the first genes isolated through the use of an enhancer trap screen. It was isolated as a lethal insertion of a *P-lacZ* transposon into a region previously defined by the lethal complementation group *ck16.* Because members of this group died as embryos, its eye phenotype had not been recognized. However, one copy of the enhancer trap insert into *seven-up* provided a provocative staining pattern in both the embryo and the eye. In the eye, the *seven-up* insert stained R1, R3, R4, and R6 specifically (Mlodzik *et al.,* 1990).

The *seven-up* gene encodes at least two transcripts, giving rise to protein products of 543 and 746 amino acids. The sequence of *svp* places it in the steroid receptor superfamily, a family of proteins containing both steroid-hormone-binding and DNA-binding domains. Members of this family include the receptors for glucocorticoid and retinoic acid. The smaller protein's amino acid sequence is 75% identical to the human transcription factor COUP. This homology is intriguing because it suggests a possible role for diffusible cues in regulating cell–cell interactions.

The name for *seven-up* comes from its eye phenotype. Although mutations at the *svp* locus are embryonic lethal, its role in the eye could be examined in mosaic patches generated by mitotic recombination. Most genotypically *svp* ommatidia had the proper number of R cells, though some contained an additional cell. What was unusual was the number of small rhabdomeres with respect to large ones (Fig. 10D). Recall that in a normal ommatidum near the apical surface, R1, R2, R3, R4, R5, and R6 have large rhabdomeres, whereas only R7 has a small one. Thus, each ommatidium should have only one small rhabdomere near the surface of the eye. Typical *svp* ommatidia have 3–5. Furthermore, these cells with small rhabdomeres express the R7-specific rhodopsin Rh4. Thus, *svp* ommatidia appear to have too many R7 cells.

To determine which cells might be transformed into R7 cells, Mlodzik *et al.* (1990) examined genotypically mixed ommatidia at the edge of mosaic patches. Normal ommatidia were found only when R1, R3, R4, and R6 were svp^+, the very cells in which the enhancer trap was expressed. Apparently, loss of *svp* activity has misdirected these cells into the R7 pathway. Counting R7 itself, this would account for the five R7-like cells seen in many *svp* ommatidia. Mlodzik *et al.* suggested that *svp* is required for R1/R3/R4/R6 fate. Perhaps the role of *svp* is to repress the R7 pathway in R1, R3, R4, and R6. When *svp* activity is removed, this repression is removed and the cells enter the R7 pathway. Surprisingly, only some of these R7-like cells require *sevenless.* When *svp* clusters were produced in a *sevenless* background, generally only three of the five R7-like cells were removed. The other two R7-like cells appeared to be unaffected, and remained in the ommatidium. The significance of this observation will be considered in Section VI.

VI. Perspective

Although study of the *Drosophila* eye is a relatively young field, an intriguing picture of cell choice and patterning is beginning to emerge. Lineage and disc culturing studies indicate that local information directs cell fate. Careful morphological studies reveal that cell–cell contacts are remarkably stereotyped, suggesting that they could be used to provide the information needed to direct cell fate. Isolating and manipulating some of the molecules that carry this information has begun to refine this picture, and promises to further elucidate the mechanisms involved. Many of the genes discussed in this chapter, when mutated, switch a particular cell fate into another, a process referred to by Bateson as "homeosis" (1894). Examining the interactions among various genes involved in specific pathways should provide important information on the basis of their action in driving the development of the eye. Some of these experiments have been presented in previous sections. In this section we consider three issues: (1) the initiation of ommatidial cluster formation; (2) an assessment of the sequential induction model; and (3) the specification of the R7 cell fate.

A. Initiating Ommatidial Cluster Formation

Events at the morphogenetic furrow represent a somewhat unusual example of neural patterning since ommatidial clusters appear at the furrow in a line (Figs. 3, 4). Thus the eye can be viewed as being built in a one-dimensional pattern, a process that could simplify formation of the reiterated pattern of ommatidia. This special precision is needed because, unlike many higher neural systems that rely on extensive neuronal plasticity during development, the acuity of the eye is directly related to the precise organization of the cells that compose it.

Little is known about the initial events of cluster formation. In Section III,A we discussed the possibility that each ommatidium contains a founder cell that, in addition to recruiting cells to form a cluster, prevents formation of nearby clusters. R8 is perhaps the best candidate for this role: it is the first R cell to differentiate, and is found at the center of the ommatidial cluster where it contacts all other R cells. Unfortunately, as with the other cells in the eye disc, the small apical profile of R8 does not easily permit cell ablation studies, which would critically address whether R8 serves a founder cell function.

If R8 is indeed the founder cell, then its identity must be determined before cluster formation, presumably in the morphogenetic furrow. However, although many antibodies recognize R8 early, none do so before the second or third row after the furrow. This is true of antibodies directed generally toward neurons, such as anti-HRP, Mab 22C10, and anti-elav, as well as of more specific antibodies directed toward the *chaoptin* and *boss* gene products. Thus it remains unclear whether cluster formation requires proper R cell determination.

Recent studies with *glass,* a site-specific DNA binding protein (K. Moses and G. Rubin, personal communication), suggest the processes of cluster formation and R cell identity may indeed be separable. Ommatidial clusters in genotypically *glass* eyes express neural-specific antigens but fail to express R-cell-specific ones. For example, in normal eyes antibodies to the boss protein stain R8 early in its development; in *glass* eyes this staining is absent (H. Krämer, personal communication). The loss of R-cell-specific staining has been interpreted as a failure of cells in *glass* eyes to make the transition from neuron to R cell (Ready *et al.,* 1986; Moses *et al.,* 1989). Nevertheless, cluster formation is relatively unaffected (Moses *et al.,* 1989). Thus, what appears to be affected in *glass* eyes is not the initial clustering event but the subsequent appearance of R cell identities in the cluster.

A view of early clustering events as visualized with cobalt sulfide also supports a separation of cluster formation and R cell identity. As can be seen in Fig. 3, the first clusters to arise from the morphogenetic furrow usually contain 6–8 cells, generally with a central cell ("mystery cell," see Tomlinson and Ready, 1987a; Cagan and Ready, 1989a) surrounded by 5–7 cells on its posterior face. Although in the second row 2–3 cells often show heavy staining among these 5–7 cells, by the third row often only the fuure R8 will remain heavily stained. Interestingly, the third row is about the stage at which many of the neural (e.g., HRP) and R-cell (e.g., boss) specific antigens are first expressed in R8. Thus, currently available reagents only recognize R-cell specific differentiation after cluster formation.

Based on this evidence, we propose that cluster formation occurs before R cell determination, and does so in a stochastic manner. In this view, cluster formation is initiated either by a nonneural founder cell such as the central mystery cell or perhaps by aggregation of cells with no single founder. Once the cluster is formed, interactions between cells in the cluster could then decide R8's identity. For example, the initial heavy staining with cobalt sulfide of 2–3 cells seen in row 2 of Fig. 3, which resolves to heavy staining of R8, could reflect a stochastic process by which one of these cells becomes R8. In other words, after the cluster is formed, competition between cells on the posterior face of the central mystery cell could decide which cell becomes R8. One prediction of this model is that, because cell identities are not produced *a priori,* the initial cluster should contain an excess of cells and later discard those that are not needed, allowing regulation of cell identities in the cluster. As described in Section III,B and Fig. 3, this is just what is seen.

Ommatidial formation also bears a striking resemblance to development of other sensory organs in the fly. For example, bristles in the thorax have been proposed to derive from "proneural" groups that bear a remarkable resemblance to ommatidial preclusters. These proneural groups are defined by the combined actions of several identified genes (for reviews, see Ghysen and Dambly-Chaudiere, 1988; Simpson, 1990). After these initial groups are defined, individual cells in the group are selected to be bristle precursors. This selection requires genes such as *Notch,* which, as we have seen, play an apparently similar role in the eye. Interestingly, no single precursor cell is proposed to be involved in spacing these proneural groups, suggesting that ommatidial precursors in the developing eye may not require a single founder cell either.

The determination of R8 appears rather similar to heterocyst development in the blue-green alga *Anabaena. Anabaena* is composed mainly of a long string of vegetative cells with morphologically distinct nitrogen-fixing heterocysts spaced at regular intervals (Wilcox, 1970). Often more than one precursor cell, or proheterocyst, arises in an interval; later all but one will eventually regress back to the vegetative state. Experiments by Wilcox *et al.* (1973a,b,1975) suggest that competition between proheterocysts decide which cell becomes the heterocyst. A similar mechanism could decide which among the cells in the precluster becomes R8. Another feature of this model is that, if interactions do indeed occur among the line of cells at the posterior face of the central mystery cell, once R8 is determined it has only two neighbors in this line: the future R2 and R5. Similarly, only two cells are in contact with R2/R5, and these cells are the future R3 and R4 (Figs. 3B,11). Thus, this

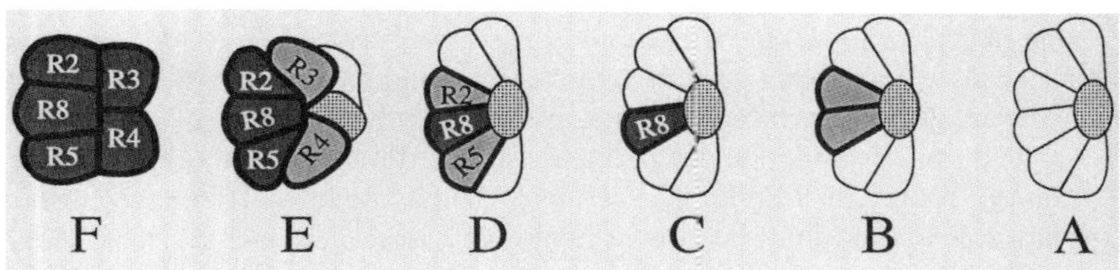

Figure 11. A model for determination of the first five R cells near the morphogenetic furrow (see Section VI). A. The initial clustering of cells next to the morphogenetic furrow typically contains 5–7 cells on the posterior face of a central "mystery cell." We propose that specific cell identities have yet to be determined. B. The heavy staining with cobalt sulfide of 2–3 cells, often seen in slightly more mature clusters, could reflect the stochastic determination of R8 (see Fig. 3A). C. Competition between these cells could result in a single R8, which can be uniquely recognized with currently available antibodies after it reaches the third row after the furrow. D. If only the cells along the posterior face of the cluster are competent to differentiate into R cells, then only two potential R cells are in contact with R8. These cells will, in fact, differentiate as R2 and R5. E. In a similar manner, R3 and R4 could receive their initial determinative cues from R2 and R5. F. R3 and R4 move together to produce the initial 5-cell precluster (see Fig. 3B, Rows 2,3).

model predicts that, once R8 is determined, the constraints of its neighbors' positions lead naturally to the required cell types.

B. Assessing the Sequential Induction Model

Using antibodies specific to neurons, Tomlinson and Ready (1987a) found that photoreceptors arise in each ommatidium in a stereotyped sequence: first R8, then R2/R5, R3/R4, R1/R6, and finally R7. This sequence of differentiation led them to propose a sequential induction model in which each R cell was induced by contact with previously determined R cells. This model, later extended to include the pigment cells and cell death (Cagan and Ready, 1989b), is discussed more fully in Section II,C. What is the evidence for the sequential induction model?

Three lines of evidence support the importance of interactions between cells for the specification of cell fates. First, the *sevenless* gene encodes a protein with a large extracellular domain and an intracellular protein tyrosine kinase motif. This structure is consistent with a role for *sevenless* in both receiving information from a neighboring cell and transducing that information into a cytoplasmic signal. Furthermore, the sevenless protein has been reported to be localized in the portion of R7's membrane that is adjacent to R8, suggesting that the *sevenless*-dependent signal for R7 development is received from R8. Second, the *boss* gene encodes a transmembrane protein that is both localized (Krämer *et al.*, 1991) and required (Reinke and Zipursky,

1988) solely in R8 for the development of the adjacent R7. Recent studies indicate that it functions as a ligand of the sevenless receptor. Third, although *rough* gene activity is required in R2 and R5, the development of R3 and R4 is also affected.

The importance of the sequential nature of inductive interactions in the eye is underscored by studies examining *Notch*'s role in ommatidial assembly (Cagan and Ready, 1989a; see Section IV,A). When *Notch* activity was reduced at each step in ommatidial development, cell types that normally appeared at that stage were misrouted into other developmental pathways. The simplest interpretation of these results is that *Notch* plays a permissive role in cell fate decisions: failure to express *Notch* may block a cell's ability to effectively communicate with its neighbor. Interestingly, when *Notch* activity was returned to the eye disc a few hours later, cells differentiated as a cell type appropriate for the new developmental time. For example, early temperature shifts of N^{ts1} flies blocked cone cell differentiation; restoring *Notch* activity produced a primary pigment cell from a cell that would normally become a cone cell. Notice that the *position* of the cell has not changed, since it is in contact with the same cells as before the shift began. Thus timing appears to be crucial and the ommatidium has irreversibly lost a cone cell. The simplest model to account for these observations is that information is presented on the surface of a neighboring cell for a limited period of time. If the cell does not respond to this signal in the allotted time, it must await the next signal.

C. Induction of R7

R7 development presents one of the first opportunities to study induction of a single cell type in a developing nervous system. Several genes have already been isolated that play a role in its development. Studies with *boss* suggest that R8 plays a key role in specifying the R7 fate. Studies with the *sevenless* tyrosine kinase gives an indication of one mechanism through which this external information is conveyed. In addition, other genes important for R7 development have been isolated. For example, mutations in the gene *sevenless in absentia (sina)* block R7 development in much the same way as *boss* and *sevenless*. The *sina* gene, which unlike *boss* and *sevenless* has subtle effects on other adult structures, encodes a nuclear protein (Carthew and Rubin, 1990). Other genes are currently being characterized from enhancer trap lines that are expressed in R7.

Despite the remarkable specificity of *sevenless* for R7 induction, recent studies suggest that it may play a permissive, rather than instructive, role in R7 development. For instance, removing *seven-up* activity produced several ectopic R7s in each ommatidium, one or two of which remained in a *sevenless* background. Thus, not only is expression of *sevenless* not sufficient to induce an R7 fate, it appears that in certain genetic backgrounds it is not absolutely required (Mlodzik *et al.*, 1990). Another experiment also suggests that *sevenless*'s role may be more permissive. Recall that when *rough* was ectopically expressed in the cell normally destined to become R7, that cell became an R1–R6 type. This transformation was dependent on normal *sevenless* activity: in a *sevenless* background the transformed cell was missing. In other words, if a cell can join the cluster in the position of R7, *rough* expression can reroute it to a different fate. Apparently activation of the *sevenless* kinase is required for a cell to be responsive to internal cues that actually specify its fate. Similarly, one might expect that ectopic expression of *seven-up* in the prospective R7 would repress expression of the R7 fate, and an R1–R6 type cell should arise in the position of R7. Despite is altered fate, development of this cell should still be *sevenless* dependent.

Several genetic approaches have been used to identify other interacting components of the R7 inductive pathway. For instance, an allele-specific suppressor of *sevenless* called *Son of sevenless (Sos)* has been isolated (U. Banerjee, personal communication). A single copy of the dominant suppressor *Sos* restores R7s to 18% of the ommatidia in the *sevenless* allele *sev^{E4}*. Since *Sos* only suppresses a specific allele of *sevenless,* it may represent a compensatory mutation that restores a functional interaction with *sev^{E4}*. Deleting the *Sos* locus gave rise to recessive lethal mutations; mosaic patches in the eye showed disturbances in ommatidial development. Simon and Rubin (personal communication) have made use of a different strategy to isolate enhancers of *sevenless.* The *sevenless* gene was mutagenized *in vitro* to produce a temperature-sensitive allele, *sev^{ts}*. This construct was especially useful for isolating interacting genes because it showed an intermediate *sevenless* activity at 23°C so a subset of ommatidia contained R7s. Mutagenized flies were examined in a *sev^{ts}* background for a change in the number of ommatidia with R7s. Seven enhancers were found, of which one was allelic to *Sos.* The roles these genes may play in R7 determination is currently being assessed. In addition, further genetic screens and molecular characterization of the genes defined by mutations will provide insight into the mechanisms by which the inductive interactions between cells are translated into cell fate.

References

Baker, N., and Rubin, G. (1989). Effect on eye development of dominant mutations in *Drosophila* homologue of the EGF receptor. *Nature (London)* **340,** 150–153.

Banerjee, U., Renfranz, P. J., Pollack, J. A., and Benzer, S. (1987). Molecular characterization and expression of *sevenless*, a gene involved in neuronal pattern formation in the *Drosophila* eye. *Cell* **49**, 281–291.

Basler, K., and Hafen, E. (1988). Control of photoreceptor cell fate by the *sevenless* protein requires a functional tyrosine kinase domain. *Cell* **54**, 299–311.

Basler, K., and Hafen, E. (1989). Ubiquitous expression of *sevenless*: Position-dependent specification of cell fate. *Science* **243**, 931–934.

Basler, K., Yen, D., Tomlinson, A., and Hafen, E. (1990). Reprogramming cell fate in the developing *Drosophila* retina: Transformation of R7 cells by ectopic expression of *rough*. *Genes Devel.* **4**, 728–739.

Basler, K., Christen, B., and Hafen, E. (1991). Ligand-independent activation of the sevenless receptor tyrosine kinase changes the fate of cells in the developing Drosophila eye. *Cell* **64**, 1069–1081.

Bateson, W. (1894). *Materials for the Study of Variation.* London: Macmillan.

Becker, H. (1957). Über Röntgenmosaikflecken und Defektmutationen am Auge von *Drosophila* und die Entwicklungsphysiologie des Auges. *Z. Induk. Abst. Vererb. Lehre* **88**, 333–373.

Bernard, F. (1937). Recherches sur la morphogénèse des yeux composés d'arthropodes. *Bull. Biol. Fr. Belg. (Suppl.)* **23**, 1–162.

Bier, E., Vaessin, H., Shephard, S., Lee, K., McCall, K., Barbel, S., Ackerman, L., Carretto, R., Uemura, T., Grell, E., Jan, L., and Jan, Y. (1989). Searching for pattern mutations in the *Drosophila* genome with a P-*lac-Z* vector. *Genes Devel.* **3**, 1273–1287.

Bowtell, D., Simon, M., and Rubin, G. (1988). Nucleotide sequence and structure of the *sevenless* gene of *Drosophila melanogaster*. *Genes Devel.* **2**, 620–634.

Bowtell, D., Kimmel, B., Simon, M., and Rubin, G. (1989). Ommatidia in the developing *Drosophila* eye require and can respond to *sevenless* for only a restricted period. *Cell* **56**, 931–936.

Cagan, R., and Ready, D. (1989a). *Notch* is required for successive cell decisions in the developing *Drosophila* retina. *Genes Devel.* **3**, 1099–1112.

Cagan, R., and Ready, D. (1989b). The emergence of order in the *Drosophila* pupal retina. *Dev. Biol.* **136**, 346–362.

Campos-Ortega, J. A. (1980). On compound eye development in *Drosophila melanogaster*. *In* "Current Topics in Developmental Biology" (A. A. Moscona and A. Monroy, eds.), Vol. 15, pp. 346–371. New York: Academic Press.

Campos-Ortega, J. A., Jurgens, G., and Hofbauer, A. (1979). Cell clones and pattern formation: Studies on *sevenless*, a mutant of *Drosophila melanogaster*. *Roux's Arch. Dev. Biol.* **186**, 27–50.

Carthew, R., and Rubin, G. (1990). *seven-in-absentia*, a gene required for specification of R7 cell fate in the *Drosophila* eye. *Cell* **63**, 561–577.

De Robertis, E., Oliver, G., and Wright, C. (1990). Homeobox genes and the vertebrate body plan. *Sci. Am.* 46–52.

Dietrich, U., and Campos-Ortega, J. A. (1984). The expression of neurogenic loci in imaginal epidermal cells of *Drosophila melanogaster*. *J. Neurogen.* **1**, 315–332.

Doe, C., and Goodman, C. (1985). Early events in insect neurogenesis. II. The role of cell interactions and cell lineage in the determination of neuronal precursor cells. *Dev. Biol.* **3**, 206–219.

Felder, S., Miller, K., Moehren, G., Ullrich, A., Schlessinger, J., and Hopkins, C. R. (1990). Kinase activity controls the sorting of the epidermal growth factor receptor within the multivesicular body. *Cell* **61**, 623–634.

Garcia-Bellido, A., and Merriam, J. (1969). Cell lineage of the imaginal discs in *Drosophila* gynandromorphs. *J. Exp. Zool.* **170**, 61–76.

Ghysen, A., and Dambly-Chaudiere, C. (1988). From DNA to form: The *achaete–scute* complex. *Genes Devel.* **2**, 495–501.

Hafen, E., Basler, K., Edstroem, J. E., and Rubin, G. (1987). *sevenless,* a cell-specific homeotic gene of *Drosophila* encodes a putative transmembrane receptor with a tyrosine kinase domain. *Science* **236**, 55–63.

Hart, A., Krämer, H., Van Vactor, D., Paidhungat, M., and Zipursky, S. L. (1990). Induction of cell fate in the *Drosophila* retina: *bride of sevenless* is predicted to contain a large extracellular domain and seven transmembrane segments. *Genes Devel.* **4**, 1835–1847.

Hartenstein, V. and Campos-Ortega, J. A. (1984). Early neurogenesis in wild-type Drosophila melanogaster. *Roux's Arch. Dev. Biol.* **193**, 308–325.

Hedgecock, E. M., Sulston, J. E., and Thomson, J. N. (1983). Mutations affecting programmed cell deaths in the nematode *Caenorhabditis elegans. Science* **220**, 1277–1279.

Hunter, T., and Cooper, J. (1986). Viral oncogenes and tyrosine phosphorylation. *In* "The Enzymes" (P. Boyer and E. Krebs, eds.), pp. 191–246. Orlando, Florida; Academic Press.

Karpilow, J., Lolodkin, A., Bork, T., and Venkatesh, T. (1989). Neuronal development in the *Drosophila* compound eye: *rap* gene function is required in photoreceptor cell R8 for ommatidial pattern formation. *Genes Devel.* **3**, 1834–1844.

Kidd, S., and Young, M. (1986). Transposon-dependent mutant phenotypes at the *Notch* locus of *Drosophila. Nature (London)* **323**, 89–91.

Kimmel, B., Heberlein, U., and Rubin, G. (1990). The homeo domain protein *rough* is expressed in a subset of cells in the developing *Drosophila* eye where it can specify cell subtype. *Genes Devel.* **4**, 712–727.

Krämer, H., Cagan, R., and Zipursky, S. L. (1991). Interaction of bride of sevenless membrane-bound ligand and the sevenless tyrosine kinase receptor. *Nature* **352**, 207–212.

Lawrence, P. A., and Green, S. M. (1979). Cell lineage in the developing retina of *Drosophila. Dev. Biol.* **71**, 142–152.

Lebovitz, R., and Ready, D. F. (1986). Ommatidial development in eye disc fragments. *Dev. Biol.* **71**, 663–671.

Lehmann, R., Jimenez, F., Dietrich, U., and Campos-Ortega, J. (1983). On the phenotype and development of mutants of early neurogenesis in *Drosophila melanogaster. Roux's Arch. Dev. Biol.* **192**, 62–74.

Markopoulou, K., Welshons, W., and Artavanis-Tsakonis, S. (1989). Phenotypic and molecular analysis of the *facets,* a group of intronic mutations at the *Notch* locus of *Drosophila melanogaster* which affect post-embryonic development. *Genetics* **122**, 417–428.

Mlodzik, M., Hiromi, Y., Weber, U., Goodman, C., and Rubin, G. (1990). The *Drosophila seven-up* gene, a member of the steroid receptor gene superfamily, controls photoreceptor cell fates. *Cell* **60**, 211–224.

Moses, K., Ellis, M., and Rubin, G. (1989). The *glass gene* encodes a zinc-finger protein required by *Drosophila* photoreceptor cells. *Nature (London)* **340**, 531–536.

O'Kane, C., and Gehring, W. (1987). Detection *in situ* of genomic regulatory elements in *Drosophila. Proc. Natl. Acad. Sci. U.S.A.* **84**, 9123–9127.

Poulson, D. (1937). Chromosomal deficiencies and the embryonic development of *Drosophila melanogaster. Proc. Natl. Acad. Sci. U.S.A.* **23**, 133–137.

Ready, D. F., Hanson, T. E., and Benzer, S. (1976). Development of the *Drosophila* retina, a neurocrystalline lattice. *Dev. Biol.* **53**, 217–240.

Ready, D., Tomlinson, A., and Lebovitz, R. (1986). Building an ommatidium: Geometry and genes. *In* "Development of Order in the Visual System" (S. Hilfer and J Sheffield, eds.), pp. 97–125. New York: Springer.

Reinke, R., and Zipursky, S. L. (1988). Cell–Cell interaction in the *Drosophila* retina: The *bride of sevenless* gene is required in photoreceptor cell R8 for R7 cell development. *Cell* **55**, 321–330.

Roux, W. (1888). Beiträge zur Entwicklungsmechanik des Embryo. 5. Über die künstliche Hervorbringung "halber" Embryonen durch zerstörung einer der beiden ersten Furchungszellen, sowie über die Nachentwicklung (postgeneration) der fehlenden Körperhälfte. *Virchows Arch. 114 Ges. Abb.* **2**, 419–521.

Saint, R., Kalionis, B., Lockett, T., and Elizur, A. (1988). Pattern formation in the developing eye of *Drosophila melanogaster* is regulated by the homeobox gene *rough*. *Nature (London)* **334**, 151–154.

Shellenbarger, D. L., and Mohler, J. D. (1975). Temperature-sensitive mutations of the *Notch* locus in *Drosophila melanogaster*. *Genetics* **81**, 143–162.

Simon, M., Bowtell, D., and Rubin, G. (1989). Structure and activity of the sevenless protein: A protein tyrosine kinase receptor required for photoreceptor development in *Drosophila*. *Proc. Natl. Acad. Sci. U.S.A.* **86**, 8333–8337.

Simpson, P. (1990). Lateral inhibition and the development of the sensory bristles of the adult peripheral nervous system of *Drosophila*. *Development* **109**, 509–519.

Spemann, H. (1928). Die Entwicklung seitlicher und dorso-ventraler Keimhälften bei verzögerter Kernversorgung. *Z. Wiss. Zool.* **132**, 105–134.

Sulston, J., Albertson, D., and Thomson, J. (1980). The *Caenorhabditis elegans* male: Postembryonic development of nongonadal structures. *Dev. Biol.* **78**, 542–576.

Sulston, J., Schierenberg, E., White, J., and Thomson, J. (1983). The embryonic cell lineage of the nematode *Caenorhabditis elegans*. *Dev. Biol.* **100**, 64–119.

Tomlinson, A. (1985). The cellular dynamics of pattern formation in the eye of *Drosophila*. *J. Embryol. Exp. Morph.* **89**, 313–331.

Tomlinson, A., and Ready, D. F. (1986). *sevenless:* A cell–specific homeotic mutation of the *Drosophila* eye. *Science* **231**, 400–402.

Tomlinson, A., Bowtell, E., Hafen, E., and Rubin, G. M. (1987). Loclaization of the *sevenless* protein, a putative receptor for positional information, in the eye imaginal disc of *Drosophila*. *Cell* **51**, 143–150.

Tomlinson, A., and Ready, D. F. (1987a). Neuronal differentiation in the *Drosophila* ommatidium. *Dev. Biol.* **120**, 336–366.

Tomlinson, A., Kimmel, B., and Rubin, G. (1988). *rough,* a *Drosophila* homeobox gene required in photoreceptors R2 and R5 for inductive interactions in the developing eye. *Cell* **55**, 771–784.

Turner, D., and Cepko, C. (1987). A common progenitor for neurons and glia persists in rat retina late in development. *Nature (London)* **328**, 131–136.

Ullrich, A., and Schlessinger, J. (1990). Signal transduction by receptors with tyrosine kinase activity. *Cell* **61**, 203–212.

Van Vactor, D. I., Cagan, R. L., Krämer, H., and Zipursky, S. L. (1991). Induction in the developing compound eye of Drosophila: multiple mechanisms restrict R7 induction to a single retinal precursor cell. *Cell.* In press.

Waddington, C. (1962). "New patterns in genetics and development" New York: Columbia University Press.

Welshons, W. (1965). Analysis of a gene in *Drosophila*. *Science* **150**, 1122–1129.

Wieschaus, E., and Gehring, W. (1976). Clonal analysis of primordial disc cells in the early embryo of *Drosophila melanogaster*. *Dev. Biol.* **50**, 249–263.

Wilcox, M. (1970). One-dimensional pattern found in blue-green algae. *Nature (London)* **228**, 686–687.

Wilcox, M., Mitchison, G., and Smith, R. (1973a). Pattern formation in the blue-green algae *Anabaena*. I. Basic mechanisms. *J. Cell Sci.* **12**, 707–723.

Wilcox, M., Mitchison, G., and Smith, R. (1973b). Pattern formation in the blue-green algae *Anabaena*. II. Controlled heterocyst regression. *J. Cell Sci.* **13,** 637–649.

Wilcox, M., Mitchison, G., and Smith, R. (1975). Mutants of *Anabaena cylindrica* altered in heterocyst spacing. *Arch. Microbiol.* **103,** 219–223.

Wyllie, A. H., Kerr, J. F., and Currie, A. R. (1980). Cell death: The significance of apoptosis. *Int. Rev. Cytol.* **68,** 251–306.

Development of the Peripheral Nervous System in *Drosophila*

Alain Ghysen
Laboratoire de Neurobiologie
Départment de Biologie Moléculaire
Université Libre de Bruxelles
Rhode-Saint-Genèse, Belgium

Christine Dambly-Chaudière
Laboratoire de Génétique
Départment de Biologie Moléculaire
Université Libre de Bruxelles
Rhode-St-Genèse, Belgium

I. Introduction

A. The Genetic Approach

One of the most challenging riddles of biology is the ability of living organisms to generate progeny. This implies the existence of a set of mechanisms that can instruct a single cell, the zygote, to build up reproducibly the diversity and complexity that are found in the adult organism. How are we to identify these mechanisms?

One way is to challenge the system with unexpected inputs and assess its reactions. This "classical" approach has led to the considerable series of grafts, ablations, transplantations, and other surgical operations that form the bulk of experimental embryology. A major conclusion from these experiments is that cell interactions (e.g., induction) play a major role in the process of development. In the fly, examples of the role and importance of cell interactions are seen in the development of the compound eye (see Chapter 7) and the singling out of neuronal precursors (see Chapter 6; see also Section IV). On the other hand, the experimental approach has produced disappointingly few results about how these interactions are integrated in a general program. Part of the reason may be that every experiment asks a question, but the question the experimenter has in mind may be quite different from the question the system answers. The problem is illustrated well by the discrepancy between Driesch's and Roux's results about the developmental potential of each cell at the 2-cell stage of development: depending on exactly how they isolated one of the two cells, Driesch regenerated entire embryos whereas Roux obtained only half-embryos; the inspired misinterpretation by

Roux of his own experiment may be considered the founding blunder of experimental embryology.

A rather different approach, based on the idea that the program of development is of necessity genetic in nature, was pioneered in the case of *Drosophila* by E. B. Lewis and, more recently, by C. Nüsslein-Volhard and E. Wieschaus. This second approach recognizes that we must disassemble the system itself before we can attempt to understand how it works. Since we have no clue nor idea about what drives development, the problem is to find a way to disassemble the system into its constitutive parts. The method that has proved most suitable so far is to disable elements of the system by means of mutations, and see how the system comes apart. In this approach, the mutation is much like the geologist's hammer that reveals the fracture planes of the crystal, from which it is then possible to infer the structure of the crystal unit.

The two papers that mark the coming of age of this approach (Lewis, 1978; Nüsslein-Volhard and Wieschaus, 1980) were devoted to the antero-posterior organization of the embryo. We have probably gained enough perspective to state with some confidence that, more than a breakthrough, we have witnessed a revolution in the analysis of development. The explosive growth of the studies on the basic organization of the fly embryo, and their immediate relevance for the antero-posterior organization of all animals, undoubtedly played a major role in the current interest in this field. However, the most novel aspect of the mutational approach lies in its intellectual restraint: refusing to assume anything, the pioneering work relied on no preconception about how development proceeds, except that it is somehow controlled by genes.

In this chapter we intend to summarize what is presently known of the development of the sensory system of the fly, from the initial decision to form a sense organ to the final specification of the synaptic connections in the central nervous system (CNS). Ideally we want to describe development in terms of its generative operations. Much like in the case of the antero-posterior organization of the embryo, then, our tool is the analysis of mutations that disrupt these generative operations; the final aim is to disassemble the developmental system into its constitutive elements. We are still far from that goal, yet what we have learned so far suggests that the system features a bizarre mixture of robust common sense and extreme sophistication, but who would expect less from the work of a billion-year-old craftsman?

B. Structure of Fly Sense Organs

The reader is referred to one of several excellent reviews for a general introduction to the structure and development of insect sense organs (Wigglesworth, 1972; Bate, 1978; Zacharuk, 1985). Here we will only mention the most salient features of the fly sense organs that will be discussed in this chapter.

I. TYPES AND FUNCTIONS OF SENSE ORGANS

a. External Sense Organs

External sense organs (es organs) typically contain two external elements: an external process inserted into a socket. The external process comes under various forms, the most abundant of which in the fly are the pointed bristles of mechanosensory organs, the open-tipped bristles of chemosensory organs, and the flat dome of the campaniform sensilla. Other types of es organs are also found, most notably on the antenna (e.g., Hodgkin and Bryant, 1978), but will not be considered in this chapter.

Figure 1 illustrates the three major types of es organs found in the body segments of the adult fly. The campaniform sensilla respond to strains in the cuticle (and mediate proprioception), the mechanosensory bristles respond to the deflection of the shaft (and therefore mediate touch), the chemosensory bristles respond to chemical stimulation of the dendrite (and mediate taste or smell). The first two types of organs contain only one neuron (m-es, *m*onoinnervated *e*xternal *s*ense organs) whereas the chemosensory bristles are innervated by 2–4 neurons (p-es, *p*olyinnervated *e*xternal *s*ense organs). All es organs contain an inner support cell that surrounds the dendrite(s), the thecogen cell. The external process and the socket are formed by the two outer support cells, called, respectively, the trichogen and the tormogen. Each neuron extends an axon toward and into the CNS. There the axon will reach and contact appropriate targets, forming the central projection of the sense organ.

b. Internal Sense Organs

Whereas all organs share basically the same structure, internal sense organs are more diverse (Fig. 1) Some of them, the stretch-sensitive chordotonal organs (ch organs), resemble the es organs because they comprise four cells: the neuron, a thecogen cell surrounding its dendrite, and two additional support cells. Furthermore, in both ch and es organs, the sensory neuron is a bipolar cell with a simple dendrite opposite the axon. Because of this similarity, the neurons that underlie the ch organs (ch neurons) and the neurons that innervate es organs (es neurons) are considered to belong to a common category, the type 1 neurons.

A second group of internal sense organs differs from those described previously by consisting of a single neuron, without any support cell. These neurons differ from the bipolar neurons just described by the presence of more than one dendrite, and have been called multiple dendrite neurons (md neurons). They correspond to the type 2 neurons described in other insects.

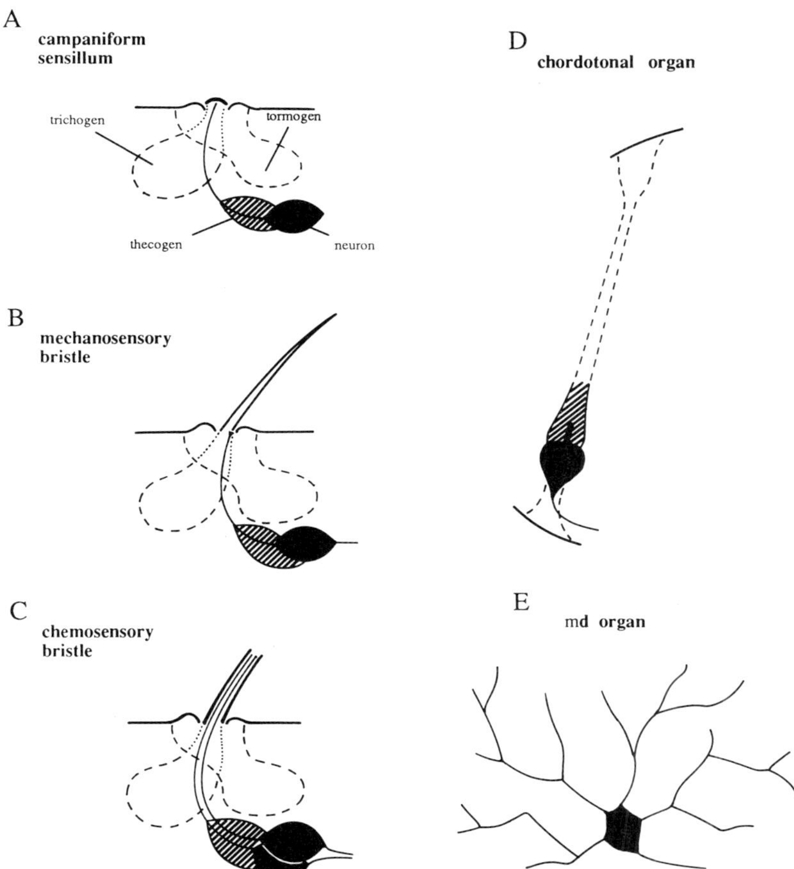

Figure 1. The major types of sense organs in *Drosophila*. A. The campaniform sensillum contains one type I neuron, is located externally, and performs a proprioceptive function. B. The mechanosensory bristle contains one type I neuron, is located externally, and performs an exteroceptive function. C. The chemosensory bristle contains at least two type I neurons, is located externally, and performs an exteroceptive function. D. The chordotonal organ contains one type I neuron, is located internally, and performs a proprioceptive function. E. The type 2 organ contains one type 2 neuron, is located internally, and may be both proprioceptive and exteroceptive. The monoinnervated external sense organs (A and B) are abbreviated m-es, the polyinnervated external sense organs (C) are abbreviated p-es, the chordotonal organs (D) are abbreviated ch, and the type 2 neurons (E) are abbreviated md.

The md neurons are common in the fly larva, in which they account for about half the entire complement of neurons in the body segments. The majority of md neurons has profuse dendritic arborization (Bodmer and Jan, 1987). Similar md neurons are abundant in other soft-skinned insect larvae, in which their naked endings extending under the epidermis are thought to act as touch-receptors. Other md neurons have less extensive dendritic arborizations and are associated to tissues other than epidermis, for example, the tracheal system. Very little is known of these, and they will not be considered further.

2. ORIGIN OF SENSE ORGANS

It has been shown in many insects that the different cells that form an es organ are related by lineage, since they all derive from a common ancestor called the sensory mother cell (SMC). One might object to the use of " mother cell" in this case, since the name is suggestive of a stem-cell type lineage: mothers, after all, remain mothers after they have produced their progeny. Thus, "precursor cell" might be more appropriate or, even better, "progenitor cell" (Y. N. Jan, personal communication). In this chapter, however, we have used the traditional terminology (Bate, 1978).

SMCs that form mechanosensory organs (bristles and campaniform sensilla) undergo two consecutive mitoses to generate the four constitutive cells of the sense organ. The formation of multiply innervated chemosensory organs involves one or more additional mitoses of the neuronal precursor to generate two or more neurons, depending on the organ. In the fly, lineage analysis based on patterns of 5-bromodeoxyuridene (BUdR) incorporation (Truman and Bate, 1988) has confirmed that larval and adult sense organs are formed by sibling cells (Bodmer *et al.*, 1989; Hartenstein and Posakony, 1989). The analysis has also revealed slight differences in the pattern of mitoses among ch, m-es, and p-es organs. It is important to point out that these results are simply observations of normal development. To what extent lineage relations are necessary, or determinant, for the daughter cells to assume their appropriate fate is not known.

In the case of the es organs of the adult fly, there is good evidence that the SMC originates from the epidermis and forms close to the position at which the sense organ will eventually differentiate (Garcia-Bellido and Merriam, 1971a); in other words, cell migration does not play a major role in the process. Short-range migration may, however, be responsible for the fine tuning of the final pattern, at least in the abdomen (Garcia-Bellido and Merriam, 1971b) and in the legs (Held and Bryant, 1984).

The evidence is more limited in the case of chordotonal organs, and even more so in the case of the md neurons, but in any case there is little doubt that all sense organs originate from the epidermis.

3. LARVAL AND ADULT SENSE ORGANS

The larval sense organs are formed during embryogenesis and persist unchanged during the entire larval life (Hertweck, 1931; Kankel *et al.*, 1980; Campos-Ortega and Hartenstein, 1985; Dambly-Chaudière and Ghysen, 1986). They are lost early during metamorphosis, at the time when the larval epidermis and most other larval tissues are lysed. The adult sense organs differentiate during metamorphosis (Murray *et al.*, 1984; Hartenstein and Posakony, 1989). All adult es organs originate from nests of undifferentiated cells set apart early during embryogenesis (Bate and Martinez-Arias, 1991; Cohen *et al.*, 1991). These undifferentiated cells keep dividing during all larval life, contrary to the larval epidermal cells, which never divide after the larva has hatched. Many of these nests of cells form disc-like structures called imaginal discs. Each imaginal disc gives rise to a well-defined part of the adult epidermis: for example, each of the six leg discs differentiates one leg and the surrounding ventral thorax, whereas two discs called wing discs each provide one wing and half the dorsal and lateral thorax.

The major types of es organs are similar in the larva and adult. The morphology of the external process may, however, differ somewhat. For example, the external process of the adult bristles is a straight shaft, whereas that of the larval sensory hairs is sinuous and often branched. Some types of es organs described in the larva have no known homologs in the adult fly, for example, the doubly innervated papilla, p6, of the abdominal segments (Figs. 2B,3). This, however, may be due to a much more limited knowledge of the adult sense organs. With the exception of the chordotonal organs, virtually nothing is known about the internal sense organs of the adult.

C. Patterns of Sense Organs

I. THE ADULT

One remarkable feature of the sense organs of the fly is that many of them form at constant positions. For example, the large bristles (macrochaetes) that are located on the thorax and head each occupy a fixed position (Fig. 2A). This pattern is so conserved that each macrochaete has been given a name; the presence or absence of particular macrochaetes is a reliable taxonomic trait. The same is true of several campaniform sensilla located on the wing blade (Bryant, 1975) and of the chemosensory bristles located on the leg (Held and Bryant, 1984). Other types of patterns are also observed in the adult. The small bristles (microchaetes) on the notum are more or less regularly spaced but do not have constant positions. This type of pattern is very common and is found

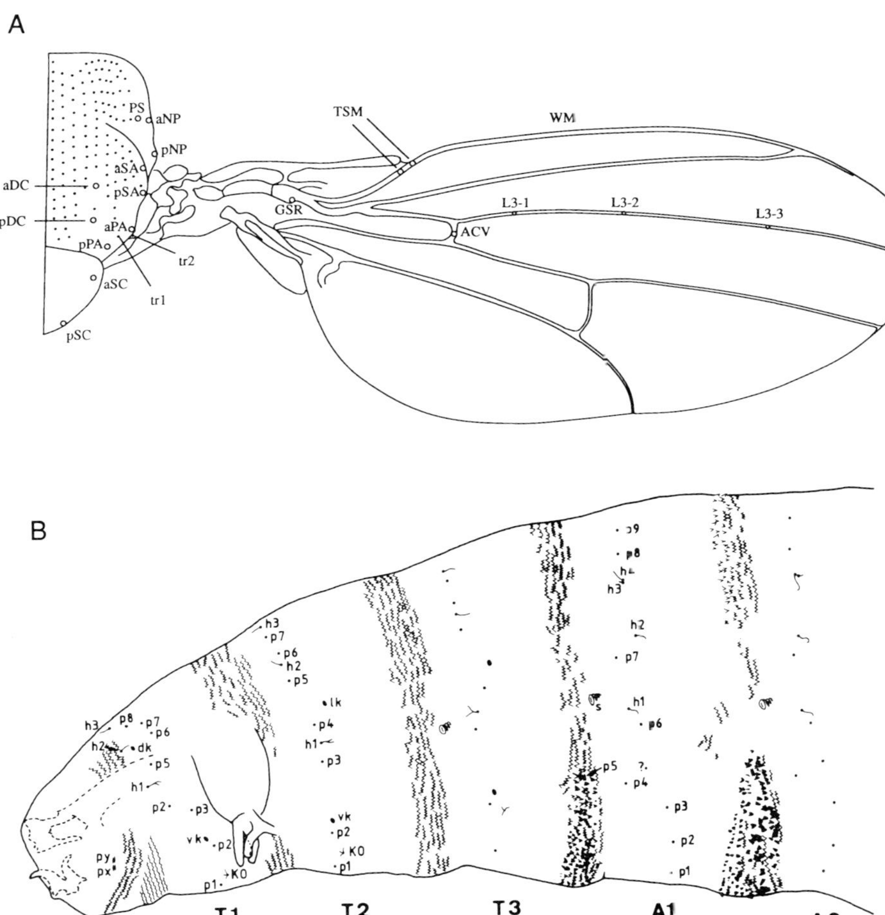

Figure 2. Pattern of sense organs on the thorax and wing of the adult fly (A), and on the anterior segments of the larva (B). A. Right side of the thorax and wing of *Drosophila*. ACV, campaniform sensillum of the anterior crossvein; DC, dorsocentral bristles (anterior and posterior); GSR, giant sensillum of the radius; L3-1, L3-2, L3-3, campaniform sensilla of the third wing vein; NP, notopleural bristles (anterior and posterior); PA, postalar bristles (anterior and posterior); PS, presutural bristle; SA, supraalar bristles (anterior and posterior); SC, scutellar bristles (anterior and posterior); tr1, tr2, trichoid sensilla 1 and 2; TSM, twin campaniform sensilla of the margin; WM, chemosensory bristles of the anterior wing margin. B. Anterior end of a third instar larva. Each sense organ is labeled in T1, T2, and A1. The patterns in T3 and in A2–A7 are identical to those in T2 and A1, respectively. dk, dorsal kölbchen; h, hair; KO; Keilin organ; p, papilla; s, residual spiracles that are detected in all segments from T3 to A7; vk, ventral kölbchen. The question mark labels a very small pit of unknown origin and function. (Reproduced from Dambly-Chaudière and Ghysen, 1986, with permission.)

in many insects. Other sense organs are grouped in clusters. For example, at the base of the wing is a cluster of about 24 campaniform sensilla, and chordotonal organs form large clusters at the base of the femur of all legs.

2. THE LARVA

In the larva, all es organs have fixed positions (Dambly-Chaudière and Ghysen, 1986; Fig. 2B). All internal organs also can be uniquely identified (Ghysen *et al.*, 1986; Bodmer and Jan, 1987). In Fig. 3, we have compiled these results by showing separately the pattern of neurons, the pattern of es organs, and the relationship between neurons and es organs in the case of the thoracic pattern (present in the second and third thoracic segments) and the abdominal pattern present in the first seven abdominal segments. The neuronal patterns in T1, A8, A9, and A10 are given in Ghysen *et al.* (1986); the pattern in the gnathal segments is given in Campos-Ortega and Hartenstein (1985).

The relative simplicity of the larval pattern (41 neurons, 13 es organs per abdominal hemisegment), its richness (5 different types of neurons, 3 types of es organs), and its complete reproducibility make this pattern uniquely suitable for the identification of patterning genes (Jan *et al.*, 1987). On the other hand, the larval sensory neurons are much more difficult to backfill than adult neurons, and almost nothing is known of their central projections. This restriction is most unfortunate, since the larval sensory system typifies to the extreme one of the major advantages of studies on insect nervous systems: that one can work with uniquely identifiable neurons. In retrospect, the ability to recognize individual neurons may have been the most crucial feature of the work on invertebrate systems, because it made it possible to consider each identifiable neuron as unique, to follow its particular development or properties, and only then to see if general features could be extracted from the analysis of many independent cases. The alternative possibility, to work with supposedly homogeneous populations of cells, is, of course, open to the problem that one can never know for sure whether the assumption of homogeneity is valid.

Current attempts to generate enhancer-trap lines (see subsequent text) in which the product of the reporter gene would be transported down the axon might solve the problem of tracing the axon, and make the larva a good system for the genetic dissection of axonal pathfinding and connectivity (E. Giniger, personal communication). The already impressive achievement of the fly larva as a model developmental system could then be extended to the analysis of a central problem of neurobiology, an amusing turn of events, since the larval stage was completely ignored for more than 50 years after the adult fly had become the geneticist's pet.

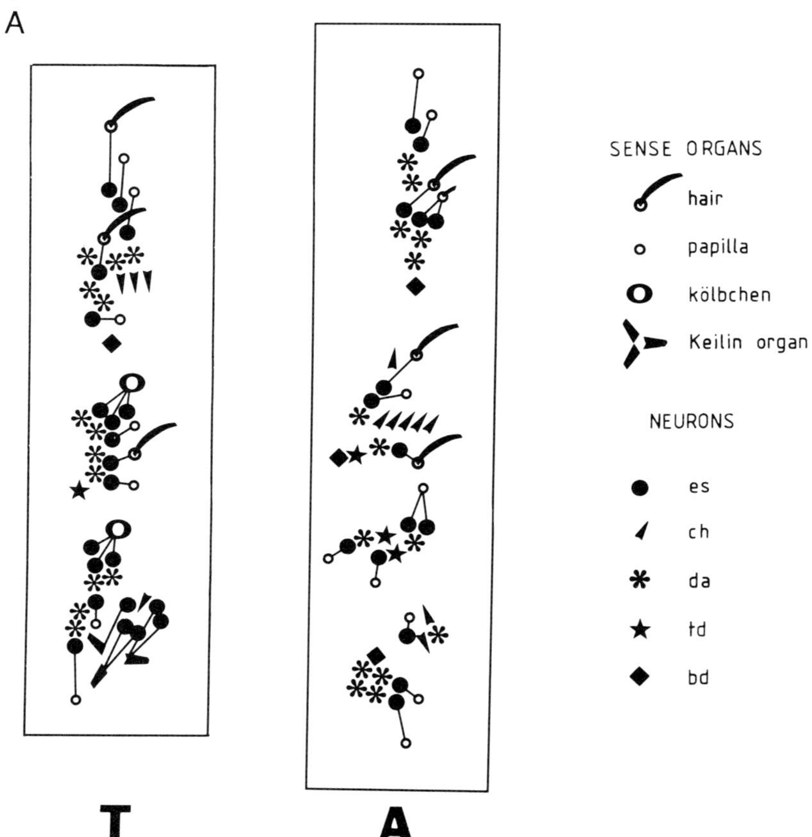

Figure 3. The sensory system of the larva. The thoracic (T) and abdominal (A) patterns of sensory neurons and external sense organs, represented in three complementary diagrams, in which dorsal is up and anterior is to the left. A. Schematic diagram of the entire complement of sensory neurons and external sense organs (da,td, and bd are three types of md neurons.) (Reproduced from Ghysen and Dambly-Chaudière, 1990, with permission.) B. The pattern of peripheral neurons. v, v', l, and d are the two ventral, the lateral, and the dorsal clusters of neurons. p4, p5, p8, and p9 show the location of four abdominal papillae, at the tip of the corresponding es dendrites. ch neurons are in black, es neurons are shaded. (Reproduced from Ghysen and O'Kane, 1989, with permission.) C. Diagram of the pattern of external sense organs showing the neural clusters to which the corresponding es neurons belong. (Reproduced from Ghysen and Dambly-Chaudière, 1990, with permission.)

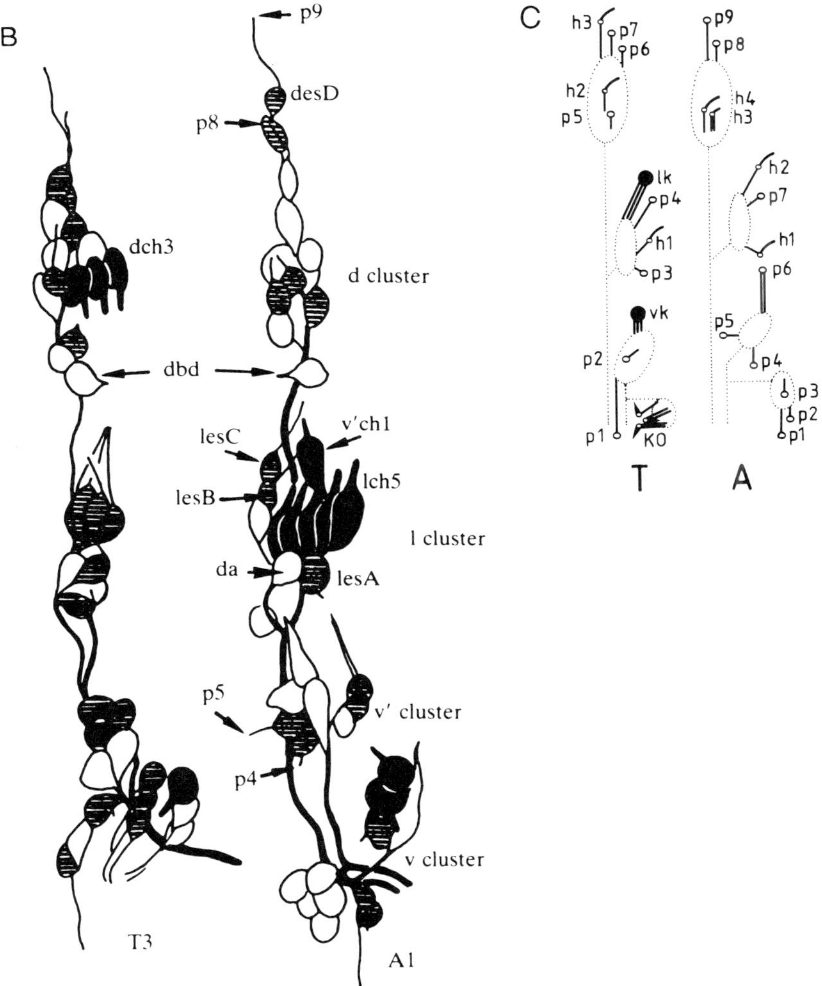

Figure 3 *(continued)*

3. THE SENSORY MOTHER CELLS

Until recently, studies of the development of the sense organs were mostly restricted to the detection and analysis of the differentiating cells, that is, to the very last step of the process. This is because it was generally not possible to visualize any of the steps that precede the final differentiation, so that previous studies had to resort to indirect means to assess the temporal dimension of pattern formation. The situation has now changed completely, thanks to the advent of the method known as enhancer trapping (O'Kane and Gehring, 1987; see Appendix). Enhancer trapping has led to the generation of an ever-increasing number of useful transgenic lines, each of which displays a highly specific pattern of expression of the bacterial gene *lacZ* (Bellen *et al.*, 1989; Bier *et al.*, 1989). In some of these lines, *lacZ* is expressed not only in all the cells that will form the sense organs but also in their mother cell.

We will summarize the pattern of expression of *lacZ* in one of these lines, A37, for two reasons: first, as an illustration of the power of enhancer-trap lines as cell markers, and second, because it will be used later in this chapter. In this line, *lacZ* is expressed in all cells that form the sense organs, both in the larva and in the adult. Furthermore, *lacZ* expression can be detected in the progenitor cells as well, allowing for the first time the visualization of the SMCs themselves (Ghysen and O'Kane, 1989). Figure 4 shows that the earliest SMCs appear in a defined and reproducible sequence. A comparison of the A37 pattern with the pattern of *lacZ* expression in A18, another enhancer-trap line in which only ch organs are labeled, reveals that the P cells will give rise to ch organs, whereas the A cells will give rise to es organs. Another enhancer-trap line, A101, is more sensitive than A37 in the imaginal discs, where it reveals not only the SMCs but also the cells that are about to become SMCs (Huang *et al.*, 1991). Here again, the emergence of the SMCs follows a reproducible sequence that extends over more than 40 hr, a considerable fraction of the entire larval life (4 days at 25°C). With the help of these and other lines, a detailed analysis of the emergence of the final pattern in normal and mutant flies has now become feasible.

II. A Progressive Process

In the following sections, we will show how the genetic methods described in the appendix have been applied to the problem of the origin and connectivity

Figure 4. Pattern of early *lacZ* expression in an embryo of the A37 enhancer-trap line. a. Prior to the formation of SMCs in the body segments, *lacZ* is expressed in a small group of epidermal cells in the posterior region of all segments (*arrows*). b. One SMC forms in the posterior region of each segment: the P cell (*arrowheads*). c. A second SMC appears in each segment, anterior to the P cell: the A cell (*arrows*). d. An anterior pair of SMCs is found in some segments: the A pair (*arrows*). e. Pairs of A cells are present in all segments; pairs of P cells are found in some segments (*arrows*). f. All segments contain an A pair and a P pair, most segments also contain one or more dorsal (D) cells and ventral (V) cells. At this time of embryonic development (5–7 hr after fertilization), the embryo is in the "extended germband stage," that is, the embryo is doubled up on itself and assumes a horizontal U shape. G, gnathal segments; T, thoracic segments; A, abdominal segments. (Reproduced from Ghysen and O'Kane, 1989, with permission.)

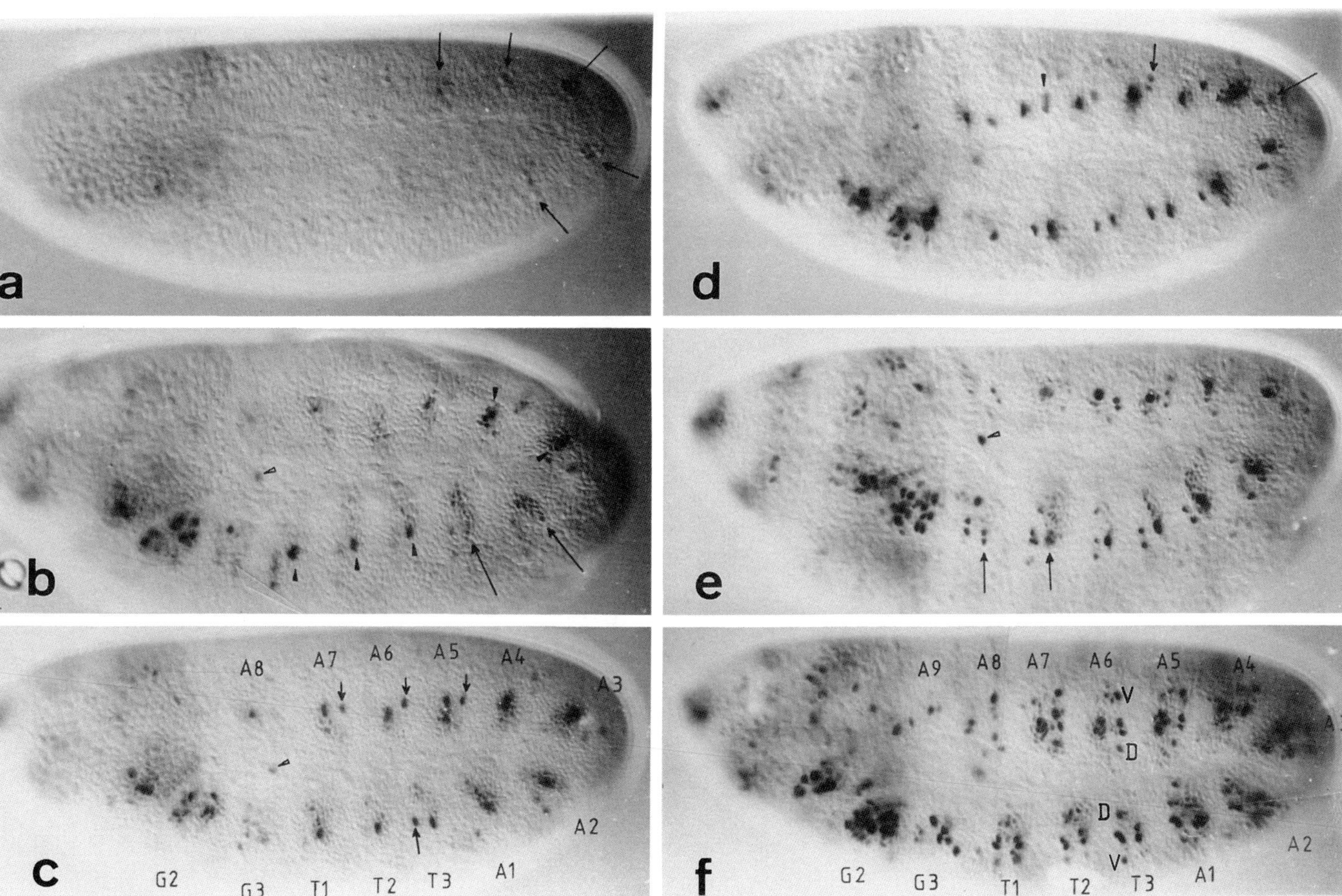

a
b
c
d
e
f
A8
A7
A6
A5
A4
A3
A2
A1
G2
G3
T1
T2
T3
A9
V
D

of the fly sensory neurons. Here we will summarize what we have learned so far, in order to provide a general framework in which each particular result can find its place.

One major principle that arises from these studies is that the development of the peripheral nervous system (PNS) is a progressive process, the early steps of which are depicted in Fig. 5. First, groups of ectodermal cells become endowed with the capability to form a sense organ precursor. Then, three events occur almost simultaneously: one cell of each group becomes a precursor, that is, assumes the fate of SMC; this precursor now prevents the other competent cells from becoming SMCs; and the precursor becomes further specified toward the type of sense organ that it will form. The precursor then undergoes a fixed pattern of mitoses, producing four (or more) daughter cells. One of the daughter cells, the neuron, will extend its axon along defined paths up to the CNS. Once in the CNS, the axon recognizes and follows specific guides. Finally, the axon identifies its targets and establishes the appropriate synaptic connections.

The second principle of interest is that each of the steps just summarized appears to involve a limited number of genes acting as a team (what A. Garcia-Bellido calls a "syntagma," 1981, 1984). Thus a first set of genes defines the competent state, a second set of genes mediates the lateral inhibition, and a third set specifies the precursor. One of the last steps, the recognition of specific guides in the CNS, also involves a specific family of genes. Little is known yet of the genetics of the remaining steps, although these steps are now coming under vigorous investigation in several laboratories. A most interesting feature of these teams of genes is that there is a clear tendency for the different genes of a given team to share a particular sequence. For example, most of the genes that define the competence to form SMCs share a particular helix-loop-helix motif, several of the genes that are involved in lateral inhibition share a multiple EGF motif, and several of the genes involved in pathway recognition contain the immunoglobulin super-family motif.

Both principles appear generally valid in the programming of fly development. For example, the extensive analysis of embryonic segmentation has shown that the definition of segments is also a progressive process involving four distinct groups of zygotic genes. The first group (gap genes) transforms the maternally derived antero-posterior polarization of the oocyte into a crude partitioning of the zygote. The second group (pair-rule genes) transforms this crude partitioning into a metamerically repeated organization. The third group (segment polarity genes) transforms the metameric repeat in a segmental pattern. The fourth group (homeotic genes) transforms the serially repeated segments into a set of unique segments, each with its specific attributes such as legs, wings, or mouthpieces. Here again is a tendency for the

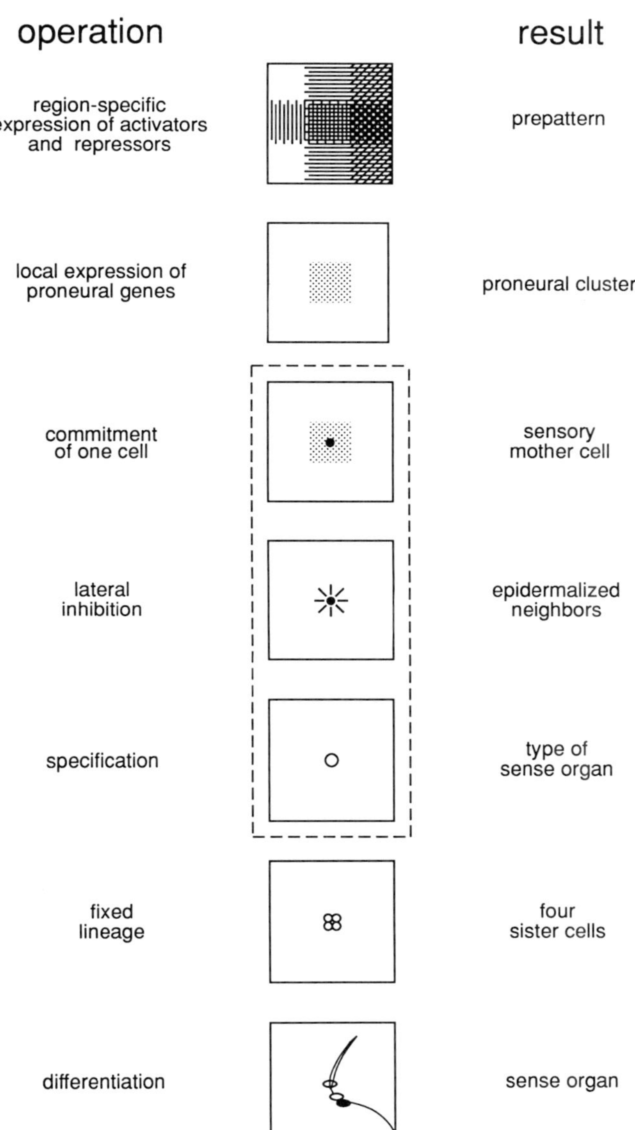

Figure 5. The early steps in the formation of a sense organ. Several operations are involved in the formation of sense organs. The order in which the middle three operations (dashed box) occur is somewhat uncertain. In addition to the 7 operations illustrated, the differentiation of the axon involves the establishment of the appropriate path up to and in the CNS, and the establishment of the appropriate synaptic connections. Many variations of this flow chart can be imagined and probably exist. For example, an array of previously formed sense organs may act as an element of the prepattern for the development of later sense organs; the commitment of a SMC may alter the local expression of the proneural genes; a SMC may divide to generate several SMCs; a SMC may induce or recruit additional SMCs from its neighbors; elements of the lineage may be deleted to generate isolated neurons or noninnervated organules. (Reproduced from Ghysen and Dambly-Chaudière, 1989, with permission.)

genes of a given syntagma to share a given motif. For example, most of the gap genes encode proteins with zinc fingers, many of the pair-rule genes have a divergent homeobox-like sequence, and all homeotic genes share the strongly conserved homeobox motif.

III. Acquisition of Competence

A. Original Observations

The existence of a local competence to form sense organs was originally inferred by Stern (1954) in the case of adult bristles. He studied a mutation, *achaete (ac)*, that removes a pair of large bristles on each side of the thorax. Using mosaics, he showed that, if the region where the bristle should have formed is mutant, no bristle would be present; however, if the boundary between mutant and normal cells runs close to the expected position of the bristle, then a bristle may be formed by normal cells at a slightly displaced position. This strongly suggests that the cells in the region around the expected position are all competent to form a sense organ, although only one will normally do so.

Quantitative simulations based on Stern's data suggested that the gene *ac* itself might be the factor conferring competence to groups of epidermal cells (Ghysen and Richelle, 1979). This implied that the *ac* gene should be locally expressed in regions where bristles will form, as was later confirmed by studying the distribution of *ac* transcripts in the imaginal disc (Romani *et al.,* 1989). Data similar to Stern's are not available for other sense organs. However, the observation that the expression of *ac* and the related genes occurs in clusters of epidermal cells prior to the formation of the SMC suggests that the acquisition of competence is a general feature in the formation of sense organs (and probably of neuroblasts as well; see Chapter 5).

B. The Genetics of Competence

I. THE *ACHAETE–SCUTE* COMPLEX

The gene *ac* is part of a gene complex called *achaete–scute* complex (AS-C; reviewed in Ghysen and Dambly-Chaudière, 1988). The complex comprises four genes: *ac, scute (sc), lethal of scute (lsc),* and *asense (ase).* The genes *ac* and *sc* are required for the formation of two nearly complementary subsets of adult sense organs (Garcia-Bellido, 1979). For example, of the 11 pairs of large bristles on the dorsal thorax, 2 depend on *ac,* 8 depend on *sc,* and 1 requires both *ac* and *sc.* Likewise, many campaniform sensilla on the wing blade depend on *sc,* some others depend on *ac,* and two clusters of sensilla require both genes (Leyns *et al.,* 1989). As expected from these phenotypes, the double mutant *ac sc* lacks virtually all external sense organs. Among the few sense organs that remain in the double mutant are a row of bristles on the anterior margin of the wing (Garcia-Bellido and Santamaria, 1978). These bristles depend on the fourth gene of the complex, *ase* (M. Ruiz-Gomez, personal communication).

All mutations mentioned so far are fully recessive loss-of-function (LOF) mutations. In addition, there exists a class of AS-C dominant mutations called *Hairy-wing (Hw).* As their name suggests, *Hw* mutations form supernumerary sense organs [bristles on the thorax (Gottlieb, 1964); bristles and campaniform sensilla on the wing blade (Lees, 1942)]. The analysis of different *Hw* mutations demonstrated that they are gain-of-function (GOF) mutations of either *ac* or *sc* (Garcia Alonso and Garcia-Bellido, 1986). The comparison of the LOF and GOF phenotypes of AS-C (see Appendix, Section 3) strongly supports the notion that *ac* and *sc* are responsible for the initial decision that leads to the formation of a sense organ.

2. AS-C AND THE LARVAL SENSE ORGANS

Because all larval sense organs are formed by the end of embryogenesis, and because all sensory neurons can be detected in whole mount preparations of late embryos, the larval PNS is a convenient system in which to assess the requirements for AS-C genes for all types of sense organs. A deletion of the entire complex removes all es organs (Fig. 6A, upper panel; Dambly-Chaudière and Ghysen, 1987). Most or all type 2 neurons are also absent; therefore, they also require AS-C function. The ch organs, however, are all present, as are some of the other types of larval peripheral neurons.

As in the case of the adult sense organs, two genes in the complex are required for the formation of two complementary subsets of es organs in the larva (Fig. 6B, lower panel; Dambly-Chaudière and Ghysen, 1987). For the larval sense organs, however, the relevant genes are *ac* and *ase,* with *sc* playing only a minor role. The third AS-C gene, *lsc,* plays an essential role in the formation of the CNS (Jimenez and Campos-Ortega, 1979,1987) but does not seem to be of major importance in the PNS.

The use of the enhancer-trap line A37, in which the SMCs (and all their progeny) express the reporter gene *lacZ,* showed that among the first SMCs that are detected, only those that correspond to ch organs are present in

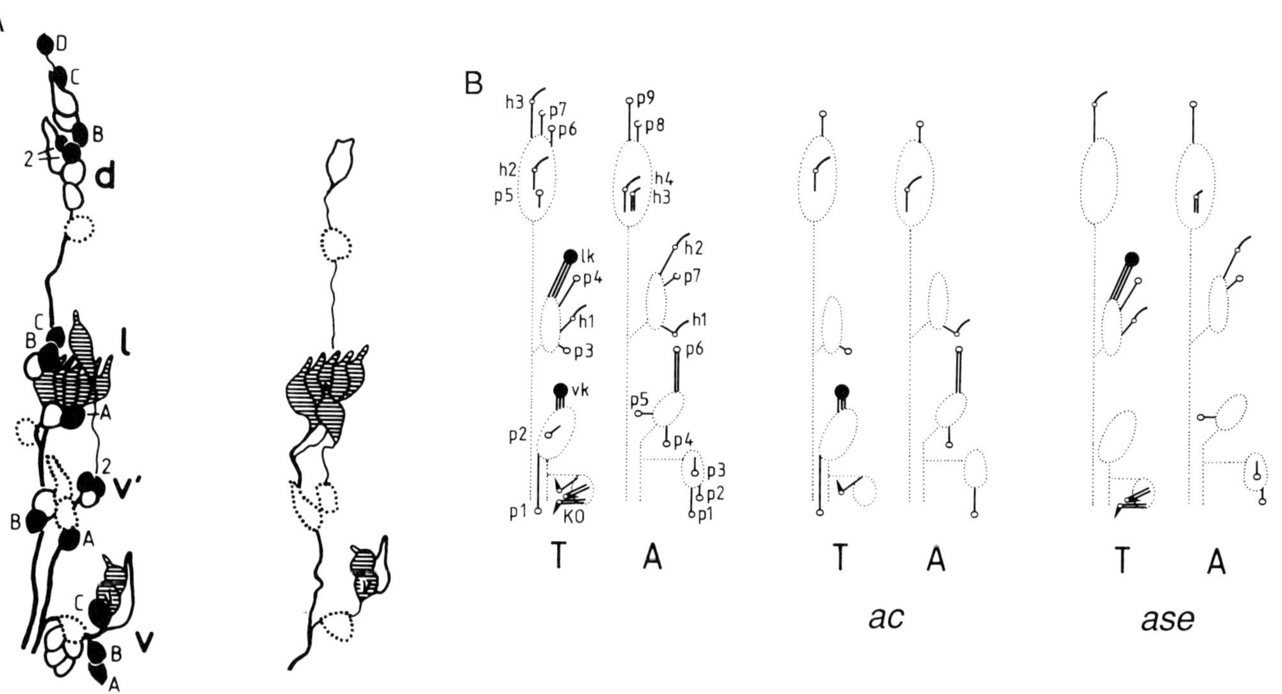

Figure 6. Requirement for the AS-C genes in the formation of the larval PNS. A. The peripheral neurons in an abdominal segment of a normal embryo (*left*) and of an embryo deleted for AS-C (*right*). The es neurons are black; the ch neurons are striped. Among the type 2 neurons, the da neurons are white, the td and bd neurons have a dotted outline. The dendrites of es and ch neurons have been omitted for clarity (Reproduced from Dambly-Chaudière and Ghysen, 1987, with permission.) B. The two subpatterns of sense organs defined by the different AS-C genes. (*Left*) Diagram of the complete pattern of external sense organs. The subset of sense organs that depend, respectively, on the left part of AS-C (*ac* and, to some extent, *sc*) and on the right part of the complex (*ase* and possibly *lsc*). (Reproduced from Ghysen and Dambly-Chaudière, 1990, with permission.)

embryos deficient for AS-C (Fig. 7; Ghysen and O'Kane, 1989). This demonstrates that the formation of the SMCs that will give rise to es organs (as detected by *lacZ* expression in this line) requires the previous expression of AS-C.

These results indicate that as early as the competent stage, that is, before the SMCs exist as such, differences already exist between competent clusters. In other words, competence imposes a first element of specificity onto the process of sense organ formation, depending on which AS-C gene is involved: cells in which the *ac* gene is active become competent to form one subset of sense organs, cells in which *ase* is active will form SMCs of another subset, and cells in which neither *ac* nor *ase* is active will form yet a third subset of sense organs.

3. A GENE THAT INTERACTS POSITIVELY WITH AS-C

Mutations in the gene *daughterless (da)* were first detected by their maternal effect on sex determination: female embryos from mothers homozygous for the hypomorphic allele *da*[1] die—hence, the name of the gene (Bell, 1954). This is because the product of the gene, which is expressed during oocyte formation, is necessary in XX zygotes to establish the appropriate genetic path for female sex determination (Cline, 1984); therefore, XX embryos from *da* mothers die because of inappropriate dosage compensation of X-linked genes (Sanchez and Nöthiger, 1983). Complete LOF mutations are embryonic lethals in both sexes (Cronmiller and Cline, 1987) and result in the absence of all sense organs in the embryo (Caudy *et al.*, 1988a). Thus the normal gene must be expressed in the mother to ensure the proper sex determination of female embryos, and in the zygote to ensure the formation of sense organs. The latter requirement concerns not only all the sense organs that depend on AS-C, but also the AS-C independent sense organs, in particular the chordotonal organs.

The analysis of the A37 enhancer-trap line showed that no SMC ever appears in homozygous *da* embryos, confirming that *da* is indeed required for the formation of all sense organs, and demonstrating that *da* is required for, or prior to, the formation of the SMCs (Fig. 7; Ghysen and O'Kane, 1989). A dosage analysis (see Appendix, Section D) revealed that *da* interacts with at least some of the AS-C genes: adult flies that are doubly hemizygous for *da* and AS-C (that is, have only one copy of each locus) have a reduced number of bristles (Dambly-Chaudière *et al.*, 1988). Thus we can conclude that the formation of the SMCs for the es organs requires the cooperation of *da* and AS-C.

Interestingly, one of the AS-C genes, *sc*, was subsequently found also to be involved in sex determination (Torres and Sanchez, 1989). Whether the

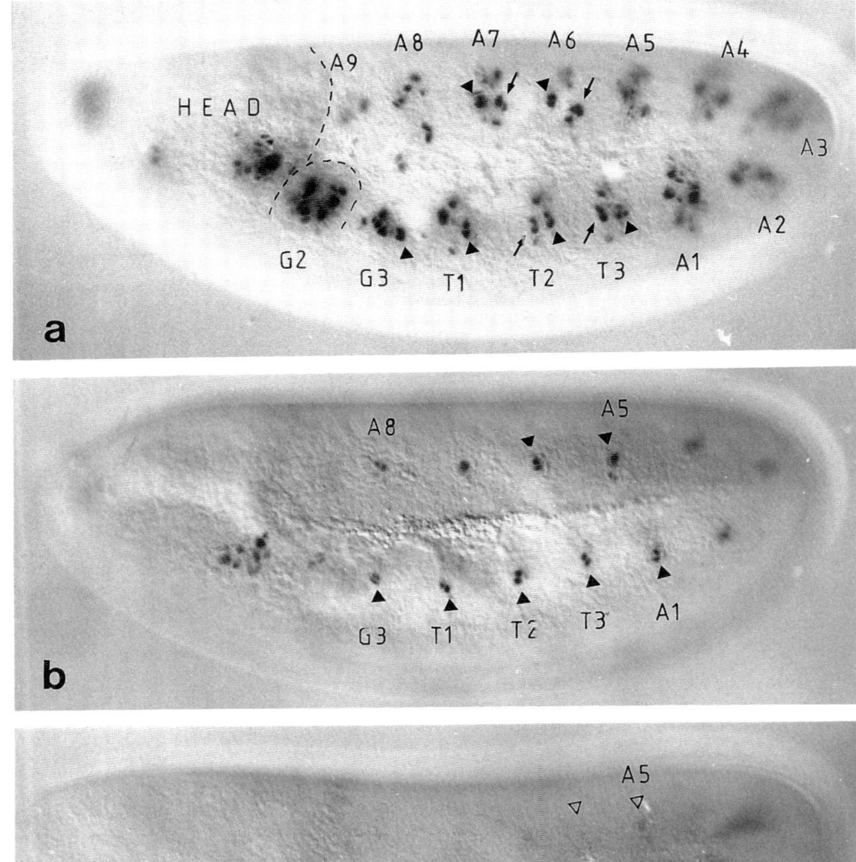

Figure 7. The emergence of the early SMCs in A37 embryos. a. Normal embryo. Arrows point to the A pairs, arrowheads indicate the P pairs. b. Embryo deleted for all AS-C genes. Arrowheads indicate the P pairs. c. Embryo deleted for the gene da. Empty arrowheads point to the sites at which P pairs should be present at this stage. (Reproduced from Ghysen and Dambly-Chaudière, 1990, with permission.)

dual involvement of *da* and *sc* in both sense organ formation and sex determination is evolutionary opportunism, just coincidence, or has some deep meaning is, for the moment, a matter of conjecture.

4. GENES THAT INTERACT NEGATIVELY WITH AS-C

Two genes that interact negatively with AS-C have been identified: *hairy (h;* Sturtevant, 1970) and *extramacrochaetae (emc,* Botas *et al.,* 1982). LOF mutations in either gene result in the formation of supernumerary sense organs in the adult, suggesting that the function of the normal gene is somehow to repress or antagonize AS-C activity in the corresponding regions.

A preliminary analysis suggests that neither *h* nor *emc* mutations show clear defects in the formation of the larval PNS (C. Dambly-Chaudière, unpublished observations). Whether this lack of effect is real or due to some complication, such as an important maternal contribution (see Appendix) or a problem of allele specificity, cannot yet be decided.

Using the method of dosage analysis, Garcia-Bellido showed that both *h* and *emc* interact directly with the AS-C genes: *h* mostly with *ac* and *emc* mostly with *sc* (Moscoso del Prado and Garcia-Bellido, 1984). The simplest explanation at that time was that *h* and *emc* act as transcriptional repressors of *ac* and *sc,* respectively. The distribution of *ac* and *sc* transcripts is not altered in *emc* mutants, however (Romani *et al.,* 1989), and it now seems more likely that the *h* and *emc* products interact directly with the AS-C products to prevent them from conferring competence (see subsequent text).

C. The Molecular Biology of Competence

I. STRUCTURAL ANALYSIS OF AS-C, *da, h,* AND *emc*

The major structural feature of the products of the genes just mentioned is that they all share a motif, called helix-loop-helix (HLH; Murre *et al.,* 1989a), formed by two amphipathic helices joined by a loop (AS-C; Villares and Cabrera, 1987; Alonso and Cabrera, 1988; *da:* Caudy *et al.,* 1988b; *h:* Rushlow *et al.,* 1989; *emc:* Ellis *et al.,* 1990; Garrell and Modolell, 1990). Most of them also contain, adjacent to the first helix, a basic region with potential to bind DNA. The two helices are involved in the formation of dimers, possibly by direct interaction between their hydrophilic moieties (Lassar *et al.,* 1989; Murre *et al.,* 1989a; Davis *et al.,* 1990). A most interesting feature of these proteins is that the HLH motif can mediate the formation of hetero- as well as homodimers (Murre *et al.,* 1989b; Davis *et al.,* 1990).

The details of the interactions between HLH proteins, and of their effect on DNA recognition, are likely to be extremely complex. Nevertheless, the preliminary data now available suggest that at least some heterodimers are much more efficient to promote the expression of a given gene than either of the two homodimers (Murre *et al.*, 1989b). Furthermore it seems that the DNA sequence that is recognized may also differ for different heterodimers. Finally the two HLH proteins that act as "repressors" of AS-C genes have an interrupted (*h*) or nonexistent (*emc*) basic region, suggesting that they may antagonize the AS-C products either by competing with them or by forming inactive heterodimers.

These results fully support the genetic arguments suggesting the existence of direct interactions between the AS-C genes, *da, h,* and *emc.* They are also consistent with the idea that the differential expression of the various AS-C genes already confers specificity to the very first step of sense organ formation, the acquisition of competence.

2. REGULATION OF AS-C EXPRESSION

Different *sc* mutations remove different subsets of bristles in the adult (Serebrovsky and Dubinin, 1930; Agol, 1931). This observation led to the idea that each bristle depends on a particular domain of the *sc* gene, and that each mutation inactivates one or more contiguous domains (Dubinin, 1932). The molecular analysis of a large number of *sc* mutations (Campuzano *et al.*, 1985) suggests that these domains are part of an extensive *cis*-acting control region that spans a surprisingly large 40-kb region, and is also unusual because it is located mostly downstream of the *sc* gene (though a few bristles depend on upstream control sites, Ruiz-Gomez and Modolell, 1987).

The gene *sc* is also required for the formation of most campaniform sensilla on the wing. The phenotypic analysis of mutations in and around *sc* shows that, much as in the case of bristles, each position at which sensilla will form depends on a particular domain of the gene, presumably containing a particular control site (Leyns *et al.*, 1989). In contrast to the control sites involved in the formation of bristles, however, those involved in the formation of campaniform sensilla are located mostly upstream of the coding region, with only a few of them downstream.

The simplest interpretation of these results is that the coding region of *sc* is embedded in a long array of control sites, each of which acts as an enhancer to promote the expression of *sc* in response to local cues (Fig. 8; Ruiz-Gomez and Modolell, 1987; Ghysen and Dambly-Chaudière, 1988). The pattern of expression of *sc* in the imaginal wing disc fits well with the idea of multiple control sites, since transcripts are found in clusters of cells in positions at which adult sense organs will eventually form (Balcells *et al.,* 1988). Further-more, a *sc* mutation that specifically affects one bristle strongly reduces the expression of *sc* in the corresponding region of the disc, but not elsewhere (Romani *et al.,* 1989).

Although the nature of the local cues that may act on the *sc* enhancers is still unknown, reasonable guesses can now be made. Several segment polarity

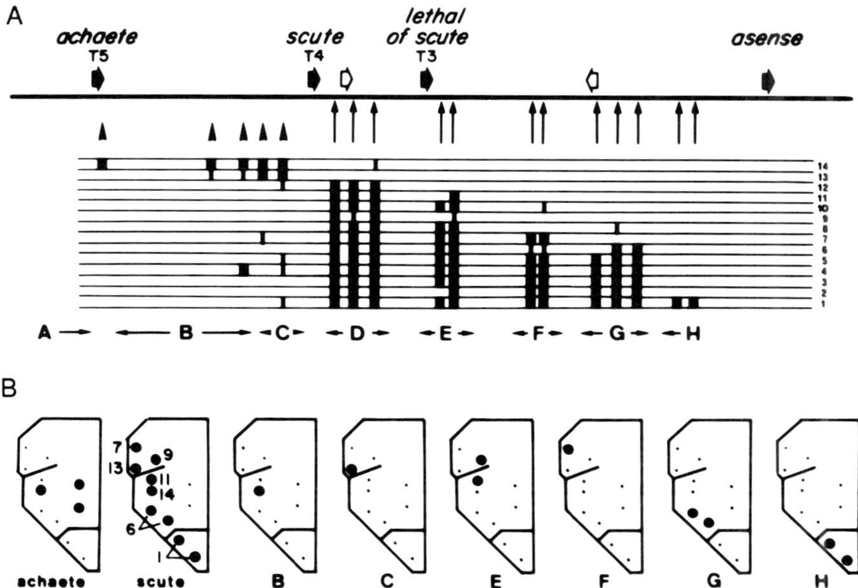

Figure 8. Molecular and phenotypic map of the *achaete–scute* complex. A. The upper line shows the chromosome segment of interest, which is 100 kb long. Distal is to the left, proximal to the right. The plain arrows above the line represent the four transcripts that share the HLH sequence. The vertical arrows under the line mark the location of *scute* breakpoints (inversions, translocations). The arrow-heads mark the breakpoints of five terminal deletions. The middle of the panel represents the *scute* phenotype of each mutant. The numbers at the right represent the different *scute* bristles on the head and notum, ordered according to their sensitivity to *scute* mutations. Wide bars represent a suppres-sion of more than 50%, thin bars, more than 10%. The data on the terminal deletions are from heterozygotes for a deletion of the *scute* gene, so only the *scute* phenotype is seen. At the bottom of the panel, the complex is divided into seven regions, A–H, according to the variations in phenotype. B. Diagram of the left half of the thorax, showing the location of the 11 precisely located macrochaetes (dots). Bristles are numbered as in A. The complementary sets of bristles that depend, respectively, on *achaete* and on *scute* are shown on the left. The *scute* bristles can be subdivided as shown in B–H, according to which region of the AS-C must be present adjacent to the coding region for the development of that particular set of bristles. (Reproduced from Ghysen and Dambly-Chaudière, 1988, with permission.)

genes (reviewed in Ingham, 1988) show a patterned expression in the imaginal discs (*engrailed* in the posterior region; Kornberg *et al.*, 1985; *patched* as a medial stripe; Phillips *et al.*, 1990; *hairy* in patches and stripes, Carroll and Whyte, 1989; *wingless* in particular regions; Baker, 1988).

As judged by the many enhancer-trap lines that show patterned expression of *lacZ* in imaginal discs (Bellen *et al.*, 1988), a number of other gene products may also be restricted to specific regions of the discs. It seems likely that each AS-C enhancer will respond to a particular combination of some of these gene products, and trigger AS-C expression in the limited region where this particular combination is achieved (Ghysen and Dambly-Chaudière, 1989).

We have so far confined the analysis of AS-C *cis*-regulation to the origin of the adult sense organs. Much less is known for the larval sense organs, because the system has been explored only recently. The analysis of the expression of AS-C during embryogenesis shows that, here again, AS-C genes are expressed locally in clusters of cells (M. Ruiz-Gomez, personal communication) and suggests that this expression makes these cells competent to form SMCs. In the case of the embryo, it is probable that specific combinations of the segment polarity and dorso-ventral genes are responsible for the local activation of the AS-C genes.

The study of the expression of AS-C in the embryo also reveals that the regulation of AS-C expression is extremely dynamic, raising the possibility that time may play a role in the process. Specifically, it may be that the same few cells become transiently competent at two or more consecutive times, and that the two or more resulting SMCs follow different fates because they were born at different times (and therefore in different contexts).

D. Other Elements of Competence

I. UNKNOWN HLH GENES

It seems likely that other HLH genes await identification. One reason to think so is that the absence of all AS-C genes leaves unaffected several types of sense organs, most notably the ch organs. Yet the absence of *da* eliminates all SMCs (Caudy *et al.*, 1988a). This suggests that the different types of sense organs require different heterodimers containing the *da* product. Unless *da* homodimers are sufficient by themselves to promote the formation of ch organs, it follows that at least one additional HLH gene must exist to give rise to the SMCs of ch organs. Furthermore, *da* is ubiquitously expressed [like its mammalian counterparts, the human E12 and E47 immunoglobulin activators (Lenardo *et al.*, 1987), which are more similar to *da* than to any other HLH gene presently known (Murre *et al.,* 1989a)], supporting the idea that other HLH genes are probably required to localize the AS-C-independent SMCs.

Attempts to detect other HLH genes by crosshybridization with AS-C probes have failed to detect anything, including *da* (Beamonte and Modolell, 1988), demonstrating that this method is of little use in this case, in part because of the variability of the loop region. Since the two helices are better conserved, PCR amplification with degenerate primers corresponding to the two helices may be more suitable. Indeed, this approach has led to the identification of mammalian homologs to AS-C genes that are specifically expressed in neural cell types (Johnson *et al.,* 1990). New HLH genes are now being isolated in the fly by this method, one of which displays an expression pattern suggestive of a role in the determination of ch organs (Y. Grau and Y. N. Jan, personal communication).

2. OTHER FACTORS INVOLVED IN THE FORMATION OF SENSORY MOTHER CELLS

Several arguments suggest that the AS-C genes are not the only determinants of SMC formation. One is based on the phenotype of *Hw* mutations, which are GOF mutations in AS-C leading to the formation of supernumerary sense organs (Garcia Alonso and Garcia-Bellido, 1986). At least some *Hw* mutations lead to the generalized expression of *sc* on the wing disc (Balcells *et al.,* 1988), yet additional sense organs are formed only in defined regions: around the normally formed bristles (Gottlieb, 1964) and in regions where the formation of sense organs is normally suppressed by the activity of the *h* and *emc* genes (Garcia Alonso and Garcia-Bellido, 1986).

The generalized expression of *sc* can also be achieved by introducing into flies a construct in which *sc* has been put under the control of a heat-shock promoter (hsp). The expression of *sc* can then be induced in all cells at any developmental time by heat-pulsing the transformant flies. The results confirm the observations on *Hw* flies, and also indicate that, for every region where supernumerary sense organs can be produced, the heat shocks will only be effective at a particular time of development (Rodriguez *et al.,* 1990).

The most likely interpretation of the results is that the products of AS-C genes can act only in cells that satisfy another condition. Although we do not know what the nature of this second condition could be, several cues suggest that it might be related to some aspect of the cell cycle. First, the spatial pattern of cell divisions during embryogenesis is remarkably constant (Foe, 1989); therefore, the phase of cells may itself be a patterning feature. Second, the distribution of mitosis in the developing wing imaginal disc is far from homogeneous, in particular along the dorso-ventral compartment boundary, as early as mid-larval life (O'Brochta and Bryant, 1985). Third, the spatial distribution of dividing cells in at least some regions of the late imaginal discs is also highly patterned, in particular in the prospective veins (Schubiger and Palka, 1987) and notum (Hartenstein and Posakony, 1989). Fourth, the pattern of the last divisions in the wing disc is largely synchronized (Garcia-Bellido and Merriam, 1971a).

Finally, we must mention two puzzling observations for which we presently have no adequate explanation. The first is based on experiments made with a construct in which the coding sequence of the gene *h* has been put under the control of a hsp promoter. The generalized expression of the gene *h* will suppress the formation of supernumerary microchaetes formed in *h* mutants, as well as of some of the microchaetes formed in *Hw* mutants, but has no effect on the formation of the normal microchaetes (Rushlow *et al.,* 1989). The second observation is based on the hsp–*sc* construct mentioned earlier. When this construct is used in a fly that is doubly mutant for *ac* and *sc,* and therefore forms virtually no sense organs, heat shocks occasionally results in the formation of a bristle. Whenever this happens, the bristle is always found at one of the 11 normal sites, suggesting again that the localized expression of AS-C genes is not the only spatial determinant involved in the positioning of bristles (Rodriguez *et al.,* 1990).

In conclusion, there are several indications that factors other than the distribution of AS-C products also play an important role in the formation of SMCs. The nature and number of these other factors is presently unknown. As a final note, it may be worth keeping in mind the pleasant caveat of Eddington: "It is also a good rule not to put overmuch confidence in experimental results that have not been confirmed by the theory."

V. Singling out the Sensory Mother Cell

A. Lateral Inhibition and Bristle Spacing

The acquisition of competence endows a cluster of cells with the ability to form a sense organ. How is it that only a defined number of cells, usually one, will become sensory mother cells? A simple answer is that whichever cell first turns into a SMC will prevent the other cells from undergoing the same change. This explanation is based on the classical work of Wigglesworth on the regular arrangement of bristles in another insect, *Rhodnius* (Wigglesworth, 1940). He demonstrated that a regular pattern can be accounted for by assuming that randomly located epidermal cells become SMCs, and that the surrounding cells then become incapable of undergoing the same transition.

The simple mechanism of lateral inhibition may explain the formation of regular patterns in a range of organisms (Claxton, 1964,1967), and was also proposed to account for the fact that a single SMC will be formed by a cluster of competent cells (Richelle and Ghysen, 1979). In this view, the singling out of the SMC, that is, the final decision of which cell will form the sense organ, depends on cell interactions among competent cells (reviewed in Simpson, 1990).

In the fly CNS, Doe and Goodman (1985) have demonstrated that neuroblasts do exert an inhibitory influence on the surrounding epidermal cells, each of which has the capability to also become a neuroblast. Thus the singling out of SMCs and central neuroblasts are probably very similar processes, and also resemble the process of fate selection in the equivalence groups in worms (Greenwald, 1989).

B. The Genetics of Singling out

Several genes are required to achieve the selection of a single SMC from among the competent cluster. Mutations in any of them are homozygous lethals and lead to a characteristic hypertrophy of the CNS (Lehmann *et al.*, 1981,1983), hence their generic name of "neurogenic" mutations. By extension, the normal genes were also, somewhat unfortunately, collectively called "neurogenic." Let it be clear, therefore, that the "neurogenic" genes are required to restrict, not to promote, neurogenesis. In addition to hypertrophy of the CNS, "neurogenic" mutations also lead to a parallel effect on the peripheral nervous system, by which the number of sensilla is increased by a factor of about 4 (Hartenstein and Campos-Ortega, 1986).

This set of genes has been the subject of intense genetic analysis. The cell autonomy of several of the mutations has been assessed by either genetic (Hoppe and Greenspan, 1986) or transplantation methods (Technau and Campos-Ortega, 1987), sometimes with conflicting results (see Chapter 6); the existence and nature of genetic interactions between them has been examined by gene dosage analysis and by studies of the modifications of dominant phenotypes (Vässin *et al.*, 1985; de la Concha *et al.*, 1988). The results of these analyses suggest that the different genes of this group form a functional chain, which extends from the inhibiting cell to its inhibited neighbors (reviewed in Campos-Ortega, 1985).

Several other mutations are known that result in the formation of supernumerary sense organs near the normal ones. Two of these mutations have been examined in some detail: *lethal (1) zeste-white 3 [l(1)zw3],* renamed *shaggy (sgg),* and *scabrous (sca).* The role played by either gene in the process of singling out remains rather obscure. The first one is a kinase

(Bourouis *et al.*, 1990; Siegfried *et al.*, 1990) and might be involved in a feedback mechanism in which the more a cell is inhibited, the less inhibitory it becomes (Heitzler and Simpson, 1991; see Section IV,D,3). The second one, *sca*, appears to encode a secreted protein that might play a role in the process of lateral inhibition (Mlodzik *et al.*, 1990). Alternatively, *sca* might be involved in the averaging process (Richelle and Ghysen, 1979) that insures that the expression of AS-C genes is usually higher near the center of the proneural clusters than at their periphery (Cubas *et al.*, 1991; M. Ruiz-Gomez, personal communication).

C. The Molecular Biology of Singling out

In spite of the virtually identical phenotypes resulting from their loss of function, the "neurogenic" genes form a structurally diverse group. Two of them, *Notch* (Wharton *et al.*, 1985; Kidd *et al.*, 1986) and *Delta* (Vässin *et al.*, 1987), are membrane proteins with a large number of EGF-like repeats in the extracytoplasmic domain, supporting a role for this group of genes in cell–cell interactions. A third one, *big brain*, resembles a channel protein, again indicating a role in cell contacts (Rao *et al.*, 1990) Another gene of this set, *neuralized*, has features that suggest a role as a transcriptional regulator (Y.N. Jan, personal communication). Yet another of the "neurogenic" genes, *Enhancer of split*, was initially defined by a dominant GOF phenotype in the adult eye, and was included among the "neurogenic" genes because a deletion of the region produces a typical neurogenic phenotype (Knüst *et al.*, 1987a). However the molecular analysis has been complicated by the discovery that the smallest deletion with a strong neurogenic phenotype contains about 10 transcriptional units, none of which by itself produces the strong phenotype when deleted (Knüst *et al.*, 1987b). Among these transcripts, one contains features typical of a G-protein (Hartley *et al.*, 1988), whereas four others contain a sequence reminiscent of the HLH motif (Klämbt *et al.*, 1989). Interestingly, the hinge between the first helix and the flanking basic region is disrupted by a proline, as is the case for the product of the gene *hairy*. The *Espl* HLH products may therefore be one focal point at which the machinery of lateral inhibition impinges directly on the capability of cells to become a SMC.

In combination, these results suggest that the different "neurogenic" genes are involved in a particular system of cell communication that includes membrane proteins, signal transducing gene(s), and transcriptional regulator(s) (reviewed in Campos-Ortega, 1988). This neural cell communication system would mediate the cell interactions that are required to restrict the number of cells that enter the neural pathway: in its absence all competent cells become neuroblasts (in the ventral neurectodermal region) or SMCs (in the lateral and dorsal clusters of competent cells).

The exact nature of these interactions, and their immediate effect, is not known. The radius of inhibition can be estimated from the distance between microchaetes on the notrum to extend over about three to four cell diameters in that case. The clusters of AS-C expressing cells that will give rise to the thoracic macrochaetes contain about 20–30 cells, suggesting that here again the radius of inhibition might cover about three to four cell diameters. Interestingly, this is exactly the distance covered by the "feet" or "strands" that form long extensions around the basal region of each epidermal cell (Wigglesworth, 1977; Locke and Huie, 1981). It may therefore be that the lateral inhibition is mediated by direct contact between the SMC and all of its 40 or so closest neighbors (assuming an extension of the feet of about three cell diameters). Alternatively, of course, it may be that the inhibitory cell contacts are self-propagating, but then one should invoke some additional reason for the tapering of this propagation after a few cell diameters.

D. The Function of the "Neurogenic" Genes

I. THE EMBRYO

In the embryo, the "neurogenic" genes are involved in restricting the number of SMCs that will be formed by a competent cluster. This was shown by using the enhancer-trap line A37, in which the SMC (and all their progeny) express the reporter gene *lacZ*. In "neurogenic" mutants, the first *lacZ*-expressing cells appear at the appropriate times and location in each body segment (Fig. 9). Soon after, however, clusters of *lacZ*-positive cells are observed at these positions, leading to the characteristic early "neurogenic" phenotype (Ghysen and Dambly-Chaudière, 1990, unpublished results). Figure 9 shows that, at this stage, each segment contains irregular anterior and posterior clusters of about 10 SMCs instead of the highly regular pattern of an anterior and a posterior pair of SMCs in all segments. The absence of AS-C reduces the neurogenic phenotype of the mutants (Brand and Campos-Ortega, 1989). This is as expected, since in embryos deficient for AS-C the hypertrophy of the PNS will be confined to the chordotonal SMCs.

2. THE ADULT

All strong "neurogenic" mutations are embryonic lethal. The adult phenotype of the "neurogenic" mutations therefore must be assessed in clones of homozygous cells obtained in heterozygous (viable) flies by somatic recombination (see Appendix, Section C). The general conclusion from the clonal analysis is that homozygous clones may show either a large excess of sense organs or an absence thereof, depending on the time at which the clone is

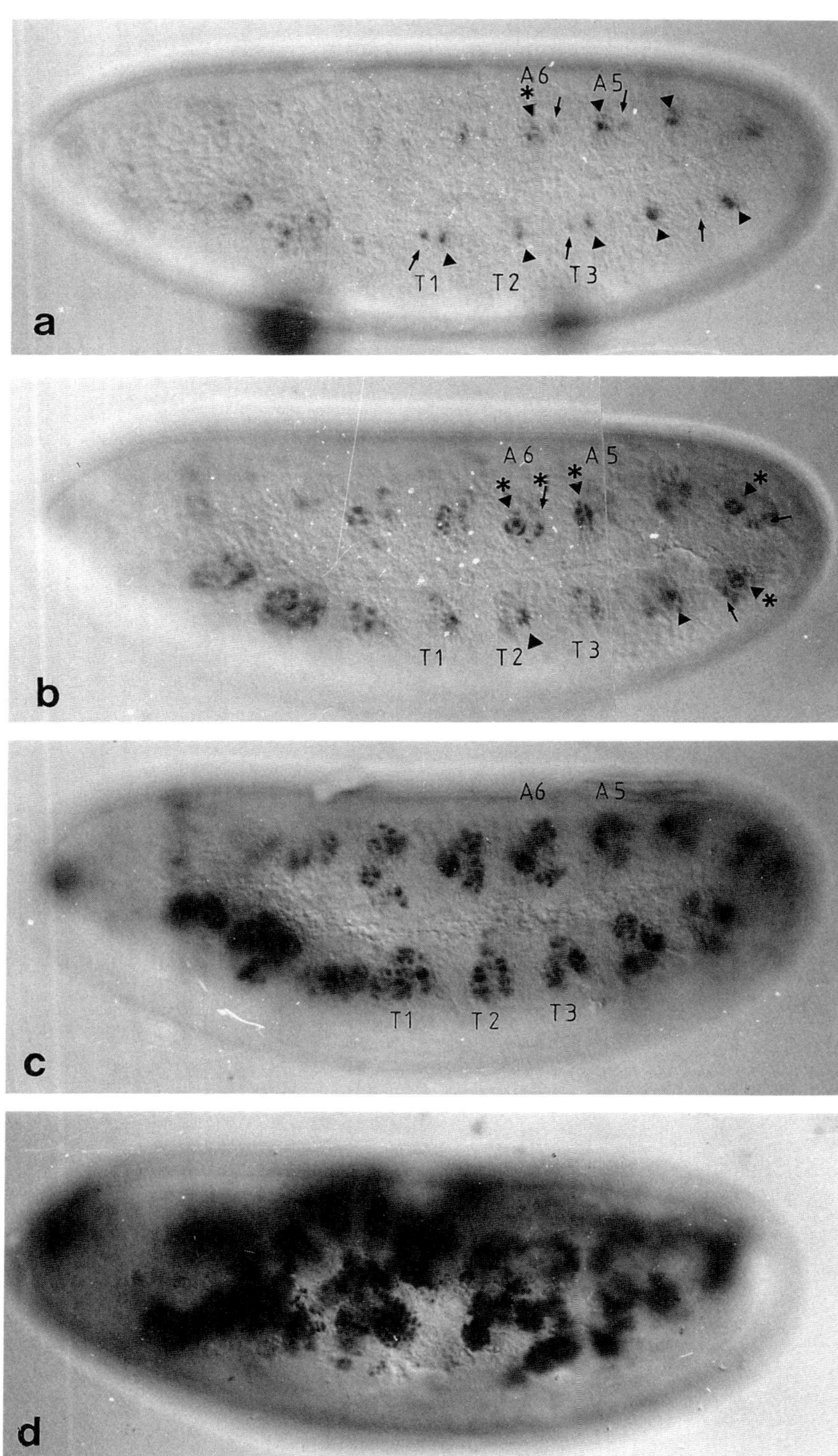
A6
A5
*
T1
T2
T3
a
A6
A5
*
*
*
*
*
T1
T2
T3
b
A6
A5
T1
T2
T3
c
d

induced, the strength of the allele, and so forth (Dietrich and Campos-Ortega, 1984). This conclusion is most clearly demonstrated by the use of one conditional allele, the thermosensitive mutation N^{ts1} (Shellenbarger and Mohler, 1978; Hartenstein and Posakony, 1990). Temperature shift experiments have shown that an early shift toward the restrictive temperature results in a large excess of sense organs, presumably because the inactivation of N results in too many competent cells becoming SMCs. In contrast, a late shift results in an apparent lack of sense organs. The latter result is due to the fact that all the progeny of the SMC become neurons, so the external derivatives of the sense organ (e.g., the bristle and socket) are not formed. Thus N is involved not only in the early process by which one cell among a competent group is singled out to become the SMC, but also in the subsequent process by which one cell among the progeny of the SMC is singled out to become a neuron.

In the eye, it has been shown that *Notch* is also required to restrict the number of cells that enters specific developmental pathways at different stages of eye development. Depending on the stage, the restriction will concern neuronal or nonneuronal developmental pathways, indicating that this gene is not exclusively involved in neural–epidermal decisions (Cagan and Ready, 1989).

3. DEVELOPMENTAL FUNCTION

The "neurogenic" loci are required to limit the number of competent cells that will become SMCs. This might be achieved in two ways. One way is that, once a SMC has formed, it produces an inhibitory signal mediated by the "neurogenic" loci. Under these circumstances the products of the loci would play no role before the first SMC is formed. Only then would they begin to function to prevent the neighboring cells from adopting the same fate. An alternative possibility is that the role of the "neurogenic" loci is to set up a system of mutual inhibition that is already active before the SMC emerges. Provided that there is a feedback mechanism by which the level of inhibitory signal emitted by one cell is inversely related to the level of inhibitory signal

---

Figure 9. The effect of a deletion of *N* on the emergence of early SMCs in an A37 embryo. Shown are four developmental stages of A37 embryos deleted for the *Notch* gene. a. The earliest pattern of *lacZ* expression is normal; most-segments contain a large P cell (*arrowheads*); in some segments the A cell is also beginning to express *lacZ*. This is very similar to the pattern in a normal embryo at the same developmental stage (e.g., see Fig. 4c). b. A and P cells are present in all segments; however, in several cases the posterior cluster already contains three or more cells (*asterisks*), whereas in the wild type there is only one pair of cells until after the appearance of the dorsal and ventral cells (see Fig. 4f). c. Large clusters of *lacZ*-expressing cells are now present in all segments. d. After the retraction of the germ band, the PNS is much hypertrophied and disorganized. (Reproduced from Ghysen and Dambly-Chaudière, 1990, with permission.)

received by that cell (in other words, if a cell is less capable of inhibiting its neighbors the more it is inhibited), then the system will amplify small differences so one cell will become fully inhibitory while its neighbors become fully inhibited (Heitzler and Simpson, 1991). In the nematode, the choice of one cell among a particular equivalence group involves a reinforcement mechanism by which small differences between neighboring cells are amplified into a "one cell on–one cell off" situation (Greenwald, 1989). Interestingly, one of the genes involved in this reinforcement mechanism, *lin-12*, shows a marked homology to the fly neurogenic gene *Notch*. If the nematode interpretation can be extrapolated to the fly, it suggests that the singling out might be the outcome of the conflict between competence and inhibition in all cells of the cluster, and that the commitment of one cell and the inhibition of its neighbors are two aspects of the same process.

Recent support to this view came from a careful re-examination of the adult and embryonic effects of neurogenic mutations. In the adult, extensive mosaic analyses have shown that whenever a proneural cluster includes cells with two or three copies of N^+, the cells with more copies of N^+ invariably become epidermal (Heitzler and Simpson, 1991), demonstrating that the choice of which cell will become the SMC obviously involves N. These and other results suggest that *Dl* is the inhibitory signal and N its receptor (de Celis *et al.*, 1991; Simpson, 1991; see Chapter 6). The choice of the SMC also responds to the dosage of the AS-C genes: in a competent cluster, cells with two doses of AS-C have a much higher probability of being chosen as SMCs than cells with only one dose (Cubas *et al.*, 1991). Thus competence may also be a graded property, in the sense that, the more competent a cell is, the more likely it is to become the SMC.

In the embryo, a detailed analysis of the early phenotype of neurogenic mutants has shown that the first SMCs appear at the appropriate locations and in the appropriate sequence, but at earlier times than in normal embryos (Goriely *et al.*, 1991). This result also agrees with the view that the appearance of a SMC is the outcome of a conflict between competence and inhibition in all cells of the proneural cluster. A reinforcement system of this type would guarantee that not more than one cell of the cluster will ever become a SMC, maybe not a very serious problem in the PNS, but certainly a crucial one in the CNS.

V. Differentiating the Sensory Mother Cell

To what extent do neuronal precursors differ from each other? This question is central to the problem of defining neuronal identity, yet remains most mysterious. In the case of the fly SMCs, some progress has been made recently (reviewed in Jan and Jan, 1990). We will consider successively (1) the differentiation between type 1 and type 2 neurons, (2) the differentiation between es and ch organs, (3) the differentiation between monoinnervated and polyinnervated organs, and (4) the differentiation between bristles and campaniform sensilla. A largely hypothetical "choice tree" is represented in Fig. 10. The most interesting aspect of this tree is that most of the genes mentioned are now available both in LOF and GOF condition (see Appendix, Section A,3), opening the way to a detailed dissection of the hierarchical relationships hypothesized in the figure.

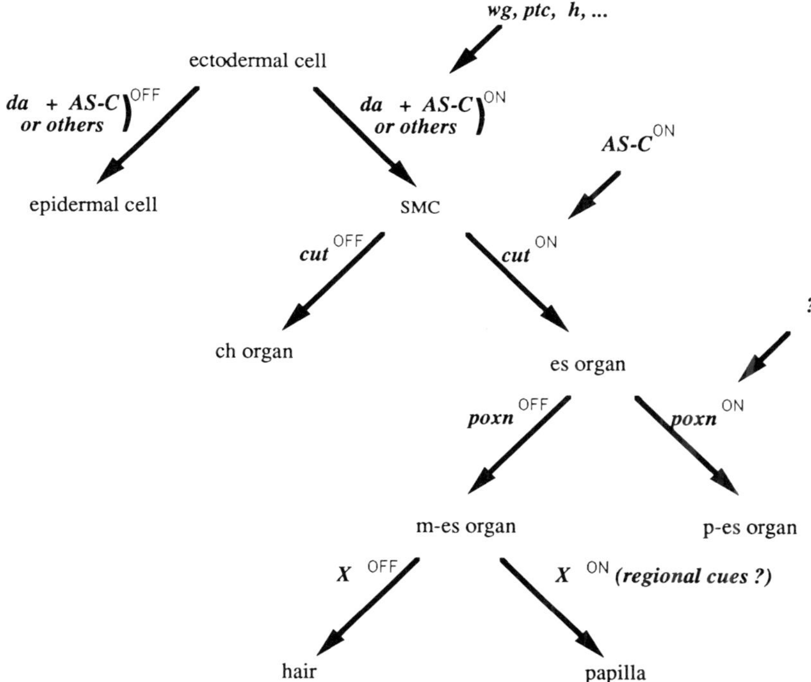

Figure 10. The specification of a sensory mother cell. For the sake of simplicity, the choices have been shown as sequential. It is quite possible, however, that the choices are made in parallel instead, as suggested by the fact that the expression of *poxn* is normal in embryos that are deficient for *cut*. The hypothetical gene *X*, responsible for the choice between hair and papilla, is supposed to be "on" in the papillae because (1) papillae are probably evolutionarily derived from hairs and (2) papillae may (rarely) develop as hairs in normal flies, possibly a phenocopy of an *X* mutation. The controls of AS-C by *h, wg, ptc*, etc.; of *cut* by AS-C; and of gene *X* by regional cues are still largely speculative. They are shown to provide a plausible, if schematic, view of the type of network that might control specification.

A. Type-1 versus Type-2

Type-1 sense organs include all es organs and ch organs; they are formed by a fixed lineage and comprise three support cells and one or more neurons, each of which has a single dendrite. Type-2 sense organs are single neurons with no identified support cell; most of them form multiple extended dendrites (Zawarzin, 1912). Very little is known about the larval type-2 neurons, other than their spatial distribution (Bodmer and Jan, 1987), and nothing is known about adult type-2 neurons. In the larva, many type-2 neurons are found associated to es neurons (Ghysen *et al.*, 1986), suggesting that the formation of some type-2 neurons may be somehow linked to that of the es organs. Furthermore, in the absence of the AS-C genes not only all es organs, but also most type-2 neurons, fail to form (Dambly-Chaudière and Ghysen, 1987), supporting the idea of an association between the two types of sense organs. Type-2 cells are born before the SMC of the associated es organ undergoes its first division (Bodmer *et al.*, 1989), as expected if the type-2 cell and SMC were formed at about the same time. The association between es SMCs and type-2 neurons might result from a common origin for the two cells or from the induction (recruitment) of one by the other. In either case, this early interaction could specify the fate of the two cells, one as type 2 and the other as the es SMC.

B. es Organs versus ch Organs

The difference between es and ch SMCs is due to the expression of the gene *cut*. The product of this gene is present only in the cells that form es organs (Blochlinger *et al.*, 1988). Complete LOF mutations in *cut* transform es into ch organs in homozygous embryos, as well as in clones of homozygous cells in the adult (Bodmer *et al.*, 1987). Thus the expression of *cut* is required for the formation of es organs as opposed to ch organs.

The GOF phenotype of *cut* was determined by using a construct in which the coding sequence of *cut* is put under the control of a heat-shock promoter. Overexpression of *cut* during embryogenesis results in the conversion of all ch into es organs (Blochlinger *et al.*, 1991). Thus *cut* is the key gene that differentiates es from ch organs. Not surprisingly, the *cut* gene product contains a DNA binding motif that may mediate its regulatory function (Blochlinger *et al.*, 1988).

The lineage of an es organ differs slightly from that of a ch organ (Bodmer *et al.*, 1989); therefore one would expect *cut* to be already expressed in the SMCs that will form es organs, and not in ch SMCs, as was indeed observed (Blochlinger *et al.*, 1990). What, then, is the factor that triggers *cut* expression in the es SMCs? Good candidates are the AS-C products, since all SMCs that will express *cut* arise from cells expressing AS-C genes, whereas SMCs that do not depend on AS-C do not express *cut.*

C. p-es Organs versus m-es Organs

The difference between monoinnervated external sense organs (m-es) and polyinnervated organs (p-es) is related to the expression of the gene *pox-neuro (poxn).* This gene was isolated by homology with a motif called "paired box," which is thought to mediate DNA binding (Bopp *et al.,* 1989). *poxn* is specifically expressed in the cells that will form p-es organs, both in the embryo and in the imaginal discs (C. Dambly-Chaudière *et al.,* 1992). Removing the gene results in the transformation of p-es organs into m-es organs or, in some cases, in their absence. Thus the gene is required for the formation of a p-es as opposed to a m-es organ. Overexpression of the gene was obtained, as in the case of *cut,* by using a hsp-*poxn* construct. Heat-shocking transgenic flies showed that the GOF phenotype of *poxn* is an excess of p-es organs (in the thoracic segments, where the p-es organs are most readily detected because of their massive external process). Thus *poxn* is a good candidate for a gene involved in the choice between m-es and p-es.

The most obvious difference between the m-es and p-es lineages occurs late, when one of the four daughter cells forms one neuron in the m-es lineage, but keeps dividing to generate several neurons in the case of the p-es lineage. However, a BUdr lineage analysis of adult p-es indicates that the lineages may differ earlier, possibly as early as the first division of the SMC (Hartenstein and Posakony, 1989). An early difference between the two lineages is also suggested by the observation that m-es organs are absent in embryos that are mutant for the gene encoding cyclin, whereas p-es organs are formed normally in such embryos (E. Giniger, personal communication). One would therefore expect that *poxn* be expressed early in the lineage, much like *cut.* Expression of *poxn* is indeed observed early, probably as soon as the SMC is singled out, remains high in all the progeny of the SMC and disappears shortly before the onset of differentiation (C. Dambly-Chaudière *et al.,* 1992). This temporal pattern of expression is entirely consistent with the idea that *poxn* is necessary to specify the particular pattern of mitoses involved in the generation of p-es organs.

We do not know what factor causes the expression of *poxn* in a small subset of embryonic SMCs. It may be worth pointing out that, in the embryo, in which each body segment contains two p-es organs, the two essential AS-C genes *ac* and *ase* encode one p-es each (Dambly-Chaudière and Ghysen, 1987).

D. Hairs versus Papillae

The two major types of m-es organs are the hairs or bristles (sensilla chaetica), in which the trichogen support cell produces an elongated shaft, and the papillae or campaniform sensilla (sensilla campaniformia), in which the trichogen forms a dome-shaped structure. Large and small bristles are called, respectively, macrochaetae and microchaetae in the adult; in the larva all monoinnervated bristles are about the same size.

In the embryo, each of the two essential AS-C genes, *ac* and *ase,* is required for both hairs and papillae in each segment. In the adult also, the AS-C genes involved (*ac* and *sc)* are required for the formation of both bristles and campaniform sensilla. It seems, therefore, that whether a SMC is formed by one or another AS-C gene does not specify the type of es organ that will be produced. An indication of how the type of sense organ might be selected comes from the analysis of supernumerary sense organs produced in different ways. In the wing, bristles are normally formed only along the margin. Several morphologically distinct types of bristles are found in successive regions of the margin. When clones of cells homozygous for the mutation *sgg* are induced in the wing blade, they exclusively form bristles. For each clone, the type of bristle formed resembles the type present on the wing margin at the same antero-posterior level, suggesting that the wing blade is divided in four or five stripes along the antero-posterior axis, each of which specifies a given type of bristle (Ripoll *et al.,* 1988). Thus the succession of the different types of bristles along the wing margin would reflect the successive intersection of these stripes by the prospective margin.

Clones of *emc* cells also produce supernumerary sense organs in the wing blade (Garcia Alonso and Garcia-Bellido, 1988). These may be either bristles or campaniform sensilla. The compilation of a large number of clones suggests a graded variation from proximal to distal along the wing blade, so clones in the most proximal region almost invariably contain campaniform sensilla, whereas clones in the most distal region contain mostly bristles.

In conjunction, these results suggest that, independent of their role in the local activation of AS-C expression, regionally expressed genes are used to further determine the type of sense organ the SMC will form.

VI. Differentiating the Neuron

We will first summarize the basic principles of axonal guidance as a background for the section on the mechanisms of path choice.

A. The Scaffold

1. PERIPHERAL PATHWAYS: CONTACT GUIDANCE AND PIONEERING

One essential component of the centripetal growth of peripheral axons is guidance by pre-existing nerves. Basically, the idea is that sooner or later the growing axon will meet other axons which can then be used as guides to help the growing axon home in on the right place (Wigglesworth, 1953). Before the developing axon can follow an older axon, however, it has to find it, implying that the growth cone must be capable of oriented growth in the absence of axonal guidance. This is particularly crucial in the case of the very first axons that have to find their course in uncharted territory; indeed, the long lonesome journey of such pioneers is particularly suited for the analysis of guiding cues.

The question of pioneering in the insect embryo was first focused on, with characteristic foresight, by Bate (1976). His and a large amount of subsequent work suggests that oriented axonal growth relies on orienting cues laid down by the epidermis along which the growth cone progresses, on the basal lamina formed by this epidermis (Nardi, 1983; Blair *et al.,* 1987), or on "stepping stones," cells that are located along the prospective path of the axon toward the CNS (Bate, 1976; Ho and Goodman, 1982; Bentley and Caudy, 1983; Keshishian and Bentley, 1983a).

In the fly embryo, the first guides are axons sent dorsally into the periphery by motor neurons at the same time as the first peripheral axons are extended ventrally toward the CNS (Ghysen *et al.,* 1986; Hartenstein, 1988). The two growth cones will meet somewhere on their way and thereby establish the first peripheral nerve. Since both sensory and motor neurons are segmentally repeated, one fascicle will be formed in each segment. Another set of pioneers will establish a second fascicle, slightly posterior to the first one. Later, developing peripheral neurons send axons along either of these pioneer tracts to form the larval peripheral nerves. During metamorphosis, the guides for the developing adult axons are the larval peripheral nerves themselves (Ghysen and Deak, 1978). Before they find their larval guide, however, adult axons have to travel some distance in the discs. The basic ingredients of oriented growth seem to be the same in the discs as in the embryo: differential affinity for the epidermis or its basement membrane, selective recognition of guidepost cells, and fasciculation with pre-existing axons (Blair and Palka, 1985). The relative importance of orienting cues and of strategically located stepping stones depends very much on the particular situation a given axon will meet. Imaginal discs expand at very different rates after the onset of metamorphosis, and the spacing between sense organs can also vary enormously: each disc has its particular solution to the problems of the pioneers (Jan *et al.*, 1985), which is different again from the system used in the fly embryo or in the grasshopper limb.

It must be realized that all peripheral axons, by virtue of their having to reach a pre-existing nerve fiber, make their own contribution to the establishment of the final network. The progressive construction of a complex network is nicely illustrated in the case of the grasshopper limb, in which each component of the final scaffold has been pioneered in turn by a newly developing axon (Ho and Goodman, 1982; Keshishian and Bentley, 1983b). Some of these contributions may later turn out to be essential, whereas others will be of lesser importance, but only further development will tell which is which. Thus, the progressive elaboration of the peripheral nerve net is a vivid metaphor of the progressive elaboration of science itself.

2. CENTRAL PATHWAYS: PATH RECOGNITION

The ability to form long precise projections relies on the ability of the growing axon to specifically recognize and follow pre-existing pathways (Ghysen, 1978). Thus, as in the case of the peripheral pathways, guidance along pre-existing axons plays a central role in the establishment of connectivity, with one major difference between peripheral and central guidance. In the CNS, each sensory axon is able to recognize and follow one or a few among the many existing fiber tracts (Ghysen, 1978; Ghysen and Janson, 1980). This selective fasciculation, which does not seem to exist in the PNS (Palka and Ghysen, 1982), implies that the different tracts in the CNS must be differentially tagged [hence the names of "substrate" pathways (Katz and Lasek, 1980) or "labeled" pathways (Raper *et al.*, 1983)]. Recent work on the nature of the tags that differentiate the fiber tracts one from another indicates that some of them belong to the immunoglobulin superfamily, which also includes vertebrate cell adhesion molecules, whereas others are novel homophilic cell adhesion molecules (reviewed in Grenningloh *et al.*, 1990).

The establishment of the scaffold of pathways in the CNS is based on principles similar to these seen in the periphery: simple orienting cues laid down by the epidermis (Bate and Grunewald, 1981), presence of stepping stones (Jacobs and Goodman, 1989a), and fasciculation with pre-existing fibers (Jacobs and Goodman, 1989b). It is worth mentioning that only two types of orienting cues need be discriminated, because the entire scaffold is built as an orthogonal net. In other words, all the early tracts run either longitudinally (connectives) or transversely (commissures). Thus, all pioneers follow either the antero-posterior or the dorso-ventral axis. (Since the axons grow along the basal surface of the ectoderm, the medio-lateral direction is effectively dorso-ventral.)

The second aspect of the ontogeny of CNS tracts, as mentioned in the previous section, is the differential labeling of parallel fibers in the connectives and commissures. This aspect, which provides the molecular basis for selective fasciculation (Bastiani *et al.,* 1985), is probably achieved quite simply by reiteration. Reiteration allows the same orienting cues to be used again and again by consecutive axons carrying different tags, thereby leading to the successive formation of a set of parallel fascicles, each of which will express a particular marker or combination of markers.

Slight differences between the establishment of the early tracts in grasshopper and fly (Jacobs and Goodman, 1989b) illustrate the flexibility of the system of reiteration–differentiation, as well as its constraints: only parallel fascicles will be formed. What may vary is their number and differential labeling. This process of reiteration and differentiation of parallel fascicles may explain the complexity of the longitudinal connectives, which comprise at least 20 anatomically distinct parallel bundles (Thomas *et al.,* 1984), or of the anterior and posterior commissures (Raper *et al.,* 1983; Teugels and Ghysen, 1985). At least some of these bundles remain differentially labeled as judged from the fact that growing axons can unerringly discriminate one of them from the others (Bastiani *et al.,* 1984,1986). Due to addition of new elements during growth, maturation, and distortion of the tissue, many of these bundles will subsequently drift away from each other, leading to the adult situation in which the different longitudinal and transverse tracts are widely separated (Power, 1948). Here again the behavior of sensory axons strongly suggests that each of these tracts remains differentially labeled and can therefore be uniquely recognized by the growing axons (Ghysen, 1978).

The complication of the initially simple structure is strikingly illustrated by the transition between the embryonic and the adult patterns of commissures (Fig. 11). This transition transforms a simple periodic pattern into something so complicated that both the orthogonal structure of the tracts and their segmentally repeated nature become completely undetectable.

3. ORIGIN OF THE SCAFFOLD: PHYLOGENY

As mentioned previously, the early pattern of connections in the CNS is remarkably simple, since it consists solely of longitudinal connectives and transverse commissures. Later, pattern appears more complex, but this is most likely to result from passive distortion. The same is true in the periphery, where the early pattern comprises the segmentally repeated anterior and posterior nerves (transversely oriented) and the lateral nerve (extending longitudinally, Hertweck, 1931; Bodmer and Jan, 1987). Here again this simple

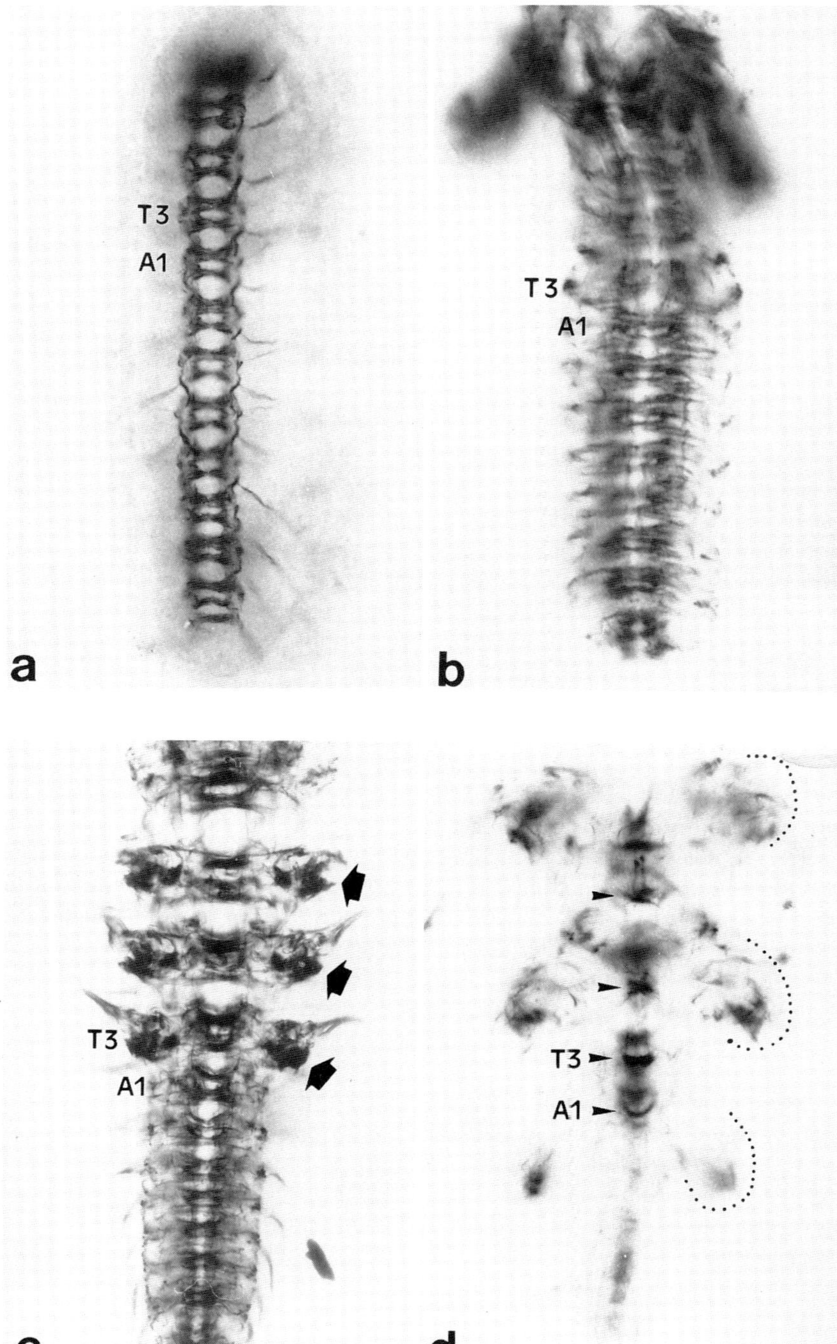

scaffold is progressively complicated by the addition of side branches and displacement of extent stretches by the growth of other tissues, until in the adult the pattern has become so distorted and so different from one segment to the next, that its basic simplicity goes unnoticed, yet there is no doubt that the adult pattern is basically grounded on the larval pattern.

We imagine that the common features of the fly PNS and CNS reflect the early stages of nervous system development, when the major achievement was to establish a regular pattern of connectivity. Presumably, the same basic methods that still are used in the fly were developed early; the reliance on whatever cue might be derived from the existence of a longitudinal and a transverse axis to establish longitudinal and transverse connections. The appearance of metamerization (or periodicity) turned out to be a major simplifying principle and, as such, may have been directly correlated to the increasing complexity of neural development. Thus the basic structure of a periodically organized orthogonal system has most likely predated the major phylogenetic explosion that led to the separate lineages that would in due time produce the vertebrates and the diptera.

Evidence in support of this view comes from the observation that an orthogonal periodic nervous system is already present in several types of flatworms (Bullock and Horridge, 1965). In some of them, for example *Bothrioplana*, the orthogonal periodic system still shows the eight-fold radial

---

Figure 11. Transformation of the simple pattern of the embryonic CNA into the complex pattern of adult tracts. The ventral CNS at different developmental stages is labeled with antibody 5D12 (isolated in the laboratory of Dr. Y. N. Jan at UCSF). This antibody recognizes a subset of tracts in the connectives and commissures. a. Regular pattern of commissures and connectives in a late embryo. The labeled tracts define two commissures in each segment except A9. b. The pattern is still very regular in a first or second instar larva. C. In a third instar larva, the pattern becomes distorted in the thoracic segments with the development of the prospective leg neuromeres *(arrows)*; minor differences can be observed between the tracts of T1, T2, T3, and A1. d, e, f. Three focal planes, from dorsal to ventral, in an adult ganglion, to illustrate the complexity arising from the segmental diversification of the commissures. d. Homologous dorsal tracts in T1, T2, T3, and A1 are marked by arrowheads. e. Homologous anterior tracts in T1, T2, T3, and A1 are marked by arrowheads; homologous posterior tracts in T2 and T3 are marked by arrows. This particular posterior tract has no detectable homolog in T1 and A1. f. Homologous anterior tracts are marked by an arrow; homologous posterior tracts are marked by an arrowhead. Neither the anterior nor the posterior tract has a detectable homolog in A1. g, h. Two focal planes similar to those of d and e in an adult ganglion of a *bithoraxoid* mutant. The inactivation of this homeotic gene prevents the segmental diversification that normally depends on this gene. As a result, the tracts in the affected region retain the shape of their homolog in the anterior segment. g. The dorsal tract in A1 (which belongs to the anterior commissure) remains similar to that of T3; compare the mutant (A1') with the normal (A1 in d) tracts. h. The posterior tract of T3 has retained the shape of its T2 homolog; compare the mutant (T3) with the normal (T3 in e) tracts. The domains of action of homeotic genes in the central nervous system are parasegmental rather than segmental, since the region affected by the mutation includes posterior T3 as well as anterior A1 tracts. (Reproduced from Teugels and Ghysen, 1985, and Weinzierl *et al.*, 1987, with permission.) Figure continues.

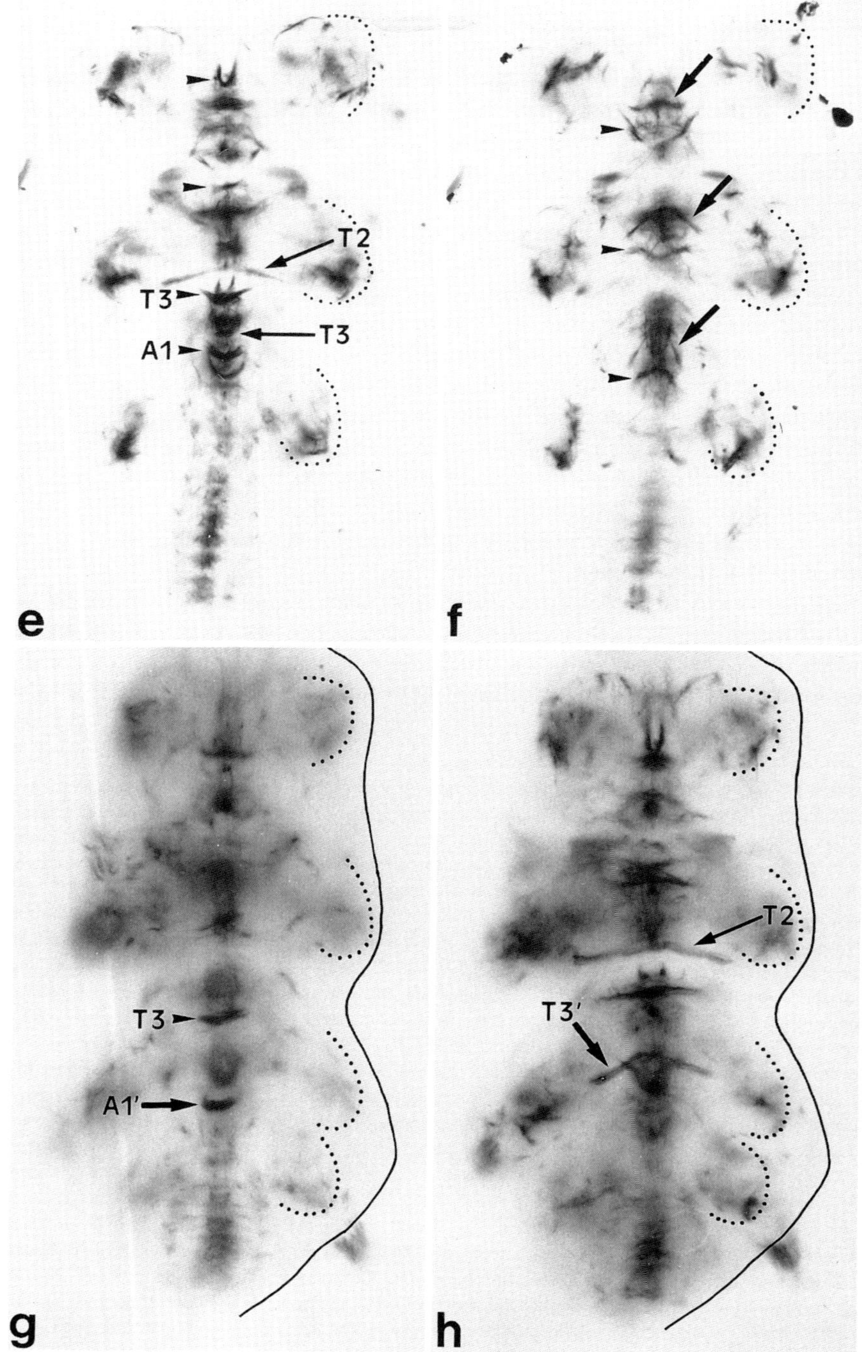

T2
T3
A1
T3
e
f
T2
T3
A1'
T3'
g
h

symmetry typical of the more primitive ctenarians. Elision or fusion of some of the longitudinal nerve cords may have subsequently generated all presently known types of nervous systems. Remarkably, the eight-fold symmetry typical of the most primitive flatworms is still obvious in annelid larvae, although the adult forms only show the two ventral cords that are supposed to be typical of their phylum (Bullock and Horridge, 1965). Likewise prochordates have both a dorsal and a ventral nerve cord, suggesting that the strictly dorsal nerve cord diagnostic of the chordate lineage is a rather late design.

We further imagine that once this basic structural design was attained and, therefore, once the tools to establish such a scaffold existed, the development of specific tags allowed the reiteration of the same basic plan to produce a much more complex nervous system than previously attainable, and opened the way to an unprecedented sophistication in connectivity and, hence, behavior. We think that this second breakthrough also predates the Cambrian explosion.

Consistent with this view is the growing evidence that molecules crucial for the differential tagging and spatial organization of the insect nervous system are highly conserved in the vertebrates, for example, the cell adhesion molecules of the immunoglobulin superfamily (Harrelson and Goodman, 1988). The family itself is proposed to have originated as neural cell recognition molecules, and only later to have become more widely used in other cell types. Much along the same line, we believe that the periodic organization and segment determination originated as advances to handle the need for an increasingly complex neural connectivity, and were later extended to other cell types. Here again the striking molecular conservation of the homeobox motif between mammalia and diptera, the fact that in both cases these genes are organized in clusters in which the order of the genes in the cluster parallels their order of deployment along the antero-posterior body axis, and finally the observation that there is a gene-by-gene homology between fly and mammalian clusters (reviewed in Holland, 1990), argues in favor of the idea that the primitive cluster of homeobox genes (and presumably its spatial pattern of deployment in the nervous system) predated the separation of the two lineages.

If this view is correct, it implies that the basics of neural development are universal (a view also supported by the remarkable conservation of the neural HLH motif from the AS-C genes of the fly to the MASH genes in the rat; Johnson *et al.*, 1990) and that each animal species represents only one way of exploiting the potential of the highly regular, primitive system. It also implies that the development of the nervous system has been, more than that of any other tissue, subject to structural constraints (Thomas *et al.*, 1984; Meier *et al.*, 1991), and, therefore, that it may be a better indicator of true evolutionary relationships than generally recognized.

B. Mechanisms of Path Choice

Based on the small number of projections that have been studied, there are at least three types of factors that may influence the pathway followed by an axon: the type of sense organ, its developmental history, and the time at which the neuron differentiates. The importance of position also must be stressed in the case of the projections from the bristles on the notum and on the legs. However, in both cases position seems to affect the extent of the projection, rather than the choice of the pathway itself; therefore, the effect of position will be discussed separately.

I. TYPE OF SENSE ORGAN

This is probably the most obvious factor that determines the projection. Bristles and campaniform sensilla, for example, always follow different pathways, even if they are located near each other. In a particular fly strain, Palka observed that one of a uniquely recognizable pair of campaniform sensilla on the wing, the twin sensilla of the margin (TSM), occasionally develops as a bristle. He found that the underlying neuron establishes a projection typical of the nearby bristles, very different from the normal projection of a TSM neuron (Palka, 1986).

The case of the chemosensory bristles is interesting, since those bristles are innervated by several neurons, one of which is usually mechanosensory whereas the others are chemosensory. Nevertheless, all neurons seem to establish the same projection, both in the case of the wing and in the case of the ieg chemosensory bristles. If this result could be confirmed, it would open the possibility that the choice of the projection is already decided before the neuron precursor divides, possibly as early as the SMC.

2. DEVELOPMENTAL HISTORY

Graft experiments have demonstrated that the projection of a sensory neuron depends on its developmental history (Anderson and Bacon, 1979). What we call developmental history of a neuron includes the different genetic tags that were consecutively imposed on the progenitors of the SMC, such as compartment and segment identity (Garcia-Bellido *et al.*, 1973; Lewis, 1978).

The importance of segmental identity for the establishment of the projection by serially homologous neurons has been demonstrated in the case of wing and haltere campaniform sensilla, and of the bristles on the different abdominal segments (Fig. 12; Ghysen *et al.*, 1983). The segmental determination of the epidermis of these segments depends on genes of the Bithorax Complex (Lewis, 1978; reviewed in Akam, 1987), which also controls seg-

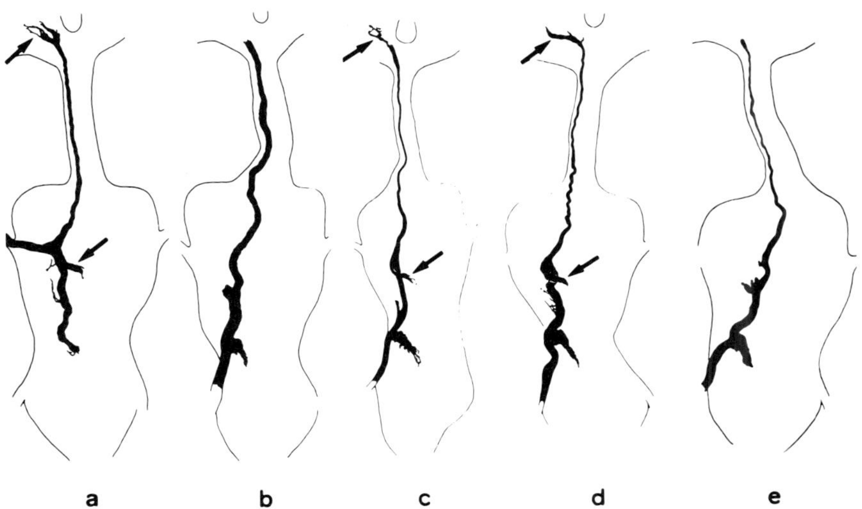

Figure 12. Segmental transformation of a sensory projection. a. The normal projection from the proximal campaniform sensilla of the left wing. The axons, which have been filled with horseradish peroxidase and can therefore easily be visualized in the CNS, enter the thoracico-abdominal ganglia (*outlined*) through the wing nerve and establish a typical projection that includes a contralateral branch (*lower arrow*). The anterior branch of the projection extends through the cervical connective (which runs in the neck) into the suboesophageal ganglion, where it arborizes deeply (*upper arrow*). b. A normal projection from the proximal campaniform sensilla of the left haltere. The axons enter the thoracico-abdominal ganglion through the haltere nerve and follow the same antero-posterior path that is recognized by the wing axons, with two differences: the axons do not establish the contralateral branch and they do not extend deeply into the suboesophageal ganglion. c, d. The projections from halteres partly transformed into wings due to a mutation in a regulator of the bithorax complex, *trithorax (trx)*. The flies were respectively homozygous (c) and hemizygous (d) for a hypomorphic allele of *trx*. The axons enter the ganglion at the position appropriate for haltere axons, but they establish a projection that is typical of wing axons (*arrows*). e. The projection from a haltere that has been entirely transformed into a wing due to an extreme *bithorax* mutation (bx^3). In spite of the complete transformation of the epidermis and the external part of the sensilla (which have slightly different morphologies on the haltere and wing), the neurons project as normal haltere axons. (Reproduced from Ghysen *et al.*, 1983, with permission.)

mental differences in axonal pathways. Early results suggested that segmental identity might depend on different gene products in epidermis and in neurons, since some Bithorax mutations that have an extreme effect on epidermal cells leave the underlying neurons apparently unaffected (Fig. 12e; Palka and Schubiger, 1980; Ghysen *et al.*, 1983). These results can now be reinterpreted in the light of the molecular analysis of the complex (Bender *et al.*, 1983). The tissue specificity of *bithorax* mutations is due not to the presence of different genes but to differential splicing of the transcripts so that different products of the same gene act in epidermis and in neurons (Weinzierl *et al.*, 1987; Mann and Hogness, 1990). Indeed, the Bithorax Complex mutations that have no effect on the axonal projections are clustered near a microexon (Peifer and Bender, 1986) that is apparently not used in adult neurons (Weinzierl *et al.*, 1987).

3. TIME OF NEURAL DIFFERENTIATION

All sense organs differ from each other not only in position but also in birth time. In the case of the 11 thoracic macrochaetes, for example, the earliest SMC originates about 35 hr before the latest one, a surprisingly long interval considering that the entire larval development spans no more than 4 days (Huang *et al.*, 1991). There is no overall gradient or progression in the pattern of birth times. For example, the very first and the very last SMCs correspond to bristles that are not very far from each other. The temporal sequence observed in the formation of the SMCs is retained during the ensuing divisions and differentiation steps up to axonogenesis.

A correlation between projection and time of origin (or of neuronal differentiation) has been demonstrated in the case of the distal campaniform sensilla of the wing. The distal sensilla may follow either of two parallel pathways in the CNS (Ghysen, 1980). One pathway is invariably preferred by the earliest four sensilla, the other by all later developing sensilla (Palka *et al.*, 1986). This rule is respected even if the number of sensilla is vastly reduced or increased, suggesting that it is not a reflection of competitive effects. Interestingly, the time of origin of the sensilla correlates not only with the pathway but also with the physiological properties of the neurons (Dickinson and Palka, 1987).

Among the distal sensilla of the wing, three deserve a special comment because they illustrate, by comparison with the thoracic bristles, the multiplicity of mechanisms that may operate in the choice of a pathway. Of the three sensilla that are aligned along the third vein, one is formed first; the other two are formed about 10 hr later, one on each side of the first one (Huang *et al.*, 1991). All three probably depend on the same AS-C control region (Leyns *et al.*, 1989). As mentioned earlier, in this case the choice of a pathway depends strictly on time: the early sensillum consistently elects one path, the late ones the other path (Palka *et al.*, 1986). This stands in contrast to the case of the thoracic bristles. The two scutellar bristles, for example, also depend on a common AS-C control region (Campuzano *et al.*, 1985), and their SMCs appear with an interval of about 20 hr (Huang *et al.*, 1991). In this case, however, the projection of the two bristles is largely similar (Ghysen, 1980). Furthermore, the differences between the projections of the most anterior and the most posterior thoracic macrochaetes are progressive, and vary continuously with position, not with the time of formation of the SMC.

4. POSITION AND THE TERMINAL ARBOR

That the position of a sense organ affects the central connections made by the axon is easily demonstrated by behavioral assays (Van der Vorst and Ghysen, 1980; Corfas and Dudai, 1989). Nearly nothing is known of the factors that determine the distribution of synaptic contacts in any sensory system other than the eye. As a first step to an analysis of the connectivity, we may examine how position affects the projection and the terminal arbor of sensory neurons.

One system in which the position of the sense organ plays a role in the shaping of the projection is the large dorsal bristles on the thorax (Ghysen, 1980). All bristle neurons follow the same longitudinal pathway, but the extent of the anterior and posterior branches varies according to the position of the bristle. This variation is not due to competition or other interactions among axons, because each neuron behaves according to the position of the bristle that it innervates, irrespective of the presence and number of other bristles around. Presumably, the neuron is using the same positional information that was used to determine the SMC in the first place. How this information is conveyed from the SMC to its daughters, and then to the local control of the growth cone, is not at all understood.

The role of position in determining the final shape of the projection has been most extensively studied in local projections, such as the projections from leg or cercal bristles in crickets, most of which arborize in the corresponding segmental ganglion (Murphey *et al.*, 1983). This type of projection differs from those discussed so far in the relative role of pathway choice and target recognition (Teugels and Ghysen, 1983). In all cases in which the axon projects to a distant part of the CNS, the choice of a particular pathway is probably important to bring the axon near its prospective target. Whenever the axon projects locally, however, the pathway that it follows does not matter too much and, indeed, axons may follow abnormal trajectories yet form normal terminal arbors (Murphey *et al.*, 1983).

The importance of position in defining the shape and position of the terminal arbor has been documented in the leg bristles of the fly (Murphey *et al.*, 1989) as well as in the leg, cercal, and dorsal bristles of the cricket (Johnson and Murphey, 1985). In the leg and cercal bristles, there is a gradual change in the central position of the terminal arbor as the position of the sense organ varies around the circumference of the appendage. This gradual change does not depend on interaction between neurons or axons, at least not in the leg of the fly, since the removal of many bristles by AS-C mutations in mosaic animals (see Appendix) does not affect the projection of the remaining bristles (Murphey *et al.*, 1989). In the cricket, in which many more sensory organs are present, competitive interactions between sensory fibers affect the extent of the arbor (Murphey and Lemere, 1984), but apparently not its position. In this animal, the analysis of sensory projections after epidermal transplantations (Murphey *et al.*, 1983; Walthall and Murphey, 1984) also led to the conclusion that the effect of position on projection is mediated by the same mysterious system of positional information that allows morphogenesis and regeneration to proceed (Malacinski and Bryant, 1984).

So far, therefore, we have no clue to how position determines axonal behavior, yet the relationship between position and projection is one of the great unanswered questions in the CNS. Answering this question may benefit from our growing understanding of the genetics of positional signaling and epidermal patterning, questions that seemed equally intractable and elusive not long ago. Thus it may be that *Drosophila* is just the animal in which an astute tap of the hammer referred to in the introduction would finally break open the position–projection mystery (M. Bate, personal communication).

5. CORRELATION BETWEEN CONTROLLING FACTORS

The pattern of sense organs is extremely constant, both in the embryo and in the adult fly. This constancy is clearly an advantage because it allows the reproducible analysis of uniquely identifiable neurons. On the other hand, invariant patterns have their drawbacks when it comes to the analysis of the control factors. Indeed most of the factors that are correlated to path choice are also correlated with each other. It is extremely difficult, then, to assess which of the correlated factors is instrumental in achieving the control of path choice. For example, a sense organ at a given position will always be of a given type and develop at a given time. In theory it should be possible to uncouple the various factors by using appropriate mutations. Many mutations are now available that may help to manipulate the pattern, type, time of origin, and segmental identity of sense organs. A systematic analysis of their effect on the projections may establish which is the crucial controlling feature in each case.

VII. Programming Diversity

Ideally we should now reconsider the formation of sense organs from the point of view of the developmental program. In other words, we should try to understand what instructions provide the different aspects examined in the previous sections, and how these instructions are integrated in an operating system, a problem A. Garcia-Bellido calls "the genetic grammar of development" (1984). Our knowledge of the different steps of the process and of their genetics is, of course, much too scattered to allow a serious attempt at understanding the program itself. However, this limited knowledge already establishes without doubt that the decision to differentiate a particular neuron is the outcome of several distinct choices. We will now extract, from the available data, tentative answers about the following two questions. What is the relative importance of intrinsic and extrinsic factors in determining cell fates? Is the genetics of developmental decisions based on binary switches or on multiple choice systems?

A. Intrinsic versus Extrinsic Factors

The growth of identified fly neurons has not been studied yet *in vitro*. In other animals, it has been shown that identified neurons differentiating in isolation express specific morphological features (Acklin and Nicholls, 1990). By analogy to the case reported by these two authors, it seems plausible that the morphological difference between type-1 and type-2 neurons is intrinsic to the neuron. This specific repertoire, however, appears limited to a few basic options. Thus a lot of what happens during neural differentiation depends on cell interactions.

Cell interactions may affect the differentiation of the neuron in very different ways. For example, the growth of an axon along a given pre-existing fiber obviously requires that the guiding fiber be present, yet the presence of the pre-existing fiber plays no role in defining the recognition properties of the growing neuron; it is active in allowing and shaping its manifestation. Different is the case in which the fasciculation with a given fiber induces a modification in the recognition properties of the growing axon (Bastiani and Goodman, 1984). Here the absence of the guide will not only prevent the phenotypic expression of part of the program but alter the unfolding of the program itself.

When discussing the nature of the program, we should restrict the discussion to those cell interactions that are instrumental in defining the future fate of the cell. In other words, we should distinguish between the type of cell interactions that may be called permissive, in the sense that they are necessary for the developing neuron to express its specificity, and interactions that maybe called instructive in the sense that they are necessary for the cell to acquire or refine its specificity. This is more easily written than done. There is no simple way to distinguish permissive from instrumental interactions; in the following discussion we are at great risk of falling into semantic traps because, in most cases, we lack strict operational definitions of the words we use.

A first task is to assess to what extent the program is written in terms of an orderly deployment of gene activity in each cell, and to what extent it is written in terms of providing the tools that will allow a cell to take advantage of nearby cells to define its own fate. In theory, this question is easily answered by relying on mosaic analysis (see Appendix) to define the cell autonomy of a particular process. However, mosaic analysis is not without its problems, both conceptual (what is actually observed is the cell autonomy of a mutant phenotype, not of the normal process) and experimental (irradiating larvae to change the genotype of some cells, or transplanting cells of one genotype into animals of another genotype, may affect development in many different ways, not all of which are easily controlled). In practice, therefore, it is not surprising that a number of mosaic analyses led to conflicting results (see Chapter 6) or erroneous conclusions (references will be provided upon request).

Based on our present knowledge, we are tempted to argue that both intrinsic and extrinsic determinants play essential roles in assigning cell fates. It appears that, in the case of es versus ch or m-es versus p-es organs, the final morphology of the structural cells depends not on interactions with their neighbors but on whether or not their mother cells expressed the genes *cut* and *poxn,* respectively. Likewise, the projection pattern of an abdominal bristle neuron depends on the state of expression of the Bithorax Complex, which it inherited from its mother cell, not on the segment in which it develops. On the contrary, the final choice between SMC and epidermal cell depends on the cell interactions mediated by a particular chain of genes; it may be that the allocation of the different fates among its progeny also depends on specific cell interactions.

The next problem, then, is to understand the interplay between the two sets of genes, those that mediate transcriptional regulation and those that mediate intercellular signaling. This is a crucial aspect of development in many organisms that is still completely obscure (although revealing clues are emerging from the analysis of the development of the fly eye; reviewed in Ready, 1989). The data on the fly PNS give a few hints about how genetic regulations and cell interactions are combined in a meaningful program. In the formation of the SMCs, the two systems may interact on at least one occasion: the singling out of the SMC and the correlative lateral inhibition of its neighbors. The interplay between the two systems seems to depend on *Espl,* one of the "neurogenic" loci involved in lateral inhibition and in the singling out of SMCs. The locus comprises several genes with a potential HLH structure, indicating a possible role as transcriptional regulators. The locus also contains a gene probably involved in signal transduction. The problem here is that the developmental funcions of the individual genes of the locus remain mysterious, since the "neurogenic" phenotype is observed only when all these genes are removed simultaneously.

The easiest interpretation of these results is that cell contact through specific membrane molecules triggers a specific chain of events that leads eventually to the modification of a defined set of transcriptional regulators. This would imply that different developmental operations have their own cell contact and signaling system, so the response of the cell may be adapted to the particular contact it has made.

In this interpretation, both intrinsic and external determinants are intimately connected. Instructive interactions can only occur if the cell to be instructed has the appropriate membrane proteins, the appropriate signal transducing machinery, and the appropriate targets (e.g., transcriptional receptors that are sensitive to particular kinases). This "preparedness" may well be identical to competence. Instructive interactions also require making contacts with the appropriate other cell to trigger the right chain, a process akin to what students of vertebrate embryology call induction. The data on the formation of the fly PNS are entirely consistent with the idea that specific changes in genetic regulations may modify the capability of the cell to respond to a specific interaction, which can further change the genetic regulations in the cell, and so forth. This punctuated progression through the developmental processes may facilitate the ordered unfolding of the program and, at the same time, insure that the different sections of the program are read in phase throughout the tissue.

B. Binary Switches and Multiple Choices

It has been demonstrated that, in order to generate more than one stationary state, a regulatory system must include a positive loop (such loops may include negative as well as positive steps as long as there is an even number of negative steps) (Thomas and d'Ari, 1990). A single positive loop is sufficient to account for a situation in which the number of states is only two: either the loop is stably active or it is stably silent. The easiest way to achieve a positive loop is by self-activation (autocatalysis), which may explain why many developmentally important genes act on their own expression (*Sex-lethal*: Cline, 1984; *Ultrabithorax*: Beachy, 1990; *fushi-tarazu*: Pick *et al.*, 1990; *cut*: Blochlinger *et al.*, 1991).

In order to provide several stationary states, a regulatory system must, of necessity, comprise several such loops. One obvious way to generate several regulatory loops is to duplicate one and to allow for some divergence. An interesting outcome of this simple evolutionary scheme is that duplicated autoregulatory genes (or, more generally, regulatory loops) will regulate each other as well. Thus the development of self-regulating genes or gene loops will almost inevitably lead to the development of regulatory networks in which slight divergences among the duplicated genes or control sequences will create complex regulatory relationships. The number of stationary states that can be generated by such networks is, for all practical purposes, infinite. More interestingly, the interactions in the network can be tuned in such a way that the network will, by itself, generate temporal or spatial order. The most illustrious example of this scheme is given by the homoeotic gene family, a set of highly homologous genes that, in the fly, regulate each other in a way that directly affects their spatial pattern of expression (Struhl and White, 1985). The analysis of regulatory interactions among groups of structurally related genes is still in its infancy, yet the available data suggest that they may be a widespread tool to achieve the simultaneous definition of a number of states in a spatially and temporally ordered manner.

We can now address the particular case of the sense organs and see whether we can provide an answer to the original question of binary or multiple choices. The acquisition of competence most likely belongs to the multiple choice type, as indicated by the dependence on a battery of homologous transcriptional regulators and the diversity of output. Furthermore, there are indirect indications that at least one of the AS-C genes activates its own expression, and that *ac* and *sc* activate each other (Martinez and Modolell, 1991). Other choices, however, seem to correspond to the binary type. For example, the decision to form a ch or an es sense organ is a binary choice between expression and nonexpression of the gene *cut*. Thus, both multiple and binary choices play a role in the program. Based on the preliminary evidence we now have in this as well as in other systems such as segmentation (Ingham, 1988), segmental determination (Akam, 1987), and sex differentiation (Nöthiger and Steinmann-Zwicky, 1985), one might form the impression that spatial organization is often achieved by a multiple choice system based on a complex regulatory network (i.e., a network comprising several interacting loops), whereas binary choices based on simple switches are more related to cell type specification.

Appendix: Genetic Methods and Tools

Much of the recent progress in the field has come from the development of new genetic methods. Since all of them turn out to be essential at one point or another in this chapter, yet some of them may not be familiar to the reader, we will briefly describe their rationale, use, and effectiveness.

A. Mutation Analysis

I. LOF VERSUS GOF

How can one move from the defect due to a mutation to an understanding of the normal function of the gene? After all, mutations leading to the formation of abnormal embryos have been known for a long time in many animals, yet none of them led to much understanding of anything. Among the analytical tools developed by Lewis, one of the most helpful is the description of a given mutation as either a loss-of-function (LOF) or a gain-of-function (GOF) mutation.

LOF mutations correspond to the inactivation of a gene or to its deletion. They are, in general, recessive, indicating that one copy of the normal gene is sufficient to fulfill the function. GOF mutations may correspond to a deregulation of the gene leading to overexpression or ectopic expression, or to a modification of the gene product so it will display some new properties. Contrary to the LOF mutations, GOF mutations will always be dominant, since one copy of the mutated gene will show its effect irrespective of whether the second copy is also mutant or is normal. Not all dominant mutations are GOF, however. If one copy of the normal gene is not sufficient to carry out the function, then the gene is said to be haplo-insufficient and mutations in the gene will be dominant by haplo-insufficiency. Dominance due to haplo-insufficiency is easily distinguished from dominance due to GOF mutations, since the former will also be observed when one copy of the gene is deleted.

In short, recessive mutations are likely to represent a LOF whereas dominant mutations are usually GOF, unless they are dominant by haplo-insufficiency (meaning that two active copies of the gene are required to fulfill the function, so only one copy will result in an abnormal phenotype).

2. LOF MUTATIONS AND GENE FUNCTION

If a mutant phenotype results from a loss of function, it follows that the normal function of the gene can be inferred, at least tentatively, from the analysis of the mutational defect. However, one must consider that the loss of function due to a mutation can be complete or incomplete, depending on the nature and site of the mutation. Whether a given mutation results in a complete loss of function (amorph) or only in a reduction of activity (hypomorph) can be asserted by the simple genetic tests devised by Müller. It is at once obvious that the most appropriate mutation to define the function of a gene is the amorph, whereby the gene is completely inactivated (or, better still, removed althogether). The different levels of hypomorphy may in turn yield interesting information, as long as one knows that they do not represent the complete lack of function. Indeed, in several cases the analysis of such an allelic series (set of alleles of varying levels of hypomorphy) has yielded valuable information about particular aspects of the function of the gene.

3. GOF MUTATIONS AND CONTROL GENES

The phenotype of GOF mutations is more difficult to analyze because there are several ways in which such gain can be achieved. Müller elaborated a number of simple genetic tests to assess the nature of dominant mutations: hypermorphs, in which the normal function is overexpressed; neomorphs, in which a new function is expressed; and antimorphs, in which the mutant product antagoizes the normal product. Clearly these different cases will lead to very different inferences about the normal function of the gene. An additional problem is that GOF mutations are much rarer than the molecularly simple inactivating mutations. Yet in spite of their rarity and intrinsic difficulty, GOF mutations are a key element in Lewis' strategy to infer function from mutational analysis. The argument is based on the analysis of LOF and GOF mutations affecting the same gene. The phenotype of LOF mutations allows one to define the operation for which the gene is needed. The existence of GOF mutations affecting the same gene indicates that the overexpression or ectopic expression of the gene is just as detrimental for normal development as its inactivation, and points to the conclusion that this gene is not simply needed for, but actually controls, the operation.

More recently, the search for, and analysis of, GOF mutations of the hypermorph type has been largely replaced by the use of transformant lines containing constructs in which the gene of interest is ectopically expressed. Misexpression can be achieved by putting a gene under the control of a heat-shock promoter, leading to generalized expression of the gene after a heat-shock. Alternatively the gene can be put under the control of the promoter region of another gene with a different pattern of expression, again leading to ectopic expression.

B. Saturation Analysis

Mutagenesis has long been considered a means to isolate potentially interesting mutations. Therefore the general trend was to screen for mutations that alter a given process, and to concentrate on the one that seemed most promising. A major contribution of Nüsslein-Volhard and Wieschaus was to shift the focus from the search for hypothetical "key" genes to a systematic dissection of the system. In this approach, the aim is to access all (or a vast majority of) the genes involved in the process under scrutiny. The search for mutations is therefore continued not until many genes have been mutationally identified but until many alleles have been isolated for each gene, indicating that the genome has effectively been saturated and that very few genes have escaped detection. In their classical work on segmentation, Nüsslein-Volhard, Wieschaus, and coworkers screened about 27,000 mutagenized lines to identify 120 genes with an average of 5 alleles per gene. The amount of work involved is truly enormous. This leads to an important aspect of this new method, which is that one needs a simple and fast assay to screen tens of thousands of mutagenized chromosomes; therefore, the scope of the analysis is defined not by a specific question but by a specific phenotype.

C. Mosaic Analysis

1. SOMATIC RECOMBINATION AND MOSAIC ANALYSIS

The mutation analysis just described implies that one can detect the phenotype due to the loss of function of the gene. More often than not, however, only part of the phenotype can be readily observed. For example, if a gene is required at different developmental stages, the earliest defect will usually cause lethality and, therefore, defects in subsequent steps will remain undetected. Likewise, if a gene is involved in different processes, the failure of one process may mask the defects in the others.

One way out of this problem is to rely on mosaic analysis, that is, on the possibility to induce clones of cells homozygous for the mutation in an otherwise heterozygous fly. Such clones can be produced at any time of development as a result of radiation-induced somatic recombination. In general, somatic recombination is achieved by X irradiation of flies at the appropriate age of the embryonic, larval, or pupal stage. In cells that are in the G_2 phase of the cell cycle, the chromosome damages resulting from the X rays may occasionally lead to a recombination between homologous chromatids, so after mitosis one daughter cell will contain the two mutant copies of the gene whereas the other daughter cell will end up with the two normal copies. The homozygous mutant cells are usually marked by linking to the mutation under scrutiny a second mutation with a readily detected phenotype, such as a change in pigmentation or in the shape of the diminutive noninnervated hairs that are produced by most epidermal cells.

The mosaic analysis has so far been most useful for the analysis of the adult epidermis and its derivatives, including the adult sense organs. The application of this analysis to internal organs is severely limited by the scarcity of marker mutations that can be used to detect and delineate the clones of homozygous cells. The application to the larval epidermis is limited for a different reason, namely, that very few cell divisions occur between blastoderm cellularization and the differentiation of the larval epidermis.

2. CELL AUTONOMY AND PERDURANCE

In addition to its usefulness in the analysis of pleiotropic mutations, mosaic analysis also provides useful information about the cell autonomy of a given mutation. If in all cells the phenotype corresponds to the genotype, then the mutation is said to be cell autonomous. In the case of LOF mutations, cell autonomy of the mutation implies cell autonomy of the normal gene; the implications of cell autonomy are fully discussed in Chapter 6.

Other information that can be derived from mosaic analysis is the time at which a given gene must be expressed in order for its function to be executed. After that time, the gene will not be required any more; therefore, the complete inactivation of the gene in homozygous mutant clones will have no effect on the cell phenotype, a phenomenon called perdurance. The interpretation of perdurance is unfortunately complicated by several problems, among which are the facts that the clone is founded not by the irradiated cell itself but by one of its daughters and that gene products present in the irradiated cell may be transmitted to its progeny.

D. Dosage Analysis and Gene Interactions

Developmental processes depend on the orderly activity of many genes. This patterned activity presumably involves complicated networks or cascades of interacting genes. The detection and analysis of gene interactions is therefore crucial to understand the genetic basis of development.

One of the most efficient ways to detect gene interaction relies on gene dosage analysis. The approach is based on the observation that the overwhelming majority of LOF mutations are fully recessive, implying that in most cases one copy of a gene is sufficient to produce a normal fly. Let us consider two of the many genes involved in a particular developmental process. The argument is as follows. If one copy of gene A is sufficient to produce a normal fly, then whatever step or operation gene A is required for can be realized with half the normal dose of that gene. Genes that act at other steps have, therefore, no way of assessing that gene A is present in only one copy, since they cannot "see" the amount of gene A, only whether the operation that required gene A has been realized. The same is true for gene B. Thus, goes the argument, flies with only one copy of A and one copy of B should also be normal, unless genes A and B are involved in the very same step. Therefore, if flies doubly heterozygous for mutations in A and B are abnormal, we can conclude that genes A and B are functioally related and probably interact with each other. In other words, any abnormal phenotype present in a fly doubly heterozygous for two recessive mutations is evidence that the corresponding genes act together. A similar reasoning can be used when the dose of one of the genes is increased, rather than decreased; the analysis of flies with either one or three copies of a particular gene has, indeed, been used successfully to reveal interactions between genes in different systems (Botas *et al.,* 1982).

The double-heterozygote method has been used to isolate mutations in interacting genes, as well as to demonstrate the existence of interactions between known genes. This method is all the more interesting when one takes into consideration the problem of genes acting at different stages or being required in different processes. Indeed the method may allow one to detect the involvement of a gene in a particular process, whether or not the gene acts at other times or in other processes.

E. Maternal Effects

A potential problem in the analysis of mutations affecting embryonic development is that many maternal genes are expressed during oocyte formation; therefore, gene product will be present in the egg even if the zygotic gene is completely inactivated. In this case, the LOF phenotype will reflect the amount of product with which the mother provided the embryo, and will be very different from the defect that would result from a complete loss of function. One obvious solution would be to use mothers homozygous for the mutation, but most mutations (in particular those that affect the development of the nervous system) are lethal at one stage or another.

Two methods have been devised to eliminate the maternal effect. One of them relies on the fact that the germ cells of the adult are entirely derived from a small number of cells set aside before the onset of gastrulation, the pole cells. Pole cells are easily recognized very early during embryonic development, and can be transferred to another embryo where they will contribute to the germ line. The host embryo is derived from a homozygous *grand-childless* mother and therefore lacks the ability to form its own pole cells. The germ cells of the resulting adult will then originate entirely from the transplanted mutant cells.

The other method involves the formation of homozygous mutant cells during the development of the germ line, by somatic recombination (see previous text). In order to detect which progeny derive from a homozygous mutant germ cell, the homolog carries a dominant mutation that prevents the formation of an oocyte. Heterozygous germ cells will be unable to form oocytes, and therefore the only eggs that will form derive from germ cells that have undergone a somatic recombination in which they have lost the dominant sterile mutation. Such cells have necessarily become homozygous for the mutation to be studied.

F. Enhancer Trapping

The expression of eukaryotic genes is controlled by *cis*-acting regulatory elements, the enhancers, that can act in either orientation and over distances of several kilobases. One way to visualize the regulatory activity of an enhancer is to flank it with a reporter gene provided with a weak ubiquitous promoter. In theory, this method can be used to probe for the presence of unknown enhancers by inserting the reporter gene at random in the genome. Occasionally, the expression of the reporter gene will have come under the control of a nearby enhancer and will show a defined temporal or spatial pattern.

This method of *in situ* enhancer detection (soon dubbed "enhancer trapping") was pioneered by O'Kane and Gehring. They used as a reporter gene the bacterial gene *lacZ* which encodes β-galactosidase, an enzyme that is easily visualized in tissues by a simple histochemical reaction giving rise to an insoluble blue product, inserted in the transposable element P in replacement of the transposase. This has the advantage that *lacZ* is now under the control of the weak ubiquitous promoter of the transposase, and that the entire construct can be mobilized by providing transposase to the cell. Within a year, the method was extensively used in many laboratories to generate thousands of individual insertion lines.

The immediate popularity of the enhancer-trap system was due to four facts. First, the production of very large numbers of independent insertions has been enormously facilitated by the development of a highly efficient system of gene transposition derived from the study of the P element. Second, it turns out that the fly genome contains very few silent regions: the integration of the reporter gene at a given location almost invariably brings it under the control of some nearby enhancer(s). Third, the reporter gene provides an excellent starting point for the recovery and cloning of the surrounding region whenever the pattern of expression suggests the presence of an interesting gene nearby (or rather, of a gene with an interesting regulation). Fourth, the large collection of independent inserts now available, each with its own pattern of expression of the reporter gene, provides an extremely elaborate array of specific cell markers. Particularly interesting, in the context of this chapter, are the enhancer-trap lines in which the reporter gene is specifically expressed in the PNS.

Acknowledgments

We thank Michael Bate, Yuh-Nung Jan, Marty Shankland, and our students for critical comments and valuable suggestions; Y.N. Jan, J. Modolell, A. Garcia-Bellido, and P. Simpson for communicating results and ideas prior to publication; and Ms. Henriette Preszow for typing the reference list. A.G. is chercheur qualifié of the Fonds National de la Recherche Scientifique (Belgium).

References

Acklin, S. E., and Nicholls, J. G. (1990). Intrinsic and extrinsic factors influencing properties and growth patterns of identified leech neurons in culture. *J. Neurosci.* **10**, 1082–1090.

Agol, I. J. (1931). Step allelomorphism in *Drosophila* melanogaster. *Genetics* **16**, 254–266.

Akam, M. (1987). The molecular basis for metameric pattern in the *Drosophila* embryo. *Development* **101**, 1–22.

Alonso, M. C., and Cabrera, C. V. (1988). The *achaete–scute* gene complex of *Drosophila melanogaster* comprises four homologous genes *EMBO J.* **7**, 2589–2591.

Anderson, H., and Bacon, J. (1979). Developmental determination of neuronal projection patterns from wind-sensitive hairs in the locust, *Schistocerca gregaria. Dev. Biol.* **72**, 364–373.

Baker, N. E. (1988). Transcription of the segment-polarity gene *wingless* in the imaginal discs of *Drosophila,* and the phenotype of a pupal-lethal *wg* mutation. *Development* **102**, 489–497.

Balcells, L., Modolell, J., and Ruiz-Gomez, M. (1988). A unitary basis for different *Hairy-wing* mutations of *Drosophila melanogaster. EMBO J.* **7**, 3899–3906.

Bastiani, M. J., and Goodman, C. S. (1984). Neuronal growth cones: Specific interactions mediated by filopodial insertion and induction of coated vesicles. *Proc. Natl. Acad. Sci. U.S.A.* **81**, 1849–1853.

Bastiani, M. J., Raper, J. A., and Goodman, C. S. (1984). Pathfinding by neuronal growth cones in grasshopper embryos. III. Selective affinity of the G growth cone for the P cells within the A/P fascicle. *J. Neurosci.* **4**, 2311–2328.

Bastiani, M. J., Doe, C. Q., Helfand, S. L., and Goodman, C. S. (1985). Neuronal specificity and growth cone guidance in grasshopper and *Drosophila* embryos. *Trends Neurosci.* **8**, 257–266.

Bastiani, M. J., du Lac, S., and Goodman, C. S. (1986). Guidance of neuronal growth cones in the grasshopper embryo. I. Recognition of a specific axonal pathway by the pCC neuron. *J. Neurosci.* **6,** 3518–3531.

Bate, C. M. (1976). Pioneer neurons in an insect embryo. *Nature (London)* **260,** 54–56.

Bate, C. M. (1978). Development of sensory systems in arthropods. In "Handbook of Sensory Physiology" (M. Jacobson, ed.), Vol. IX. New York: Springer.

Bate, C. M., and Grunewald, E. B. (1981). Embryogenesis of an insect nervous system. II. A second class of neuron precursor cells and the origin of the intersegmental connectives. *J. Embryol. Exp. Morph.* **61,** 317–330.

Bate, C. M., and Martinez-Arias, A. (1991). The embryonic origin of imaginal discs in *Drosophila. Development* **112,** 755–762.

Beachy, P. A. (1990). A molecular view of the *Ultrabithorax* homeotic gene of *Drosophila. Trends Genet.* **6,** 46–51.

Beamonte, D., and Modolell, J. (1989). Search for *Drosophila* genes encoding a conserved domain present in the *achaete-scute* complex and *myc* protein. *Mol. Gen. Genet.* **215,** 281–285.

Bell, A. E. (1954). A gene in *Drosophila melanogaster* that produces all male progeny. *Genetics* **39,** 958–959.

Bellen, H., Grossniklaus, U., O'Kane, C., Kurth Pearson, R., Wilson, C., and Gehring, W. (1988). "The Little Blue Book." (A xeroxed manual sent to Drosophila researchers.)

Bellen, H., O'Kane, C. J., Wilson, C., Grossniklaus, U., Kurth Pearson, R., and Gehring, W. (1989). P-element-mediated enhancer detection: A versatile method to study development in *Drosophila. Genes Devel.* **3,** 1288–1300.

Bender, W., Akam, M., Karck, F., Beachy, P. A., Peifer, M., Spierer, P., Lewis, E. B., and Hogness, D. S. (1983). Molecular genetics of the Bithorax Complex in *Drosophila melanogaster. Science* **221,** 23–29.

Bentley, D., and Caudy, M. (1983). Pioneer axons lose directed growth after selective killing of guidepost cells. *Nature (London)* **304,** 62–65.

Bier, E., Vaessin, H., Shephard, S., Lee, K., McCall, K., Barbel, S., Ackerman, L., Carretto, R., Uemura, T., Grell, E., Jan, L. Y., and Jan, Y. N. (1989). Searching for pattern and mutation in the *Drosophila* genome with a P-*lacZ* vector. *Genes Devel.* **3,** 1273–1287.

Blair, S. S., and Palka, J. (1985). Axon guidance in the wing of *Drosophila Trends Neurosci.* **8,** 284–288.

Blair, S. S., Murray, M. A., and Palka, J. (1987). The guidance of axons from transplanted neurons through aneural *Drosophila* wings. *J. Neurosci.* **7,** 4165–4175.

Blochlinger, K., Bodmer, R., Jack, J., Jan, L. Y., and Jan, Y. N. (1988). Primary structure and expression of a product from *cut,* a locus involved in specifying sensory organ identity in *Drosophila. Nature (London)* **333,** 629–635.

Blochlinger, K., Bodmer, R., Jan, L. Y., and Jan, Y. N. (1990). Pattern of expression of Cut, a protein required for external sensory organ development in wild type and *cut* mutant *Drosophila* embryos. *Genes Devel.* **4,** 1322–1331.

Blochlinger, K., Jan. L. Y., and Jan, Y. N. (1991). Transformation of sensory organ identity by ectopic expression of Cut in *Drosophila. Genes Dev.* **5,** 1124–1135.

Bodmer, R., Barbel, S., Sheperd, S., Jack, J. W., Jan, L. Y., and Jan, Y. N. (1987). Transformation of sensory organs by mutations of the *cut* locus of *D. melanogaster. Cell* **51,** 293–307.

Bodmer, R., and Jan, Y. N. (1987). Morphological differentiation of the embryonic peripheral neurons in *Drosophila. Roux's Arch. Dev. Biol.* **196,** 69–77.

Bodmer, R., Carretto, R., and Jan, Y. N. (1989). Neurogenesis of the peripheral nervous system in *Drosophila* embryos: DNA replication patterns and cell lineages. *Neuron* **3,** 21–32.

Bopp, D., Jamet, E., Baumgartner, S., Burri, M., and Noll, M. (1989). Isolation of two tissue-specific *Drosophila* paired box genes, *Pox meso* and *Pox neuro*. *EMBO J.* **8,** 3447–3457.

Botas, J., Moscoso del Prado, J., and Garcia-Bellido, A. (1982). Gene-dose titration analysis in the search of trans-regulatory genes in *Drosophila*. *EMBO J.* **1,** 307–310.

Bourouis, M., Moore, P., Ruel, L., Grau, Y., Heitzler, P., and Simpson, P. (1990). An early embryonic product of the gene *shaggy* encodes a serine/threonine protein kinase related to the CDC28 cdc2+ subfamily. *EMBO J.* **9,** 2877–2884.

Brand, M., and Campos-Ortega, J. A. (1989). Two groups of interrelated genes regulate early neurogenesis in *Drosophila melanogaster*. *Roux's Arch. Dev. Biol.* **197,** 457–470.

Bryant, P. J. (1975). Pattern formation in the imaginal wing disc of *Drosophila melanogaster*: Fate map, regeneration and duplication. *J. Exp. Zool.* **193,** 49–78.

Bullock, T. H., and Horridge, G. A. (1965). "Structure and Function in the Nervous System of Invertebrates," Vol. 1. San Francisco: Freeman.

Cagan, R. L., and Ready, D. F. (1989). *Notch* is required for successive cell decisions in the developing *Drosophila* retina. *Genes Devel.* **3,** 1099–1112.

Campos-Ortega, J. A. (1985). Genetics of early neurogenesis in *Drosophila melanogaster*. *Trends Neurosci.* **8,** 245–250.

Campos-Ortega, J. A. (1988). Cellular interactions during early neurogenesis of *Drosophila melanogaster*. *Trends Neurosci.* **11,** 400–405.

Campos-Ortega, J. A., and Hartenstein, V. (1985). "The Embryonic Development of *Drosophila melanogaster*." New York: Springer-Verlag.

Campuzano, S., Carramolino, L., Cabrera, C. V., Ruiz-Gomez, M., Villares, R., Boronat, A., and Modolell, J. (1985). Molecular genetics of the *archaete–scute* gene complex of *D. melanogaster*. *Cell* **40,** 327–338.

Carroll, S. B., and Whyte, J. S. (1989). The role of *hairy* gene during *Drosophila* morphogenesis: Stripes in imaginal discs. *Genes Devel.* **3,** 905–916.

Caudy, M., Grell, E. H., Dambly-Chaudière, C., Ghysen, A., Jan, L. Y., and Jan, Y. N. (1988a). The maternal sex determination gene *daughterless* has zygotic activity necessary for the formation of peripheral neurons in *Drosophila*. *Genes Devel.* **2,** 843–852.

Caudy, M., Vässin, H., Brand, M., Tuma, R., Jan, L. Y., and Jan, Y. N. (1988b). *daughterless,* a *Drosophila* gene essential for both neurogenesis and sex determination, has sequence similarities to *myc* and the *achaete–scute* complex. *Cell* **55,** 1061–1067.

Claxton, J. H. (1964). The determination of patterns with special reference to that of the central primary skin follicles in sheep. *J. Theoret. Biol.* **7,** 302–317.

Claxton, J. H. (1967). Patterns of abdominal tergite bristles in wild-type and *scute Drosophila melanogaster*. *Genetics* **55,** 525–545.

Cline, T. W. (1984). Autoregulatory functioning of a *Drosophila* gene product that establishes and maintains the sexually determined state. *Genetics* **107,** 231–277.

Cohen, B., Wimmer, E. A., and Cohen, S. M. (1991). Early development of leg and wing primordia in the *Drosophila* embryo. *Mech. Devel.* **33,** 229–240.

Corfas, G., and Dudai, Y. (1989). Habituation and dishabituation of a cleaning reflex in normal and mutant *Drosophila*. *J. Neurosci.* **9,** 56–62.

Cronmiller, C., and Cline, T. W. (1987). The *Drosophila* sex determination gene *daughterless* has different functions in the germline versus the soma. *Cell* **48,** 479–487.

Cubas, P., de Celis, J. F., Campuzano, S., and Modolell, J. (1991). Proneural clusters of *achaete–scute* expresion and the generation of sensory organs in the *Drosophila* imaginal disc. *Genes Dev.* **5,** 996–1008.

Dambly-Chaudière, C., and Ghysen, A. (1986). The pattern of sense organs in the *Drosophila* larva and its relation to the embryonic pattern of sensory neurons. *Roux's Arch. Dev. Biol.* **195,** 222–228.

Dambly-Chaudière, C., and Ghysen, A. (1987). Independent subpatterns of sense organs require independent genes of the *achaete–scute* complex in *Drosophila* larvae. *Genes Devel.* **1,** 297–306.

Dambly-Chaudière, C., Jamet, E., Burri, M., Bopp, D., Basler, K., Hafen, E., Dumont, N., Spielmann, P., Ghysen, A., and Noll, M. (1992). Role of the paired box gene *pox neuro* as an early determinant of poly-innerved sense organs in *Drosophila. Cell* (in press).

Dambly-Chaudière, C., Ghysen, A., Jan, L. Y., and Jan, Y. N. (1988). The determination of sense organs in *Drosophila:* Interaction of *scute* with *daughterless. Roux's Arch. Dev. Biol.* **197,** 419–423.

Davis, R. L., Cheng, P. F., Lassar, A. B., and Weintraub, H. (1990). The MyoD DNA binding domain contains a recognition code for muscle-specific gene activation. *Cell* **60,** 733–746.

de Celis, J. F., Mari-Beffa, M., and Garcia-Bellido, A. (1992). Cell-autonomous role of the *Notch* gene, an epidermal growth factor homolog, in sensory organ differentiation in *Drosophila. Proc. Natl. Acad. Sci. U.S.A.* **88,** 632–636.

de la Concha, A., Dietrich, U., Weigel, D., and Campos-Ortega, J. A (1988). Functional interactions of neurogenic genes of *Drosophila melanogaster. Genetics* **118,** 499–508.

Dickinson, M. H., and Palka, J. (1987). Physiological properties, time of development, and central projection are correlated in the wing mechanoreceptors of *Drosophila. J. Neurosci.* **7,** 4201–4208.

Dietrich, U., and Campos-Ortega, J. A. (1984). The expression of neurogenic loci in imaginal epidermal cells of *Drosophila melanogaster. J. Neurogenet.* **1,** 315–332.

Doe, C. Q., and Goodman, C. S. (1985). Early events in insect neurogenesis. II. The role of cell interactions and cell lineage in the determination of neuronal precursor cells. *Dev. Biol.* **111,** 206–219.

Dubinin, N. P. (1932). Step-allelomorphism and the theory of centers of the gene, *achaete–scute. J. Genet.* **26,** 443–464.

Ellis, H. M., Spann, D. R., and Posakony, J. W. (1990). *Extramacrochaetae,* a negative regulator of sensory organ development in *Drosophila,* defines a new class of helix-loop-helix proteins. *Cell* **61,** 27–38.

Foe, V. E. (1989). Mitotic domains reveal early commitment of cells in *Drosophila* embryos. *Development* **107,** 1–22.

Frigerio, G., Burri, M., Bopp, D., Baumgartner, S., and Noll, M. (1986). Structure of the segmentation gene *paired* and the *Drosophila* PRD gene set as part of a gene network. *Cell* **47,** 735–746.

Garcia Alonso, L., and Garcia-Bellido, A. (1986). Genetic analysis of *Hairy-wing* mutations. *Roux's Arch. Dev. Biol.* **195,** 259–264.

Garcia Alonso, L. A., and Garcia-Bellido, A. (1988). Extramacrochaetae, a trans-acting gene of the *achaete–scute* complex of *Drosophila* involved in cell communication. *Roux's Arch. Dev. Biol.* **197,** 328–338.

Garcia-Bellido, A. (1979). Genetic analysis of the *achaete–scute* system of *Drosophila melanogaster. Genetics* **91,** 491–520.

Garcia-Bellido, A. (1981). The Bithorax syntagma. *In* "Advances in Genetics, Development, and Evolution of *Drosophila,*" VII European *Drosophila* Conference (S. Lakovaara, ed.), pp. 135–148. New York: Plenum.

Garcia-Bellido, A. (1984). Hacia una gramatica genetica. Real Academia de Ciencias Exactas, Fisicas y Naturales: Madrid.

Garcia-Bellido, A., and Merriam, J. R. (1971a). Parameters of the wing imaginal disc development of *Drosophila melanogaster. Dev. Biol.* **24,** 61–87.

Garcia-Bellido, A., and Merriam, J. R. (1971b). Clonal parameters of tergite development in *Drosophila. Dev. Biol.* **26,** 264–276.

Garcia-Bellido, A., Ripoll, P., and Morata, G. (1973). Developmental compartmentalisation of the wing disk of *Drosophila*. *Nature New Biol.* **245**, 251–253.

Garcia-Bellido, A., and Santamaria, P. (1978). Developmental analysis of the *achaete–scute* system of *Drosophila melanogaster*. *Genetics* **88**, 469–486.

Garrell, J., and Modolell, J. (1990). The *Drosophila extramacrochaetae* locus, an antagonist of proneural genes that, like these genes, encodes a helix-loop-helix protein. *Cell* **61**, 39–48.

Ghysen, A. (1978). Sensory axons recognize defined pathways in *Drosophila* central nervous system. *Nature (London)* **274**, 869–872.

Ghysen, A. (1980). The projection of sensory neurons in the central nervous system of *Drosophila:* Choice of the appropriate pathway. *Dev. Biol.* **78**, 521–541.

Ghysen, A., and Deak, I. I. (1978). Experimental analysis of sensory nerve pathways in *Drosophila*. *Roux's Arch. Dev. Biol.* **184**, 273–283.

Ghysen, A., and Richelle, J. (1979). Bristle determination and pattern formation in *Drosophila*. II. The *ac–sc* locus. *Dev. Biol.* **70**, 438–452.

Ghysen, A., and Janson, R. (1980). Sensory pathways in *Drosophila* central nervous system. *In* "Development and Neurobiology of *Drosophila*" (O. Siddiqi, P. Babu, L. Hall, and J. C. Hall, eds.), pp. 247–265. New York: Plenum.

Ghysen, A., Janson, R., and Santamaria, P. (1983). Segmental determination of sensory neurons in *Drosophila*. *Dev. Biol.* **99**, 7–26.

Ghysen, A., Dambly-Chaudière, C., Aceves, E., Jan, L. Y., and Jan, Y. N. (1986). Sensory neurons and peripheral pathways in *Drosophila* embryos. *Roux's Arch. Dev. Biol.* **195**, 281–289.

Ghysen, A., and Dambly-Chaudière, C. (1988). From DNA to form: The *achaete–scute* gene complex. *Genes Devel.* **2**, 495–501.

Ghysen, A., and Dambly-Chaudière, C. (1989). The genesis of *Drosophila* peripheral nervous system. *Trends Genet.* **5**, 251–255.

Ghysen, A., and O'Kane, C. (1989). Detection of neural enhancer-like elements in the genome of *Drosophila*. *Development* **105**, 35–52.

Ghysen, A., and Dambly-Chaudière, C. (1990). Early events in the development of *Drosophila* peripheral nervous system. *J. Physiol. (Paris)* **84**, 11–20.

Goriely, A., Dumont, N., Dambly-Chaudière, C., and Ghysen, A. (1991). The determination of sense organs in *Drosophila:* effect of the neurogenic mutations in the embryo. *Development* (in press).

Gottlieb, F. J. (1964). Genetic control of pattern determination in *Drosophila*. The action of *Hairy-wing*. *Genetics* **49**, 739–760.

Greenwald, I. (1989). Cell–cell interactions that specify certain cell fates in *C. elegans* development. *Trends Genet.* **5**, 237–241.

Grenningloh, G., Bieber, A., Rehm, J., Snow, P., Traquina, Z., Hortsch, M., Patel, N., and Goodman, C. S. (1990). Molecular genetics of neuronal recognition in *Drosophila:* Evolution and function of immunoglobulin superfamily cell adhesion molecules. *Cold Spring Harbor Symp. Quant. Biol.* **55**, 327–340.

Harrelson, A., and Goodman, C. S. (1988). Growth cone guidance in insects: Fasciclin II is a member of the immunoglobulin superfamily. *Science* **242**, 700–708.

Hartenstein, V. (1988). Development of *Drosophila* larval sensory organs: Spatiotemporal pattern of sensory neurones, peripheral axonal pathways and sensilla differentiation. *Development* **102**, 869–886.

Hartenstein, V., and Campos-Ortega, J. A. (1986). The peripheral nervous system of mutants of early neurogenesis in *Drosophila melanogaster*. *Roux's Arch. Dev. Biol.* **195**, 210–221.

Hartenstein, V., and Posakony, J. W. (1989). The development of adult sensilla on the wing and notum of *Drosophila melanogaster*. *Development* **107**, 384–405.

Hartenstein, V., and Posakony, J. W. (1990). A dual function of the *Notch* gene in *Drosophila* sensillum development. *Dev. Biol.* **142**, 13–30.

Hartley, D. A., Preiss, A., and Artavanis-Tsakonas, S. (1988). A deduced gene product from the *Drosophila* neurogenic locus, *Enhancer-of-split*, shows homology to mammalian G-protein B subunit. *Cell* **55**, 785–795.

Heitzler, P., and Simpson, P. (1991). The choice of cell fate in the epidermis of *Drosophila. Cell* **64**, 1083–1092.

Held, L. I., Jr. and Bryant, P. J. (1984). Cell interactions controlling the formation of bristle patterns in *Drosophila. In* "Pattern Formation" (G. M. Malacinski and S. V. Bryant, eds.), pp. 291–322. McMillan.

Hertweck, H. (1931). Anatomie und Variabilität des Nervensystems und der Sinnesorgane von *Drosophila melanogaster* (Meigen). *Z. Wiss. Zool.* **139**, 560–663.

Ho, R. K., and Goodman, C. S. (1982). Peripheral pathways are pioneered by an array of central and peripheral neurons in grasshopper embryos. *Nature (London)* **297**, 404–406.

Hodgkin, N. M., and Bryant, P. J. (1978). Scanning electron microscopy of the adult of *Drosophila melanogaster. In* "The Genetics and Biology of *Drosophila*" M. Ashburner and T.R.F. Wright, eds.), Vol. 2c, pp. 337–358. New York: Academic Press.

Holland, P. W. H. (1990). Homeobox genes and segmentation: Co-option, co-evolution, and convergence. In *Seminars in Developmental Biology, Vol. 1: The evolution of segmental patterns.* (C. Stern, Ed.). (pp. 135–145). Philadelphia: Saunders.

Hoppe, P. E., and Greenspan, R. J. (1986). Local function of the *Notch* gene for embryonic ectodermal pathway choice in *Drosophila. Cell* **46**, 773–783.

Huang, F., Dambly-Chaudière, C., and Ghysen, A. (1991). The emergence of sense organs in the wing disc of *Drosophila. Development* **11**, 1087–1095.

Ingham, P. M. (1988). The molecular genetics of embryonic pattern formation in *Drosophila. Nature (London)* **335**, 25–34.

Jacobs, J. R., and Goodman, C. S. (1989a). Embryonic development of axon pathways in the *Drosophila* CNS. I. A glial scaffold appears before the first growth cones. *J. Neurosci.* **9**, 2402–2411.

Jacobs, J. R., and Goodman, C. S. (1989b). Embryonic development of axon pathways in the *Drosophila* CNS. II. Behavior of pioneer growth cones. *J. Neurosci.* **9**, 2412–2422.

Jan, Y. N., Ghysen, A., Christoph, I., Barbel, S., and Jan, L. Y. (1985). Formation of neuronal pathways in the imaginal discs of *Drosophila. J. Neurosci.* **5**, 2453–2464.

Jan, Y. N., Bodmer, R., Ghysen, A., Dambly-Chaudière, C., and Jan, L. Y. (1987). Mutations affecting the peripheral nervous system in *Drosophila* embryos. *In* "Molecular Entomology" (J. H. Law, ed.), pp. 45–56. New York: Liss.

Jan, Y. N., and Jan, L. Y. (1990). Genes required for specifying cell fates in *Drosophila* embryonic sensory nervous system. *Trends Neurosci.* **13**, 493–498.

Jiménez, F., and Campos-Ortega, J. A. (1979). A region of the *Drosophila* genome necessary for CNS development. *Nature (London)* **282**, 310–312.

Jiménez, F., and Campos-Ortega, J. A. (1987). Genes in subdivision 1B of the *Drosophila melanogaster* X-chromosome and their influence on neural development. *J. Neurogenet.* **4**, 179–200.

Johnson, J. E., Birren, S. J., and Anderson, D. J. (1990). Two rat homologues of *Drosophila achaete–scute* specifically expressed in neuronal precursors. *Nature (London)* **346**, 858–860.

Johnson, S. E., and Murphey, R. K. (1985). The afferent projection of mesothoracic bristle hairs in the cricket, *Acheta domesticus. J. Comp. Physiol.* **156**, 369–379.

Kankel, D. R., Ferrus, A., Garen, S. H., Harte, P. J., and Lewis, P. E. (1980). The structure and development of the nervous system. *In* "The Genetics and Biology of *Drosophila*" M. Ashburner and T.R.F. Wright, eds.), Vol. 2D, pp. 295–368. New York: Academic Press.

Katz, M. J., and Lasek, R. (1980). Guidance cue patterns and cell migration in multicellular organisms. *Cell Motil.* **1,** 141–157.

Keshishian, H., and Bentley, D. (1983a). Embryogenesis of peripheral nerve pathways in grasshopper legs. I. The initial nerve pathway to the CNS. *Dev. Biol.* **96,** 89–102.

Keshishian, H., and Bentley, D. (1983b). Embryogenesis of peripheral nerve pathways in grasshopper legs. II. The major nerve routes. *Dev. Biol.* **96,** 103–115.

Kidd, S., Kelley, M. R., and Young, M. W. (1986). Sequence of the *Notch* locus of *Drosophila melanogaster:* Relationship of the encoded protein to mammalian clotting and growth factors. *Mol. Cell. Biol.* **6,** 3094–3108.

Klämbt, C., Knust, E., Tietze, K., and Campos-Ortega, J. A. (1989). Closely related transcripts encoded by the neurogenic gene complex *Enhancer of split* of *Drosophila melanogaster. EMBO J.* **8,** 203–210.

Knüst, E., Bremer, K. A. L., Vassin, H., Ziemer, A., Tepass, U., and Campos-Ortega, J. A. (1987a). The *Enhancer of Split* locus and neurogenesis in *Drosophila melanogaster. Dev. Biol.* **122,** 262–273.

Knüst, E., Tietze, K., and Campos-Ortega, J. A. (1987b). Molecular analysis of the neurogenic locus *Enhancer of split* of *Drosophila melanogaster. EMBO J.* **6,** 4113–4123.

Kornberg, T., Siden, I., O'Farrell, P., and Simon, M. (1985). The *engrailed* locus of *Drosophila: In situ* localization of transcripts reveals compartment specific expression. *Cell* **40,** 45–53.

Lassar, A. B., Buskin, J. N., Lockshon, D., Davis, R. L., Apone, S., Hauschka, S. D., and Weintraub, H. (1989). Myo is a sequence-specific DNA binding protein requiring a region of *myc* homology to bind to the muscle creatine kinase enhancer. *Cell* **58,** 823–831.

Lees, A. D. (1942). Homology of the campaniform organs on the wing of *Drosophila melanogaster. Nature (London)* **150,** 375.

Lehmann, R., Dietrich, U., Jiménez, F., and Campos-Ortega, J. A. (1981). Mutations of early neurogenesis in *Drosophila. Roux's Arch. Dev. Biol.* **190,** 226–229.

Lehmann, R., Jiménez, F., Dietrich, U., and Campos-Ortega, J. A. (1983). On the phenotype and development of mutants of early neurogenesis in *Drosophila melanogaster. Roux's Arch. Dev. Biol.* **192,** 62–74.

Lenardo, M., Pierce, J. W., and Baltimore, D. (1987). Protein-binding sites in Ig enhancers determine transcriptional activity and inducibility. *Science* **236,** 1573–1577.

Lewis, E. B. (1978). A gene complex controlling segmentation in *Drosophila. Nature (London)* **276,** 565–570.

Leyns, L., Dambly-Chaudière, C., and Ghysen, A. (1989). Two different sets of *cis* elements regulate *scute* to establish two different sensory patterns. *Roux's Arch. Dev. Biol.* **198,** 227–232.

Locke, M., and Huie, P. (1981). Epidermal feet in insect morphogenesis. *Nature (London)* **293,** 733–735.

Malacinski, G. M., and Bryant, S. V. (eds.) (1984). "Pattern Formation." McMillan.

Mann, R. S., and Hogness, D. S. (1990). Functional dissection of *Ultrabithorax* proteins in *D. melanogaster. Cell* **60,** 597–610.

Martinez, C., and Modolell, J. (1991). Cross-regulatory interactions between the proneural *achaete* and *scute* genes of *Drosophila. Science* **250,** 1485–1487.

Meier, T., Chabaud, F., and Reichert, H. (1991). Homologous patterns in the embryonic development of the peripheral nervous system in the grasshopper *Schistocerca gregaria* and the fly *Drosophila melanogaster. Development* **12,** 241–253.

Mlodzik, M., Baker, N. E., and Rubin, G. (1990). Isolation and expression of *scabrous,* a gene regulating neurogenesis in *Drosophila. Genes Devel.* **4,** 1848–1861.

Moscoso del Prado, J., and Garcia-Bellido, A. (1984). Genetic regulation of the *achaete–scute* complex of *Drosophila melanogaster. Roux's Arch. Dev. Biol.* **193,** 242–245.

Murphey, R. K., Johnson, S. E., and Sakaguchi, D. S. (1983). Anatomy and physiology of supernumerary cercal afferents in crickets: Implications for pattern formation. *J. Neurosci.* **3,** 312–325.

Murphey, R. K., and Lemere, C. A. (1984). Competition controls the growth of an identified axonal arborization. *Science* **224,** 1352–1355.

Murphey, R. K., Possidente, D. R., Vandervorst, P., and Ghysen, A. (1989). Compartments and the topography of leg afferent projections in *Drosophila. J. Neurosci.* **9,** 3209–3217.

Murray, M. A., Schubiger, M., and Palka, J. (1984). Neuron differentiation and axon growth in the developing wing of *Drosophila melanogaster. Dev. Biol.* **104,** 259–273.

Murre, C., McCaw, P. S., and Baltimore, D. (1989a). A new DNA binding and dimerization motif in immunoglobulin enhancer binding, *daughterless,* MyoD and myc proteins. *Cell* **56,** 777–783.

Murre, C., McCaw, P. S., Vaessin, H., Candy, M., Jan, L. Y., Jan, Y. N., Cabrera, C. V., Buskin, J. N., Hauschka, S. D., Lassar, A. B., Weintraub, H., and Baltimore, D. (1989b). Interactions between heterologous helix-loop-helix proteins generate complexes that bind specifically to a common DNA sequence. *Cell* **58,** 537–544.

Nardi, J. B. (1983). Neuronal pathfinding in developing wings of the moth *Manduca sexta. Dev. Biol.* **95,** 163–174.

Nöthiger, R., and Steinmann-Zwicky, M. (1985). Sex determination in *Drosophila. Trends Genet.* **1,** 209–215.

Nüsslein-Volhard, C., and Wieschaus, E. (1980). Mutations affecting segment number and polarity in *Drosophila. Nature (London)* **287,** 795–801.

O'Brochta, D. A., and Bryant, P. J. (1985). A zone of non-proliferating cells at a lineage restriction boundary in *Drosophila. Nature* **313,** 138–141.

O'Kane, C. J., and Gehring, W. (1987). Detection *in situ* of genomic regulatory elements in *Drosophila. Proc. Natl. Acad. Sci. U.S.A.* **84,** 9123–9127.

Palka, J. (1986). Factors influencing neural differentiation in the periphery. *In* "Modes of Communication in the Nervous System" (M.J. Cohen and F. Strumwasser, eds.), pp. 7–24. Wiley.

Palka, J., and Schubiger, M. (1980). Formation of central patterns by receptor cell axons in *Drosophila. In* "Development and Neurobiology of *Drosophila*" (O. Siddiqi, P. Babu, L.M. Hall, and J.C. Hall, eds.), pp. 223–246. New York: Plenum Press.

Palka, J., and Ghysen, A. (1982). Segments, compartments and axon paths in *Drosophila. Trends Neurosci.* **5,** 382–386.

Palka, J., Malone, M. A., Ellison, R. L., and Wigston, D. J. (1986). Central projections of identified *Drosophila* sensory neurons in relation to their time of development. *J. Neurosci.* **6,** 1822–1830.

Peifer, M., and Bender, W. (1986). The anterobithorax and bithorax mutations of the bithorax complex. *EMBO J.* **5,** 2293–2303.

Phillips, R. G., Roberts, I. J. H., Ingham, P. W., and Whittle, J. R. S. (1990). The *Drosophila* segment polarity gene *patched* is involved in a position-signalling mechanism in imaginal discs. *Development* **110,** 105–114.

Pick, L., Schier, A., Affolter, M., Schmidt-Glenewinkel, T., and Gehring, W. J. (1990). Analysis of the *ftz* upstream element: Germ layer-specific enhancers are independently autoregulated. *Genes Devel.* **4,** 1224–1239.

Power, M. E. (1948). The thoracico-abdominal nervous system of an adult insect, *Drosophila melanogaster. J. Comp. Neurol.* **88,** 347–409.

Rao, Y., Jan, L. Y., and Jan, Y. N. (1990). Similarity of the *Drosophila* neurogenic gene *big brain* to transmembrane channel proteins. *Nature (London)* **345,** 163–167.

Raper, J. A., Bastiani, M., and Goodman, C. S. (1983). Pathfinding by neuronal growth cones in grasshopper embryos. II. Selective fasciculation onto specific axonal pathways. *J. Neurosci.* **3**, 31–41.

Ready, D. (1989). A multifaceted approach to neural development. *Trends Neurosci.* **12**, 102–109.

Richelle, J., and Ghysen, A. (1979). Bristle determination and pattern formation in *Drosophila*. I. A model. *Dev. Biol.* **70**, 418–437.

Ripoll, P., El Massal, M., Laran, E., and Simpson, P. (1988). A gradient of affinities for sensory bristles across the wing blade of *Drosophila melanogaster*. *Development* **103**, 757–767.

Rodriguez, I., Hernandez, R., Modolell, J., and Ruiz-Gomez, M. (1990). Competence to develop sensory organs is temporally and spatially regulated in *Drosophila* epidermal primordia. *EMBO J.* **9**, 3583–3592.

Romani, S., Campuzano, S., Macagno, E., and Modolell, J. (1989). Expression of *achaete* and *scute* genes in *Drosophila* imaginal discs and their function in sensory organ development. *Genes Devel.* **3**, 997–1007.

Ruiz-Gomez, M., and Modolell, J. (1987). Deletion analysis of the *achaete–scute* locus of *Drosophila melanogaster*. *Genes Devel.* **1**, 1238–1246.

Rushlow, C. A., Hogan, A., Pinchin, S. M., Howe, K. M., Landelli, M., and Ish-Horowicz, D. (1989). The *Drosophila hairy* protein acts in both segmentation and bristle patterning and shows homology to N-*myc*. *EMBO J.* **8**, 3095–3103.

Sanchez, L., and Nöthiger, R. (1983). Sex determination and dosage compensation in *Drosophila melanogaster*: Production of male clones in XX females. *EMBO J.* **2**, 485–491.

Schubiger, M., and Palka, J. (1987). Changing spatial patterns of DNA replication in the developing wing of *Drosophila*. *Devel. Biol.* **123**, 145–153.

Serebrovsky, A. S., and Dubinin, N. P. (1930). X-ray experiments with *Drosophila*. *J. Heredity* **21**, 259–265.

Shellenbarger, D. L., and Mohler, J. D. (1978). Temperature-sensitive periods and autonomy of pleiotropic effects of $l(1)N^{ts1}$, a conditional *Notch* lethal in *Drosophila*. *Dev. Biol.* **62**, 432–446.

Siegfried, E., Perkins, L. A., Capaci, T. M., and Perrimon, N. (1990). Putative protein kinase product of the *Drosophila* segment polarity gene *zeste-white3*. *Nature (London)* **345**, 825–829.

Simpson, P. (1990). Lateral inhibition and development of sensory bristles of the adult peripheral nervous system of *Drosophila*. *Development* **109**, 509–519.

Stern, C. (1954). Tow or three bristles. *Am. Scientist* **42**, 213–247.

Struhl, G., and White, R. A. H. (1985). Regulation of the *Ultrabithorax* gene by other Bithorax Complex genes. *Cell* **43**, 507–519.

Sturtevant, A. H. (1970). Studies on the bristle pattern of *Drosophila Devel. Biol.* **21**, 48–61.

Technau, G. M., and Campos-Ortega, J. A. (1987). Cell autonomy of expression of neurogenic genes of *Drosophila melanogaster*. *Proc. Natl. Acad. Sci. U.S.A.* **84**, 4500–4504.

Teugels, E., and Ghysen, A. (1983). Two mechanisms for the establishment of sensory projections in *Drosophila*. *Progr. Brain Res.* **58**, 305–312.

Teugels, E., and Ghysen, A. (1985). Domains of action of *bithorax* genes in *Drosophila* central nervous system. *Nature (London)* **314**, 558–561.

Thomas, J. B., Bastiani, M. J., Bate, M., and Goodman, C. S. (1984). From grasshopper to *Drosophila*: A common plan for neuronal development. *Nature (London)* **310**, 203–207.

Thomas, R., and D'Ari, R. (1990). "Biological Feedback." Boca Raton, Florida: CRC Press.

Torres, M., and Sanchez, L. (1989). The *scute* (T4) gene acts as a numerator element of the X:A signal that determines the state of activity of *Sex-lethal* in *Drosophila*. *EMBO J.* **8**, 3079–3086.

Truman, J. W., and Bate, M. (1988). Spatial and temporal patterns of neurogenesis in the central nervous system of *Drosophila melanogaster*. *Dev. Biol.* **125**, 145–157.

Van der Vorst, P., and Ghysen, A. (1980). Genetic control of sensory connections in *Drosophila*. *Nature (London)* **266**, 65–67.

Vässin, H., Vielmetter, J., and Campos-Ortega, J. A. (1985). Genetic interactions in early neurogenesis of *Drosophila melanogaster*. *J. Neurogenet.* **2**, 291–308.

Vässin, H., Bremer, K. A., Knust, E., and Campos-Ortega, J. A. (1987). The neurogenic gene *Delta* of *Drosophila melanogaster* is expressed in neurogenic territories and encodes a putative transmembrane protein with EGF-like repeats. *EMBO J* **6**, 3431–3440.

Villares, R., and Cabrera, C. V. (1987). The *achaete–scute* gene complex of *D. melanogaster*: Conserved domains in a subset of genes required for neurogenesis and their homology to *myc*. *Cell* **50**, 415–424.

Walthall, W. W., and Murphey, R. K. (1984). Rules for neural development revealed by chimaeric sensory systems in crickets. *Nature (London)* **311**, 57–59.

Weinzierl, R., Axton, M. J., Ghysen, A., and Akam, M. (1987). *Ultrabithorax* mutations in constant and variable regions of the protein coding sequence. *Genes Devel.* **1**, 386–397.

Wharton, K. A., Johansen, K. M., Xu, T., and Artavanis-Tsakonas, S. (1985). Nucleotide sequence from the neurogenic locus *Notch* implies a gene product that shares homology with proteins containing EGF-like repeats. *Cell* **43**, 567–581.

Wigglesworth, V. B. (1940). Local and general factors in the development of "pattern" in *Rhodnius prolixus* (Hemiptera). *J. Exp. Biol.* **17**, 180–200.

Wigglesworth, V. B. (1953). The origin of sensory neurons in an insect, *Rhodnius prolixus* (Hemiptera). *Quarto. J. Micr. Sci.* **94**, 113–124.

Wigglesworth, V. B. (1972). "The Principles of Insect Physiology," 7th Ed. New York: John Wiley & Sons.

Wigglesworth, V. B. (1977). Structural changes in the epidermal cells of *Rhodnius* during tracheole capture. *J. Cell Sci.* **26**, 161–174.

Zacharuk, R. Y. (1985). Antennae and sensilla. *In* "Comprehensive Insect Physiology, Biochemistry and Pharmacology" (L.I. Gilbert and G.A. Kerkut, eds.), Vol. 6, pp. 1–69. Oxford: Pergamon Press.

Zawarzin, A. (1912). Histologische Studien über Insekten. II. Das sensible Nervensystem der Aeschne Larven. *Z. Wiss. Zool.* **100**, 245–286.

Endocrine Influences on the Postembryonic Fates of Identified Neurons during Insect Metamorphosis

Janis C. Weeks
Institute of Neuroscience and
Department of Biology
University of Oregon
Eugene, Oregon

Richard B. Levine
Arizona Research Laboratories
Division of Neurobiology and
Department of Physiology
University of Arizona
Tucson, Arizona

I. Introduction

In most nervous systems, structural and functional plasticity peaks during the embryonic and early postnatal periods. In contrast, the nervous systems of animals that undergo metamorphosis exhibit remarkable postembryonic plasticity that can continue for a lifetime. Metamorphosis, whether it occurs in invertebrates or vertebrates, typically involves a developmental progression through two or more life stages during which the animal has different body forms, occupies different environments, and performs different behaviors. Accordingly, many embryonic capabilities such as neurogenesis, programmed neuronal death, and the remodeling of neuronal arbors and synaptic connections are retained postembryonically. However, a key feature of metamorphosis that distinguishes it from embryonic development is that much of the plasticity involves neurons that appear, by structural and functional criteria, to be already fully differentiated. At a cell biological level, this situation raises obvious questions about how neurons that have undergone an initial differentiation during embryogenesis can, during metamorphosis, redifferentiate to carry out very different roles.

Metamorphosis is controlled hormonally, which provides the additional opportunity to ask fundamental questions about how hormones affect neurons and behavior. In insects, a class of steroid hormones (the ecdysteroids) plays a major role in orchestrating the remodeling of the nervous system during metamorphosis (see Section II). The actions of these hormones on neural circuits and behavior in insects strongly parallel the actions of gonadal steroids on the developing vertebrate nervous system (*e.g.*, Arnold and Gorski, 1984). However, in contrast to the vertebrate nervous system, steroid effects on the less complex insect nervous system can be studied at the level of individually identified neurons. During metamorphosis, individual neurons show remarkably stereotyped, cell-specific fates; for instance, in response to a particular hormonal cue, a specific subset of identified neurons may undergo programmed death, another subset may initiate process outgrowth, another subset may retract their processes, and yet another subset remains unchanged. Observations such as these indicate that neurons must possess cellular identities that regulate the access of hormonal cues to particular developmental programs. In keeping with the theme of this volume, we will review selected examples from our own research on the hawkmoth, *Manduca sexta*, that provide insight into how hormonal signals interact with intrinsic and extrinsic factors to orchestrate the dramatic postembryonic reorganization of the nervous system and behavior that accompanies metamorphosis.

II. Description of the Life Cycle and Hormones of *Manduca*

When *Manduca* are reared under controlled laboratory conditions, developmental events are well synchronized (Fig. 1). Three days after an egg is laid, the caterpillar hatches as a first instar larva. Over the subsequent 2 wk, the caterpillar feeds and grows, and undergoes four molts to produce successively larger larvae. Metamorphosis begins during the fifth (final) instar, when the insect ceases feeding, burrows underground, and molts into a pupa. The development of the adult moth in the pupal case takes about 3 wk; after emergence the moth lives for 1–2 wk.

A brief consideration of the temporal fluctuations in the hemolymph levels of developmental hormones during the *Manduca* life cycle, and of the effects of these hormonal changes on epidermal cells (which secrete the cuticular exoskeleton), provides useful insights into potential molecular mechanisms by which these hormones influence neuronal form and function during metamorphosis. Each molt is initiated by the release of a peptide, prothoracicotropic hormone (PTTH), from brain neurosecretory neurons (Bollenbacher and Granger, 1985). PTTH acts on prothoracic glands located

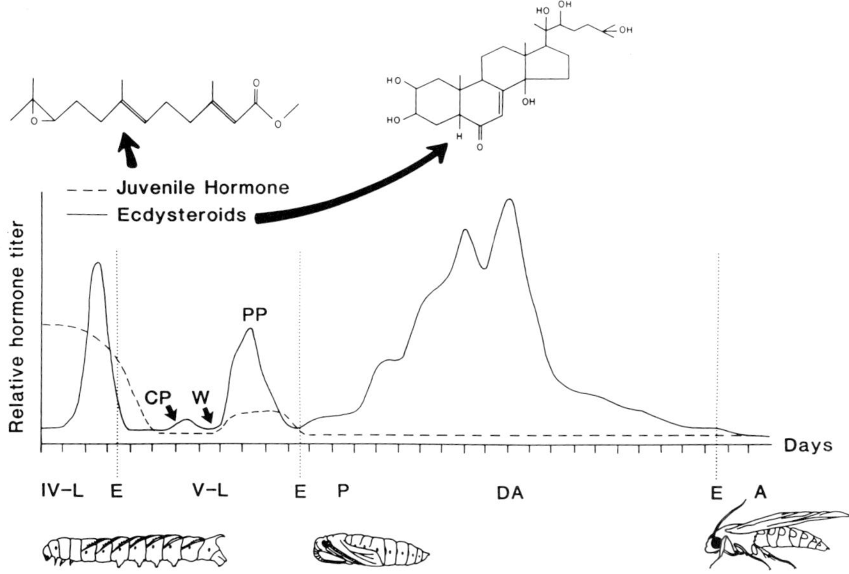

Figure 1. Endocrinology of metamorphosis in *Manduca*. The structures of juvenile hormone (JH) and 20-HE are shown at the top. The time line (in days) indicates developmental changes in the hemolymph levels of JH (---) and 20-HE (–); the curves are meant to portray the relative timing of endocrine events and not absolute levels. Abbreviations: IV-L, 4th larval instar; V-L, 5th larval instar; E, ecdysis (the shedding of the old cuticle); CP, commitment pulse; W, wandering; PP, prepupal peak; P, pupa; DA, developing adult; A, adult. Hormone titers are from Bollenbacher *et al.* (1981) and Riddiford (1985). (Reprinted with permission from Levine and Weeks, 1990; copyright © 1990 by John Wiley & Sons, Inc.)

in the thorax to induce the synthesis and release of ecdysone into the hemolymph. Ecdysone is then hydroxylated to the biologically more active form, 20-hydroxyecdysone (20-HE), in target issues. (The term "ecdysteroids" is used when the two hormones are not distinguished.) The type of molt is determined by the level of juvenile hormone (JH) present in the hemolymph during the ecdysteroid surge. JH originates from gland cells in the corpora allata, neuroendocrine organs associated with the brain. During molts from one larval instar to the next, the hemolymph level of JH is high during each ecdysteroid surge (Fig. 1), insuring that larval structures are produced. For instance, when epidermal cells from intermolt fourth instar larvae are exposed to ecdysteroids and JH, the cells synthesize mRNAs for larval-specific cuticle proteins and secrete a new larval cuticle (Riddiford, 1986).

This pattern of JH and ecdysteroid secretion changes at the larval–pupal transformation, when two ecdysteroid elevations occur. The first of these, the small *commitment pulse* (Fig. 1), occurs in the absence of JH and commits tissues to subsequent pupal development. In epidermal cells, the commitment pulse permanently shuts off the transcription of mRNAs for larval-specific cuticle proteins and induces the expression of a novel set of cuticular genes (Riddiford, 1985; Horodyski and Riddiford, 1989). The commitment pulse also triggers a 24-hr period of intense locomotory behavior called wandering, culminating in the excavation of an underground pupation chamber (Dominick and Truman, 1985). The next ecdysteroid elevation, the larger and more prolonged *prepupal peak*, stimulates the development of pupal structures. Epidermal cells respond to the prepupal leak by initiating the transcription of mRNAs for pupal-specific cuticle proteins, and secreting a pupal cuticle (Riddiford, 1986). There is a small reappearance of JH during the prepupal peak, but most tissues, with the notable exception of the imaginal discs, are refractory to the juvenilizing effects of JH at this time (*e.g.*, Kiguchi and Riddiford, 1978; Weeks and Truman, 1986). The development of the adult moth during the pupal stage is driven by a prolonged rise and fall of ecdysteriods in the absence of JH (Fig. 1). Hormone titers throughout metamorphosis are similar in male and female insects.

III. Metamorphic Fates of Identified Neurons

The most conspicuous feature of metamorphosis is the dramatic external transformation of the body from that of a vermiform larva to that of a winged adult. Internally, an equally remarkable reorganization of the nervous system takes place. The metamorphic transformation of the nervous system features many developmental processes that, in other animals, are more typically restricted to the embryonic period. These processes include neurogenesis, programmed neuronal death, the outgrowth or regression of dendritic and axonal arbors, and the establishment or elimination of specific synaptic connections. As described in the following sections, these events underlie the stage-specific reorganization of neural circuits that produce behavior, and are controlled by precise endocrine cues. Metamorphosis thus provides a particularly illuminating system in which to examine how hormones affect neuronal differentiation and plasticity. The metamorphic fates of individual neurons have been followed in several orders of holometabolous insects [*e.g.*, beetles (Breidbach, 1990); flies (Truman, 1990)], but because the endocrinology of metamorphosis is so well understood in *Manduca* we will restrict most of our discussion to this species.

A. Embryonic and Postembryonic Neurogenesis

The central nervous system (CNS) of the larva is produced during embryogenesis by the mitotic division of segmental arrays of neuroblasts, in a pattern similar to that described in other insects (Thomas *et al.*, 1984). In hemimetabolous (nonmetamorphosing) insects, such as the grasshopper, neurogenesis in the CNS appears to be complete by hatching, whereas in holometabolous insects, such as *Drosophila* or *Manduca*, neurogenesis continues into the postembryonic period (Booker and Truman, 1987a; Truman and Bate, 1988). This prolongation of the period of neurogenic potential may provide more flexibility in the determination of neuronal number and phenotype in metamorphosing insects. In *Manduca*, segmental arrays of neuroblasts in the abdominal and thoracic ganglia produce undifferentiated progeny (imaginal nest cells) throughout the postembryonic larval period. The relationship between the embryonic and postembryonic neuroblasts is not certain, but a reasonable hypothesis is that the postembryonically active neuroblasts are a subset of those neuroblasts that were active during the embryonic period (Truman and Bate, 1988; Prokop and Technau, 1991).

Beginning at the wandering stage, some imaginal nest cells differentiate into neurons while others die (Booker and Truman, 1987a; Witten and Truman, 1991). Because it has not yet been possible to follow the fates of individual imaginal nest cells, it is not known if the identities of the doomed cells are as precise as they are for the programmed deaths of larval motoneurons (see Section III,C). The programmed death or differentiation of the imaginal nest cells is controlled by the levels of ecdysteroids and JH in the hemolymph (Booker and Truman, 1987b). Postembryonic neurogenesis also plays a major role in the massive enlargement of the brain that accompanies adult development as the visual and olfactory processing centers develop (Edwards, 1969; Hildebrand, 1985).

It will be of great interest to investigate how these postembryonically derived neurons, most of which appear to be interneurons, are incorporated into pre-existing neural circuits. An intriguing finding reported by Truman and Booker (1986) was that chemical ablation of the imaginal nest cells by hydroxyurea treatment during the larval stage produced only minimal behavioral deficits in adult moths (although only a few behaviors were examined). Postembryonic neurogenesis also raises a number of interesting cell biological questions. For instance, do hormones stimulate differentiation of the immature progeny through direct actions or by their effects on presynaptic neurons? Do neurons differentiating in a mature CNS confront different challenges than they would encounter in an embryo? For instance, do the same substrate guidance cues that direct axon outgrowth in embryos (*e.g.*, Bastiani *et al.*, 1987) persist in the postembryonic CNS, or are new cues or strategies employed?

In contrast to the generation of central neurons from neuroblasts, insect sensory neurons derive almost exclusively from precursor cells located peripherally in the epidermis (Bate, 1978). In both hemi- and holometabolous insects, new sensory neurons and their associated cuticular structures arise at each molt, a pattern that permits the density of sensory receptors to be maintained as the surface area of the body increases. During metamorphic molts, the sensory neurons of the previous stage may degenerate, persist unchanged (Levine and Truman, 1983), or be modified for a different use (Section III,D; Levine *et al.*, 1986) while new sensory neurons and sensilla appropriate for the next stage are generated (Kent and Griffin, 1990). Mitosis of the epidermal precursors of sensory neurons, as well as the metamorphic reorganization of pre-existing sensory neurons, is tied to the molt cycle and is under the control of ecdysteroids and JH (*e.g.*, Levine *et al.*, 1986; Levine, 1989).

B. Reidentification of Neurons during Metamorphosis

With the exception of the imaginal nest cells and a limited number of other late-differentiating cells (Tublitz and Truman, 1985), the majority of larval neurons that have been examined appear to be fully differentiated by numerous criteria. For instance, larval motoneurons form well-developed functional neuromuscular junctions on specific muscle fibers, have profuse central arbors that receive and integrate excitatory and inhibitory synaptic inputs, and exhibit an array of voltage-activated and neurotransmitter-activated ion channels (*e.g.*, Trimmer and Weeks, 1989a,b; Truman, 1989;

Waldrop and Levine, 1989; Levine and Hayashi, 1990). At pupation, each larval neuron has one of three options: to die, to persist unchanged, or to be respecified for a new function. The population of larval neurons is again modified after emergence of the adult moth, primarily by programmed death. As will be discussed in subsequent sections, the expression of these cell-specific fates is controlled hormonally at precise times during development.

To study the metamorphic fates of neurons, it is essential that individual neurons be reidentifiable in the different life stages. The most easily followed neurons are motoneurons, which have large cell bodies located in stereotyped positions in the ganglia and can be stained by backfilling the axon with cobalt or by introducing cobalt via an intracellular recording electrode. By staining motoneurons at closely timed developmental intervals, it has been possible to follow most of the larval abdominal motoneurons through metamorphosis (Taylor and Truman, 1974; Levine and Truman, 1985; Weeks and Ernst-Utzschneider, 1989). Cell fate information derived from cobalt backfilling can be confirmed by injecting the fluorescent tracer Fluro-Gold or the carbocyanine dye Di-I into a larval muscle to retrogradely stain the motoneuron; the motoneuron is subsequently visualized *in situ* at a later developmental stage and impaled with a microelectrode for electrophysiological study and intracellular staining. This approach has been used to follow thoracic leg motoneurons from the larval to the adult stage (see Section III,D,3; Kent and Levine, 1988b,c).

In addition to motoneurons, it has been possible to follow the metamorphic fates of neurosecretory cells and sensory neurons by using cobalt or immunocytochemical staining in conjunction with physiological studies (Levine *et al.*, 1985, 1986; Levine, 1989; Tublitz and Sylwester, 1990). A slightly more difficult problem is presented by neurons that lack peripheral axons that can be backfilled, that is, interneurons. However, it has recently proven possible to reidentify some larval interneurons in the early pupal stage by comparing anatomical and electrophysiological properties at closely spaced intervals (Sandstrom and Weeks, 1988,1991).

C. **Programmed Neuronal Death**

Programmed neuronal death functions in many developing systems to eliminate superfluous or outmoded neurons (*e.g.*, Hamburger and Oppenheim, 1982; Truman, 1984). The most detailed studies of programmed neuronal death in *Manduca* have been carried out on abdominal motoneurons. The death of specific motoneurons is monitored by backfilling nerves to reveal missing neurons or by staining ganglia to visualize degenerating neurons (*e.g.*, Truman, 1983; Giebultowicz and Truman, 1984; Weeks, 1987).

During metamorphosis, the musculature of the abdomen becomes less complex, so fewer motoneurons are needed in the pupal and adult stages than in the larva. For instance, most of the abdominal muscles degenerate at pupation, leaving the majority of the motoneurons targetless. Of these motoneurons, a specific subset that constitutes approximately 16% of the total dies within the first few days of pupal life; the survivors are respecified to innervate new adult muscles that arise later (see Section III,D; Taylor and Truman, 1974; Levine and Truman, 1985). During the first few days after adult emergence, the few remaining larval muscles and many of the newly formed adult muscles degenerate. These muscles participate in emergence behavior, when the moth sheds the pupal cuticle and digs out from underground, but then are no longer needed. The postemergence muscle degeneration is accompanied by the death of approximately 50% of the motoneurons and interneurons in the abdominal ganglia (Taylor and Truman, 1974; Truman, 1983).

A great deal is known about the endocrine cues that trigger these waves of motoneuron death. Weeks and collaborators (Weeks and Truman, 1985, 1986; Weeks, 1987; Weeks *et al.*, 1992) have studied the programmed death of motoneurons innervating retractor muscles of the larval prolegs, which are locomotory appendages unique to the larval stage. Motoneurons PPR and APR (Fig. 2) both innervate proleg retractor muscles that degenerate at pupation (Weeks and Truman, 1984). The PPRs in all proleg-bearing segments (abdominal segments A3–A6) and the APRs in segments A5 and A6 die on the second day of pupal life (Fig. 2; Weeks and Ernst-Utzschneider, 1989). To examine the role of ecdysteroids and JH in these events, hormone levels were manipulated experimentally. The influence of the ecdysteroid-secreting prothoracic glands was removed by ligating abdomens at the thoracic–abdominal junction; some of the isolated abdomens received treatment with 20-HE and/or JH to replace the missing hormones. The results of a series of endocrine manipulations revealed that the rising phase of the prepupal peak of ecdysteroids (Fig. 1) triggers the degeneration of the proleg muscles and the regression and death of the proleg motoneurons (Weeks and Truman 1985, 1986; Weeks, 1987; Weeks *et al.*, 1992). These responses require a prior exposure to ecdysteroids in the absence of JH, a signal that is normally provided by the commitment pulse. Interactions between the muscles and motoneurons are not necessary for these events, because larval motoneurons whose target muscles are surgically ablated, or larval muscles that are denervated, do not initiate metamorphic changes until exposed to the appropriate endocrine cues, at which time they respond normally (Weeks and Truman, 1985).

The endocrine signal for the wave of neuron death that follows adult emergence is a *decline* in the hemolymph ecdysteroid titer (Truman and Schwartz, 1984), in contrast to the *rise* in ecdysteroids that triggers neuron

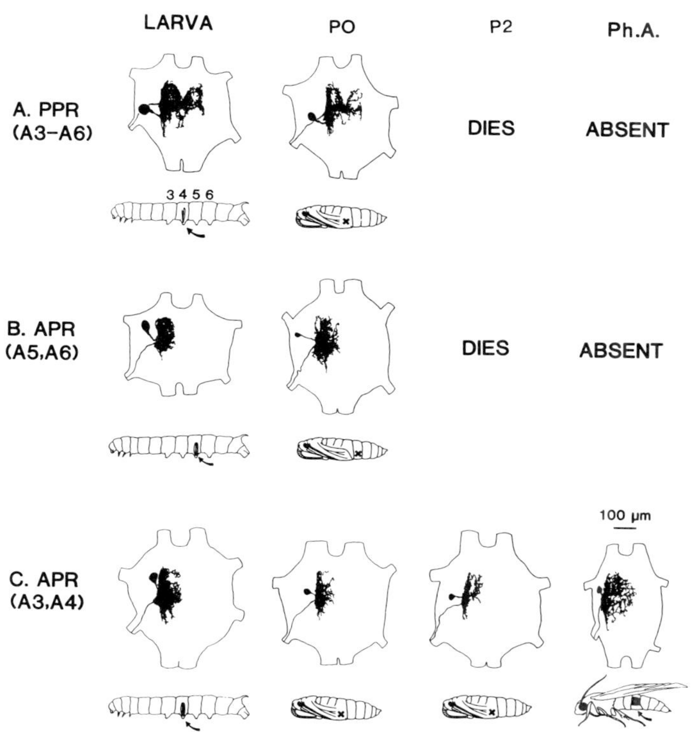

Figure 2. Cell-specific and segment-specific fates of proleg motoneurons during metamorphosis. In this and subsequent figures, *camera lucida* drawings show the outline of ganglia in whole-mount (dorsal view), with anterior to the top. The morphology of motoneurons PPR and APR, and the status of their target muscles, is shown during the early 5th larval instar (Larva), the first day of the pupal stage (day P0), the second day of the pupal stage (Day P2), and in the pharate (pre-emerged) adult (Ph. A.). Motoneurons were stained by intracellular ionophoresis of cobalt followed by silver intensification. The location of the motoneurons' target muscles in each stage is indicated by an arrow on the drawing beneath the ganglion; an "X" indicates a degenerated muscle. Morphometric studies indicate that the dendrites of PPR and APR are regressed by day P0 (**A, B, C**). The PPRs in all proleg-bearing segments (A3–A6), and the APRs in segments A5 and A6, die on day P2 (**A, B**). In contrast, the APRs in segments A3 and A4 survive, reexpand their dendritic arbors, and innervate new tergosternal muscles of the adult moth (**C**). The APRs in segments A3 and A4 do eventually die, in the wave of neuron death that occurs during the first few days of adult life (not shown). Data from Weeks and Truman (1985), Weeks and Ernst-Utzschneider (1989), and Sandstrom and Weeks, unpublished observation. (Reprinted with permission from Levine and Weeks, 1990; copyright © 1990 by John Wiley & Sons, Inc.)

death at pupation. As the ecdysteroid level falls during the final day of pupal life (Fig. 1), individual motoneurons and interneurons become committed to die in a particular sequence. The time course of neuron death can be altered predictably by endocrine manipulations. For instance, injection of 20-HE to keep the ecdysteroid levels elevated delays motoneuron death, whereas ligation of the abdomen to cause a premature fall in the ecdysteroid titer advances the time of motoneuron death (Truman and Schwartz, 1984). Similar effects were found *in vitro*; when ganglia from moths 1 day before emergence were placed in culture, addition of 20-HE to the culture medium prevented motoneuron death whereas omission of the 20-HE permitted the normal pattern of death to occur (Bennett and Truman, 1985). Thus, just as was found for the wave of neuron death at pupation, the hormonally triggered death of motoneurons after adult emergence does not require interactions with target muscles.

These observations raise obvious questions about the mechanisms by which neuronal death is triggered. Many lines of evidence suggest that programmed neuronal death in *Manduca*, just as in the nervous systems of other animals (*e.g.*, Ellis and Horvitz, 1986; Martin *et al.*, 1988; Oppenheim *et al.*, 1990), is caused by the activation of intrinsic cellular programs that involve changes in mRNA and protein synthesis; that is, the neurons commit suicide. This scenario is supported by findings that changes in mRNA and protein synthesis occur coincident with neuronal death (Montemayor *et al.*, 1990; Schwartz *et al.*, 1990a,b) and that motoneuron death can be blocked by treatment with protein or mRNA synthesis inhibitors (Fahrbach and Truman, 1987a, 1988; Weeks *et al.*, 1991). A direct hormone action on motoneurons is supported by the autoradiographic demonstration that, prior to the two waves of programmed neuron death, some motoneurons accumulate the ecdysteroid analog, ponasterone A, in their nuclei; the motoneurons do not accumulate the hormone at other times when they are unresponsive to ecdysteroids (Fahrbach and Truman, 1989; Fahrbach, 1991). In some cases, the ganglionic positions of autoradiographically labeled neuronal profiles allowed them to be identified as motoneurons known to die from previous studies (*e.g.*, motoneuron MN-12). However, other motoneurons (*e.g.*, those that innervate intersegmental muscles) did not show nuclear accumulation prior to their deaths at adult emergence. The authors point out that this finding is not inconsistent with a hormonally mediated death, because the developmental *disappearance* of ecdysteroid receptors could trigger death if motoneuron survival had become dependent on ecdysteroid receptor occupancy during adult development (Fahrbach and Truman, 1989).

Although a direct hormone action is certainly implicated in neuronal degeneration during metamorphosis, it is equally clear that other factors may intervene. Many of the motoneurons that die after adult emergence first participate in emergence behavior, when the moth sheds the pupal cuticle and digs out of the soil. Truman (1983) found that, if emerging moths were restrained in small vials that forced them to prolong their digging efforts, motoneuron degeneration was delayed. This finding suggests that behavioral activity may alter the time course of cell death. The possible involvement of descending neural influences was demonstrated by Fahrbach and Truman (1987b), who found that severance of the abdominal nerve cord could prevent the death of MN-12, which normally dies after emergence in response to the falling ecdysteroid titer. MN-12 shows nuclear accumulation of hormone at this time and is a good candidate for being a direct ecdysteroid target (previous text). These findings raise the intriguing possibility that neural inputs may somehow be able to interfere with or block the endocrine-mediated biochemical cascade that would normally lead to neuronal suicide. It is now possible to place individually identified *Manduca* motoneurons in cell culture under varying endocrine conditions (see Section III,D,4), a technique that may help determine the relative contribution of endocrine and neural influences to programmed neuronal death during metamorphosis.

A key principle of metamorphosis that is well illustrated by the phenomenon of neuronal death is that the interpretation of a particular hormonal signal depends critically on the previous endocrine exposure of a neuron. Notably, the ecdysteroid titer rises and falls repeatedly during metamorphosis, yet individual neurons degenerate in response to a specific rise or fall and ignore other fluctuations. For instance, the proleg motoneurons experience an ecdysteroid rise at each larval molt, but only after the small commitment pulse of ecdysteroids in the absence of JH do they respond to the *next* ecdysteroid rise, the prepupal peak, by degenerating. In contrast, the intersegmental muscle motoneurons experience a fall in ecdysteroid levels at each larval molt, as well as at the commitment pulse and prepupal peaks, but die only after the fall in ecdysteroids at the end of adult development. Based on work with *Manduca* epidermal cells (*e.g.*, Riddiford, 1985), one would expect these neuron-specific and stage-specific response patterns to be based on hormonally controlled access to particular developmental programs that are encoded in the genome. How, at the molecular level, endocrine events gate the subsequent access of the same hormones to developmental programs is a fundamental question in metamorphosis.

One final issue is raised by programmed neuronal death in this system. During metamorphosis, individually identified neurons show essentially invariant fates from animal to animal. This contrasts with a stochastic pattern of programmed death, as occurs in the vertebrate spinal cord, in which a certain percentage of neurons from a uniform starting population dies (*e.g.*, Oppenheim, 1985). The individualized metamorphic fates of *Manduca* neurons indicate that the cells somehow know their own identities. In other systems, cellular identity can derive from factors such as position in a lineage or early interactions with other cells (*e.g.*, Doe and Goodman, 1985). Although the cellular determinants of neuronal identity are virtually unexplored in *Manduca*, experimental observations have provided information about two factors that may contribute. First, the finding of Giebultowicz and Truman (1984) that apparently homologous motoneurons in the terminal abdominal ganglion show sexually dimorphic patterns of cell death at pupation suggests that genes involved in sex determination may influence neuronal fate. Second, Weeks and Ernst-Utzschneider (1989) found that the pupal fate of proleg motoneuron APR is segment-specific; as shown in Fig. 2, the motoneuron dies in segments A5 and A6, whereas it survives in segments A3 and A4. Furthermore, the deaths of the APRs in segments A5 and A6 have different hormonal thresholds (Weeks *et al.*, 1992). Thus, segmental identity also contributes to neuronal fate. It would be interesting to use autoradiographic techniques to examine whether the fates of these motoneurons are related to ecdysteroid receptor levels. For example, does a female motoneuron that is fated to die have ecdysteroid receptors whereas its male counterpart does not? Do APR motoneurons contain ecdysteroid receptors only in the segments in which they are fated to die? An interesting twist on the APR story is that the motoneurons that survive at pupation do eventually die after adult emergence (Weeks and Ernst-Utzschneider, 1989). Thus, these motoneurons do not lack an intrinsic degeneration program, but its expression requires a different hormonal signal from that which triggers the death of their homologs in other segments.

D. Respecification of Neurons during Metamorphosis

As already mentioned, most motoneurons lose their target muscles at pupation but the majority of these persist to carry out a different role in the adult moth. This structural and functional remodeling of differentiated neurons during metamorphosis is termed *respecification*. Respecification is not limited to motoneurons, but involves all classes of central and peripheral neurons. As will be discussed, respecification is associated with the remodeling of neural arbors; a typical pattern in motoneurons is an initial regression of larval dendrites to eliminate outmoded synaptic connections, followed by the re-expansion of the dendritic arbor to permit new adult-specific synaptic connections to form. These structural and functional changes in neurons provide an excellent opportunity to examine how hormones can modify neural circuits and behavior during postembryonic life.

1. NEURONS THAT ARE NOT RESPECIFIED

It is useful to first consider the life history of neurons that are *not* respecified during metamorphosis, for example, the motoneurons that innervate intersegmental muscles. These motoneurons innervate the same target muscles throughout metamorphosis, and do not exhibit any major structural changes (Levine and Truman, 1985). After adult emergence, the intersegmental muscles and their motoneurons degenerate together (Truman and Schwartz, 1984). Although motoneurons that are not respecified appear structurally stable, they may, nevertheless, undergo more subtle changes in their electrophysiological properties (Waldrop and Levine, 1989).

2. REMOVAL OF RESPECIFIED MOTONEURONS FROM LARVAL CIRCUITS

Larval motoneurons that do undergo respecification are faced, in theory, with two sequential or overlapping tasks: first, to extricate themselves from outmoded larval neural circuits, and second, to become integrated into the appropriate pupal or adult circuits. The first process, removal from larval circuits, has been best studied in proleg motoneurons. The prolegs (Fig. 3A) play a dominant role in larval locomotion and also exhibit local responses including a withdrawal reflex. The tip of each proleg, the planta, bears an array of approximately 50 mechanosensory hairs termed the planta hairs (PHs), each of which is innervated by a single peripheral sensory neuron that sends an axon into the CNS (Peterson and Weeks, 1988). Tactile stimulation of the PHs causes retraction of the proleg (Fig. 3B) due to contraction of proleg retractor muscles, including those innervated by PPR and APR. The excitation of the proleg motoneurons by PH stimulation is mediated by monosynaptic excitatory connections from individual PH sensory neurons (Fig. 3C), as well as by parallel polysynaptic pathways (Weeks and Jacobs, 1987; Trimmer and Weeks; 1989a; Jacobs and Weeks, 1990).

The loss of the prolegs at pupation renders proleg withdrawal behavior obsolete; in fact, the reflex can no longer be evoked on or after the second day after wandering. However, because the proleg retractor muscles degenerate during this time (Weeks and Truman, 1985), the behavioral change does not necessarily reflect a change in central neural circuits. To examine the efficacy of the sensory-to-motoneuron pathways more directly, the nerve carrying the PH sensory neuron axons was stimulated electrically while recording from the nerve that carries the proleg retractor motoneuron axons, in isolated ganglia removed on different days of development (Fig. 3D). In premetamorphic 5th instar larvae (day L3), and through the second day after wandering (day W2), the sensory stimulation evoked a burst of motor activity

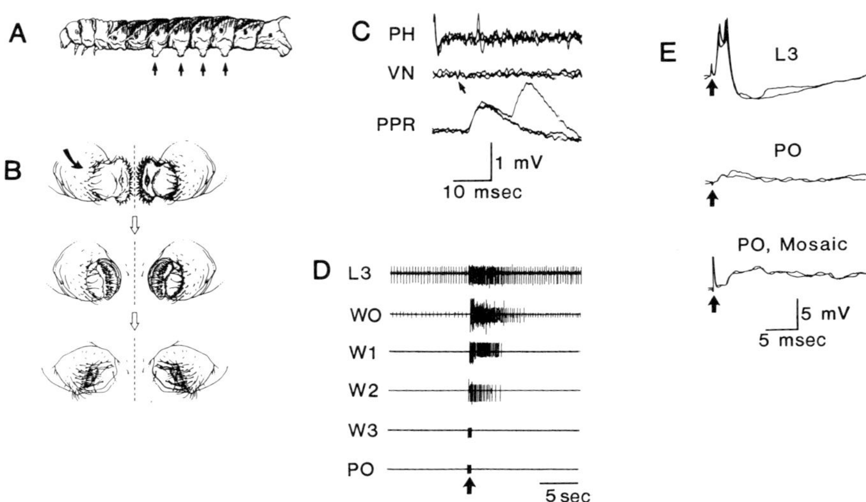

Figure 3. Metamorphic dismantling of the proleg withdrawal reflex circuit. **A.** The location of the prolegs is indicated by arrows. **B.** A pair of prolegs is shown in ventral view; the midline is indicated by a dashed line. The array of planta hairs (PHs) is indicated by a black arrow. Tactile stimulation of the PHs causes contraction of the proleg retractor muscles and retraction of the prolegs, as shown in the successive panels. **C.** Monosynaptic connections from PH sensory neurons to proleg moto-neurons. Oscilloscope sweeps were triggered by action potentials recorded in a PH sensory neuron (*top*). The sensory neuron action potentials were recorded *en passant* in the ventral nerve (VN; *arrow*), and they produced time-locked EPSPs in the ipsilateral PPR (*bottom*). In one sweep the sensory neuron fired twice, producing two EPSPs. **D.** Developmental decrease in the strength of the sensory-to-motoneuron pathway. Each trace is an extracellular recording of the nerve that carries proleg retractor motoneuron axons, from ganglia removed on consecutive days of development indicated at left (L3, third day of the 5th larval instar; W0–W3, the day of, or number of days after, wandering; P0, first day of the pupal stage.) At the time indicated by the arrow, a train of electrical stimuli was delivered to a different nerve that carries the PH sensory neuron axons. The strength of the motor response evoked by the sensory stimulus decreased during development; after day W3 the stimulus was ineffective in evoking motoneuron spikes. **E.** Intracellular recordings of motoneuron responses to PH stimulation. Each trace is a recording from PPR (held at −50 mV) during application of a single shock to the PH sensory nerve, on day L3 (*top*), day P0 (*middle*), or day P0 in a mosaic hemisegment of a pupa with a retained proleg (*bottom*; see text for details.) On day L3, the evoked compound EPSP was large and suprathreshold, whereas on day P0 the response was small and subthreshold in both normal or mosaic hemisegments. Thus, retention of the PH afferents in the larval state did not prevent the developmental weakening of the reflex pathway. [Data reprinted by permission of Springer-Verlag from Weeks and Jacobs (1987) and by permission of the *Journal of Neuroscience* from Jacobs and Weeks (1990).]

that would normally cause the proleg to retract. After day W2, however, the sensory stimulation was no longer able to bring the motoneurons to threshold (Fig. 3D). The diminished ability of PH sensory neurons to excite proleg motoneurons was further examined by recording intracellularly from motoneurons. In PPR, the amplitude of the compound excitatory postsynaptic potential (EPSP) evoked in response to a single shock applied to the sensory nerve declined by 78% between days L3 and P0 (Fig. 3E; Jacobs and Weeks, 1990); a similar decline was seen in motoneuron APR (Levine and Weeks, 1990). The finding that the motoneurons' input resistances *increased* during this period of development indicated that the decreased synaptic effect was not caused by electrical shunting. Experiments in which the ionic composition of the saline was modified indicated that the reduced sensory effect was largely attributable to the developmental weakening of the monosynaptic component of the reflex pathway (Jacobs and Weeks, 1990).

What might cause the sensory-to-motoneuron synapses to weaken? On the presynaptic side, anatomical studies suggested that the number of PH sensory neurons, and the extent of their central projections, decreased during the larval–pupal transformation (Jacobs and Weeks, 1990). Both factors might reduce the synaptic effect of sensory nerve stimulation. On the postsynaptic side, a potentially important factor was the extensive regression of proleg motoneuron arbors that occurs during the final days of larval life (Fig. 2). In the case of PPR, morphometric studies indicated that the motoneuron first shows significant regression on day W1 and loses approximately 40% of its arbor by day W3 (Weeks and Truman, 1985). PPR's regression is triggered by the prepupal peak of ecdysteroids, subject to prior exposure to ecdysteroids in the absence of JH (Weeks and Truman, 1985, 1986; Weeks, 1987; Weeks *et al.*, 1992). The regression of dendritic processes might be expected to interrupt synaptic contacts on the motoneurons, and thereby cause pre-existing inputs to be weakened or lost. To test the relative contribution of developmental changes in the presynaptic sensory neurons and postsynaptic motoneurons to the loss of the proleg withdrawal reflex, Jacobs and Weeks (1990) used endocrine manipulations to generate *heterochronic mosaic* pupae that bore a single retained larval proleg. The technique used was adapted from that of Levine *et al.* (1986), who applied a synthetic JH analog (methoprene) to a small region of the body surface during the commitment pulse of ecdysteroids to block the pupal commitment of the underlying epidermal cells and sensory neurons. During the subsequent prepupal peak, the treated area undergoes a supernumerary larval molt while the remainder of the body becomes pupal. Anatomical studies indicated that, in pupal hemisegments that bore a retained larval proleg, the sensory neurons were retained in normal numbers and continued to project correctly in the CNS whereas the proleg motoneurons underwent pupal development and their dendrites regressed normally (Jacobs and Weeks, 1990). The synapses in the treated hemisegments thus appeared to be mosaic, with larval sensory neurons and pupal (regressed) motoneurons.

Electrophysiological experiments (Fig. 3E) indicated that, in the mosaic hemisegments, the compound EPSP evoked in PPR by sensory nerve stimulation was reduced to the same extent as in normal pupae (Jacobs and Weeks, 1990). This finding suggested that the status of the PH sensory neurons was irrelevant to the developmental loss of the proleg withdrawal reflex. Instead, it appeared that the important locus of change occurred postsynaptically, in the motoneurons. The working hypothesis, that the regression of motoneuron dendrites physically disconnects the cell from PH sensory neuron synapses, is under continuing investigation. An additional conclusion that may be drawn from these experiments is that sensory neuron degeneration, with the resultant deafferentation of proleg motoneurons, does not appear to be a major factor in directing the regression of motoneuron dendrites (see subsequent text).

Thus, in at least one instance, it has been possible to correlate the endocrine-triggered regression of neuronal processes with the elimination of synaptic inputs involved in a behavior that is no longer needed. Interestingly, not all synaptic inputs to proleg motoneurons weaken at pupation. Notably, monosynaptic EPSPs produced in motoneuron APR by some identified interneurons maintain their amplitude, or even increase in amplitude, during the larval–pupal transformation (Sandstrom and Weeks, unpublished observations). Thus, dendritic regression does not cause the indiscriminate weakening of all inputs. The behavioral roles of these interneurons have not yet been determined, but one can speculate that they may contribute to pupal or adult behaviors involving the respecified proleg motoneurons. This question could be addressed in the APR motoneurons in segments A3 and A4, which persist for the first few days of adult life. These motoneurons show a re-expansion of their dendritic arbors during adult development (Fig. 2) in response to the elevated ecdysteroid titer (Weeks and Ernst-Utzschneider, 1989). Their new targets, the tergosternal muscles, cause abdomen extension during behaviors such as emergence, copulation, and oviposition; the new dendritic growth may provide sites for synaptic inputs appropriate for these behaviors.

3. INCORPORATION OF RESPECIFIED MOTONEURONS INTO NEW CIRCUITS

Insights into the relationship between dendritic growth and the acquisition of new synaptic inputs and behaviors have already been obtained in other studies of respecified motoneurons. In the larval stage, motoneuron MN-1 innervates a muscle that causes dorsolateral bending of the body; the motoneuron has a unilateral dendritic field that is located ipsilateral to the target muscle (Truman and Reiss, 1976; Levine and Truman, 1985). The larval MN-1 receives apparently monosynaptic excitatory input from an ipsilateral stretch receptor sensory neuron, an arrangement that produces postural reflexes appropriate for lateral abdominal movements (Levine and Truman, 1982). At pupation, MN-1's target muscle degenerates. During adult development the motoneuron grows new contralateral processes to produce a bilateral dendritic arbor, and innervates a new muscle that produces dorsal flexion of the abdomen. The transformation from a unilateral to bilateral dendritic arbor is a common characteristic among respecified *Manduca* abdominal motoneurons (Levine and Truman, 1985; Weeks and Ernst-Utzschneider, 1989). The new dendrites of MN-1 overlap with the terminal processes of the *contralateral* stretch receptor sensory neuron, which forms a new excitatory connection with MN-1 during adult development (Levine and Truman, 1982). The resulting neural circuit, in which MN-1 is excited by both ipsi- and contralateral stretch receptor sensory neurons, contributes to the postural reflexes of the moth abdomen. Thus, dendritic outgrowth provides the anatomical substrate for the development of a new adult-specific reflex pathway.

Another example of neuronal respecification is provided by motoneurons innervating thoracic leg muscles. Like the abdominal proleg motoneurons, these motoneurons undergo pronounced regression of their dendritic processes when the legs degenerate at the end of larval life (Fig. 4; Kent and Levine, 1988b,c). Unlike the abdominal prolegs, the thoracic legs are replaced by adult counterparts. As the new adult thoracic legs form from imaginal tissue, the motoneurons are respecified to innervate the new leg muscles, and begin to grow new dendritic processes (Fig. 4). The growth of new dendritic processes is correlated in time with the ingrowth into the CNS of axons from sensory neurons generated *de novo* during the development of the adult leg (Kent and Griffin, 1990) and with the differentiation of new interneurons that are born postembryonically (Booker and Truman, 1987a); both the sensory neurons and the interneurons may provide direct or indirect synaptic input to the motoneurons. It is likely that the expansion of the dendritic processes of the respecified leg motoneurons during metamorphosis provides postsynaptic space for new synaptic inputs that contribute to the reorganization of circuits involved in the control of leg movements.

Just as for programmed motoneuron death and dendritic regression (see previous text), specific endocrine cues have been identified as triggering the growth of dendritic processes during metamorphosis. Ligation of abdomens to separate them from the source of ecdysteroids early during the pupal stage prevents the dendritic growth of APR and other respecified proleg motoneurons (Weeks and Ernst-Utzschneider, 1989). Similarly, the dendrites of respecified abdominal motoneurons fail to grow in diapausing pupae, in

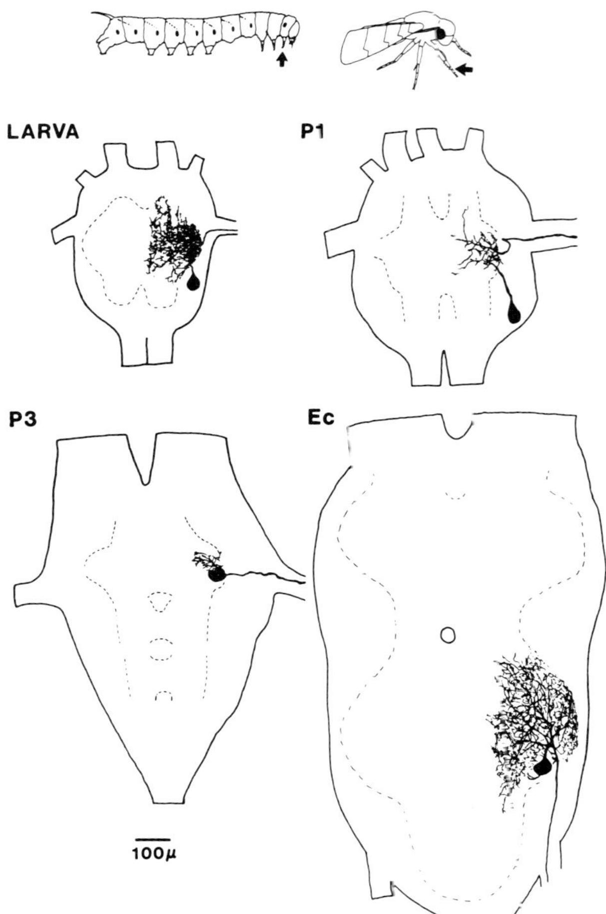

Figure 4. Dendritic remodeling of an identified thoracic leg motoneuron. The top of the figure shows a larva and an adult moth, with a prothoracic leg indicated by arrows. Each *camera lucida* drawing shows the morphology of a metathoracic leg motoneuron at different developmental stages (the neuropil outline is indicated by dashed lines). Note that the metathoracic ganglion fuses with other ganglia during adult development. In each case the motoneuron was retrogradely labeled in the larval stage by injecting Di-I into its target muscle, the femoral flexor. At later developmental stages, the motoneuron was visualized under fluorescence illumination penetrated with a microelectrode, identified physiologically, and stained with lucifer yellow or hexamine–cobalt to visualize dendritic processes and verify the double labeling. In the adult stage, the motoneuron innervates a femoral extensor muscle. Note that the larval arbor undergoes severe dendritic regression by the early pupal stage, followed by reexpansion during adult development. Abbreviations: Larva, early 5th larval instar; P1, P3, stages of pupal development roughly corresponding to days of development; Ec, eclosed (emerged) adult moth. (Reprinted with permission from Levine and Weeks, 1990; copyright © 1990 by John Wiley & Sons, Inc.)

which ecdysteroid titers remain at low levels, but expansion is initiated following the infusion of 20-HE (Levine and Truman, 1985; Truman and Reiss, 1988). Interestingly, although JH is not normally present during adult development, the dendritic growth of respecified abdominal motoneurons can be prevented by treatment with the JH analog methoprene during the first few days of pupal life (Truman and Reiss, 1988).

Hormonal cues during adult development cause cell-specific dendritic outgrowth in respecified motoneurons; although some features are common to many motoneurons (*e.g.*, the elaboration of bilateral arbors), the morphological characteristics of the dendritic expansion are unique for each individual motoneuron that has been examined. For instance, the new contralateral processes of respecified motoneurons are concentrated in different regions of neuropil (Levine and Truman, 1985; Weeks and Ernst-Utzschneider, 1989). Thus, although dendritic growth *per se* is triggered hormonally, the exact characteristics of the growth may be guided by internal developmental programs or external cues in the CNS. These observations illustrate a point that was already discussed earlier with respect to neuronal death, that is, that the same hormonal environment can have different effects on dendritic morphology at different developmental stages. Thus, 20-HE in the absence of JH during the prepupal peak triggers dendritic regression, but the same conditions cause dendritic growth *in the same motoneuron* during the early pupal stage. Similarly, exogenous JH analogs introduced during the early pupal surge of ecdysteroids prevent the growth of adult dendrites, but do not cause a return to the larval dendritic morphology. One possible explanation for this difference, as suggested in the discussion of neuronal death, is that the set of genes expressed in response to a particular hormonal context is influenced by prior hormonal experience. An additional factor may be that different conditions exist in the CNS at different developmental stages. Cues derived from JH and the ecdysteroids could interact with stage-specific cellular or other humoral signals to produce a unique morphological response.

4. SITES OF HORMONE ACTION IN TRIGGERING MOTONEURON RESPECIFICATION

What cellular mechanisms contribute to the observed structural changes in motoneuronal arbors? These morphological changes could be caused by direct hormone action mediated by ecdysteroid receptors in the affected neurons. Alternatively, interactions with pre- or postsynaptic partners has been shown to influence neuronal structure in many systems (*e.g.*, Murphey *et al.*, 1975; Kimmel *et al.*, 1977); this would provide a mechanism for indirect effects on neurons that are not themselves hormone targets. Some data are available on the possible role of cellular interactions in neuronal remodeling in *Manduca*. In the case of the proleg motoneurons, motoneuron regression and muscle degeneration normally proceed simultaneously. However, ablation of a proleg motoneuron's target muscle (Weeks and Truman, 1985), or preservation of the muscle by endocrine manipulations (Weeks, 1987), does not interfere with dendritic regression. Also, as described earlier, retention of larval PH sensory neurons in the pupal stage does not interfere with the regression of proleg motoneurons in heterochronic mosaics (Jacobs and Weeks, 1990).

The role of neuromuscular interactions for dendritic *outgrowth* was tested by Kent and Levine (1988c) using motoneurons that innervate thoracic leg muscles. Removal of an adult leg primordium in the larval stage, which deletes both the new muscle targets and the new sensory inputs, had only a minor effect on the form of the new adult-specific arbors that subsequently formed. Whether this apparent indifference of respecified motoneurons to their target muscles is a general rule, or is peculiar to the two systems that have been examined, remains to be determined. Cellular interactions do play key roles in other contexts during metamorphosis. For instance, the proper elaboration of the interneuronal visual and olfactory processing areas of the adult brain depends critically on the ingrowth of primary sensory neurons from the eyes or antennae (Maxwell and Hildebrand, 1981; Oland and Tolbert, 1987).

One approach to determining the relative importance of direct and indirect hormonal cues in the development of neuronal properties is to place identified neurons in primary cell culture, where the hormonal and cellular environment can be controlled precisely. Using techniques modified from those developed for interneurons from the antennal lobes of *Manduca* (Hayashi and Hildebrand, 1990), it has been possible to isolate and maintain thoracic leg motoneurons in culture (Griffin and Levine, 1989; R. B. Levine, unpublished results). To label the motoneurons so they can be identified in culture, individual or groups of larval leg muscles are injected with the fluorescent dye DiI (Honig and Hume, 1986; Kent and Levine, 1988b,c). At different stages during metamorphosis, the thoracic ganglia are dissociated and the cells plated at low density. The labeled motoneurons survive for up to 2 mo, grow extensive processes (Griffin and Levine, 1989), and express voltage-dependent ion channels (Levine and Hayashi, 1990).

To determine whether ecdysteroids have a direct influence on the growth of motoneuron processes, thoracic leg motoneurons were dissociated from new pupae, at which time dendritic regression is maximal and the cells are poised to begin the growth of adult dendrites in response to the next elevation of ecdysteroids. As shown in Fig. 5, leg motoneurons maintained in the absence of 20-HE grew long, but relatively unbranched, processes in culture, whereas those exposed to physiological levels of 20-HE grew extensive highly

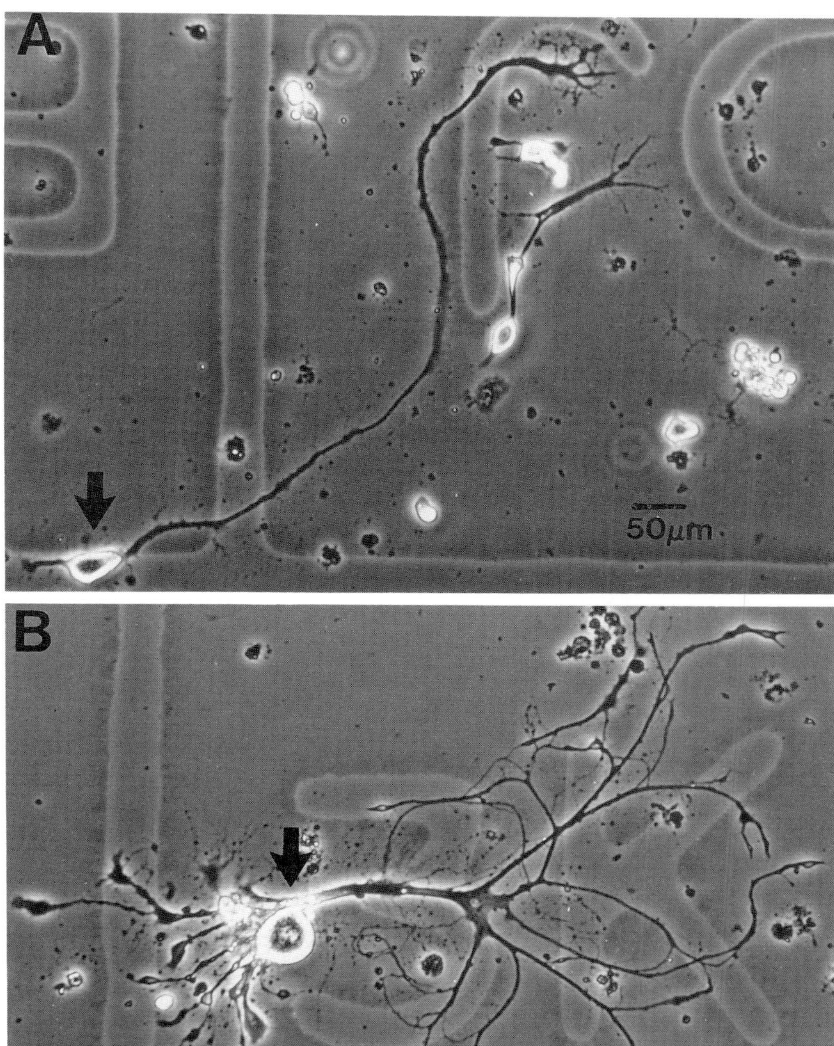

Figure 5. Effect of ecdysteroids on the morphology of thoracic leg motoneurons *in vitro*. Thoracic leg motoneurons were retrogradely labeled by injecting Di-I into the larval leg muscles. The thoracic ganglia were dissociated on the first day of the pupal stage (day P0), when the motoneuron dendrites were regressed. The subsequent outgrowth of processes was examined after 4 days in culture. **A.** Motoneuron (*arrow*) grown in medium lacking ecdysteroids. **B.** Motoneuron (*arrow*) from the same plating, but grown in medium containing 1 μg/ml 20-HE. Note that both neurons appear healthy, but that the elaboration of higher-order processes was much more extensive in the motoneuron grown in the presence of 20-HE. Data from R. B. Levine.

branched processes (Griffin and Levine, 1989; R. B. Levine, unpublished results). Thus, the characteristic induction of process outgrowth in response to the pupal ecdysteroid surge can be mimicked *in vitro*.

When interpreting these results it is necessary to bear in mind that conditions in culture differ substantially from those that the motoneurons encounter *in vivo*. Most notably, the dissociated motoneurons have been cleaved of processes and are forced to regenerate. Also, the culture dish does not provide external cues that normally influence the precise three-dimensional growth of dendrites. Nevertheless, these experiments show that motoneurons can respond appropriately to hormonal cues *in vitro*; further use of this promising approach should facilitate the investigation of the cellular and molecular mechanisms of hormone action during dendritic outgrowth, as well as the related processes of dendritic regression and programmed motoneuron death.

5. RESPECIFICATION OF SENSORY NEURONS

Another example of the relationship between the growth of neuronal processes and the formation of new behavioral circuits comes from mechanosensory neurons that innervate tactile hairs on the body surface. In the larval stage, mechanosensory hairs cover the abdominal and thoracic surfaces. Each is innervated by a single sensory neuron that projects topographically into the CNS (Levine *et al.*, 1985; Kent and Levine, 1988a; Peterson and Weeks, 1988). Thus, as has been described in other insect sensory systems (*e.g.*, Murphey, 1981), there is a rather precise somatotopic map of the body surface in the larval CNS; the central arborization pattern of each sensory neuron is correlated with the position of its cell body in the periphery. This arrangement presumably promotes the observed specificity of reflex movements evoked by stimulating hairs that have different locations on the body (Levine *et al.*, 1985; Weeks and Jacobs, 1987). Although most of the larval mechanosensory neurons die at the end of the larval stage, a small number in specific locations survives to innervate new sensilla on the pupal surface (Levine *et al.*, 1985). For example, the posterior abdominal segments of pupae bear pairs of sensory pits termed in *gin traps*, each of which contains approximately 20 mechanosensory hairs that are innervated by respecified larval sensory neurons. The central processes of these sensory neurons undergo a pronounced expansion during the last 3–4 days of larval life, and the sensory neurons evoke quite different reflex responses in the larval and pupal stages. Stimulation of the sensory neurons in larvae evokes a leisurely bending reflex, whereas the same neurons mediate a rapid and powerful defensive closing of the gin trap in pupae (Bate, 1973a,b; Levine *et al.*, 1985; Waldrop and Levine, 1989).

The relationship between the expansion of the central processes of the sensory neurons and the appearance of the new reflex response was investigated using hormonal manipulations to generate heterochronic mosaic animals. Topical treatment of the presumptive gin trap region with methoprene during the commitment pulse of ecdysteroids caused the development of otherwise normal pupae with a patch of larval cuticle and hairs in the place of one gin trap. In these animals, sensory neurons that were not exposed to the JH analog showed the normal expansion of their central projections, and they evoked normal pupal gin trap reflexes. In contrast, the JH-treated sensory neurons retained small larval-like aborizations, and continued to evoke only the larval reflex response (Fig. 6A; Levine *et al.*, 1986; Levine *et al.*, 1989). Thus, the expansion of the central processes of the sensory neurons appeared to be a necessary element in the production of the new reflex response.

In a complementary set of experiments, abdomens were ligated to remove the source of ecdysteroids prior to the commitment pulse or prepupal peak, and 20-HE was applied topically to one presumptive gin trap region. Whereas untreated sensory neurons in these animals retained larval-like arborizations in the CNS, those treated with exogenous 20-HE grew expanded central processes (Levine, 1989). However, despite their expanded terminal aborizations, the treated sensory neurons did not evoke a pupal reflex response (Fig. 6B; Levine *et al.*, 1989). This finding suggests that the growth of the sensory neuron arbors is not by itself sufficient to produce the new pupal reflex, but that other changes in the nervous system must also be required.

Several factors must interact to determine the metamorphic phenotypes of the mechanosensory neurons. One factor is positional information related to the location of the sensory neuron in the periphery. Not only is the central arborization pattern of each sensory neuron related to its position, but the very decision to live or die at the end of larval life is correlated with peripheral location (Levine *et al.*, 1985). As discussed earlier with respect to the segmental identity of motoneurons, we have no information at present about how body location is encoded in *Manduca* neurons. However, it is reasonable to assume that the same types of genes that have been described in *Drosophila* to determine sensory neuron type (Bodmer *et al.*, 1987) or endow neurons with positional information (Doe and Scott, 1988) could also operate in *Manduca* to confer cellular identity. This genetic information could promote the position-specificity of central arbors by directing intrinsic growth programs in the neurons or by priming them to respond to specific guidance cues encountered in the CNS.

A second important factor that influences sensory neurons is the hormonal environment that is experienced by the cell body. Hormonal cues interact with the positional identity of the neuron to determine cell fate. For

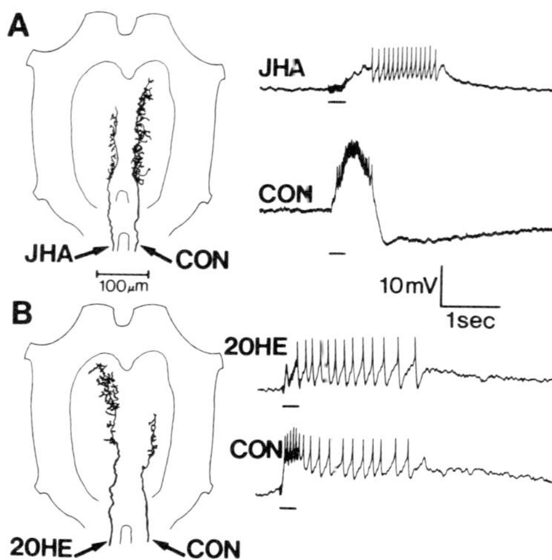

Figure 6. The relationship between gin trap sensory neuron morphology and reflex responses. **A.** Heterochronic mosaic pupae were formed by treating the presumptive gin trap region on the left side of segment A5 with the JH analog (JHA) methoprene during the commitment pulse of ecdysteroids. The *camera lucida* drawing shows the outline of ganglion A4 and the cobalt-stained terminal processes of JHA-treated (JHA; *left*) and a control (CON, *right*) gin trap sensory neuron stained early in the pupal stage. (The sensory neurons in segment A5 project into ganglion A4.) The control sensory neuron exhibited the normal pattern of terminal expansion characteristic of the pupal stage, whereas the JHA-treated neuron remained in the simpler larval form. The traces (*right*) show the intracellularly recorded responses of intersegmental muscle motoneurons to electrical simulation (*bar*) of treated or control sensory neurons (from different preparations). In each instance, the motoneuron innervated a muscle in segment A4 that would have participated in the gin trap reflex evoked by the stimulated sensory neuron. The control sensory neuron evoked the characteristic strong pupal response in the motoneuron, whereas the JHA-treated sensory neuron evoked only the weak larval-like response. **B.** Same format as **A**, except that mosaic animals were produced by ligating larvae early in the 5th instar to prevent pupal development (CON); the presumptive gin trap region on the left side of segment A5 was treated topically with 20-HE (20-HE). The untreated sensory neuron retained its small larval arbor (CON; *right*), whereas the terminals of the hormone-treated neuron (20-HE; *left*) underwent pupal-like growth. In either case, however, stimulation of the sensory neuron evoked larval-like motoneuron responses (traces at right), indicating that terminal outgrowth was not sufficient to elicit the pupal reflex. (Reprinted with permission from Levine and Weeks, 1990; copyright © 1990 by John Wiley & Sons, Inc.)

instance, most sensory neurons on the larval body surface respond to the prepupal peak of ecdysteroids by dying, whereas the small minority in the presumptive gin trap regions survive and initiate axon terminal outgrowth. This implies that hormonal access to specific developmental programs (*e.g.*, to die, to extend processes) is regulated by the positional identity of a sensory neuron. Significantly, in every permutation of the mosaic technique that has been performed, the central projection of a sensory neuron was correlated with the hormonal environment of its *cell body*, rather than that of its synaptic terminals (Levine *et al.*, 1986; Levine, 1989; Jacobs and Weeks, 1990). Thus, sensory neurons treated with a JH analog during the commitment pulse retain a larval aborization pattern despite projecting into an otherwise pupal CNS, and sensory neurons exposed prematurely to 20-HE grow processes typical of the pupal stage in a larval CNS. These results demonstrate dramatically that information available to the cell body of the sensory neurons predominates over information that the cell derives from the local hormonal environment in the CNS. Although the hormonal environment of the CNS appears irrelevant to the stage-specific expansion of sensory neuron terminal arbors, this does not eliminate the possibility of hormone-independent cues that guide the precise growth of terminal processes and the choice of postsynaptic targets. The ability to respond to such local cues, however, must be dependent on the developmental and hormonal state of the peripheral cell body. A reasonable hypothesis, considering that JH and 20-HE act by regulating gene expression in target cells (Riddiford, 1985), is that the hormonal environment of the cell body activates intrinsic developmental programs in the sensory neurons, which are played out in the context of the cellular environment of the axon terminals in the CNS.

IV. Conclusions

Because hormones play such a paramount role in coordinating the diverse phenotypic transformations exhibited by neurons during metamorphosis, this system is particularly well suited for studies of how extrinsic (i.e., endocrine) and intrinsic factors interact to influence neuronal differentiation. The stereotyped manner by which neurons undergo specific structural and functional transformations during metamorphosis indicates that hormonal access to particular developmental programs is tightly regulated in a cell-specific and stage-specific fashion. Although almost nothing is now known about the genetic or molecular determinants of cellular identity that contribute to the specificity of hormone action in *Manduca*, the increasing use of molecular biological techniques in studying the *Manduca* nervous system (*e.g.*, Horodyski *et al.*, 1989) makes us optimistic about future progress in this area. In the meantime, continued *in vivo* and *in vitro* electrophysiological and anatomical studies of processes such as neuronal respecification ought to reveal even more of the fascinating details of nervous system metamorphosis, and will hopefully provide insights that are relevant to neuronal differentiation and plasticity in other animals as well.

Acknowledgments

The authors' research was supported by NIH grant NS23208, an NSF Presidential Young Investigator Award, and an Alfred P. Sloan fellowship awarded to J.C.W., and NIH grants NS24822 and NS28495 and NSF grant BNS 89-11174 awarded to R.B.L. We thank Dr. Andrea Novicki and David J. Sandstrom for helpful suggestions on the manuscript.

References

Arnold, A. P., and Gorski, R. A. (1984). Gonadal steroid induction of structural sex differences in the CNS. *Ann. Rev. Neurosci.* **7**, 413–442.

Bastiani, M. J., Harrelson, A. L., Snow, P. M., and Goodman, C. S. (1987). Expression of fasciclin I and II glycoproteins on subsets of axon pathways during neuronal development in the grasshopper. *Cell* **48**, 745–755.

Bate, C. M. (1973a). The mechanism of the pupal gin trap: Segmental gradients and the connections of the triggering sensilla. *J. Exp. Biol.* **59**, 95–107.

Bate, C. M. (1973b). The mechanism of the pupal gin trap: The closure movement. *J. Exp. Biol.* **59**, 109–119.

Bate, C. M. (1978). Development of sensory systems in arthropods. *In* "Handbook of Sensory Physiology" (M. Jacobson, ed.) Vol. 9, pp. 2–53. New York: Springer-Verlag.

Bennett, K., and Truman, J. W. (1985). Steroid-dependent survival of identifiable neurons in cultured ganglia of the moth *Manduca sexta. Science* **229**, 58–60.

Bodmer, R. S., Shepherd, S., Jack, J., Jan, L. Y., and Jan, Y. N. (1987). Transformation of sensory organs by mutations of the *cut* locus of *D. melanogaster. Cell* **51**, 293–307.

Bollenbacher, W. E., Smith, S. L., Goodman, W., and Gilbert, L. I. (1981). Ecdysteroid titer during the larval-pupal-adult development of the tobacco hornworm, *Manduca sexta. Gen. Comp. Endocrinol.* **44**, 302–306.

Bollenbacher, W. E., and Granger, N. A. (1985). Endocrinology of the prothoracicotropic hormone. *In* "Comprehensive Insect Physiology, Biochemistry, and Pharmacology" (G. A. Kerkut and L. I. Gilbert, eds.), Vol. 7, pp. 109–151. New York: Pergamon Press.

Booker, R., and Truman, J. W. (1987a). Postembryonic neurogenesis in the CNS of the tobacco hornworm, *Manduca sexta.* I. Neuroblast arrays and the fate of their progeny during metamorphosis. *J. Comp. Neurol.* **255**, 548–559.

Booker, R., and Truman, J. W. (1987b). Postembryonic neurogenesis in the CNS of the tobacco hornworm, *Manduca sexta.* II. Hormonal control of imaginal nest cell degeneration and differentiation during metamorphosis. *J. Neurosci.* **7**, 4107–4114.

Breidbach, O. (1990). Constant topological organization of the coleopteran metamorphosing nervous system: Analysis of persistent elements in the nervous system of *Tenebrio molitor. J. Neurobiol.* **21**, 990–1001.

Doe, C. Q., and Goodman, C. S. (1985). Early events in insect neurogenesis. II. The role of cell interactions and cell lineage in the determination of neuronal precursor cells. *Dev. Biol.* **111**, 206–219.

Doe, C. Q., and Scott, M. P. (1988). Segmentation and homeotic gene function in the developing nervous system of *Drosophila. Trends Neurosci.* **11,** 101–106.

Dominick, O. S., and Truman, J. W. (1985). The physiology of wandering behavior in *Manduca sexta.* II. The endocrine control of wandering behavior. *J. Exp. Biol.* **117,** 45–68.

Edwards, J. S. (1969). Postembryonic development and regeneration of the insect nervous system. *Adv. Insect Physiol.* **6,** 97–137.

Ellis, H. M., and Horvitz, H. R. (1986). Genetic control of programmed cell death in the nematode. *C. elegans. Cell* **44,** 817–829.

Fahrbach, S. E. (1992). Developmental regulation of ecdysteroid receptors in the nervous system of *Manduca sexta. J. Exp. Zool.* (In press).

Fahrbach, S. E., and Truman, J. W. (1987a). Mechanisms for programmed cell death in the nervous system of a moth. *In* "Ciba Foundation Symposium 126: Selective Neuronal Death," pp. 65–76. (G. Bock and M. O'Connor, eds.) Chichester: Wiley.

Fahrbach, S. E., and Truman, J. W. (1987b). Possible interactions of a steroid hormone and neural inputs in controlling the death of an identified neuron in the moth *Manduca sexta. J. Neurobiol.* **18,** 497–508.

Fahrbach, S. E., and Truman, J. W. (1988). Cycloheximide inhibits ecdysteroid-regulated neuronal death in the moth *Manduca sexta. Soc. Neurosci. Abstr.* **14,** 368.

Fahrbach, S. E., and Truman, J. W. (1989). Autoradiographic identification of ecdysteroid binding cells in the nervous system of the moth *Manduca sexta. J. Neurobiol.* **20,** 681–702.

Giebultowicz, J. M., and Truman, J. W. (1984). Sexual differentiation in the terminal ganglion of the moth *Manduca sexta:* Role of sex-specific neuronal death. *J. Comp. Neurol.* **226,** 87–95.

Griffin, L., and Levine, R. B. (1989). Hormonal influences on insect motoneurons developing in cell culture. *Soc. Neurosci. Abstr.* **15,** 87.

Hamburger, V., and Oppenheim, R. W. (1982). Naturally occurring neuronal death in vertebrates. *Neurosci. Comm.* **1,** 39–55.

Hayashi, J. H., and Hildebrand, J. G. (1990). Insect olfactory neurons *in vitro*: Morphological and physiological characterization of cells from the developing antennal lobes of *Manduca sexta. J. Neurosci.* **10,** 848–859.

Hildebrand, J. G. (1985). Metamorphosis of the insect nervous system: Influences of the periphery on the postembryonic development of the antennal sensory pathway in the brain of the moth, *Manduca sexta. In* "Model Neural Networks and Behavior" (A. I. Selverston, ed.), pp. 129–148. New York: Plenum Press.

Honig, M. G., and Hume, R. I. (1986). Fluorescent carbocyanine dyes allow living neurons of identified origin to be studied in long-term cultures. *J. Cell Biol.* **103,** 171–183.

Horodyski, F. M., and Riddiford, L. M. (1989). Expression and hormonal control of a new larval cuticular multigene family at the onset of metamorphosis of the tobacco hornworm. *Dev. Biol.* **132,** 292–303.

Horodyski, F. M., Riddiford, L. M., and Truman, J. W. (1989). Isolation and expression of the eclosion hormone gene from the tobacco hornworm, *Manduca sexta. Proc. Natl. Acad. Sci. U.S.A.* **86,** 8123–8127.

Jacobs, G. A., and Weeks, J. C. (1990). Postsynaptic changes at a sensory-to-motoneuron synapse contribute to the developmental loss of a reflex behavior during insect metamorphosis. *J. Neurosci.* **10,** 1341–1356.

Kent, K. S., and Levine, R. B. (1988a). Neural control of leg movements in a metamorphic insect: Sensory and motor elements of the larval thoracic legs in *Manduca sexta. J. Comp. Neurol.* **271,** 559–576.

Kent, K. S., and Levine, R. B. (1988b). Neural control of leg movements in a metamorphic insect: Persistence of the larval leg motor neurons to innervate the adult legs of *Manduca sexta. J. Comp. Neurol.* **276,** 30–43.

Kent, K. S., and Levine, R. B. (1988c). Reorganization of an identified leg motor neuron during metamorphosis of the moth *Manduca sexta. Soc. Neurosci. Abstr.* **14,** 1004.

Kent, K. S., and Griffin, L. M. (1990). Sensory organs of the thoracic legs of the moth, *Manduca sexta. Cell Tissue Res.* **259,** 209–223.

Kiguchi, K., and Riddiford, L. M. (1978). A role of juvenile hormone in pupal development of the tobacco hornworm, *Manduca sexta J. Insect Physiol.* **24,** 673–680.

Kimmel, C. B., Schabtach, E., and Kimmel, R. J. (1977). Developmental interactions in the growth and branching of the lateral dendrite of Mauthner's cell (*Ambystoma mexicanum*). *Dev. Biol.* **55,** 244–259.

Levine, R. B. (1989). Expansion of the central aborizations of persistent sensory neurons during insect metamorphosis: The role of the steroid hormone, 20-hydroxyecdysone. *J. Neurosci.* **9,** 1045–1054.

Levine, R. B., and Truman, J. W. (1982). Metamorphosis of the insect nervous system: Changes in morphology and synaptic interactions of identified neurons. *Nature (London)* **299,** 250–252.

Levine, R. B., and Truman, J. W. (1983). Peptide activation of a simple neural circuit. *Brain Res.* **279,** 335–338.

Levine, R. B., Pak, C., and Linn, D. (1985). The structure, function, and metamorphic reorganization of somatotopically projecting sensory neurons in *Manduca sexta* larvae. *J. Comp. Physiol.* **157,** 1–13.

Levine, R. B., and Truman, J. W. (1985). Dendritic reorganization of abdominal motoneurons during metamorphosis of the moth *Manduca sexta. J. Neurosci.* **5,** 2424–2431.

Levine, R. B., Truman, J. W., Linn, D., and Bate, C. M. (1986). Endocrine regulation of the form and function of axonal arbors during insect metamorphosis. *J. Neurosci.* **6,** 293–299.

Levine, R. B., Waldrop, B., and Tamarkin, D. (1989). The use of hormonally-induced mosaics to study alterations in the synaptic connections made by persistent sensory neurons during insect metamorphosis. *J. Neurobiol.* **20,** 326–338.

Levine, R. B., and Hayashi, J. H. (1990). Calcium channels in insect motoneurons during metamorphosis. *Soc. Neurosci. Abstr.* **16,** 177.

Levine, R. B., and Weeks, J. C. (1990). Hormonally mediated changes in simple reflex circuits during metamorphosis in *Manduca. J. Neurobiol.* **21,** 1022–1036.

Martin, D. P., Schmidt, R. E., DiStefano, P. S., Lowry, O. H., Carter, J. G., and Johnson, E. M., Jr. (1988). Inhibitors of protein synthesis and RNA synthesis prevent neuronal death caused by nerve growth factor deprivation. *J. Cell Biol.* **106,** 829–844.

Maxwell, G. D., and Hildebrand, J. G. (1981). Anatomical and neurochemical consequences of deafferentation in the development of the visual system of the moth *Manduca sexta. J. Comp. Neurol.* **195,** 667–680.

Montemayor, M. E., Fahrbach, S. E., Giometti, C. S., and Roy, E. J. (1990). Characterization of a protein that appears in the nervous system of the moth *Manduca sexta* coincident with neuronal death. *FEBS Lett.* **276,** 219–222.

Murphey, R. K. (1981). The structure and development of a somatotopic map in crickets: The cercal afferent projection. *Dev. Biol.* **88,** 236–246.

Murphey, R. K., Mendenhall, B., Palka, J., and Edwards, J. S. (1975). Deafferentation slows the growth of specific dendrites of identified giant interneurons. *J. Comp. Neurol.* **159,** 407–418.

Oland, L. A., and Tolbert, L. P. (1987). Glial patterns during early development of antennal lobes of *Manduca sexta*: A comparison between normal lobes and lobes deprived of antennal axons. *J. Comp. Neurol.* **255,** 196–207.

Oppenheim, R. W. (1985). Naturally occurring cell death during neural development. *Trends Neurosci.* **8,** 487–493.

Oppenheim, R. W., Prevette, D., Tytell, M., and Homma, S. (1990). Naturally occurring and induced neuronal death in the chick embryo *in vivo* requires protein and RNA synthesis: Evidence for the role of cell death genes. *Dev. Biol.* **138,** 104–113.

Peterson, B. A., and Weeks, J. C. (1988). Somatopic mapping of sensory neurons innervating mechanosensory hairs on the larval prolegs of *Manduca sexta. J. Comp. Neurol.* **275,** 128–144.

Prokop, A., and Technau, G. M. (1991). The origin of the postembryonic neuroblasts in the ventral nerve cord of *Drosophila melanogaster. Development* **111,** 79–88.

Riddiford, L. M. (1985). Hormone action at the cellular level. *In* "Comprehensive Insect Physiology, Biochemistry, and Pharmacology" (G. A. Kerkut, and L. I. Gilbert, eds.), Vol. 8, pp. 37–84. New York: Pergamon Press.

Riddiford, L. M. (1986). Hormonal control of sequential larval cuticular gene expression. *Arch. Insect Biochem. Physiol. Suppl.* **1,** 75–86.

Sandstrom, D. J., and Weeks, J. C. (1988). Identified interneurons in larval and pupal abdominal ganglia of the tobacco hornworm, *Manduca sexta. Soc. Neurosci. Abstr.* **14,** 1003.

Sandstrom, D. J., and Weeks, J. C. (1991). Reidentification of larval interneurons in the pupal stage of the tobacco hornworm, *Manduca sexta. J. Comp. Neurol.* **308;** 311–327.

Schwartz, L. M., Kosz, L., and Kay, B. K. (1990a). Gene activation is required for developmentally programmed cell death. *Proc. Nat. Acad. Sci. U.S.A.* **87,** 6594–6598.

Schwartz, L. M., Myer, A., Kost, L., Engelstein, M. and Maier, C. (1990b). Activation of polyubiquitin gene expression during developmentally programmed cell death. *Neuron* **5,** 411–419.

Taylor, H. M., and Truman, J. W. (1974). Metamorphosis of the abdominal ganglia of the tobacco hornworm, *Manduca sexta. J. Comp. Physiol.* **90,** 367–388.

Thomas, J. B., Bastiani, M. J., Bate, C. M., and Goodman, C. S. (1984). From grasshopper to *Drosophila:* A common plan for neuronal development. *Nature (London)* **310,** 203–207.

Trimmer, B. A., and Weeks, J. C. (1989a). Effects of nicotinic and muscarinic agents on an identified motoneurone and its direct afferent inputs in larval *Manduca sexta. J. Exp. Biol.* **144,** 303–337.

Trimmer, B. A., and Weeks, J. C. (1989b). Characterization of an afferent-induced change in the excitability of an insect motoneuron. *Soc. Neurosci. Abstr.* **15,** 26.

Truman, J. W. (1983). Programmed cell death in the nervous system of an adult insect. *J. Comp. Neurol.* **216,** 445–452.

Truman, J. W. (1984). Cell death in invertebrate nervous systems. *Ann. Rev. Neurosci.* **7,** 171–188.

Truman, J. W. (1989). Hormonal regulation of axon terminal reorganization during metamorphosis in the moth, *Manduca sexta. Soc. Neurosci. Abstr.* **15,** 65.

Truman, J. W. (1990). Metamorphosis of the central nervous system of *Drosophila. J. Neurobiol.* **21,** 1072–1084.

Truman, J. W., and Reiss, S. E. (1976). Dendritic reorganization of an identified motoneuron during metamorphosis of the tobacco hornworm, *Manduca sexta. Science* **192,** 477–479.

Truman, J. W., and Schwartz, L. M. (1984). Steroid regulation of neuronal death in the moth nervous system. *J. Neurosci.* **4,** 274–280.

Truman, J. W., and Booker, R. (1986). Adult-specific neurons in the nervous system of the moth, *Manduca sexta:* Selective chemical ablation using hydroxyurea. *J. Neurobiol.* **17,** 613–625.

Truman, J. W., and Bate, C. M. (1988). Spatial and temporal patterns of neurogenesis in the central nervous system of *Drosophila melanogaster. Dev. Biol.* **125,** 145–157.

Truman, J. W., and Reiss, S. E. (1988). Hormonal regulation of the shape of identified motoneurons in *Manduca sexta. J. Neurosci.* **8,** 765–775.

Tublitz, N. J., and Truman, J. W. (1985). Identification of neurones containing cardioacceleratory peptides (CAPs) in the ventral nerve cord of the tobacco hawkmoth, *Manduca sexta. J. Exp. Biol.* **116,** 395–410.

Tublitz, N. J., and Sylwester, A. W. (1990). Postembryonic alteration of transmitter phenotype in individually identified peptidergic neurons. *J. Neurosci.* **10,** 161–168.

Waldrop, B., and Levine, R. B. (1989). Development of the gin trap reflex in *Manduca sexta:* A comparison of larval and pupal motor responses. *J. Comp. Physiol.* **165,** 743–753.

Weeks, J. C. (1987). Time course of hormonal independence for developmental events in neurons and other cell types during insect metamorphosis. *Dev. Biol.* **124,** 163–176.

Weeks, J. C., and Truman, J. W. (1984). Neural organization of peptide-activated ecdysis behaviors during the metamorphosis of *Manduca sexta.* II. Retention of the proleg motor pattern despite loss of the prolegs at pupation. *J. Comp. Physiol.* **155,** 423–433.

Weeks, J. C., and Truman, J. W. (1985). Independent steroid control of the fates of motoneurons and their muscles during insect metamorphosis. *J. Neurosci.* **5,** 2290–2300.

Weeks, J. C., and Truman, J. W. (1986). Hormonally mediated reprogramming of muscles and motoneurons during the larval–pupal transformation of the tobacco hornworm, *Manduca sexta. J. Exp. Biol.* **125,** 1–13.

Weeks, J. C., and Jacobs, G. A. (1987). A reflex behavior mediated by monosynaptic connections between hair afferents and motoneurons in the larval tobacco hornworm, *Manduca sexta. J. Comp. Physiol.* **160,** 315–329.

Weeks, J. C., and Ernst-Utzschneider, K. (1989). Respecification of larval proleg motoneurons during metamorphosis of the tobacco hornworm, *Manduca sexta:* Segmental dependence and hormonal regulation. *J. Neurobiol.* **20,** 569–592.

Weeks, J. C., Debu, B. H. G., and Davidson, S. K. (1991). Cycloheximide blocks the steroid-mediated death of proleg motoneurons during the metamorphosis of *Manduca sexta. Soc. Neurosci. Abstr.* **17:** 229.

Weeks, J. C., Roberts, W. M., and Trimble, D. L. (1992). Hormonal regulation and segmental specificity of motoneuron phenotype during metamorphosis in *Manduca sexta. Dev. Biol.,* in press.

Witten, J. L., and Truman, J. W. (1991). The regulation of transmitter expression in postembryonic lineages in the moth *Manduca sexta.* I. Transmitter identification and developmental acquisition of expression. *J. Neurosci.* **11,** 1980–1989.

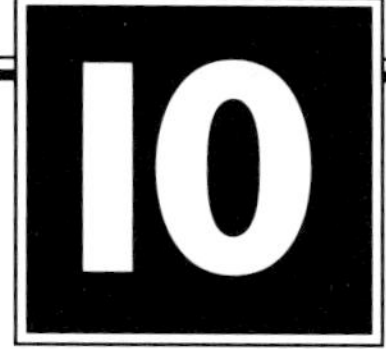

Neuron Determination in the
Ever-Changing Nervous System of *Hydra*

Hans R. Bode
Developmental Biology Center
Department of Developmental and Cell Biology
University of California, Irvine
Irvine, California

I. Introduction

In most animals, the development of the nervous system occurs during embryogenesis or larval stages, and is generally complete shortly after hatching, eclosion, or birth. By the time the animal reaches an adult stage, the nervous system is generally static in terms of development. Throughout the life of the organism, the changes that occur might involve the loss of neurons or, in a few isolated cases, the turnover of neurons such as the nasal sensory cells in some animals.

The nervous system in adult hydra is unusual and differs from most other animals in several respects. It is dynamic because it is in a steady state of production and loss of neurons. All neurons continuously change their axial or regional location in the animal. The phenotype of many neurons is only metastable because the phenotype changes with changing location. Adult hydra have many characteristics of regulative embryos because their patterning processes are based almost exclusively on cell–cell interactions. These same mechanisms probably play a role in the processes governing neuron phenotype.

The aim of this chapter is, first, to describe the nervous system of hydra and to place the question of neuronal identity in the context of the unusual tissue dynamics of this animal. Second, the current understanding of the generation of neurons and the control of neuronal phenotype will be described.

II. The Nervous System of Hydra

The body plan of hydra is simple. It is essentially a tube with a head and foot at opposite ends (see Fig. 1). The body wall consists of two epithelial layers separated by a basement membrane termed the mesoglea. The outer layer is

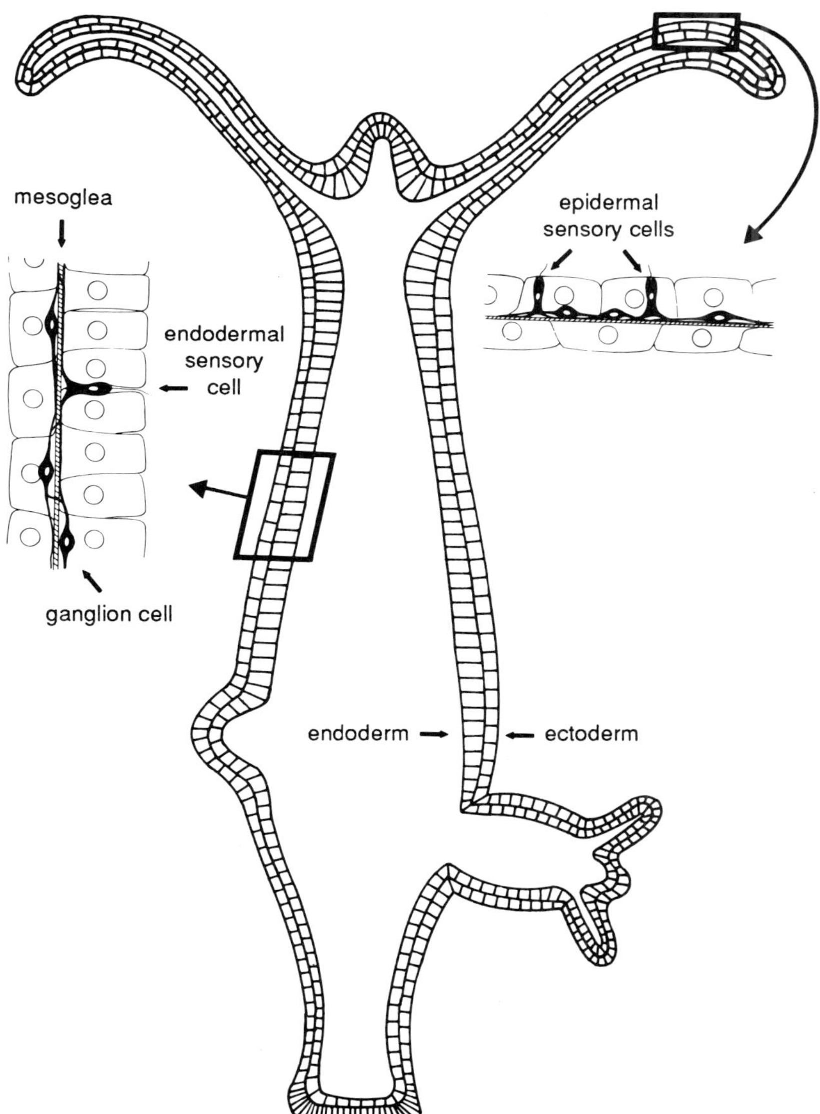

Figure 1. Longitudinal cross section of a hydra showing the two epithelial layers and the location of the nerve net. The two enlargements illustrate the location of neuron cell bodies and their neurites in the tissue layers. All cell types except neurons and epithelial cells have been omitted. The mesoglea is the basement membrane separating the two epithelia. [Reprinted from Bode *et al.*, *American Zoologist* **28**, 1053–1063 (1988b), with permission.]

known as the ectoderm (or epidermis); the inner layer is known as the endoderm (or gastrodermis). This double-layered construction extends throughout the animal.

The regions of the animal are few and also simple in organization. The head consists of two parts. The hypostome is the upper part and is a dome or cone containing the mouth at its apex. Below the hypostome is the tentacle zone, from which emerge the tentacles. The tentacles are spaced evenly around the tentacle zone and are commonly 5–7 in number. The body column is roughly divided into three regions. The upper two-thirds is the gastric region. Below this region is the budding zone where buds, the asexual progeny emerge. Below the budding zone is the peduncle, a stalk through which the body column narrows to the foot. At the basal end of the animal is the foot, which serves to anchor the animal to a substratum.

A. The Nervous System Is a Nerve Net Consisting of a Mosaic of Subsets of Neurons

Interspersed among the epithelial cells that make up the two layers are several other classes of cell types. One class of cells is the neurons. They form a net in both layers that extends throughout the animal (Hadzi, 1909). The density of neurons and, hence, the mesh size of the net, varies among the regions (e.g. Bode *et al.*, 1973; Epp and Tardent, 1978). The neuron density is fairly uniform in the body column, with one neuron for every 6–10 epithelial cells. The density rises abruptly at the apical end to a level of roughly one neuron epithelial cell. At the basal end, the neuron density begins to rise in the lower peduncle, reaching a density that is 2–3-fold higher than in the body column.

The neurons of the net are not all the same. Morphologically, there are two classes of neurons. The ganglion cells are bipolar and multipolar neurons that make up the net throughout the animal (Burnett and Diehl, 1964; Lentz and Barrnett, 1965; Davis *et al.*, 1968; Westfall, 1973). Their cell bodies are located near, but are not in contact with, the mesoglea on the basal side of both epithelia. The processes extending from the cell bodies run between epithelial cells, contacting processes of neighboring neurons in the same layer as well as crossing the mesoglea to neurons in the opposite layer.

The sensory neurons do not so much make up the nerve net as connect into the net made of the ganglion cells. Four types are known, each of which has a discrete regional distribution and slightly different morphology (Fig. 1): epidermal sensory cells are found only in the ectoderm of the head (Westfall and Kinnamon, 1978; Dunne *et al.,* 1985), two types of gastrodermal sensory cells only in the endoderm of the body column (Westfall and Rogers, 1990), and foot sensory cells only in the ectoderm of the foot (Koizumi and Bode, 1991). The cell bodies vary from elongate (epidermal sensory cell) to oval (foot sensory cell), and all have cilia extending from the apical side of the cell body toward, or into, the surrounding aqueous environment.

Antisera against known neuropeptides as well as monoclonal antibodies specific for neurons have provided additional and, in part, more refined criteria for defining subsets of neurons. Using antisera against neuropeptides isolated primarily from vertebrates, Grimmelikhuijzen and associates (summarized in Grimmelikhuijzen, 1984) identified separate subsets that expressed antigens similar to FMRFamide, neurotensin, substance P, cholecystokinin, vasopressin/oxytocin, and bombesin. Each subset has a distinct regional distribution that is usually part of the head, or foot, or both structures. As an example, the distribution of the subset stained with the antiserum against FMRFamide is shown in Fig. 2 (Grimmelikhuijzen *et al.,* 1982; Koizumi and Bode, 1986).

A number of monoclonal antibodies that recognize specific subsets of neurons have been generated. Among them, JD1 and DB5 recognize the epidermal sensory cells (ESn) of the head of *H. oligactis* (Dunne *et al.,* 1985), whereas TS33 recognizes only the ESn of the hypostome of *H. vulgaris* (formerly *H. attenuata*) (Koizumi *et al.,* 1988). RC7 recognizes a fraction of the ganglion cells throughout *H. oligactis* (Yaross *et al.,* 1986).

Not all subsets defined by antibodies are unique, nor do the neurons belong to one morphological cell type. The antiserum against FMRFamide stains both ganglion cells and sensory cells in the hypostome, but only ganglion cells in the tentacles (Koizumi and Bode, 1986). Two subsets recognized by an antiserum against bombesin and another against oxytocin overlap in part (Grimmelikhuijzen, 1983). Finally, the ESn of the hypostome are composed of at least three subsets defined by the monoclonal antibody JD1 and the antiserum against FMRFamide [FMRFamide-like immunoreactivity (FLI)]. These subsets are $JD1^+ FLI^+$, $JD1^+ FLI^-$, and $JD1^- FLI^+$ (C. J. P. Grimmelikhuijzen, personal communication).

Hence, the nerve net is a mosaic of subsets. Most of the subsets have specific regional distributions, although at least one is found throughout the animal. The number of subsets is not yet known since the existing antibodies are not likely to account for all the neurons. The nervous system appears to consist of a single nerve net, but that is not established. More complex coelenterates with a greater variety of behaviors also have more than one net. Although the nets may overlap in location, they have separate functions (Spencer, 1978; Spencer and Arkett, 1984).

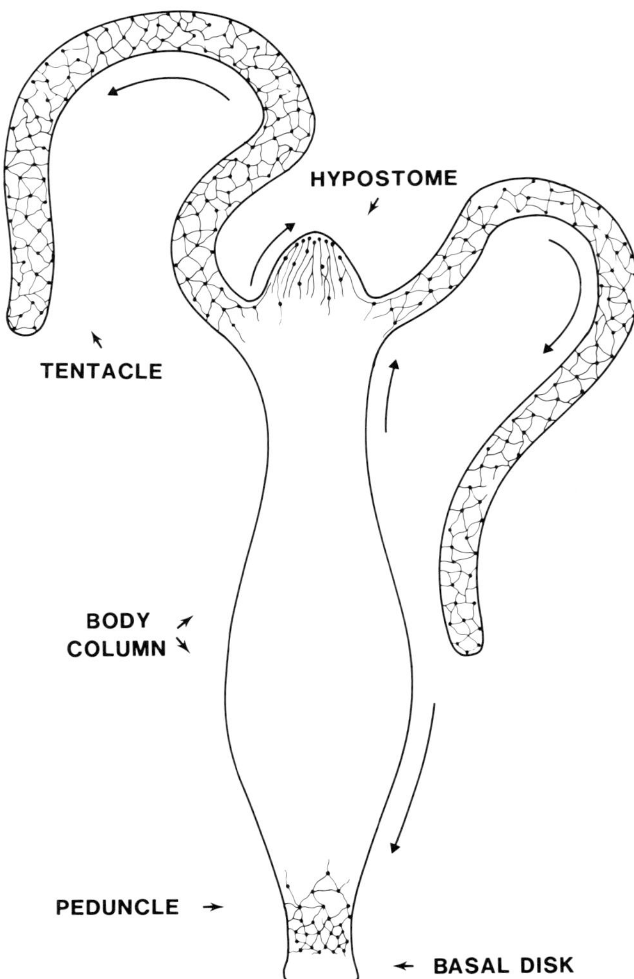

Figure 2. Overall structure of a hydra and the distribution of the subset of neurons exhibiting FMRF amide-like immunoreactivity (FLI). The regions of the animal are identified. Arrows running along the body column indicate the direction of tissue displacement. The location of FLI^+ neurons is indicated by the network of dots and connecting lines. [Reprinted from Bode *et al.*, *American Zoologist* **28**, 1053–1063 (1988B), with permission.]

III. The Nerve Net Is Dynamic

As stated at the outset, the nervous system of an adult hydra is dynamic since neurons are continuously produced and lost, and every neuron is continuously changing location. This behavior is understandable in the context of the tissue dynamics of *Hydra.*

A. Tissue Dynamics of Hydra

The epithelial cells of the body column of both layers are always in the mitotic cycle, with a cell cycle time of 3–4 days in well-fed animals (Campbell, 1967a; David and Campbell, 1972). Fewer cell divisions occur in the extremities (Campbell, 1967a). Despite this continuous production of epithelial tissue, the adult animal remains constant in size. It does so by also continuously losing tissue, which occurs in two ways. Hydra normally reproduces asexually by budding, a process in which an evagination forms on the lower part of the body column, grows in size, and develops into a small complete hydra that eventually detaches from the parent. This process accounts for 70–85% of tissue loss (Campbell, 1967b). The remainder is lost by the sloughing of cells at the extremities: the tips of the tentacles, the apex of the hypostome, and the base of the foot (Campbell, 1967b).

An important consequence of the geometry of these dynamics, in which new tissue is produced in the middle of the animal (the body column) and lost at the extremities and into buds, is that essentially every epithelial cell is continuously displaced toward an extremity (Campbell, 1967b). Cells in the upper part of the body column are displaced into the tentacle zone, and are then displaced onto the tentacles. Thereafter, they are displaced along the tentacle and finally are lost by sloughing at the end (Fig. 2). This behavior is akin to the movement of a conveyer belt. Similarly, cells in the middle or lower end of the body column are displaced down the column, either onto a developing bud or down the peduncle onto the foot to be sloughed (Fig. 2). This displacement behavior occurs roughly in tandem in the two epithelial layers (Wanek and Campbell, 1982).

Because of this geometry, there must also be a zone in the body column in which the cells are not displaced in either direction; that is, in fact, the case. However, there is nothing intrinsically different about the cells in this stationary zone since the location of the zone is readily shifted up or down the body column by the rate of feeding (Otto and Campbell, 1977).

Thus, the two epithelial layers of hydra are in a steady state in which the constant production of tissue in the form of new epithelial cells is balanced by the constant loss of these cells. Further, the maintenance of this steady state involves the continuous displacement of cells toward the extremities.

B. The Nerve Net Is Also in a Steady State of Production and Loss of Neurons

This behavior of the epithelial layers affects the nerve net since the neurons are intimately associated with the epithelial cells. To illustrate this clearly, the structure of the epithelial cells needs to be described briefly. Hydra have no muscle cells. Instead, all the epithelial cells have muscle processes on their basal sides. These processes extend under, and interdigitate with, processes of neighboring epithelial cells, and are in close apposition to the mesoglea as well (Campbell, 1980).

The cell body of most neurons is located near the basal side of each layer, and resides on the mat of muscle processes wholly enveloped by the surrounding epithelial cells (Diehl and Burnett, 1964; Lentz and Barrnett, 1965). The neuronal processes run between the neighboring epithelial cells to contact processes of other neurons. Because the neurons are intertwined among the epithelial cells, one would logically conclude that, when a region of epithelial tissue of the body column is displaced toward an extremity, the neurons of that region would be displaced with it. Thus, every neuron is also constantly displaced toward an extremity or onto a bud.

An experiment in which the displacement of epidermal sensory cells (ESn) along the tentacles was demonstrated confirms this conclusion (Yaross *et al.*, 1986). New ESn cells arise by differentiation in the tentacle zone (Dunne *et al.*, 1985; Koizumi and H. R. Bode, unpublished results), and are intercalated into the nerve net at the base of the tentacle. From there, they are displaced along the tentacle in concert with their accompanying epithelial cell. Treatment of hydra with nitrogen mustard removes all the neuron precursors (Diehl and Burnett, 1964). By staining treated animals periodically thereafter with JD1, a monoclonal antibody that specifically recognizes ESn cells (Dunne *et al.*, 1985), one finds that the distribution of JD1$^+$ cells changes. Normally JD1$^+$ ESn cells are found uniformly along the entire length of the tentacle. The outer 90% of the tentacle contains JD1$^+$ ESn cells but the tentacle base and inner 10% of the tentacle are devoid of them (see Fig. 3). By 6 days, the region without JD1$^+$ cells, or gap, has extended to the inner half of the tentacle, and by 10 days there are few stained cells at the apical tip of the tentacles. Subsequently, there are none.

Some epithelial cells at the base of the tentacles of some of these animals were marked at the time of treatment. The rate of displacement of these

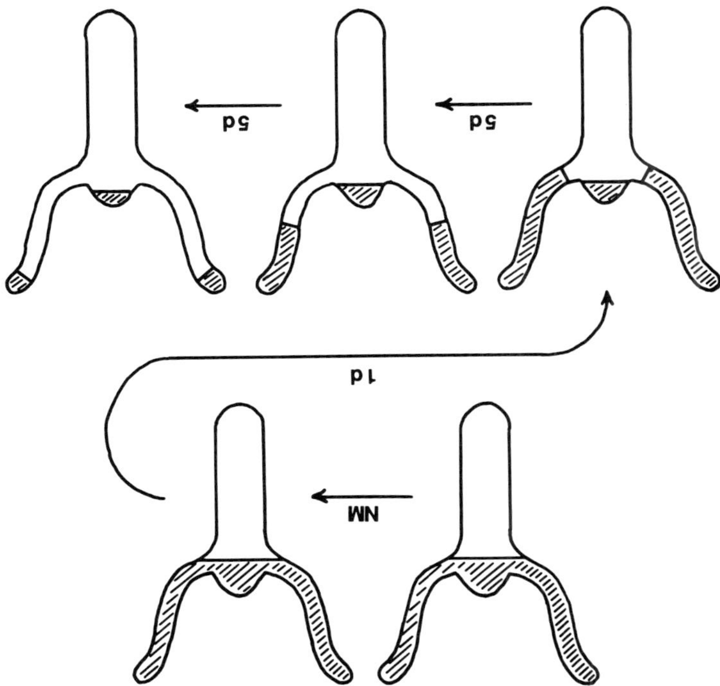

Figure 3. Alteration of the distribution of the JD1[+] subset of epidermal sensory cells in nitrogen-mustard-treated animals due to tissue displacement. Shaded areas indicate location of the JD1[+] subset of neurons. NM; nitrogen mustard treatment, 1d, 5d, 5d, time (days) between successive analyses of samples of animals after nitrogen mustard treatment.

marked cells coincided with rate of displacement of the basal boundary of the JD1[+] region (Yaross *et al.,* 1986). The simplest explanation of the ever-increasing gap is that no new ESn cells were added to the net after nitrogen mustard treatment, and the existing set was continuously displaced toward the tentacle tip. A similar, but much slower, rate of displacement of the subset of JD1[+] neurons toward the tip of the hypostome was also observed (Yaross *et al.,* 1986). This, too, is consistent with the much slower rate of epithelial cell displacement in the hypostome (Campbell, 1967b).

Although there is no direct evidence for the other regions, the data for the head, the known tissue movements, and the intimate association of neurons and epithelial cells make the continuous displacement of neurons a certainty. Therefore, neurons are lost constantly from the animal. The tissue dynamics continuously alter the nerve net in a second way. In the body column, the neuron density is fairly uniform at 1 neuron per 6–10 epithelial (e.g., Bode *et al.,* 1973). Since the epithelial cells are always in the mitotic cycle, the neuron density is being diluted constantly.

Therefore, new neurons must be produced constantly to maintain the number of neurons per animal as well as the density of the net. In fact, this production has been observed. As measured by pulse-labeling animals with ^{3}H-thymidine, neurons arise by differentiation throughout the body column as well as in the head and foot, but not in the tentacles. Further, the rate of production is higher in regions of high neuron density, such as the head, than in the body column (David and Gierer, 1974; Yaross and Bode, 1978a).

Given the steady state nature of the nerve net, and the continuous change in location of every neuron, there are two overriding questions. How are the regional differences in density maintained? And, how is the mosaic of subsets maintained? Rephrasing these questions in terms of the theme of this volume: how are neurons of the appropriate phenotype found in the right place? The information available provides partial answers that permit sketching an outline of the processes underlying the maintenance of the net. This outline will be presented in the remaining sections.

IV. Neuron Cell Lineages

A. Interstitial Cell System

In addition to the neurons, a number of other cell types are nestled among the epithelial cells of both layers. All these cell types, except for the epithelial cells, belong to the interstitial cell system. These cells fall into five classes. There are four classes of differentiation products: neurons, nematocytes (four types), secretory cells (three types), and gametes (two types) (Campbell and Bode, 1983). The fifth class, the interstitial cells, which are identified morphologically as large interstitial cells, are a heterogeneous population with respect to function. One type of interstitial cell is a multipotent stem cell that gives rise to the cell types of the four classes of differentiated cell types (David and Murphy, 1977; Bosch and David, 1987).

B. Neuronal Differentiation Pathway

Several lines of evidence collectively indicate that neurons arise by differentiation from the multipotent stem cells among the large interstitial cells.

(1) Cells that form a morphological sequence (see Fig. 4), starting with large interstitial cells through small interstitial cells to neurons, are found in regions with a high rate of neuronal differentiation (Bode *et al.*, 1990). Ultrastructural studies provide evidence consistent with this view (Davis, 1974). (2) Animals devoid of interstitial cells do not produce neurons (Marcum and Campbell, 1978). These animals, termed "epithelial animals," are also devoid of all other differentiation products of the interstitial cell system (Campbell, 1976). (3) Interstitial cells are capable of migration along the body axis (Campbell, 1967c; Heimfeld and Bode, 1984a). By grafting normal animals pulse-labeled with ^{3}H-thymidine to unlabeled epithelial animals, labeled interstitial cells (both large and small) migrate into the epithelial tissue. Subsequently, labeled neurons are found in the epithelial tissue (Heimfeld and Bode, 1984b). The only other cell types capable of migration are nematocytes (Campbell, 1967c), which are unrelated to neurons. (4) Aggregates made by centrifuging viable dissociated cells into pellets undergo the usual cell division and differentiation

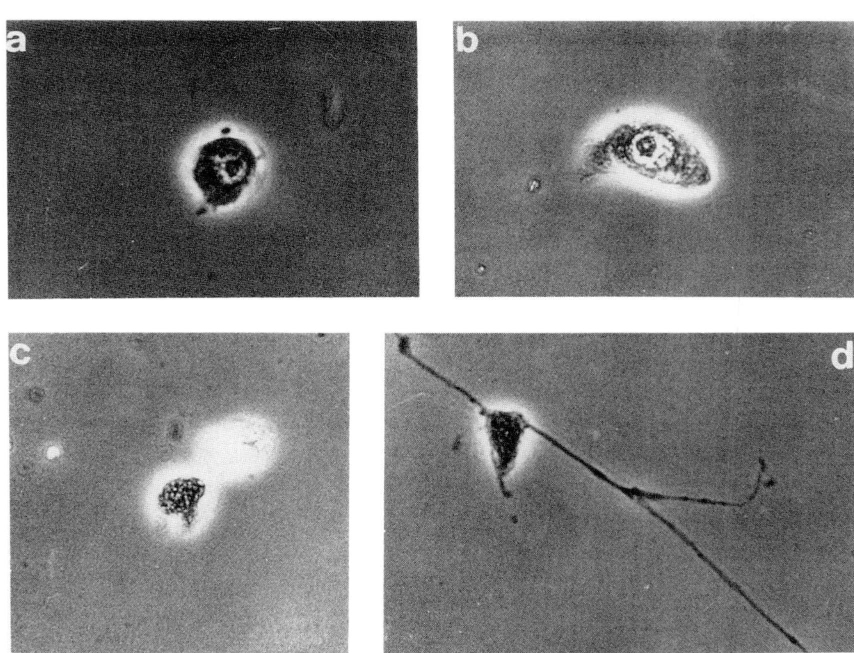

Figure 4. Morphological sequence of cells in the neuron differentiation pathway. Animals were macerated into a suspension of fixed cells and observed with phase microscopy. a,b. Large interstitial cells. c. Small interstitial cells. d. Neuron. [Reprinted from Bode *et al.*, *Developmental Biology*, **139**, 231–243 (1990), with permission.]

behavior, and develop into normal animals (Gierer *et al.,* 1972). The addition of small numbers of cells, containing statistically one multipotent stem cell, to aggregates devoid of interstitial cells results in the formation of new neurons (David and Murphy, 1977).

To the extent that it is understood, the neuronal differentiation pathway is fairly simple (see Fig. 5). The common view (Fig. 5a) has been that a multipotent stem cell (Im) becomes committed to neuron differentiation in S-phase (Bi), traverses G2 (~12 hr), and divides to form two postmitotic small interstitial cells (pSi), which differentiate into neurons in about 6 hr (David and Gierer, 1974). More recent evidence indicates that the intermediate small interstitial cells are capable of cell division (Bode *et al.,* 1990). In the lower peduncle of *H. oligactis* there are many neurons, substantial numbers of small interstitial cells, vanishingly few large interstitial cells, and no other cell types of the interstitial cell system. Pulse-labeling with ^{3}H-thymidine or 5-bromo-2'-deoxyuridine results in a variable fraction of labeled small interstitial cells, indicating that the small interstitial cells are capable of cell division. A day later, labeled neurons appear in such large numbers that their only plausible precursors are the labeled small interstitial cells. Small interstitial cells capable of cell division have also been detected in the tentacle zone in which large numbers of neurons are formed. The small interstitial cells do not appear to be stem cells since their cell division capacity is limited in these experiments. Hence, another view of the pathway is the one shown in Fig. 5b.

Which version, if either, is accurate is unclear. The small interstitial cells may be capable of more than one round of cell division, thereby extending the time to traverse the pathway. However, the small interstitial cells in the

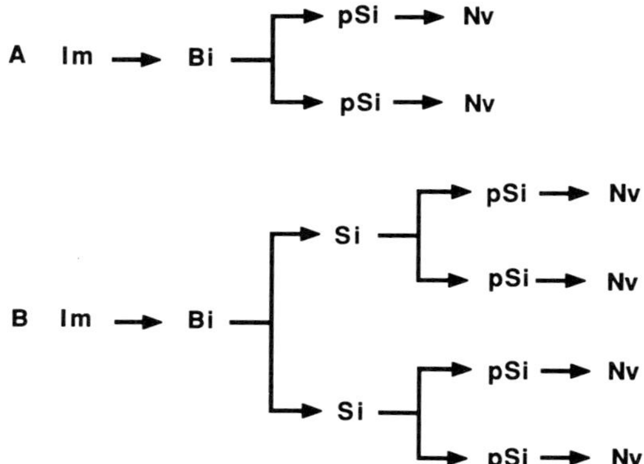

Figure 5. Proposed neuron differentiation pathways. A. The common view involving a multipotent stem cell, (Im), a committed large interstitial cell (Bi), postmitotic small interstitial cells (pSi), and differentiated neurons (Nv). B. A more recent version that also involves dividing intermediates (Si).

described experiments do not appear to be stem cells since their cell division capacity in these experiments is very limited. Conversely, other experiments suggest that the multipotent stem cells may undergo switches in morphology between large and small interstitial cell (Holstein and David, 1991).

V. Commitment of Multipotent Stem Cells to Neuronal Differentiation

Since neurons in hydra arise from multipotent stem cells an initial question in establishing neuronal phenotype concerns the number of decisions involved. Is a multipotent stem cell committed to a specific type of neuron in a single step or are there two steps involved? The first of these steps would be commitment of the stem cell to the class of neurons, while the second would be the commitment to a specific type of neuron. The evidence accumulated so far indicates that there are two steps, and possibly more. These two steps are the subject of the next two sections.

How cells capable of more than one differentiation make a decision as to which pathway to enter is poorly understood in most cases. In a few instances with a small number of differentiation pathways, such as the vulval equivalence group in *C. elegans,* a formal explanation has been achieved (e.g., Sternberg, 1988). However, for those multipotent cells that can give rise to a fairly large number (>5) of types of progeny, the understanding of the process is generally poor. The evidence concerning the multipotent stem cells in hydra indicates which mechanisms are unlikely and which are more likely. Three of these mechanisms will be considered fairly briefly. All three possibilities arise from a consideration of the regional differences in neuron density, and the fact that the rates of neuron differentiation are correlated with these densities.

A. Commitment Based on Feedback from Neurons

One possibility is that a positive feedback loop is involved, that is, the stem cells receive information from the surrounding neurons to differentiate into neurons. The higher the density of neurons, the larger the fraction of stem cells committed to neuron formation. Although inherently an explosive process, this need not be a problem. In the tentacle zone, where large numbers of neurons are made, the neurons do not accumulate because they are continuously displaced onto the tentacles and, thus, removed. The stem cells also are not all lost to the pressure of differentiation, since new ones are continuously displaced into the tentacle zone from the body column.

However, an experiment that provides a direct test renders this mechanism inadequate (Heimfeld and Bode, 1981). The approach was to raise the neuron density of the body column, and determine if the rate of neuronal differentiation increased (see Fig. 6). This was carried out by making use of hydra's ability to regenerate. Decapitation of an animal results in the regeneration of a head from the healed apical tip of the remaining animal. During the regeneration process, large numbers of neurons are formed in the apical tip during the first 24 hr (Yaross and Bode, 1978b). One day after decapitation the apical tip was excised and allowed to regenerate which resulted in the formation of a small, yet complete, well-proportioned animal (Bode and Bode, 1980). Because regeneration is morphallactic in hydra, the process involves reorganization of the existing tissue, can occur in the absence of cell division (Hicklin and Wolpert, 1973; Cummings and Bode, 1984).

Most of the neurons formed in the apical tip during the first day became part of the body column or part of the head. The neuron density of the newly formed head was similar to that observed in normal animals (0.58 and 0.51, respectively), but was 3–4-fold higher in the regenerated than in the normal body column (0.41 and 0.11, respectively) (Heimfeld and Bode, 1981). These changes in neuron density in the regenerate had no effect on the subsequent rates of neuronal differentiation. The rates were normal: high in the head and low in the body column. Thus, it is unlikely that commitment decisions of the stem cells to form neurons is influenced by previously existing neuron density.

B. Commitment Based on Position Dependence

Another obvious possibility is that the stem cells are receiving cues from the surrounding cells, most likely the epithelial cells, about their axial or

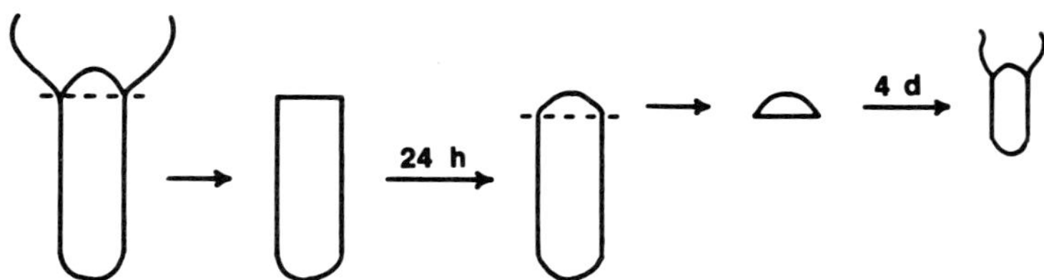

Figure 6. Experimental design to alter the neuron concentration of the body column. This design takes advantage of the ability of hydra tissue to reform complete animals from fragments of the body column.

regional location, and will differentiate accordingly. This idea is consistent with the observations, but there is no experimental evidence to provide direct support. Further, there is a difficulty with this mechanism. The multipotent stem cells form more than one differentiation product in every region (see Fig. 7). For example, neurons and mucous cells are formed in the hypostome and tentacle zone. The difficulty is even greater throughout the body column where neurons, four types of nematocytes, and gland cells are formed at every axial level (David and Gierer, 1974; Bode *et al.*, 1987). This renders unlikely the idea that a multipotent stem cell makes a decision as to type of differentiation formed by "reading" its position or regional location.

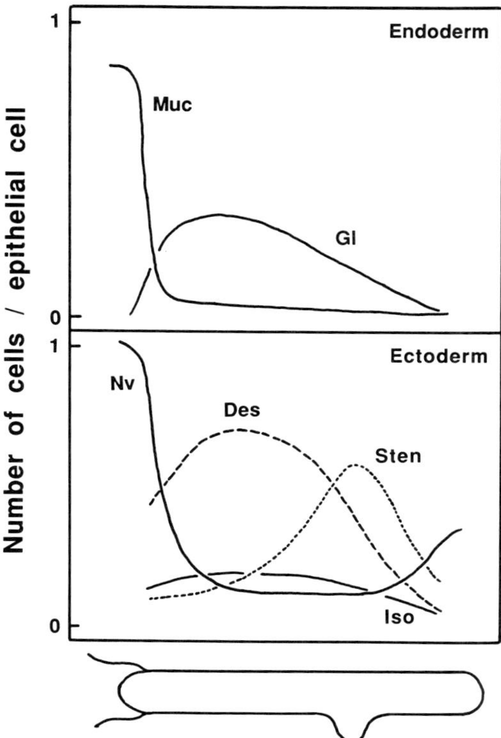

Figure 7. Axial distribution of the differentiation of each of the several somatic cell products of the multipotent stem cells. Two of the products, mucous (Muc) cells and gland (Gl) cells differentiate and are located only in the endoderm (*top*). The four nematocyte types, desmonemes (Des), stenoteles (Sten), and the two types of isorhizas (Iso) form and are found only in the ectoderm (*bottom*). Although neurons (Nv) are found in both layers, the large majority is in the ectoderm. Only that differentiation distribution is shown.

C. Commitment Based on a Stochastic Mechanism Coupled with Migration of Committed Cells

A third possibility is based on the migration behavior of small interstitial cells that are intermediates in the neuronal differentiation pathway. Individual large interstitial cells (Bi) and small interstitial cells (Si) are known to migrate in substantial numbers when the halves of two animals are grafted together (Campbell, 1967c; Heimfeld and Bode, 1984a). The extent of migration in both apical and basal directions, can be extensive. Many Si cells, but few Bi cells traverse half the length of the animal within 24 hr (Heimfeld and Bode, 1984a). Most Bi cells tend to migrate only a fraction (1/8–1/6) of the length of the body column in this period (Heimfeld and Bode, 1984a; Fujisawa *et al.*, 1990). More recent evidence indicates that the grafting process itself can influence the migration behavior of interstitial cells (Fujisawa *et al.*, 1990). Hence, it is likely that Bi cells migrate in considerable numbers in grafted animals, but in very small numbers if at all in normal hydra (Bosch and David, 1990). In contrast, Si cells migrate as well in grafted animals as in normal animals. By staining a small region in the middle of the body column with the lipophilic dye DiI (Honig and Hume, 1986) and waiting 24 hr, one finds labeled single Si cells in the head far from their original location, indicating an extensive migration capacity in intact animals (Teragawa and Bode, 1990). The numbers of migrating interstitial cells calculated from DiI-labeling experiments are consistent with the numbers of Si cells migrating in grafting experiments (Teragawa and Bode, 1990). Thus, it is likely that both Bi cells and Si cells are capable of migration, but normally only single Si cells actually migrate.

Several lines of evidence indicate that migrating cells can form neurons. (1) Using grafts in which the upper half was labeled with ^{3}H-thymidine, Berking (1980) found labeled neurons in otherwise unlabeled tissue of buds developing from the unlabeled lower half. (2) In grafts consisting of an epithelial upper half (devoid of the interstitial cell lineage products) and a normal lower half, large numbers of Si cells but few Bi cells were found in the head 24 hr after grafting. By 48 hr, large numbers of neurons were observed that could have arisen from the Si cells, but not the Bi cells since there were insufficient numbers of the latter (Heimfeld and Bode, 1984b). (3) Finally, many of the DiI-labeled interstitial cells that had migrated as described earlier formed neurons after completion of migration (Teragawa and Bode, 1990).

Thus, it is likely that single Si cells normally migrate and that they form neurons. Further, they are most likely to be neuronal differentiation intermediates, since neurons have been found in the epithelial half of epithelial animal–normal animal grafts within 8 hr of forming the graft (Fujisawa, personal communication; Heimfeld and Bode, 1984b). This rapid rate of neuron formation is hard to reconcile with the possibility that the migrating cells are uncommitted interstitial cells that must undergo commitment to neuronal differentiation, traverse the pathway, and subsequently differentiate into neurons. This process would require 18–24 hrs at least.

However, simply the ability of neuronal intermediates to migrate does not explain the regional differences in neuron density. An additional factor is that interstitial cell migration is directionally biased (Heimfeld and Bode, 1984a; Teragawa and Bode, 1990). Emigration from the budding zone region of the body column in apical and basal directions is roughly equal. The more apical the region, the larger the bias in the apical direction. The bias increases from 55:45 for the region directly above the budding zone to 70:30 for the region directly below the head (Heimfeld and Bode, 1984a). Below the budding zone the bias is in the basal direction, but it is much less pronounced (Teragawa and Bode, 1990). Coupled with the extensive migration capacity of Si cells these biases could explain the elevated neuronal differentiation rates and densities in the extremities.

How then is a multipotent stem cell committed to neuronal differentiation? Since stem cells become committed to more than one type of differentiation product in every region of the animal, the decision is unlikely to be based on the simple "reading" of position or reaction to environmental cues. This is especially true throughout the body column, where cells of all three classes of somatic cells are formed at every axial level. In addition, the commitment process for neurons must account for the uniform rate of their formation along the body column. A simple view would be that the decision is stochastic. With some probability, multipotent stem cells throughout the animal are committed to forming neurons. The committed Bi cells enter and traverse the neuron differentiation pathway, when they reach the Si stage, a fraction of them will migrate toward an extremity, eventually stop migrating, and complete neuronal differentiation. Stochastic determination coupled with biased migration would account for the observed nonuniform neuronal differentiation rates along the body column.

Invoking a stochastic mechanism is often a reflection of lack of understanding of a more complex process. As an example, the commitment of stem cells to several types of differentiation products in the same region could be caused by their response to a surrounding milieu of factors, each influencing the stem cell toward a specific differentiation. The stochastic element would enter as the random fluctuations in concentrations of such factors in the immediate vicinity of a particular stem cell. Since cell types of classes other than neurons that also are derived from the stem cells are not formed at uniform rates along the body column in *hydra* (see Fig. 7), one could imagine the concentrations of some of the determination factors to be somewhat nonuniform, thereby affecting the probabilities of stem cell commitment.

The head activator peptide isolated from *Hydra,* is often considered to be such a determination factor. The head activator is found in high concentration in the head and forms a gradient down the body column (Schaller *et al.,* 1989). When added to animals, a general increase in neuron density is observed (Holstein *et al.,* 1986; Hoffmeister and Schaller, 1987). However, given the possible existence of dividing intermediates in the neuronal differentiation pathway, it is unclear whether the head activator is affecting the stem cells or the differentiation intermediates.

VI. Neuronal Phenotype Is Position-Dependent

The foregoing provides an explanation of the commitment of multipotent stem cells to neuronal differentiation as well as for the nonuniform differentiation rates. Unanswered is the question of how a cell committed to forming a neuron acquires a specific phenotype. The available evidence indicates that acquisition of phenotype is strongly, but not solely, influenced by axial positionof the differentiating neuron. Further, the result in many cases is that the expressed phenotype is not terminal, but only metastable: with a change of location, the neuron changes phenotype. Two lines of evidence support this concept.

A. Migrating Small Interstitial Cells Are Committed to Neuronal Differentiation, but Not to a Particular Phenotype

Are the migrating Si committed only to neuronal differentiation, or also to a particular neuronal phenotype? If the latter is true, it provides a particular explanation for the directionally biased migration. For a subset of neurons found only in the head, migrating Si cells already committed to this subset would migrate apically into the head. This would suggest that the differences in apically biased migration of the body column regions reflect differences in the neuronal phenotypes to which stem cells are committed. Thus, because the apical bias is higher in the upper part of the body column, the fraction of stem cells committed to forming neuronal phenotypes found only in the head would be higher than further down the column.

A simple experiment indicates this is not so (Fig. 8). The apical bias is 70:30 in the upper region and 60:40 in the lower region (Teragawa and Bode, 1990). By replacing the lower region with an upper region and vice versa, one can determine if the apical migration bias is determined by the source of the transplanted region or by the site to which the transplant is made. The evidence clearly indicates that the transplanted region exhibits the bias of its new location: an upper region transplanted to a lower switches its normal 70:30 bias to 60:40. The reciprocal is also true (Teragawa and Bode, 1990).

The data are not easily reconciled with stem cell commitment to neuronal phenotype in a single step. If the 70:30 bias of the apical region reflects the fraction of Si cells that will be phenotypes that differentiate in the head, then those Si cells should migrate toward the head regardless of new axial location. Consequently, one would have expected the extent of the apical bias to correspond with the source of the region, not the site of implantation.

The simplest explanation is that the apical bias of migrating Si is a response to an environmental cue. One possibility would be a chemoattractant produced in the head, and transmitted to, and distributed in a gradient down, the body column. Thus, the closer to the head, the higher the concentration of the attractant resulting in a larger apical bias. The fact that excising a region and grafting it into the same location in reverse orientation does not affect the apical bias of emigration from the region supports chemotaxis rather than contact guidance as the basis of the apical bias (Teragawa and Bode, 1990).

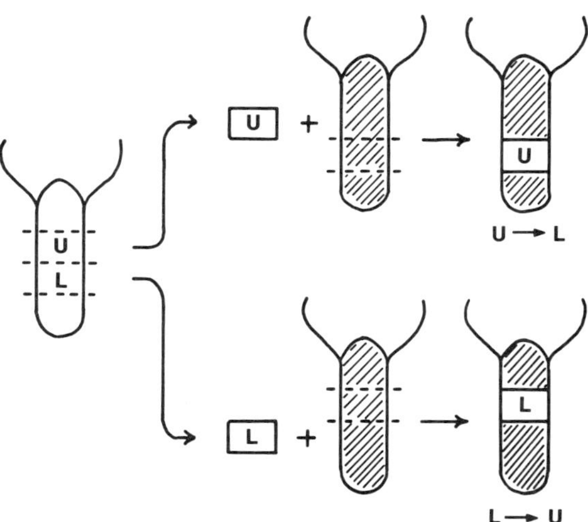

Figure 8. Experimental design for examining the basis of the regional differences in extent of apical migration of interstitial cells. U, upper region, second quarter of the body column; L, lower region, third quarter of the body column. U → L; U region of a labeled animal (white) is grafted into the L region of an unlabeled animal (shaded). L → U; the reverse procedure.

Then, as observed, the apical bias of a transplanted region would be determined by the final grafting site, not the origin of the transplant. In turn, the result indicates that migrating Si cells are committed to neuronal differentiation, but not to a particular phenotype.

B. Necessity for Position-Dependent Neuron Differentiation

A consideration of a single subset in the context of tissue dynamics illustrates why the position of a neuron, or a differentiating neuron, strongly affects the phenotype. A subset of neurons identified by staining with an antiserum against the neuropeptide FMRFamide is located in the head and in the lower peduncle just above the foot, but not in the rest of the body column (Fig. 2). Since the antigen has not been identified explicitly, the subset is defined by its FMRFamide-like immunoreactivity (FLI).

Neurons are continuously displaced from the 1-region into the tentacle zone, and subsequently onto the tentacles, yet the distribution of the FLI^+ subset remains constant. To insure that FLI^+ neurons are always found at the tentacle base, new FLI^+ neurons must be formed continuously at that location. If not, the basal border of the FLI^+ pattern would be changing location continuously as it moves toward the tentacle tip.

There are two means for maintaining the location of the basal border of the subset. New FLI^+ neurons could arise by differentiation from neuron precursors, or they could arise by conversion of FLI^- neurons that have been displaced up the body column into this location. These alternatives apply to all subsets with specific regional or axial distributions. Both alternatives occur, and an example of each will be presented.

C. The Epidermal Sensory Neuron Subset in the Tentacles Is Maintained by Differentiation

As described earlier, ESn (epidermal sensory) cells are found only in the ectoderm of the tentacles and hypostome, but do not occur in the tentacle zone (Westfall and Kinnamon, 1978; Dunne *et al.*, 1985). One ESn cell is associated with each ectodermal epithelial cell in the tentacles; the arrangement is more complex in the hypostome (Kinnamon and Westfall, 1981).

There is evidence that the ESn cells of the tentacles arise by differentiation, and only by differentiation, in the tentacle zone or at the base of the tentacle. (1) As new tentacles just begin to emerge from the developing head of a bud, each of the 5–15 epithelial cells of the young tentacle has an ESn cell associated with it, as detected with the ESn-specific antibody, JD1. As the tentacle grows, every newly added epithelial cell also has a JD1$^+$ ESn cell associated with it (Dunne *et al.*, 1985). (2) DB5, another monoclonal antibody specific for the ESn cells, also stains the differentiation intermediates from the Si stage through the young neuron with developing processes, to the final form with its elongate cell body and basal neuron processes. These intermediates are found exclusively in the tentacle zone and to a lesser extent in the tentacle base (O. Koizumi and H. R. Bode, unpublished results). (3) Finally, elimination of the neuron precursors Bi and Si results in the cessation of appearance of new JD1$^+$ or DB5$^+$ ESn cells. Any epithelial cells displaced onto the tentacle after the removal of the neuron precursors do not have ESn cells associated with them (Yaross *et al.*, 1986). Hence, these ESn cells cannot arise by conversion. They arise only by differentiation in the specific location of the tentacle zone near the base of the tentacles.

D. The FLI$^+$ Subset of Neurons in the Head Is Maintained by Conversion

In the head, the FLI$^+$ subset consists of ganglion cells found throughout the ectoderm of the tentacles and of both ganglion and ESn cells in the ectoderm of the hypostome (Koizumi and Bode, 1986). Two experiments indicate that this subset is maintained by the conversion of FLI$^-$ to FLI$^+$ neurons. (1) All the neuron precursors (Bi and Si) were removed from animals, and samples were stained periodically with an anti-FMRFamide antiserum. The regional distribution of the FLI$^+$ subset did not change over 18 days (Koizumi and Bode, 1986). In this time period, the tentacles turned over completely at least once. If FLI$^+$ neurons arise by differentiation as does the ESn subset just discussed, one would expect the distribution to change and become increasingly restricted to the outer portions of the tentacles. The constancy of the pattern indicates that new FLI$^+$ neurons are formed. Since there are no precursors present, they must have arisen by conversion from some other cell type. (2) A more direct experiment involves removal of the neuron precursors, decapitation of the animal, and subsequent regeneration. The apical tip that regenerates the head was part of the body column which was initially devoid of FLI$^+$ neurons. There are many FLI$^+$ neurons in the head after it regenerates, again indicating conversion (Koizumi and Bode, 1986).

Treatment to remove the neuron precursors leaves only neurons, nematocytes, and epithelial cells in the ectoderm. Since nematocytes are terminally differentiated, and epithelial cells in epithelial animals never form neurons (Marcus and Campbell, 1978; Littlefield and Bode, 1986), it is most likely that the appearance of FLI$^+$ neurons is due to the conversion of FLI$^-$ neurons.

Further, the conversion appears to depend on the position of the FLI⁻ neurons. When they are displaced onto the tentacles or into the hypostome, some, but not all, are converted into FLI⁺ neurons.

An alternative to position dependence is that the conversion is simply part of a time-dependent maturation process. This type of change has been observed in the neurotransmitter switch that neurons innervating the sweat gland of the developing rat embryo undergo (Landis and Keefe, 1983; Landis *et al.*, 1988). One experiment suggests that this is unlikely for the FLI⁺ neuron. Among the FLI⁺ neurons in the hypostome are ESn cells. Bisection in the middle of the body column of an animal devoid of Bi cells and Si cells results in the regeneration of a head in which some of the neurons are FLI⁺ ESn cells. Since ESn cells are confined to the head, and tissue of the middle of the body column is always displaced in a basal direction (Fig. 2), the formation of ESn cells is not a natural maturation endpoint for these cells of the mid body column. Neurons displaced onto a bud can form ESn cells, but which tissue will end up on a bud rather than being displaced onto the foot is not predetermined. Thus, the simplest explanation is that the mid-body column FLI⁻ neurons undergo a position-dependent conversion to form FLI⁺ ESn cells in the regenerated head, and that a maturation process is not involved.

E. A Subset Can Change Phenotype More than Once

If a neuron can switch phenotype by changing its location, and neurons continually change location, one might expect a neuron to change its phenotype more than once. This, in fact, is true of the part of the FLI⁺ subset located at the lower end of the body column. These neurons are ganglion cells that are confined to the lower peduncle since there are none in the upper peduncle nor in the foot.

As in the head region, position-dependent FLI⁻ to FLI⁺ conversion of neurons occurs. Removal of the lower half of an animal devoid of neuron precursors results in the regeneration of the peduncle and foot, and the subsequent reappearance of FLI⁺ neurons (Koizumi and Bode, 1986). In addition, in animals devoid of neuron precursors, the FLI⁺ pattern of the lower peduncle is unaltered over a period of time during which the entire peduncle is displaced onto the foot and subsequently sloughed. Hence, the distribution of the FLI⁺ subset in the lower peduncle is maintained by continuous neuron conversion. Further, this observation suggests that the same neurons undergo two conversions. Some of the FLI⁻ neurons displaced into the lower peduncle are converted into FLI⁺ neurons; when these are subsequently displaced onto the foot they undergo the reverse, a FLI⁺ to FLI⁻ conversion.

That the expression of this subset is strongly correlated with position is demonstrated by the following experiment. Using animals without neuron precursors, the lower peduncle of one animal was grafted in to the middle of the body column of a second animal. Three different results were obtained. In some grafts, the lower peduncle was converted into tissue of the gastric region. None of the neurons of the transplant expressed FLI. In other grafts, the lower peduncle maintained its integrity as a lower peduncle, which is clearly evident from the morphology. Here, the subset of FLI$^+$ neurons was maintained. The most interesting result was the third one. In some grafts, the lower peduncle formed a secondary axis protruding from the body column with a basal disk at the end. The part of the secondary axis corresponding to a lower peduncle exhibited FLI$^+$ neurons whereas the newly formed foot was devoid of FLI$^+$ neurons (Koizumi and Bode, 1986).

When the original lower peduncle tissue maintained its character as lower peduncle tissue, FLI$^+$ neurons were expressed. In contrast, when the tissue changed either into gastric region or foot tissue, no FLI$^+$ neurons were expressed. Again, the simplest explanation is that the FLI$^+$ neurons were responding to their position, and FLI expression was determined accordingly. The data do not exclude the possibility that the FLI$^+$ neurons died when the tissue no longer had the character of a lower peduncle. This is considered unlikely, since there is no evidence that neurons die when displaced from the lower peduncle onto the foot where the FLI$^+$ to FLI$^-$ transition normally occurs. Hence, it seems likely that neurons can undergo more than a single position-dependent conversion.

F. Some Conversions Involve More than a Single Antigen

The position-dependent changes in FLI expression could be viewed simply as modulations of the concentration of a single substance. However, the conversions that neurons undergo are often much more extensive. As described, some of the FLI$^-$ neurons were converted into FLI$^+$ ESn cells. Since there are no sensory cells in the ectoderm of the body column, these conversions must have involved converting a FLI$^-$ ganglion cell into a FLI$^+$ ESn.

A second example leads to a similar conclusion. A subset of neurons defined by staining with an antiserum against vasopressin is located in the ectoderm of the head, the lower peduncle, and the foot. The vasopressin-like-immunoreactive (VLI$^+$) neurons of the lower peduncle are all ganglion cells whereas many of the VLI$^+$ neurons of the foot are a type of sensory cell that is peculiar to the ectoderm of the foot. By carrying out the same experiments for the VLI subset that were performed for the FLI subset, it has been shown that VLI$^-$ ganglion cells of the body column are converted into VLI$^+$ foot sensory cells, (Koizumi and Bode, 1991).

These conclusions, though quite certain, are based on deduction. More direct evidence was provided using two monoclonal antibodies that stained two subsets in *H. vulgaris.* One, TS33, stained the ESn cells of the hypostome only and the other TS26 stained ganglion cells all over the animal. If conversion of TS26$^+$ TS33$^-$ ganglion cells into TS26$^-$ TS33$^+$ ESn cells takes place, one might expect to find an intermediate that stains with both antibodies. Animals devoid of neuron precursors were decapitated and allowed to regenerate. Double-staining neurons with a morphology similar to ESn cells were found in the regenerating head. With time, the number of TS26$^-$ TS33$^+$ ESn cells increased and the number of double-labeled cells remained constant, which is the result one would expect if the double-stained cell were a conversion intermediate. Careful examination of intact animals revealed small numbers of double-staining cells, indicating that the conversion process occurs normally (Koizumi *et al.,* 1988).

The conversion of ganglion cells to epidermal sensory cells involves many changes. The cell body is altered in shape from ovoid to elongate. The ESn cell develops a stereociliary complex made up of a number of components detectable at the ultrastructural level, in addition to a cilium (Westfall and Kinnamon, 1978). This implies the synthesis of an array of molecules during conversion. One is the TS33 antigen. In addition, one molecule, the TS26 antigen, either is no longer synthesized or is modified. These extensive changes indicate that the neurons are undergoing extensive alterations, not simply modulation of a single molecule, indicating a true conversion of phenotype.

G. The Decision as to Neuronal Phenotype Depends on Position and Is Often Reversible

The question of how a neuron acquires its phenotype can now be addressed more fully. It involves two known decisions. In the first, multipotent stem cells are committed to form neurons all along the body axis, most likely by some form of stochastic process. As differentiation proceeds, Si cells are formed, some of which emigrate toward the extremities. The evidence indicates that these Si cells are clearly neuronal differentiation intermediates, but are not committed to a particular phenotype. It is most likely, but unproven, that those Si cells that do not migrate far, but differentiate close to their site of generation, are also initially uncommitted to a particular phenotype.

Once the Si has settled into a location, the second decision occurs. The Si "reads" its axial position or regional location (i.e. head vs. body column) to determine the phenotype to be formed. The requirement for the differentiation of the ESn cells of the tentacles in the tentacle zone and the tentacle base, as well as the position-dependent conversion of the phenotype of several cell types, argues quite forcefully for this idea. The conversion experiments also indicate that the phenotype acquired by the Si by "reading" its position is often only metastable, since the phenotype can alter with change in location.

The fact that one subset has been shown to arise only by differentiation, and three others by conversion, could suggest that subsets acquire their phenotype by one or two mutually exclusive means. This is most likely only partly true. Some subsets may arise only by differentiation. However, there is reason to believe that others may arise by both conversion and differentiation, based on the following consideration.

The density of ganglion cells in the tentacles is 3–5-fold higher than in the body column (Bode *et al.*, 1973; H. R. Bode and L. W. Gee, unpublished results). Hence, the ganglion cells of the tentacles cannot simply arise by the displacement of ganglion cells from the body column. Many must arise by differentiation. As an example, a subset of the ganglion cells are stained with the monoclonal antibody RC9 and are found throughout the animal (Yaross *et al.*, 1986). Thus, some RC9$^+$ neurons of the tentacle arrive by displacement. Since RC9 also stains the intermediates of the RC9$^+$ neuronal differentiation pathway, one can readily show that substantial numbers of RC9$^+$ neurons are formed in the tentacle zone and the tentacle base (O. Koizumi and H. R. Bode, unpublished observations). This implies that the RC9$^+$ population of the tentacles arises by displacement as well as by differentiation. Although there is no direct evidence, it seems reasonable that the FLI$^+$ subset of the tentacles could arise both by conversion of displaced FLI$^-$ neurons and by differentiation. Most likely, both processes take place simultaneously in the tentacle zone and tentacle base.

H. Position Dependence Is Necessary but Not Sufficient to Determine Phenotype

There must be an additional mechanism of phenotype determination. The FLI$^+$ and VLI$^+$ neurons are both found in the head, and belong to non-overlapping subsets (Grimmelikhuijzen, 1984). Both can arise by conversion of FLI$^-$ VLI$^-$ neurons of the body column that have been displaced into the tentacles. How does a FLI$^-$ VLI$^-$ neuron make a choice between a FLI$^+$ or a VLI$^+$ neuron, since the conversion to either type occurs in the same location, the tentacle base? Given the ability to change the phenotype of a neuron to one that it would not normally acquire (see Section VI,D), it is less likely that the FLI$^-$ VLI$^-$ neuron is intrinsically biased toward one or the other phenotype before arriving at the tentacle base.

One reasonable possibility is that a second mechanism based on a form of lateral inhibition is involved. There is precedent for such a mechanism in neuronal determination. Experiments exploring the spacing of dopaminergic amacrine cells of the frog neural retina (Reh and Tully, 1986), the RAS and CAS neurons in leeches (Martindale and Shankland, 1990), and the formation neurons in the thorax in *Drosophila* (Doe *et al.,* 1985) all suggest such a role for lateral inhibition.

Thus, in hydra, a newly formed FLI$^+$ neuron at the tentacle base would inhibit other neurons in its immediate vicinity from expressing FLI. These other neurons would then make a choice to form another type of neuron, such as a VLI$^+$ or still another type. The newly formed VLI$^+$ neuron in turn would exert a lateral inhibition to prevent neurons among its nearest neighbors from becoming VLI$^+$. As these newly formed FLI$^+$ and VLI$^+$ neurons are displaced along the tentacles, the effect of the lateral inhibition diminishes; once again, new FLI$^+$ and VLI$^+$ neurons are formed at the tentacle base. This type of mechanism would also account for the observed fairly uniform spacing of FLI$^+$ and VLI$^+$ neurons along a tentacle. Thus, determination of phenotype would involve at least three sequential decisions for some neurons.

VII. Basis of Position-Dependent Conversion

The mechanistic basis of the position-dependent influence on neuronal phenotype is unknown. However, correlated changes in the head activation gradient, and changes in two subsets of neurons that can arise by conversion, suggest that this particular pattern-forming process governing head formation may also play a role in the position-dependent effects. To place these observations in context, the patterning processes governing head formation will be described briefly.

A. Head Patterning Processes

A pair of developmental gradients is largely responsible for the formation of a head at the apical end of an animal (e.g., MacWilliams, 1983a,b). One gradient is the head inhibition gradient, and is a lateral inhibition process. Any part of the body column is capable of forming a head, but normally does not because the existing head prevents this from occurring. As measured by grafting experiments, the ability to inhibit head formation by a head is highest near the head and decreases with distance (e.g., MacWilliams, 1983a). The controlling element, head inhibition, is produced in the head, and is most likely transmitted down the body column by diffusion (MacWilliams, 1983a) via gap junctions in the two epithelia (Fraser *et al.,* 1987).

The second gradient is the head activation gradient. Head activation is defined by the ability of an excised piece of tissue to form a secondary axis after transplantation into the body column of another animal (Wolpert, 1971). This gradient is high in the head and decreases down the body column, that is, pieces from an upper axial position form secondary axes more frequently after transplantation than do pieces from a lower axial location (MacWilliams, 1983b). The head activation gradient, which is associated with the epithelial cells (Nishimiya *et al.,* 1986), is stable despite the continuous tissue displacement.

A current view is that this gradient is a dynamic process in which a signal produced in the head (S. Chung, C. K. Teragawa, and H. R. Bode, unpublished results), and transmitted down the body column, is transduced by epithelial cells via a second messenger system involving protein kinase C (Muller, 1989). The end of the pathway is the synthesis of a molecule or molecules, plausibly transcription factors, involved in head formation. This (these) represent the stable measured head activation. Because the concentration of the signal is graded down the body column, the concentration of these molecules is presumably also graded.

If this idea is correct then, as the epithelial cells are displaced up or down the column, the head activation level would shift in accordance with the concentration of the signal. When displaced up the column, the head activation level would rise. After reaching the head, the level would be high enough for the epithelial cells to differentiate into epithelial cells of the head. They would produce head inhibition and, in *H. oligactis,* for example, express the CP8 antigen (Javois *et al.,* 1986).

B. Head Activation Affects Neuronal Phenotype Conversion

As the epithelial cells are displaced into the head, so are the accompanying neurons. As described, some of these neurons undergo phenotypic changes. These parallel changes suggest that epithelial cells and neurons are influenced by the same processes, or that the neurons are influenced by these processes via the epithelial cells. Two examples in which head activation plays a role in the position-dependent influence on neuronal phenotype provide support for this concept.

The first example concerns the formation of epidermal sensory neurons in the head. These ESn cells are found in the upper part of the head, the hypostome, but not in the lower part, the tentacle zone (Kinnamon and

Westfall, 1981; Dunne *et al.,* 1985). Ganglion cells are found in large numbers in the tentacle zone and in small numbers in the hypostome (Kinnamon and Westfall, 1981). The order of the appearance of these two cell types during head regeneration provides the evidence for the influence of the head activation gradient on neuronal phenotype development.

After decapitation, the wound closes over, and the resulting dome begins to undergo regeneration. The apex first takes on the characteristics of the tentacle zone, that is, that tentacles can form, and later develops the characteristics of the hypostome (see Fig. 9). The outer ring of the dome, which will form the tentacle zone, becomes competent to form tentacles at the time that the apex is forming the hypostome (Bode and Bode, 1987). This sequence of events is also correlated with the changing distribution of TS19, a monoclonal antibody that specifically stains the ectodermal cells of the tentacles. During regeneration, TS19 reactivity first appears at the apex, then spreads over the entire dome, and later vanishes at the apex (Bode *et al.,* 1988a). Both sets of observations are correlated with the sharp increase in head activation found only in the regenerating tip (MacWilliams, 1983b). The transition through tentacle competence to hypostome competence in the apex can be correlated with the rising level of head activation.

ESn cells and ganglion cells appear in the regenerating head in the same order. Early in regeneration, ganglion cells, typical of the tentacle zone, appear at the apex of the dome; only later do they appear in the outer ring. Once the apex has taken on the characteristics of a hypostome, ESn cells appear there and nowhere else (Bode *et al.,* 1988a). Hence, the order of appearance of the two neuron types suggest that an intermediate level of head activation is required for ganglion cell differentiation and a high level is required for ESn cell formation.

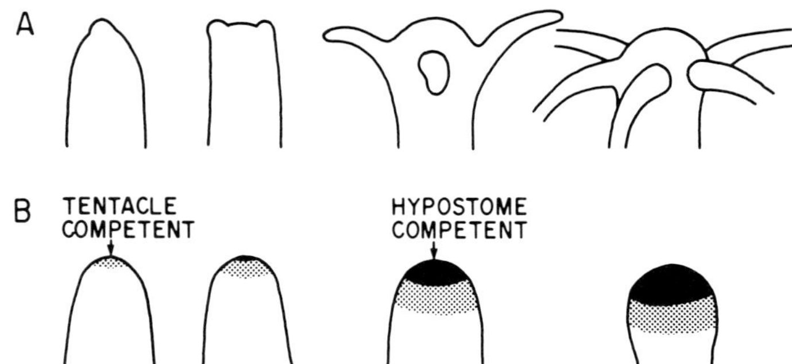

Figure 9. Development of the two-part head pattern during regeneration. A. The positions of the tentacles as they first appear. B. The development of the underlying head pattern suggested by the tentacle positions and the time-dependent changes in the TS19-staining pattern. [Reprinted from Bode and Bode, *Development* 1, 89–98 (1987), by permission of the Company of Biologists, Ltd.]

Analysis of the mutant reg-16, which is defective in head regeneration, provides additional support for this idea. After decapitation, reg-16 regenerates poorly, most often forming 0–3 tentacles and rarely forming a complete head (Sugiyama and Fujisawa, 1977). Those animals that form only a few tentacles never lose the TS19 reactivity at the apex (Koizumi *et al.,* 1991) that normally disappears when the apex forms the hypostome. Finally, the head activation level never rises to the level of a hypostome during regeneration (Achermann and Sugiyama, 1985).

Those regenerates that do not form a hypostome form ganglion cells but do not form ESns (Koizumi *et al.,* 1991). Those few regenerates that do form a hypostome also form ESn cells and lose TS19 reactivity. Thus, either the patterning defect that results in the insufficient rise in head activation level leads to the absence of hypostome formation as well as the absence of ESn cells or the formation of Esn cells is coupled with a threshold level of head activation.

The second example involves the regional distribution of the RLI$^+$ subset and its dependence on diacylglycerol (DAG). This subset is virtually identical to the FLI$^+$ subset but is identified with an antiserum against the peptide RFamide instead of FMRFamide. Treatment of hydra with DAG causes the body columns to become more head-like, a response that increases the longer the treatment. The animal elongates and forms a ring of tentacles in the middle of the body column (Muller, 1989), from which a secondary axis eventually develops (J. Lee, T. Daly, and H. R. Bode, unpublished results). Isolation of pieces of the body column results in heads regenerating at both ends (Muller, 1989). Normally a head regenerates only at the original apical end. The cell composition shifts away from that of the body column toward that of the head (J. Lee, T. Daly, and H. R. Bode, unpublished results). Finally, measurement of the head activation levels of the body column indicates that they rise with DAG treatment (Muller, 1990; Sugiyama, personal communication; J. Lee, R. Brenner, and H. R. Bode, unpublished).

Treatment of animals with DAG for 6 days also results in the displacement of the basal border of the RLI$^+$ subset of neurons of the head from the base of the head to a point about two-thirds of the way down the body column (W. A. Muller, personal communication; J. Lee, T. Daly, H. R. Bode, unpublished results). This basal movement of the border of the subset is progressive. The longer the treatment, the further down the column the border moves (J. Lee, T. Daly, H. R. Bode, unpublished results). If DAG has a direct effect on the appearance of RLI$^+$ neurons in the body column, one would expect them to appear all along the body column at the same time. Instead, the progressive appearance is what one would expect if the expression of RLI by a neuron were dependent on a specific head activation concentration. Since DAG treatment raises the head activation concentration, the general level of the gradient would rise in the body column. With time, the threshold level of head

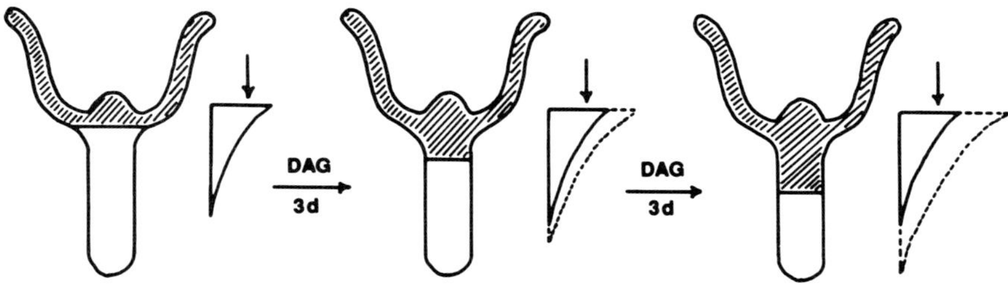

Figure 10. Change in the distribution of RLI[+] neurons after treatment with diacylglycerol (DAG). The distributions in the center and right hydra depict successive changes in the RLI[+] pattern after daily treatment for 3 days with DAG. The schematic to the right of each hydra represents the head activation gradient in normal animals. The dotted extension represents the increase in head activation caused by DAG treatment. The arrow indicates a proposed threshold concentration of head activation for RLI[+] expression.

activation would move down the column and, with it, the basal border of the RLI[+] subset, as shown in Fig. 10.

Thus, the level of head activation apparently plays a role in the position-dependent appearance of these two subsets. Whether the neurons are directly assaying a component of the head activation process or indirectly reacting to epithelial cells that have attained a threshold head activation level is not known. Since the neurons are nestled in among the epithelial cells, either possibility is reasonable. Finally, it is unlikely that axial distribution of all subsets depends on this patterning process. For example, the subset of ganglion cells defined by RC9[+] is found uniformly throughout the animal (Yaross *et al.*, 1986).

VIII. Summary

Returning to one of the original questions, how is the mosaic of subsets maintained in this steady state in which every neuron is always changing location? A first approximation to an answer can be offered, and consists of the following.

Throughout the body column, multipotent stem cells continuously give rise to interstitial cells that are committed to forming neurons but not committed to a particular phenotype. This is most likely a stochastic process. The production of neurons compensates for the continuous dilution of the density of the nerve net by epithelial cell proliferation as well as for the continuous loss of neurons. As the committed interstitial cells traverse the neuronal differentiation pathway, some of the differentiation intermediates migrate toward either extremity. This redistribution contributes substantially to, or may be solely responsible for, the observed higher neuronal differentiation and density in the head and foot.

Determination of phenotype of a neuron clearly depends very strongly on the axial location or specific region in which the differentiation process is completed. The developing neuron "reads" its location, and differentiates accordingly. For two subsets of neurons, a process involved in head pattern formation may be the signal that the neuron is "reading." Because more than one type of neuron is often formed in the same location, it is clear that position-dependent influences are important for the determination of phenotype but are not sufficient. Additional processes must be acting in concert with or subsequent to the position-dependent effects.

For many neurons in *Hydra,* the expressed phenotype represents a metastable state instead of a terminally differentiated state. A change in location results in a change in phenotype. This metastability of the differentiated state may represent an adaptation peculiar to hydra, given its unusual nervous system. It could also be that neurons in other animals are also only metastably differentiated but one does not notice this quality because the neurons do not change location.

Acknowledgments

I wish to thank Ann Grens and Douglas Fisher for a critical reading of the manuscript, and the National Institutes of Health (HD 08086) for support.

References

Achermann, J., and Sugiyama, T. (1985). Genetic analysis of developmental mechanisms in hydra. X. Morphogenetic potentials of a regeneration-deficient strain (reg-16). *Dev. Biol.* **107,** 13–27.

Berking, S. (1980). Commitment of stem cells to nerve cells and migration of nerve cell precursors in preparatory bud development in hydra. *J. Embryol. Exp. Morph.* **60,** 373–387.

Bode, H., Berking, S., David, C., Gierer, A., Schaller, H., and Trenkner, E. (1973). Quantitative analysis of cell types during growth and regeneration in hydra. *Roux Arch. Entw. Mech. Org.* **171,** 269–285.

Bode, P. M., and Bode, H. R. (1980). Formation of pattern in regenerating tissue pieces of *Hydra attenuata.* I. Head–body proportion regulation. *Dev. Biol.* **78,** 484–496.

Bode, P. M., and Bode, H. R. (1987). Formation of pattern in regenerating tissue of *H. attenuata.* IV. Three processes combine to determine the number of tentacles. *Development* **1,** 89–98.

Bode, H. R., Heimfeld, S., Chow, M. A., and Huang, L. W. (1987). Gland cells arise by differentiation from interstitial cells in *Hydra attenuata. Dev. Biol.* **122,** 577–585.

Bode, P. M., Awad, T. A., Koizumi, O., Nakashima, Y., Grimmelikhuijzen, C. J. P, and Bode, H. R. (1988a). Development of the two-part pattern during regeneration of the head in hydra. *Development* **102,** 223–235.

Bode, H. R., Heimfeld, S., Koizumi, Littlefield, C. L., and Yaross, M. S. (1988). Maintenance and regeneration of the nerve net in hydra. *Am Zool.* **28,** 1053–1063.

Bode, H. R., Gee, L. W., and Chow, M. C. (1990). Neuron differentiation in hydra involves dividing intermediates. *Dev. Biol.* **139,** 231–243.

Bosch, T., and David, C. (1987). Stem cells of *Hydra magnipapillata* can differentiate somatic cells and germ line cells. *Dev. Biol.* **121,** 182–191.

Bosch, T. C. G., and David, C. N. (1990). Cloned interstitial stem cells grow as contiguous patches in hydra. *Dev. Biol.* **138,** 513–515.

Burnett, A. L., and Diehl, N. A. (1964). The nervous system of *Hydra.* I. Types, distribution and origin of nerve elements. *J. Exp. Zool.* **157,** 217–226.

Campbell, R. D. (1967a). Tissue dynamics of steady state growth in *Hydra littoralis.* I. Patterns of cell division. *Dev. Biol.* **15,** 487–502.

Campbell, R. D. (1967b). Tissue dynamics of steady state growth in *Hydra littoralis.* II. patterns of tissue movement. *J. Morph.* **121,** 19–28.

Campbell, R. D. (1967c). Tissue dynamics of steady state growth in *Hydra littoralis.* III. Behavior of specific cell types during tissue movement. *J. Exp. Zool.* **164,** 379–392.

Campbell, R. D. (1976). Elimination of *Hydra* interstitial cells and nerve cells by means of colchicine. *J. Cell Sci.* **21,** 1–13.

Campbell, R. D. (1980). Role of muscle processes in hydra morphogenesis. *In* "Developmental and Cellular Biology of Coelenterates" (P. Tardent and R. Tardent, eds.) pp. 421–428. Amsterdam:Elsevier/North Holland.

Campbell, R. D., and Bode, H. R. (1983). Terminology for morphology and cell types. *In* "*Hydra:* Research Methods" (H. M. Lenhoff, ed.), New York:Plenum Press. pp. 5–16.

Cummings, S. G., and Bode, H. R. (1984). Head regeneration and polarity reversal in *Hydra attenuata* can occur in the absence of DNA synthesis. *Roux's Arch. Dev. Biol.* **194,** 79–86.

David, C. N., and Campbell, R. D. (1972). Cell cycle kinetics and development of *Hydra attenuata.* I. Epithelial cells. *J. Cell Sci.* **11,** 557–568.

David, C. N., and Gierer, A. (1974). Cell cycle kinetics and development of *Hydra attenuata.* III. Nerve and nematocyte differentiation. *J. Cell Sci.* **16,** 359–375.

David, C. and Murphy, S. (1977). Characterization of interstitial stem cells in hydra by cloning. *Dev. Biol.* **58,** 372–383.

Davis, L. E. (1974). Ultrastructural studies of the development of nerves in hydra. *Am. Zool.* **14,** 551–573.

Davis, L. E., Burnett, A. L., and Haynes, J. F. (1968). A histological and ultrastructural study of the muscular and nervous system in *Hydra.* II. Nervous system. *J. Exp. Zool.* **167,** 295–332.

Diehl, F. A., and Burnett, A. L. (1964). The role of interstitial cells in the maintenance of hydra. I. Specific destruction of interstitial cells in normal, asexual and nonbudding animals. *J. Exp. Zool.* **155,** 253–259.

Doe, C. Q., Kuwada, J. Y., and Goodman, C. S. (1985). From epithelium to neuroblasts to neurons: The role of cell interactions and cell lineage during insect neurogenesis. *Phil. Trans. R. Soc. London B* **312,** 67–81.

Dunne, J. F., Javois, L. C., Huang, L. W., and Bode, H. R. (1985). A subset of cells in the nerve net of *Hydra oligactis* defined by a monoclonal antibody: Its arrangement and development. *Dev. Biol.* **109,** 41–53.

Epp, L., and Tardent, P. (1978). The distribution of nerve cells in *Hydra attenuata* Pall. *Roux's Arch.* **185**, 185–193.

Fraser, S. E., Green, C. R., Bode, H. R., and Gilula, N. B. (1987). Selective disruption of gap junctional communication interferes with a patterning process in hydra. *Science* **237**, 49–55.

Fujisawa, T., David, C. N., and Bosch, T. C. G. (1990). Transplantation stimulates interstitial cell migration in hydra. *Dev. Biol.* **138**, 509–512.

Gierer, A., Berking, S., Bode, H., David, C. N., Flick, K., Hansmann, G., Schaller, H., and Trenkner, E. (1972). Regeneration of hydra from cell reaggregates. *Nature New Biol.* **239**, 98–101.

Grimmelikhuijzen, C. J. P. (1983). Coexistence of neuropeptides in hydra. *Neurosci.* **9**, 837–845.

Grimmelikhuijzen, C. J. P. (1984). Peptides in the nervous system of coelenterates. *In* "Evolution and Tumour Pathology of the Neuroendocrine System" (S. Falkmer *et al.*, eds.), pp. 39–58. Elsevier Science Publishers.

Grimmelikhuijzen, C. J. P., Dockray, G. J., and Schot, L. P. C. (1982). FMRFamide-like immunoreactivity in the nervous system of hydra. *Histochemistry* **73**, 499–508.

Hadzi, J. (1909). Über das Nervensystem von Hydra. *Arb. Zool. Inst. Univ. Wien.* **17**, 225–268.

Heimfeld, S., and Bode, H. R. (1981). Regulation of interstitial cell differentiation in *Hydra attenuata*. VI. Positional pattern of nerve cell commitment is independent of local nerve cell density. *J. Cell Sci.* **52**, 85–98.

Heimfeld, S., and Bode, H. R. (1984a). Interstitial cell migration in *Hydra attenuata*. I. Quantitative description of cell movements. *Dev. Biol.* **105**, 1–9.

Heimfeld, S., and Bode, H. R. (1984b). Interstitial cell migration in *Hydra attenuata*. II. Selective migration of nerve cell precursors as the basis for position-dependent nerve cell differentiation. *Dev. Bio.* **105**, 10–17.

Hicklin, J., and Wolpert, L. (1973). Positional information and pattern regulation in *Hydra*: The effect of radiation. *J. Embryol. Exp. Morph.* **30**, 741–752.

Hoffmeister, S. A. H., and Schaller, H. C. (1987). Head activator and head inhibitor are signals for nerve cell differentiation in hydra. *Dev. Biol.* **122**, 72–77.

Holstein, T., Schaller, H. C., and David, C. N. (1986). Nerve cell differentiation in hydra requires two signals. *Dev. Biol.* **115**, 9–17.

Honig, M. G., and Hume, R. I. (1986). Fluorescent carbocyanine dyes allow living neurons of identified origin to be studied in long-term cultures. *J. Cell Biol.* **103**, 171–187.

Javois, L. C., Wood, R. D., and Bode, H. R. (1986). Patterning of the head in hydra as visualized by a monoclonal antibody. I. Budding and regeneration. *Dev. Biol.* **117**, 607–618.

Kinnamon, J. C., and Westfall, J. A. (1981). A three-dimensional serial reconstruction of neuronal distributions in the hypostome of a *Hydra*. *J. Morph.* **168**, 321–329.

Koizumi, O., and Bode, H. R. (1986). Plasticity in the nervous system of adult hydra. I. The position-dependent expression of FMRFamide-like immunoreactivity. *Dev. Biol.* **116**, 407–421.

Koizumi, O., Heimfeld, S., and Bode, H. R. (1988). Plasticity in the nervous system of adult hydra. II. Conversion of ganglion cells of the body column into epidermal sensory cells of the hypostome. *Dev. Biol.* **129**, 358–371.

Koizumi, O., Mizumoto, H., Sugiyama, T., and Bode, H. R. (1991). Nerve net formation in the primitive system of hydra: An overview. *Neuroscience Res. Suppl.* **13**, S165–S170.

Koizumi, O., and Bode, H. R. (1991). Plasticity in the nervous system of adult hydra. 3. Conversion of neurons to expression of a vasopressin-like-immunoreactivity. *J. Neuroscience* **11**, 2011–2020.

Landis, S. C., and Keefe, D. (1983). Evidence for neurotransmitter plasticity *in vivo*: Developmental changes in properties of cholinergic sympathetic neurons. *Dev. Biol.* **98**, 349–372.

Landis, S. C., Siegel, R. E., and Schwab, M. (1988). Evidence for neurotransmitter plasticity *in vivo*. II. Immunocytochemical studies of rat sweat gland innervation during development. *Dev. Biol.* **126**, 129–140.

Lentz, T. L., and Barrnett, R. (1965). Fine structure of the nervous system of *Hydra. Am. Zool.* **5,** 341–356.

Littlefield, C. L., and Bode, H. R. (1986). Germ cells in *Hydra oligactis* males. II. Evidence for a subpopulation of interstitial stem cells whose differentiation is limited to sperm production. *Dev. Biol.* **116,** 381–386.

MacWilliams, H. K. (1983a). Hydra transplantation phenomena and the mechanism of hydra head regeneration. I. Properties of head inhibition. *Dev. Biol.* **96,** 217–238.

MacWilliams, H. K. (1983b). Hydra transplantation phenomena and the mechanism of hydra head regeneration. II. Properties of head activation. *Dev. Biol.* **96,** 239–272.

Marcum, B. A., and Campbell, R. D. (1978). Development of hydra lacking nerve and interstitial cells. *J. Cell Sci.* **29,** 17–33.

Martindale, M. Q., and Shankland, M. (1990). Neuronal competition determines spatial pattern of neuropeptide expression by identified neurons of the leech. *Dev. Biol.* **139,** 210–226.

Muller, W. A. (1989). Diacylglycerol-induced multihead formation in *Hydra. Development* **105,** 309–316.

Muller, W. A. (1990). Ectopic head and foot formation in hydra: Diacylglycerol induced increase in positional value and assistance of the head in foot formation. *Differentiation* **42,** 131–143.

Nishimiya, C. Wanek, N., and Sugiyama, T. (1986). Genetic analysis of the developmental mechanisms in hydra. XIV. Identification of the cell lineages responsible for the altered developmental gradients in a mutant strain, reg-16. *Dev. Bio.* **115,** 469–478.

Otto, J. J., and Campbell, R. D. (1977). Tissue economics of hydra: Regulation of cell cycle, animal size and development by controlled feeding rates. *J. Cell Sci.* **28,** 117–132.

Reh, T. A., and Tully, T. (1986). Regulation of tyrosine hydroxylase-containing amacrine cell number in larval frog retina. *Dev. Biol.* **114,** 463–469.

Schaller, H. C., Hoffmeister, S. A. H., and Dubel, S. (1989). Role of the neuropepide head activator for growth and development in hydra and mammals. *Development* **107,** 99–107.

Spencer, A. N. (1978). Neurobiology of *Polyorchis.* II. Structure of effector systems. *J. Neurobiol.* **10,** 95–117.

Spencer, A. N., and Arkett, S. A. (1984). Radial symmetry and the organization of central neurones in a hydrozoan jellyfish. *J. Exp. Biol.* **110,** 69–90.

Sternberg, P. (1988). Control of cell fates within equivalence groups in *C. elegans. Trends Neurosci.* **11,** 259–264.

Sugiyama, T., and Fujisawa, T. (1977). Genetic analysis of developmental mechanisms in hydra. III. Characterization of a regeneration-deficient strain. *J. Embryol. Exp. Morph.* **42,** 65–77.

Teragawa, C. K., and Bode, H. R. (1990). Spatial and temporal patterns of interstitial cell migration in *Hydra vulgaris. Dev. Biol.* **138,** 63–81.

Wanek, N., and Campbell, R. D. (1982). Roles of ectodermal and endodermal epithelial cells in hydra morphogenesis: Construction of chimeric strains. *J. Exp. Zool.* **221,** 37–47.

Westfall, J. A. (1973). Ultrastructural evidence for a granule-containing sensory-motor-interneuron in *Hydra littoralis. J. Ultrastruct. Res.* **42,** 268–282.

Westfall, J. A., and Kinnamon, J. C. (1978). A second sensory-motor-interneuron with neurosecretory granules in *Hydra. J. Neurocytol.* **7,** 365–379.

Westfall, J. A. and Rogers, R. A. (1990). A combined high-voltage and scanning electron microscope study of 2 types of sensory cells dissociated from the gastrodermis of hydra. *J. Submicro. Cytol. Pathol.* **22[2],** 185–190.

Wolpert, L. (1971). Positional information and pattern formation. *Curr. Top. Dev. Biol.* **6,** 183–224.

Yaross, M. S., and Bode, H. R. (1978a). Regulation of interstitial cell differentiation in *Hydra attenuata.* III. Effects of I-cell and nerve cell densities. *J. Cell Sci.* **34,** 1–26.

Yaross, M. S., and Bode, H. R. (1978b). Regulation of interstitial cell differentiation in *Hydra attenuata*. IV. Nerve cell commitment in head regeneration is position-dependent. *J. Cell Sci.* **34**, 27–38.

Yaross, M. S., Westerfield, J., Javois, L. C., and Bode, H. R. (1986). Nerve cells in hydra: Monoclonal antibodies identify two lineages with distinct mechanisms for their incorporation into head tissue. *Dev. Biol.* **114**, 225–237.

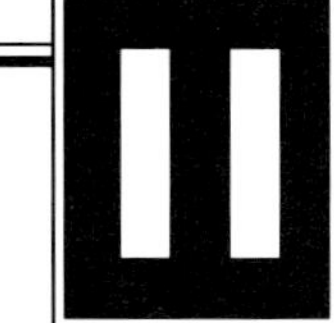

Cell Lineage Segregation in the Vertebrate Neural Crest

Marianne Bronner-Fraser
Developmental Biology Center
University of California, Irvine
Irvine, California

I. Introduction
II. Developmental Potential of Neural Crest Cell Populations
III. Evidence That Individual Neural Crest Cells Are Multipotent
IV. Evidence for Subpopulations at Stages of Neural Crest Cell Migration
V. Evidence for Neural Crest Sublineages at Postmigratory Stages
VI. Role of Growth Factors in Neural Crest Cell Differentiation
VII. Phenotypic Plasticity in Neural-Crest-Derived Ganglia
VIII. Conclusions Regarding Mechanisms of Cell-Type Segregation in the Neural Crest
References

I. Introduction

The neural crest is a cell population unique to vertebrates and higher chordates. These cells arise during neurulation as the neural folds close to form the neural tube. In most species, neural crest cells leave the apical neural tube shortly after tube closure and subsequently undergo extensive migrations. After their migratory phase, these cells come to rest at a variety of sites. Some aggregate to form sensory, sympathetic and parasympathetic ganglia, and chromaffin cells of the adrenal medulla; others populate tissues to form melanocytes in the skin, enteric neurons in the gut, and connective tissue in the face (LeDouarin, 1982). The intricate migratory patterns of neural crest cells and their extensive array of derivatives (Table 1) have intrigued developmental biologists for over a century. However, the mechanisms that control their migratory patterns and the generation of diverse phenotypes are

DETERMINANTS OF NEURONAL IDENTITY
Copyright © 1992 by Academic Press, Inc.

TABLE I
Derivatives of the Neural Crest

Peripheral nervous system
  Autonomic ganglia and plexuses
    Sympathetic ganglia—neurons and satellite cells
    Parasympathetic and enteric ganglia—neurons and satellite cells
  Sensory ganglia
    Dorsal root ganglia—neurons and satellite cells
    Cranial sensory ganglia—some neurons and satellite cells
    Ciliary ganglia—neurons and satellite cells
    Rohon beard cells(amphibian)
  Schwann cells
Pigment cells
Endocrine and paracrine cells
  Chromaffin cells of adrenal medulla
  Calcitonin-producing cells
  Carotid body type I cells
Cranial mesectodermal derivatives
  Skeleton
    Palate, visceral skeleton, otic capsule
  Connective tissue
    Dermis, smooth muscle adipose tissue of the face and neck, ciliary
    muscle, connective and muscle tissue of arteries, tooth papillae,
    cornea, meninges, glandular connective tissue
Trunk mesectodermal derivative
  Dorsal fin of lower vertebrates

only beginning to be understood. This chapter will review some of the important advances of the last decade.

As a population, the neural crest is regionalized: cells derived from different axial levels give rise to a varied array of progeny and follow distinct migratory pathways to their final destinations. The regions of the neuraxis have been designated as cranial, vagal, trunk, and lumbosacral (Fig. 1), based on differences in neural crest migratory pathways and derivatives as determined by orthotopic quail/chick grafts (LeDouarin, 1982).

1. Cranial neural crest cells depart from the neural tube after its closure in the chick, but prior to tube closure in murine embryos, and migrate subjacent to the cranial ectoderm. Some cranial neural crest cells enter the branchial arches, where they will form many of the cartilaginous elements of the facial skeleton. Others contribute to the ciliary ganglion of the eye and various cranial sensory ganglia, which also receive contributions from the ectodermal placodes. Cranial neural crest cells do not emerge from the neural tube uniformly; in the rhombencephalon, the neural tube at the level of

rhombomeres 1, 3, and 5 does not give rise to neural crest cells (A. G. S. Lumsden, personal communication).

2. Vagal neural crest cells emerge from the neural tube at the level of somites 1–7 (LeDouarin and Teillet, 1973). These cells migrate ventrally to invade the gut and then move caudally along the gut to contribute to the enteric nervous system.

3. Trunk neural crest cells, which emerge from somites 8–28, migrate along two primary pathways. The first is a ventral pathway through the rostral

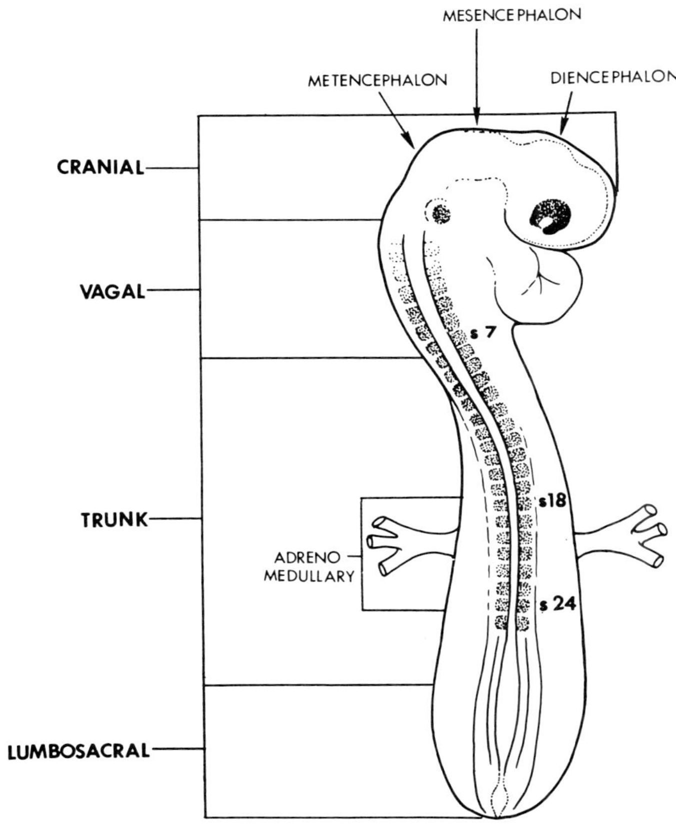

Figure I. Regions along the neural axis that differ in their range of neural crest derivatives and migratory pathways. The cranial neural crest emerges from levels of the neural axis above the otic vesicles. The vagal neural crest arises from the neural tube between somitic levels 1 and 7. The trunk neural crest emerges from axial levels between somites 8 and 28; those cells that contribute to the adrenal gland arise from somitic levels 18–24. The lumbosacral neural crest emerges from axial levels below the 28th somite. (Reprinted from Bronner-Fraser and Cohen, 1980, with permission.)

half of each somitic sclerotome (Rickmann *et al.*, 1985), with a few cells found in the intersomitic region; cells following this route contribute to the dorsal root and sympathetic ganglia, adrenal medulla, and aortic plexuses. The second pathway followed by trunk neural crest cells is a dorsal route underneath the ectoderm, along which presumptive pigment cells migrate (Fig. 2). In avian embryos, neural crest cells initiate migration along this pathway at relatively late stages of migration, whereas in the mouse, neural crest cells initiate migration along both the dorsal and ventral pathways simultaneously (Serbedzija *et al.*, 1989, 1990).

4. The lumbosacral neural crest cells, like vagal neural crest cells, contribute to the enteric nervous system in the postumbilical gut. In addition, these cells contribute to sacral dorsal root and sympathetic ganglia. They migrate ventrally through the rostral somites and invade the gut through the dorsal mesentery (Serbedzija *et al.*, 1991).

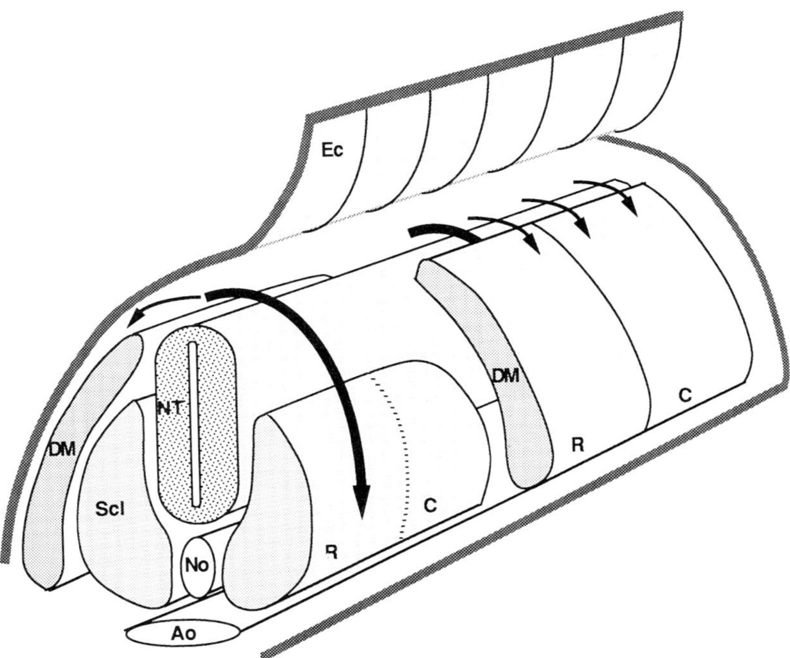

Figure 2. The early pathways of trunk neural crest cell migration. Neural crest cells emerge from the neural tube (NT) and proceed either ventrally (wide arrow) through the somitic sclerotome (Scl) or dorsolaterally (thin arrow) between the ectoderm (Ec) and dermomyotome (DM). The ventrally migrating cells only move through the rostral (R) half of each sclerotome and are not observed in the caudal (C) half. Neural crest cells avoid the region around the notochord (No). Ao, dorsal aorta.

At the onset of their migration, neural crest cells at all axial levels appear to be morphologically similar. After their migratory phase, they differentiate into widely varied cell types, as different as pigment cells, neurons, and cartilage. How is diversity generated in this apparently homogeneous population, both at a single axial level and at different axial levels? Several scenarios have been proposed to account for the diversity of neural crest derivatives. One possibility is that the neural crest is a homogeneous population of multipotent cells, each with identical developmental potential and able to give rise to a large range of phenotypes. A multipotent cell, by definition, has the ability to make a different set of descendant cell types in different conditions. Multipotent cells may migrate randomly and differentiate according to instructive cues encountered along their migratory pathway or at their final sites of localization. A second possibility is that the neural crest is composed of a heterogeneous mixture of "predetermined" (unipotent) cells, each fated to become a given derivative. These cells either migrate in a directed fashion to their proper locations and differentiate according to their prescribed fate or migrate randomly so those localized in inappropriate sites may fail to differentiate or may die. These alternatives are summarized in Fig. 3. A third possibility reconciles these two extreme and divergent views and proposes that neural crest cells represent a mixture of multipotent and predetermined cells. This chapter will summarize recent ideas about the developmental potential of neural crest cells and how this potential may become restricted with time.

II. Developmental Potential of Neural Crest Cell Populations

Transplantation experiments have been used to test the developmental potential of neural crest cell populations arising from different axial levels. By changing the environment through which populations of neural crest cells migrate, these experiments test whether the cells' migratory pathway or final resting site alters their prospective phenotype. Transplantation experiments initially were performed in amphibian embryos (Hörstadius, 1950) and more recently in birds using quail/chick chimeras (LeDouarin, 1982). In these grafts, a piece of the host neural tube is removed and substituted with a piece of donor neural tube derived from a different axial level. Because development occurs in a rostral-to-caudal sequence, neural crest migration is more advanced in more rostral regions in any given embryo. To assure that donor and

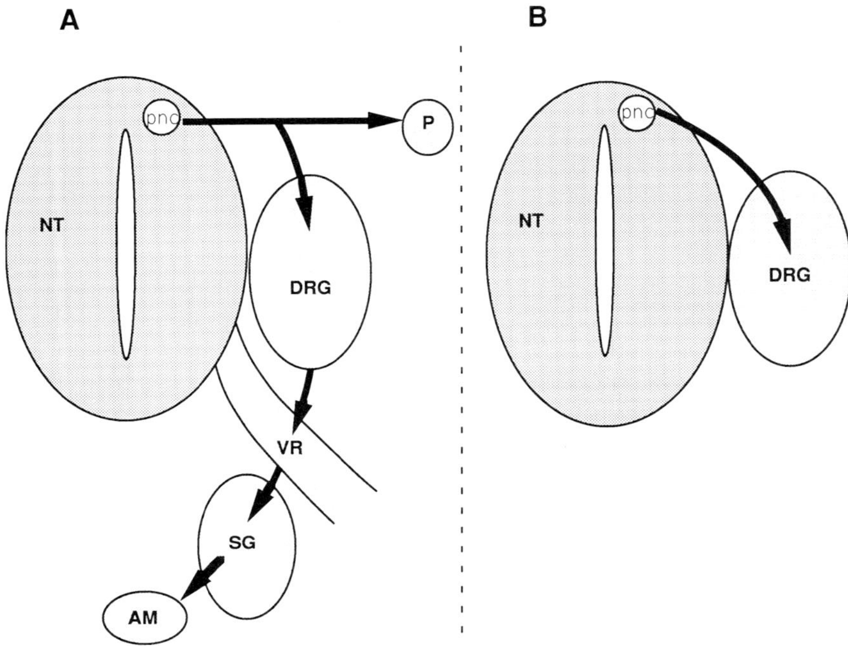

Figure 3. Two possible mechanisms to explain neural crest cell lineage in the trunk. A. Neural crest cells may be multipotent, so an individual premigratory neural crest cell (pnc) has the ability to give rise to multiple neural crest derivatives such as pigment cells (p), dorsal root ganglion cells (DRG), Schwann cells in the ventral root (VR), sympathetic ganglion cells (SG), and cells in the adrenal gland (AM). B. Alternatively, neural crest cells may be predetermined to give rise to a single cell type.

host tissue are matched in developmental age, grafts are typically made between embryos of different ages so the maturity of the grafted neural tubes is well matched. After fixation, sectioning, and staining, grafted quail tissue can be distinguished from host chick tissue by the condensed mass of heterochromatin in the quail nuclei.

Heterotopic transplantations first were used to examine the developmental potential of vagal and trunk neural crest cells, which normally give rise to parasympathetic and sympathetic derivatives, respectively, of the autonomic nervous system, as well as to other cell types. When a neural tube from the vagal region was transplanted in place of a trunk neural tube, many of the vagal neural crest cells migrated appropriately for their new environment, contributing to the dorsal root ganglia, sympathetic ganglia, and adrenal medulla of the host (LeDouarin and Teillet, 1974; Smith *et al.*, 1977). This suggests that the fate of this cell population is not fixed to give rise to enteric ganglia. However, some vagal neural crest cells did invade the gut after transplantation to the trunk, where they contributed to the enteric ganglia, although endogenous trunk neural crest cells do not normally enter this region. These results demonstrate that developmental fate is not fixed for all vagal neural crest cells; however, some vagal cells behave appropriately for their position of origin rather than for their new position. In the reciprocal experiment, trunk neural crest cells grafted to vagal regions contributed to the preumbilical enteric nervous system, appropriate for their new position (LeDouarin *et al.*, 1975).

Similar experiments have been performed using cranial and trunk level grafts. Cranial neural crest cells grafted to the trunk exhibit mixed behaviors: some cranial cells contribute to normal trunk neural crest derivatives, such as the dorsal root and the sympathetic ganglia, whereas other cranial neural crest cells do not move but differentiate into cartilage—a derivative that trunk neural crest cells never form (LeDouarin and Teillet, 1974). Thus, some cells appear to be flexible with respect to cell fate whereas others differentiate according to their level of origin. When trunk neural crest cells are transplanted into the head, some of the trunk neural crest cells contribute to normal cranial structures, but no transplanted trunk neural crest cells form cartilage (Noden, 1975). In conjunction, these experiments indicate that premigratory neural crest cells from different axial levels share some common developmental potential and, when transplanted to a new environment, can contribute to derivatives that they would not normally form. These results suggest that the developmental potential of neural crest cells is greater than their normal repertoire of fates. However, some properties appear to be intrinsic to the neural crest cells derived from a particular region and are expressed regardless of their transplantation site.

Even after neural crest cells have formed some of their derivatives, their fates are not completely fixed. LeDouarin and colleagues have performed a series of "back-transplantation" experiments (LeDouarin *et al.*, 1978; LeLievre *et al.*, 1980; Dupin, 1984) in which neural-crest-derived ganglia from 6-day-old or older embryos were grafted into the trunk region of 2-day-old host embryos at the onset of trunk neural crest cell migration. For all types of grafted ganglia, quail cells left the ganglia and migrated along the ventral neural crest migratory pathway through the somites. However, different distributions of grafted cells were observed, depending on whether the grafted tissue was obtained from sympathetic, sensory, or parasympathetic ganglia. Cells derived from sympathetic ganglia contributed to sympathoadrenal derivatives, but not to sensory ganglia. In contrast, cells derived from sensory ganglia were found in both sensory ganglia and sympathoadrenal derivatives. Finally, quail cells derived from ciliary or Remak's ganglia were found in the sympathoadrenal regions as well as in enteric ganglia of the gut (LeDouarin *et al.*, 1978). The cells that contributed to these wide-ranging derivatives are likely to have been nonneuronal cells in the ganglia, since the neurons appeared to die after this grafting procedure (Dupin, 1984). The observation of differential contributions of nonneuronal cells from different ganglia has led to the hypothesis that these cells represent two or more populations of cells with different developmental potentials. The nonneuronal cells derived from sensory ganglia have been designated S/A, or "sensory/adrenergic," precursors, which have the ability to give rise to both adrenergic and sensory derivatives; the nonneuronal cells derived from sympathetic ganglia have been designated A, or "adrenergic," precursors, which have the ability to contribute to adrenergic but not sensory derivatives (LeDouarin, 1986). Whether S/A and A precursors exist in the premigratory neural crest as well as in neural-crest-derived ganglia has not been determined. Since these cells already have completed migration and have localized in peripheral ganglia, their developmental options are likely to be fewer that those available to the developmentally younger population of emigrating or migrating neural crest cells.

A major problem in the interpretation of results from transplantation experiments is that the transplants contain large numbers of heterogeneous neural crest cells. Thus, after altering the cells' local environment, one cannot distinguish instructive from selective effects of the new environment on choice of cell fate. For example, it is unclear whether the environment at a given axial level promotes differentiation of the appropriate phenotype or simply eliminates cells with the innappropriate phenotype. A second complication is that the neural crest cells themselves, or the migratory paths available to them, may change as a function of embryonic age.

In order to test whether the time at which neural crest cells exit the neural tube contributes to the range of derivatives available to them, Weston and Butler (1966) transplanted [³H]thymidine-labeled neural tubes from the trunk region of "older" avian embryos to trunks of "younger" hosts (Weston and Butler, 1966). Their results demonstrated that the population of neural crest cells emerging from both the older and young neural tubes could give rise to all neural crest derivatives. In contrast, neural crest cells emerging from "young" neural tubes transplanted to "older" embryos contributed only to dorsal derivatives, such as dorsal root ganglia and pigment cells. We have confirmed that neural crest cells have an orderly pattern of migration using the lipophilic vital dye 1,1-dioctadecyl-3,3,3',3'-tetramethylindocarbocyanine perchlorate (DiI) (Serbedzija *et al.*, 1989). By injecting DiI into the neural tube prior to neural crest cell migration, we were able to label all neural tube cells including premigratory neural crest cells (Fig. 4). When neural tubes of "young" embryos are labeled, the DiI-labeled neural crest cells subsequently

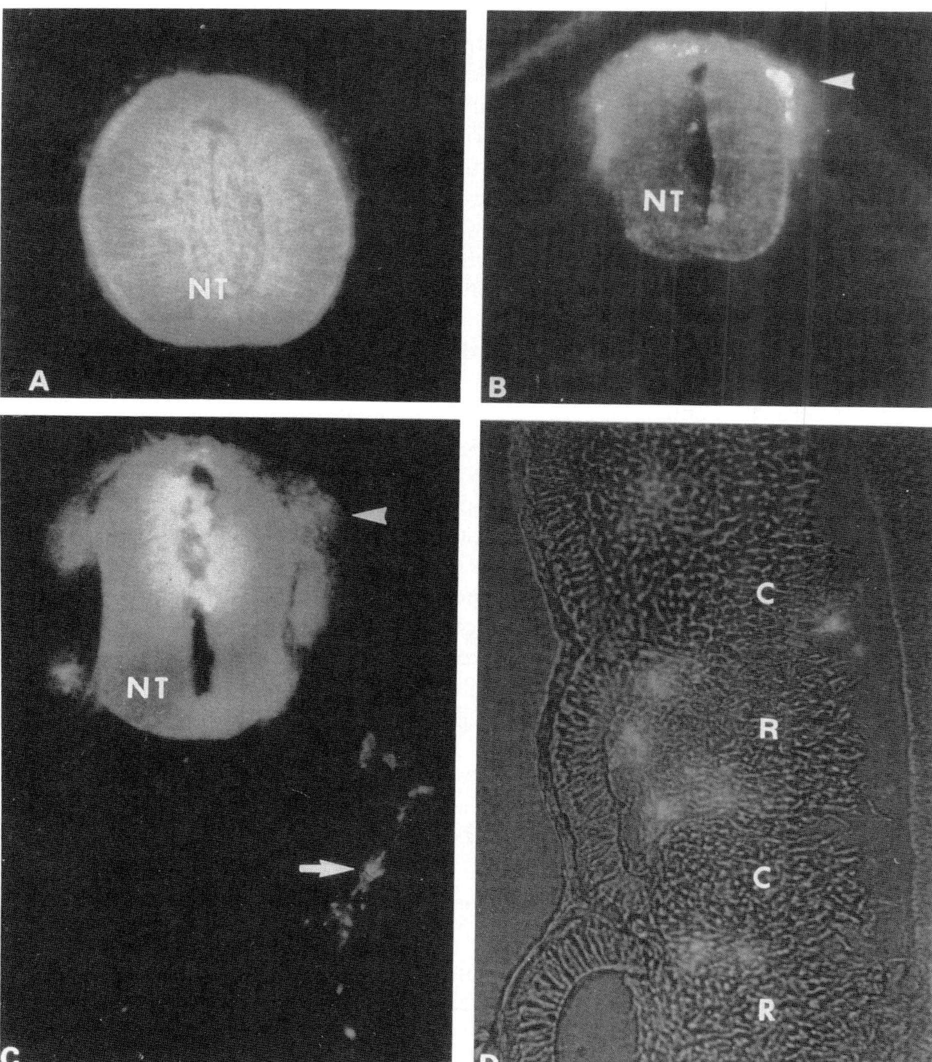

Figure 4. Sections through embryos injected with DiI at stage 12 and incubated for an additional 4, 12, or 24 hr. A. Transverse section through an embryo fixed after 4 hr. DiI-labeled cells were seen exclusively in the neural tube (NT). B. Transverse sections through an embryo fixed after 12 hr. Migrating cells were labeled with DiI (*arrowhead*). C. Transverse section through an embryo fixed after 24 hr. DiI-labeled cells were observed in the sympathetic ganglia (*arrow*) and in the region of presumptive dorsal root ganglia (*arrowhead*). D. Longitudinal section through an embryo fixed after 24 hr. DiI-labeled cells were observed in the rostral (R) half, but not the caudal (C) half, of each somitic sclerotome. Bar: 50 μm (A,D); 125 μm (B,C). (Reprinted from Serbedzija *et al.*, 1989, with permission.)

migrate out of the neural tube to form dorsal root and sympathetic ganglia, adrenomedullary cells, and chromaffin cells. By injecting DiI at progressively later stages of development, we labeled only those neural crest cells that were premigratory at the time of injection. It was determined that later emigrating cells contributed to progressively more dorsal derivatives (Fig. 5). Thus, the contribution of neural crest cells to their derivatives becomes restricted in a ventral-to-dorsal order; the precursors to pigment cells are the last ones to exit the neural tube (Serbedzija *et al.*, 1989). This orderly pattern of migration may restrict the range of derivatives open to later emigrating neural crest cells, although other factors also could contribute to the restriction of these cells' fates.

The experiments just described demonstrate that neural crest cells, as a population, have a great deal of flexibility. Not only can premigratory neural crest cells differentiate appropriately for their new environment after transplantation to a different axial level, but even neural-crest-derived ganglion cells can populate other neural crest sites after transplantation to a younger embryo. However, both neural crest cell populations and the migratory pathways available to them are changing over time. Furthermore, some populations of neural crest cells, for example, some cranial neural crest cells, appear to be somewhat restricted in prospective fate. Because transplantation experiments test the developmental potential of neural crest cell populations, they are not informative about individual neural crest cell potential and cannot distinguish between instructive and selective influences of the environment on neural crest cell differentiation.

III. Evidence That Individual Neural Crest Cells Are Multipotent

An understanding of individual cell lineage is vital for distinguishing the relative importance of the cell's inherent developmental program from the influence of the external environment on cell fate. To gain understanding of individual neural crest cell lineage, one must examine the neural crest at a single-cell level and at prescribed times in development. Two experimental approaches have emerged for studying the developmental potential of individual neural crest cells: (1) isolating single cells in tissue culture and (2) marking individual cells in the living embryo.

A number of investigators have cultured individual neural crest cells successfully (Bronner-Fraser *et al.*, 1980; Sieber-Blum and Cohen, 1980;

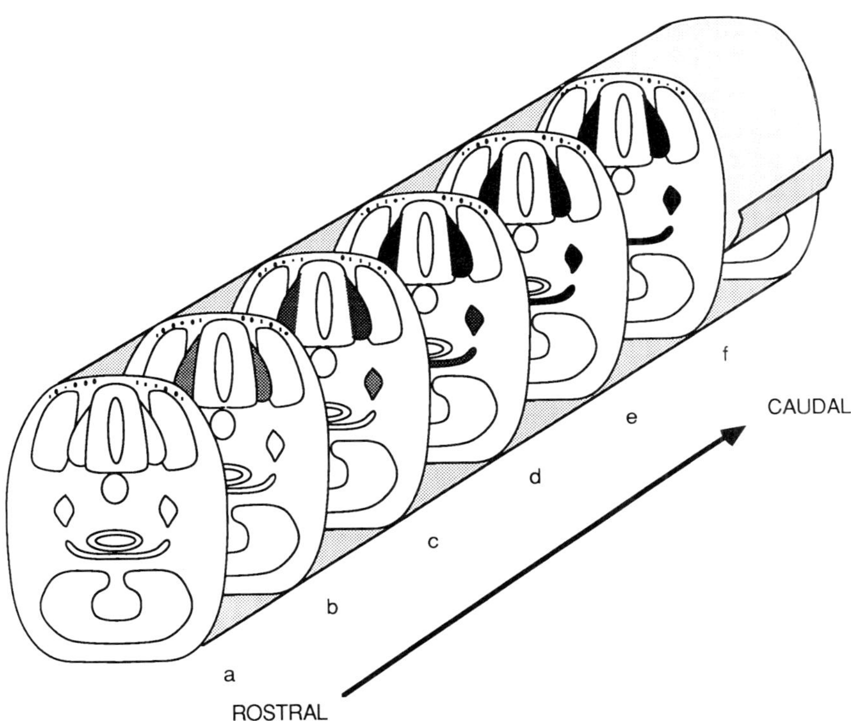

Figure 5. The rostral to caudal distribution of DiI in the neural crest derivatives of a single embryo injected at stage 19 and fixed at stage 21. a–f represent levels along the rostrocaudal axis from which transverse sections were taken. a. At the level of the 9th somite, DiI-labeled cells were observed along the dorsolateral pathway. b. At the level of the 15th somite, DiI-labeled cells were observed along the dorsolateral pathway and in the dorsal root ganglia. c. At the level of the 22nd somite, DiI-labeled cells were seen along the dorsolateral pathway, in the dorsal root ganglia, and in the sympathetic ganglia. d–f From the level of the 38th somite to the caudal end of the embryo, DiI-labeled cells were observed in all truncal neural crest derivatives. (Reprinted from Serbedzija *et al.*, 1980, with permission.)

Baroffio *et al.*, 1988; Sieber-Blum, 1989). Cohen and Konigsberg (1975) first isolated single trunk neural crest cells that proliferated in culture to form clones, in which all cells were descended from the same precursor. Under the culture conditions used in their study, they found three types of clones: all pigmented, all unpigmented, and mixed pigmented and unpigmented. Sieber-Blum and Cohen (1980) later showed that the mixed clones could give rise to both pigmented cells (melanocytes) and adrenergic cells (sympathetic neuroblasts). These results were the first to suggest that the progeny of individual neural crest cells could have more than one fate. These experiments have recently been extended to demonstrate that single neural crest cells can give rise to adrenergic, sensory-like, and pigmented cells, again supporting the notion that some premigratory neural crest cells are multipotent (Sieber-Blum, 1989).

Cranial neural crest cells also have been studied by clonal analysis *in vitro*. Baroffio *et al.* (1988) have used 3T3 feeder layers to support the survival of cloned cranial neural crest cells. Under their culture conditions, they find clones of many different sizes, as small as a few cells or as large as 20,000. Some clones contained only neural cells; others had mixed derivatives as diverse as neurons and cartilage (Baroffio *et al.*, 1991). The results suggest that some cranial neural crest cells are multipotent and can give rise to quite divergent derivatives.

These *in vitro* experiments, however, do not rule out the possibility that other neural crest cells are predetermined. One potential problem with *in vitro* experiments is that cells may behave differently in culture than they do in the intact embryo. Thus, such data can be interpreted only as a suggestive of the potential of neural crest cells *in situ* because of influences of the tissue culture environment. It is important to complement *in vitro* experiments with a prospective cell lineage analysis in the intact embryo.

Another means of testing the developmental potential of neural crest cells is to mark individual cells *in situ* so their descendants can be uniquely identified. Two methods have emerged recently for the study of cell lineage in the nervous system: (1) introduction of a marker gene by infection with limiting dilutions of a replication incompetent retrovirus (Sanes *et al.*, 1986; Turner and Cepko, 1987) and (2) microinjection of individual cells with lineage tracers such as lysinated fluorescent dextran (Gimlich and Braun, 1986) or horseradish peroxidase (HRP) (Weisblat *et al.*, 1978). Unfortunately, retroviral markers are not appropriate for a widely dispersing cell type such as the neural crest (reviewed in Lumsden, 1989), since the classification of a group of retrovirally labeled cells as clonal requires that the marked cells remain coherent. In contrast, intracellular microinjection of vital fluorescent dyes or HRP offers a method for directly labeling individual cells and their progeny in the developing vertebrate nervous system (Wetts and Fraser, 1988; Holt *et al.*, 1988). Observation of the fluorescent dye in living cells permits direct confirmation that a single cell was labeled and of the cell's position in the embryo at a variety of developmental stages (cf. Wetts and Fraser, 1988).

To analyze the developmental potential of individual neural crest cells or their precursors, we have microinjected a vital dye, lysinated rhodamine dextran (LRD), intracellularly into the dorsal portion of the neural tube that contains premigratory neural crest cells (Bronner-Fraser and Fraser, 1988,1989). Immediately after injection, it was possible to confirm that a single cell had been labeled (Fig. 6a). Embryos were allowed to survive for up to 2 days after injection (total incubation time of 4.5 days), by which time neural-crest-derived dorsal root and sympathetic ganglia had formed. The phenotypes of the descendants that inherited the LRD from the injected cells were evaluated based on their position, morphology, and neurofilament expression (Fig. 6). By 2 days after injection, the LRD-labeled clones contained from 2 to 73 cells that were distributed bilaterally in about one-third of the embryos. Individual labeled precursors gave rise to both sensory (Fig. 7) and sympathetic neurons (neurofilament-positive), cells with the morphological characteristics of Schwann cells or pigment cells (neurofilament-negative), and other nonneuronal cells (neurofilament-negative)(Table 2). Furthermore, analysis of neurofilament immunoreactivity demonstrated that a single labeled precursor contributed to both neural-crest- and neural-tube-derived neurons. These data show that (1) premigratory neural crest cells have the ability to assume multiple fates in neural crest derivatives, and (2) the neural crest is not a segregated population in the neural tube, but shares a common lineage with some neural tube cells.

These analyses have been extended to label emigrating neural crest cells with LRD as they emerge from the neural tube or migrating neural crest cells in the rostral sclerotome. About half the clones derived from emigrating or migrating neural crest cells had progeny in multiple neural crest derivatives. Even in a single derivative, both neurofilament-positive and -negative labeled cells were observed (Bronner-Fraser and Fraser, 1989; Fraser and Bronner-Fraser, 1991). These data demonstrate that both migrating, emigrating, and premigratory trunk neural crest cells can be multipotent, giving rise not only to cells in multiple neural crest derivatives, but also to both neuronal and nonneuronal elements in a given derivative. Although these studies suggest that many premigratory and migrating neural crest cells have the potential to form multiple cell types, we cannot rule out the possibility that some neural crest cells are more restricted or even predetermined in their prospective fates.

Cell death represents one mechanism by which clonally related cells in certain derivatives, some of which may have differentiated inappropriately for their sites of localization, may be eliminated. Naturally occurring cell death occurs after the stages at which embryos were fixed in our study; for example, in dorsal root ganglia, cell death takes place between days 4.5 and 9.5 (Hamburger and Levi-Montalcini, 1949; Carr and Simpson, 1978). Thus, we cannot rule out the possibility that certain LRD-labeled cells may be eliminated at relatively late stages after their overt differentiation. Alternatively, some clones containing both neuronal and nonneuronal cells may eventually become completely neuronal with continuing neurogenesis in the embryo.

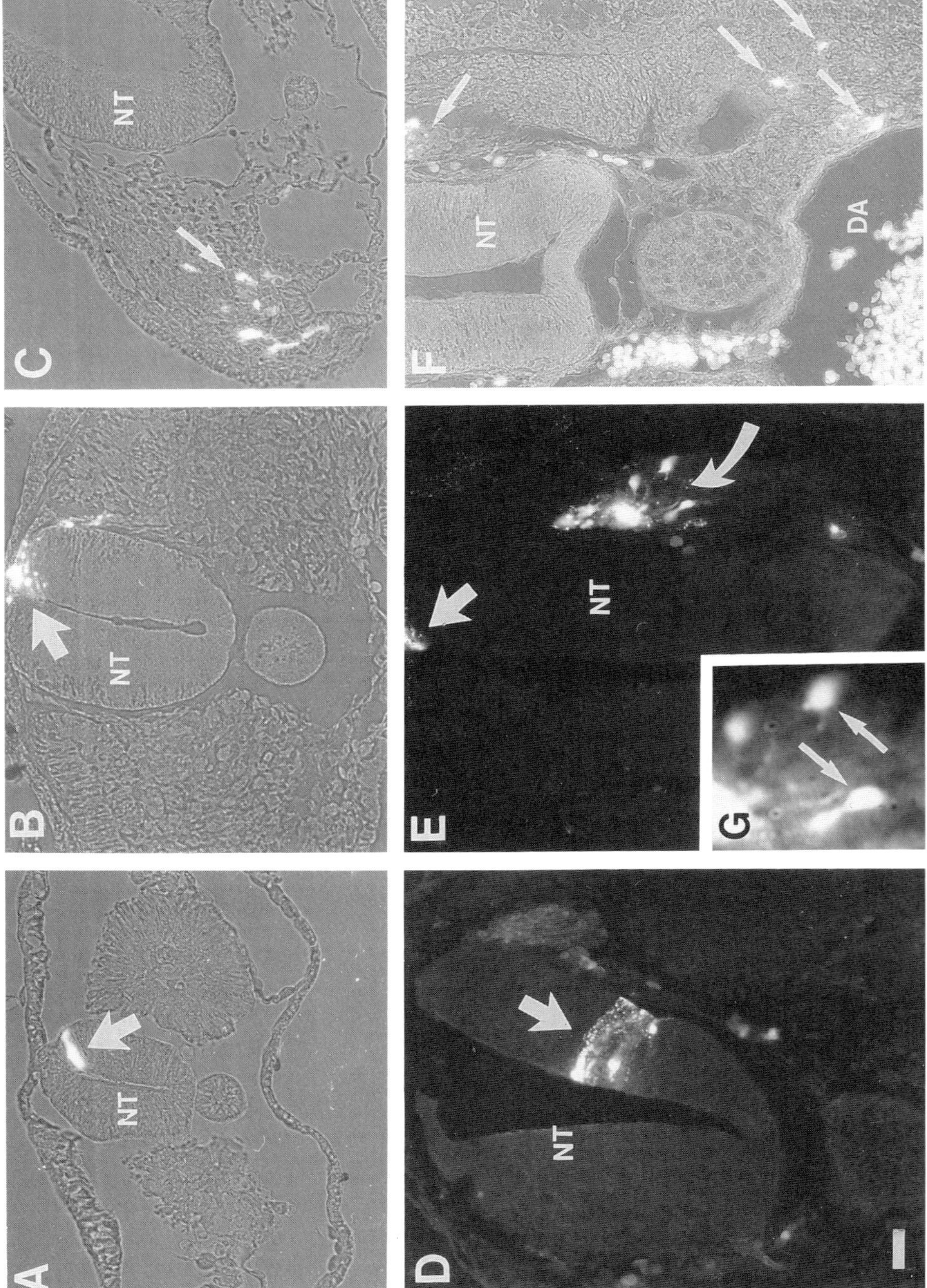

On the other hand, clones containing LRD-labeled cells in only one neural crest derivative cannot be considered "restricted" in prospective fate. First, the dye may be diluted to undetectable levels in some progeny, making it possible that apparently unlabeled cells are actually descended from the same progenitor. Second, the range of fates adopted by the descendants of a labeled cell do not necessarily reflect the full range of potential derivatives for that cell. Assuming that the sites occupied by clonal descendants is determined somewhat randomly, occasionally one would expect that all the descendants would distribute to the same site. Superimposed on this are nonrandom orderly patterns of neural-crest-cell migration, so the derivatives populated by neural crest cells become restricted in a ventral-to-dorsal order (Serbedzija *et al.*, 1989,1990). This increases the likelihood that the descendants of a single labeled cell occupy similar sites, and suggests that the descendants of any one neural crest cell (which, by definition, exit from the neural tube at a single stage) will be biased toward certain neural crest derivatives. Thus, one cannot conclude that an individual neural crest cell is "restricted" in developmental potential without perturbing the normal migration pathways or transplanting the progeny cells to a new locale to test the full set of phenotypes available to its descendants.

Figure 6. Photomicrographs of chick embryos fixed after injection of LRD into a single dorsal neural tube cell. A. Superimposed bright-field and fluorescence micrograph of an embryo fixed immediately after injection, showing a LRD-labeled neuroepithelial cell which spans the dorsal neural tube (broad arrow). B. Superimposed bright-field and fluorescence micrograph of an embryo fixed one day after injection of LRD into a trunk neural tube cell (somites 8 to 28). Some labeled cells remain in the neural tube (broad arrow), whereas others have migrated away (thin arrow). C. Superimposed bright-field and fluorescence micrograph of an embryo fixed one day after injection of LRD into a cell in the rhombencephalic neural tube (level of first somite). During the 24-h period, the labeled cell gave rise to approximately 70 progeny (thin arrow), suggesting that the injected cell had divided about 6 times; these were distributed in the cranial mesenchyme over 120 μm in rostrocaudal extent. D. Fluorescence photomicrograph of an embryo fixed two days after injection of LRD into a trunk-level dorsal neural tube cell. Labeled cells were only detected within the neural tube (thick arrow). The thickened regions of the individual cells appear to be the cell nuclei which move from the apical to basal surface and back during the cell cycle. E. Fluorescence photomicrograph of an embryo fixed two days after injection. Labeled cells were observed within the dorsal neural tube (thick arrow) and in the dorsal root ganglion (curved arrow), where many of the cells appeared neuronal, with large cell bodies and neurites. F. Superimposed bright-field and fluorescence micrograph of another section of the same embryo pictured in (E). In this section, LRD-labeled cells were observed both in the DRG (thin arrow) and around the dorsal aorta (thin arrow), where adrenergic neural crest cells localize. G. Higher power fluorescence micrograph of a portion of the DRG pictured in e, showing neurites extending from large cell bodies. The bright cells within the dorsal aorta and in other parts of the sections not marked with arrows are blood cells which autofluoresce brightly. NT, neural tube; DA, dorsal aorta. Scale bar: 25 μm in A, B, E; 30 μm in C, D, F; 10 μm in G.

TABLE 2
Distribution of Neurofilament-Immunoreactive Cells in LRD-Labeled Clones Contributing to the Neural Crest[a,b,c]

Class	Number of embryos	NT		DRG		VR		SG		Adrenal		PIGM	
		+	−	+	−	+	−	+	−	+	−	+	−
1	2			X	X								
2	6	X	X	X	X								
3	1	X	X		X								
4	1	X		X	X								
5	1	X	X	X									
6	1			X	X		X						
7	1						X	X	X				
8	1			X	X			X					
9	1				X		X	X	X				
10	2[d]			X	X		X	X	X				
11	1				X			X	X	X			
12	2		X	X	X								X
13	1		X	X	X		X	X	X				
14	1		X	X	X		X						X
15	1	X	X	X	X		X	X	X				
16	1		X	X	X		X	X	X	X			

[a]Reprinted from Bronner-Fraser and Fraser, 1989, with permission.

[b]+ indicates the presence of neurofilament-positive LRD-labeled cells; − indicates the presence of neurofilament-negative LRD-labeled cells.

[c]NT, neural tube; DRG, dorsal root ganglia; VR, ventral root; SG, sympathetic ganglia; Adrenal, adrenomedullary site; PIGM, prepigment cells underneath the ectoderm.

[d]One clone in each group was derived from an emigrating cell.

IV. Evidence for Subpopulations at Stages of Neural Crest Cell Migration

It has been suggested that some neural crest cells are restricted in their developmental potential. In culture, the heterogeneous nature of different clones has been interpreted to indicate that the precursors from which they arose were heterogeneous. Thus, clones containing multiple phenotypes were assumed to arise from precursors having a greater developmental potential than those containing single phenotypes (Baroffio *et al.*, 1988; Sieber-Blum, 1989). As described earlier, however, one cannot ascertain "restriction" of phenotype without challenging cell fate. Other evidence for "restriction" comes from the observation of molecular heterogeneity in neural crest cell populations; some neural crest cells bear different molecular markers (e.g.,

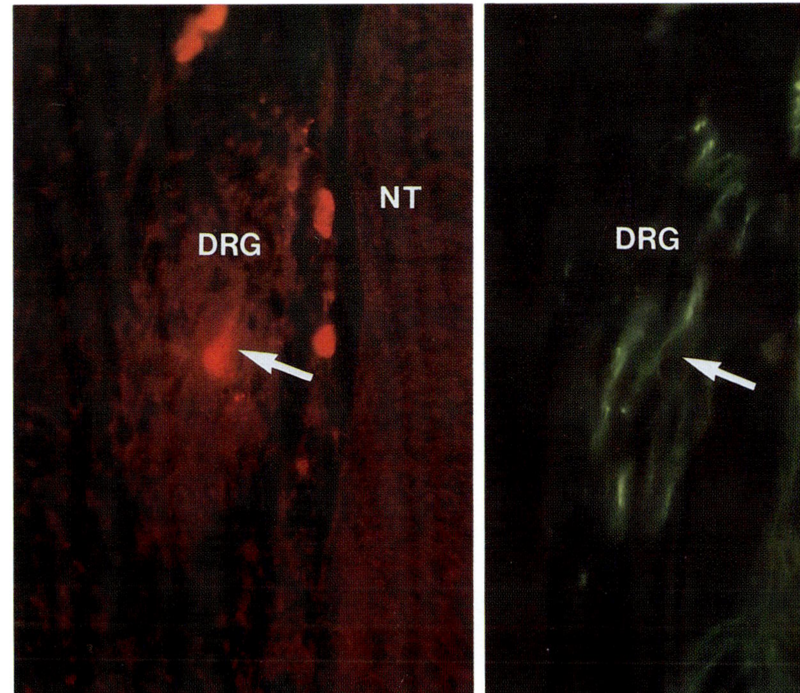

FIGURE 7. Distribution of lysinated rhodamine dextran (LRD)-labeled cells, viewed with a rhodamine filter set *(left)* and neurofilament immunoreactivity, viewed with a fluorescein filter set *(right)*. An LRD-labeled cell in the dorsal root ganglion (DRG) has a large cell body; it has a strongly neurofilament-positive axonal process as well as a few immunoreactive filaments wrapped around its nucleus. This same embryo possessed LRD-labeled cells in the neural tube, dorsal root ganglion, and presumptive pigment region. Reprinted from Bronner-Fraser and Fraser, 1989 with permission.

antigens, lectins) than other neural crest cells. However, heterogeneity of developmental potential is not necessarily equivalent to molecular heterogeneity. The possible heterogeneity in the neural crest will be explored next.

Based on the occurrence of some clones with a single cell phenotype *in vitro*, Sieber-Blum (1989) has proposed that a subpopulation of sensory neurons that retains processes connected to the neural tube may be determined quite early. This is consistent with the *in vitro* observations of Ziller *et al.* (1983), who found that sensory-like neurons develop in primary neural crest cell cultures during the first 24 hr. Because the neural-crest-cell cycle time is approximately 12 hr (Maxwell, 1976), this suggests that they may arise from neuroblasts that are postmitotic or in their last cell cycle in the neural tube. This population may be distinct from the common sensory/autonomic precursor suggested by grafting experiments (reviewed in LeDouarin, 1986). Similar clones containing a single phenotype have not been observed in the *in situ* cell lineage analyses of Bronner-Fraser and Fraser (1988,1989), although the possibility of their existence was not ruled out. Although no current cell lineage analysis can directly address the issue of predetermination of a minority of the cells, Bronner-Fraser and Fraser (1989) did find sensory neurons with central connections in the same clones as satellite cells of the dorsal root ganglion. This observation is consistent with the idea that commitment to a sensory neuron fate occurs after emigration from the neural tube.

Other evidence for heterogeneity in the cranial and trunk neural crest cell populations comes from studies using monoclonal antibodies that recognize only subpopulations of migrating neural crest cells (Ciment and Weston, 1982; Payette *et al.*, 1984; Girdlestone and Weston, 1985; Barbu *et al.*, 1986). This is particularly striking in the case of a subpopulation of mesencephalic neural crest cells that expresses an antigen characteristic of mature ciliary neurons (Barald, 1982,1988a). This antigen has been identified as the high affinity choline uptake protein and is expressed in approximately 5% of mesencephalic neural crest cells. It is not yet clear whether these cells uniquely give rise to cells of the ciliary ganglion. However, neural crest cells sorted on the basis of antibody immunoreactivity retain the antigen over several generations *in vitro*, suggesting that its expression is stable (Barald, 1988b). Neural crest cells fated to give rise to cholinergic neurons in other regions of the embryo do not express this antigen. Thus, there may be regional specificity in subpopulations committed to similar fates. Another subpopulation of migrating cranial neural crest cells expresses the NAPA-73 antigen, which is a neurofilament-associated protein (Ciment and Weston, 1985). These cells are found in the posterior, but not the anterior, branchial arches. Neural crest cells in the posterior branchial arch give rise to neurons, glia, glandular tissue, and connective tissue. In contrast, neural crest cells derived from the anterior branchial arch can only give rise to connective tissue. Neither of these populations can give rise to melanocytes (Ciment and Weston, 1985). Thus, these populations appear to be different from one another and restricted in developmental potential in comparison with early migrating cranial neural crest cells.

Selective isolations or depletions of neural crest cells bearing a particular epitope have been used to test the functional significance of subpopulations identified by particular antibodies. Such experiments have been performed on cultured neural crest cells (Vogel and Weston, 1988; Maxwell *et al.*, 1988) or their derivatives (Vogel and Weston, 1990a,b) and have led to the expression of a different range of phenotypes in neural crest cultures. The HNK-1 antibody, which recognizes a carbohydrate epitope present on many migrating neural crest cells and later primarily on neurons and neuronal support cells (Tucker *et al.*, 1984), and the A2B5 antibody, which is thought to recognize neural crest cells in a neuronal lineage (Girdlestone and Weston, 1985), have been particularly useful for these experiments. Selective cell sorting experiments with the HNK-1 antibody yield HNK-1-immunoreactive cells that can generate both melanogenic and catecholaminergic cells as well as HNK-1-negative cells that only give rise to melanogenic cells (Maxwell *et al.*, 1988). Immunoablation of neural crest cultures with the A2B5 antibody leads to depletion of catecholaminergic cells (Vogel and Weston, 1988). These experiments suggest a functional significance for the observation of subpopulations identified by particular antibodies. However, a heterogeneous antigen distribution tells little about cell fate unless it can be shown that antigenicity at early stages dictates a prescribed phenotype at later stages *in vivo*. Thus, antigenic or other molecular diversity does not necessarily indicate diversity in developmental potential.

V. Evidence for Neural Crest Sublineages at Postmigratory Stages

Although many migrating neural crest cells appear to have the potential to form multiple derivatives, their progeny eventually become committed to a single phenotype. Thus, their developmental potential must become restricted at later developmental times, perhaps in a stepwise fashion. This possibility gains support from the existence of some partially restricted neural-crest-derived sublineages at postmigratory stages.

The best-studied examples of a partially restricted neural crest sublineage is the sympathoadrenal sublineage, including sympathetic neurons, adrenomedullary chromaffin cells, and small intensely fluorescent (SIF) cells, all of which contain catecholamines (Landis and Patterson, 1981). Sympathoadrenal progenitors isolated from embryonic sympathetic ganglia or adrenal glands can differentiate into either sympathetic neurons or chromaffin cells, depending on the culture conditions. In the presence of nerve growth factor (NGF) these cells become neuronal, whereas in the presence of high levels of glucocorticoids they differentiate into chromaffin cells (Anderson and Axel, 1986). When grown in the presence of low concentrations of glucocorticoids, sympathoadrenal precursors differentiate into SIF cells (Doupe *et al.*, 1985a,b). Thus, both NGF and glucocorticoids in the local environment appear to influence the differentiation of sympathoadrenal cells. Furthermore, not only the proper molecule but also its local concentration may be important in determining cellular response.

In addition to the sympathoadrenal lineage, there may exist a glial lineage, derived from a glial precursor or a dual glial/pigment cell progenitor. Dorsal root ganglia (DRG) contain proliferating glial progenitors that are recognized by the O4 antibody (Rohrer *et al.*, 1985). Because glial cells fail to develop in DRG cultures from which O4-immunoreactive cells have been immunoablated, these antibodies may recognize a glial cell progenitor. It is not clear if this progenitor is uniquely fated to give rise to glia or if it can contribute to other derivatives as well. Some nonneuronal cells in ganglion cultures have the ability to give rise to other neural crest derivatives. For example, when DRG cells from 4-day-old avian embryos are grown in culture, some of the cells form melanocytes (Cowell and Weston, 1970; Nichols and Weston, 1977). This melanogenic ability is lost in 7-day DRG cultures. Both melanocytes and some nonneuronal cells in dorsal root ganglia possess the R24 antigen, which was originally raised against human melanoma cells (Girdlestone and Weston, 1985). These findings are consistent with the existence of a common glial/pigment cell precursor in the DRG, but we cannot rule out the possibilities that separate precursors exist for each lineage or that an undifferentiated nonneuronal cell exists that has the ability to give rise to melanocytes, glia, and perhaps other cells types as well.

The choice of final phenotype in each sublineage appears to be influenced by the cell's local surroundings. Thus, a sympathoadrenal cell becomes a chromaffin cell in the adrenal gland or a sympathetic neuron in a ganglion. Specific factors in these tissues, described in the next section, appear to direct the final differentiation of these cells.

VI. Role of Growth Factors in Neural Crest Cell Differentiation

It has been known for many years that the differentiation of neural crest cells can be influenced by surrounding tissues. The approaches for studying the role of tissues and specific tissue-derived factors in neural crest cell differentiation include embryonic microsurgical experiments, in which various tissues are grafted or ablated from regions containing neural crest cells in the intact embryo, and cell culture experiments, in which neural crest cells are grown in the presence of tissues, tissue extracts, or defined growth factors. For both paradigms, the ability of neural crest cells to differentiate into various derivatives is assessed. Microsurgical experiments have the advantage of examining factors present in the intact embryo, but are often difficult to interpret because of the complexity of the embryonic environment. Culture experiments, on the other hand, offer a more defined but less realistic environment.

Various tissues and tissue-derived factors are known to affect the expression of the adrenergic phenotype. Neural crest cell differentiation into catecholamine-containing cells can be elicited in organ culture by the ventral neural tube, notochord, and somites (Cohen, 1972; Norr, 1973); *in situ*, adrenergic differentiation appears to require signals from the periaortic region and the ventral neural tube or notochord (Stern *et al.*, 1991). The effects of these tissues can be substituted by high concentrations of chick embryo extract (Cohen, 1977; Howard and Bronner-Fraser, 1985,1986). This suggests that specific factors present in the embryo extract are sufficient to elicit adrenergic differentiation without the necessity of cell–cell contact. Extracellular matrix molecules can also enhance or stimulate differentiation of neural crest cells (Maxwell and Forbes, 1987,1990; Perris *et al.*, 1988). When axolotl neural crest cells are cultured on filters coated with extracellular matrix material derived from different regions of the embryo, pigment cells differentiate on filters coated with subepidermal extracellular matrix whereas neurons differentiate on filters coated with matrix from around the neural tube (Perris *et al.*, 1988). Because the matrix is well known to bind a number of growth factors, it is likely that these effects are the results of region-specific accumulation of growth factors associated with the extracellular matrix.

Defined growth factors are known to affect some neural crest cells and their derivatives. The best-studied growth factor, NGF, affects the maturation and survival of neural-crest-derived sympathetic and some sensory neurons (Levi-Montalcini, 1982) and can cause sympathoadrenal cells and differentiated chromaffin cells to elicit axons. However, NGF does not affect migrating neural crest cells (Anderson and Axel, 1986; Ernsberger *et al.*, 1989). What causes neural crest cells to differentiate into sympathetic neurons? There is evidence that fibroblast growth factor (FGF) may affect early neural crest cells. When immortalized sympathoadrenal progenitor cells (Birren and Anderson, 1990) or adult chromaffin cells (Claude *et al.*, 1988; Stemple *et al.*, 1988) are grown in the presence of basic FGF, they differentiate into neuron-like cells. With time, sympathoadrenal precursors change in their responsiveness to growth factors. These alterations correlate with some antigenic changes; for example, expression of the B2 cell-surface antigen in sympathetic cells occurs concomitant with a loss of sensitivity to glucocorticoids and the onset of NGF responsiveness (Anderson and Axel, 1986).

Both basic (Stemple *et al.*, 1988) and acidic (Claude *et al.*, 1988) FGF stimulate proliferation of chromaffin cells, consistent with the idea that they are mitogens for sympathoadrenal progenitors. Similarly, insulin-like growth factor (IGF) I is mitogenic for sympathetic precursor cells (DiDiccio-Bloom and Black, 1988). Other growth factors, such as ciliary neurotrophic factor (CNTF), have the opposite effect of causing withdrawal from the cell cycle (Ernsberger *et al.*, 1989).

Brain-derived neurotrophic factor (BDNF) appears to belong to the same family as NGF (Barde, 1989), based on amino acid similarity. BDNF induces sprouting of sensory ganglion neurons, an effect similar to that of NGF (Davies *et al.*, 1986). Early administration of either NGF or BDNF can prevent naturally occurring cell death in the dorsal root ganglia (Hofer and Barde, 1988), although the populations of sensory neurons supported by the two growth factors become nonoverlapping after E9. BDNF may be one of several neural-tube-derived factors that are important for the survival of precursors to sensory neurons. Removal of the neural tube from chicken embryos shortly after neural crest cells have begun their migration results in the disappearance of the dorsal root ganglion anlage, although the sympathetic ganglia differentiate normally (Teillet and LeDouarin, 1983). A similar absence of DRG precursors occurs if a silastic membrane is interposed between the neural tube and the somites (Kalcheim and LeDouarin, 1986). However, if the silastic membrane is coated with a neural tube extract (Kalcheim and LeDouarin, 1986) or with laminin and BDNF (Kalcheim *et al.*, 1987), many cells distal to the silastic membrane are rescued. Membranes coated with laminin and NGF do not rescue the sensory precursor, nor do membranes with laminin or BDNF alone. These results suggest that BDNF and laminin may partially substitute for neural-tube-derived factors in supporting survival of sensory neuron precursors.

Some factors appear to influence phenotypic expression in already differentiated neural crest derivatives. Leukemia inhibitory factor (LIF) has been shown to be equivalent to the cholinergic neuronal differentiation factor (Yamamori *et al.*, 1989). This factor is produced by a variety of nonneuronal cells, and causes adrenergic neurons to express cholinergic traits (see subsequent text).

In addition to neuronal lineages, some factors appear to enhance differentiation of other neural crest lineages. For example, α-melanocyte stimulating hormone (MSH) accelerates pigmentation in avian neural crest cultures

(Satoh and Ide, 1987) and a pigment-promoting factor (PPF) derived from fetal calf serum stimulates pigmentation in avian neural crest and mouse melanoma cell cultures (Jerdan *et al.*, 1985). Factors affecting Schwann cells have been described; although these cells are generally nondividing, they can be stimulated to divide by a factor derived from axonal membranes (Ratner *et al.*, 1985,1988) and by glial growth factor (GGF; Lemke and Brockes, 1984). Whether or not these factors affect Schwann cell precursors has yet to be established.

These experiments demonstrate that environmental factors can bias the differentiation of both early neural crest cells and neural-crest-derived sublineages. The experiments described next demonstrate that factors present in the local environment may be involved in the maintenance of the cell's phenotype in addition to influencing the cell's differentiation.

VII. Phenotypic Plasticity in Neural-Crest-Derived Ganglia

Even after overt differentiation, there is phenotypic plasticity in some neural crest derivatives; for example, the choice of neurotransmitter synthesis in neural-crest-derived neurons appears to be labile for a critical period, even in postmitotic cells (see Chapter 15). *In vitro*, superior cervical ganglion cells from newborn rats synthesize and store catecholamines under certain culture conditions; however, identical cultures grown in the presence of nonneuronal cells, or in medium conditioned by nonneuronal cells, produce acetylcholine and form cholinergic synapses (Patterson, 1978). During the adrenergic to cholinergic transition, some neurons have been shown to express both adrenergic and cholinergic properties simultaneously (Potter *et al.*, 1983). These results suggest that a factor (or factors) is capable of eliciting an adrenergic-to-cholinergic transition in these postmitotic cells. This factor has been purified from myocardial conditioned medium (Fukada, 1985) and is identical to LIF (Yamamori *et al.*, 1989).

Some evidence also exists for transmitter lability *in vivo*. In the rat footpad, the cholinergic sympathetic neurons of the sweat glands appear to undergo an adrenergic-to-cholinergic switch during development (Landis and Keefe, 1983). Early in development, the sympathetic fibers to the footpad are adrenergic; with increasing developmental age, their adrenergic properties are lost and replaced with cholinergic characteristics. A similar transition can be induced in adrenergic neurons that normally innervate the skin when a footpad is grafted ectopically into the skin (Schotzinger and Landis, 1988). In addition to alterations in norepinephrine and acetylcholine content, the levels of putative peptide neurotransmitters appear to be plastic in both embryonic and adult neural-crest-derived ganglia after denervation or explantation.

Is this phenotypic plasticity unidirectional (i.e., from adrenergic to cholinergic only) or bidirectional? As a first attempt to address this issue, LeDouarin *et al.* (1978) transplanted quail cells from the cholinergic ciliary and Remak's ganglia into the trunk of young embryos at an age at which endogenous neural crest migration was just beginning. The trunk is the normal site of origin for adrenergic sympathetic neurons and adrenal medullary cells. The transplanted ganglionic cells populated the host sympathetic ganglia and adrenal gland, and some of the cells synthesized catecholamines. Because intact ganglia contain many nonneuronal cells in addition to neurons, these experiments cannot distinguish between plasticity of phenotype and environmental selection for undifferentiated cells that may remain in the ganglia. When similar experiments were performed with chimeric nodose ganglia in which nonneuronal cells could be distinguished from the neuronal cells, it was clear that the nonneuronal cells became adrenergic neurons in the host embryos (Lelievre *et al.*, 1980). Subsequent experiments suggested that nonneuronal cells in the backtransplanted ciliary ganglia divide rapidly in the host, whereas neuronal cells do not survive (Dupin, 1984).

We have shown that cholinergic ciliary neurons can survive in the host embryo and that some of these cells become adrenergic in their new environment (Coulombe and Bronner-Fraser, 1986). The neurons were retrogradely labeled with fluorescent latex microspheres, the ciliary ganglia were dissociated, and the ganglion cell suspension was microinjected into the trunk region of 2.5-day-old chick embryos. The labeled neurons survived in the host and, 4 or 5 days after injection, some of them were found incorporated into host adrenergic structures such as the sympathetic ganglia or adrenomedullary cords (Coulombe and Bronner-Fraser, 1986). Similar results recently have been obtained with DiI-labeled ciliary ganglion cells (Sechrist *et al.*, 1989). A small number of the labeled cells contained catecholamine histofluorescence, demonstrating that previously cholinergic neurons acquired the ability to accumulate catecholamines in their new location (Fig. 8). Thus, some cholinergic neurons can "switch" to the adrenergic phenotype under the proper environmental conditions.

The phenotypic plasticity observed in several neural-crest-derived cell types suggests that a cell's lineage is not fixed but, at least in some cases, remains plastic during development and perhaps into adulthood. Factors present in the local environment are important for both directing and maintaining the differentiation of these cell types.

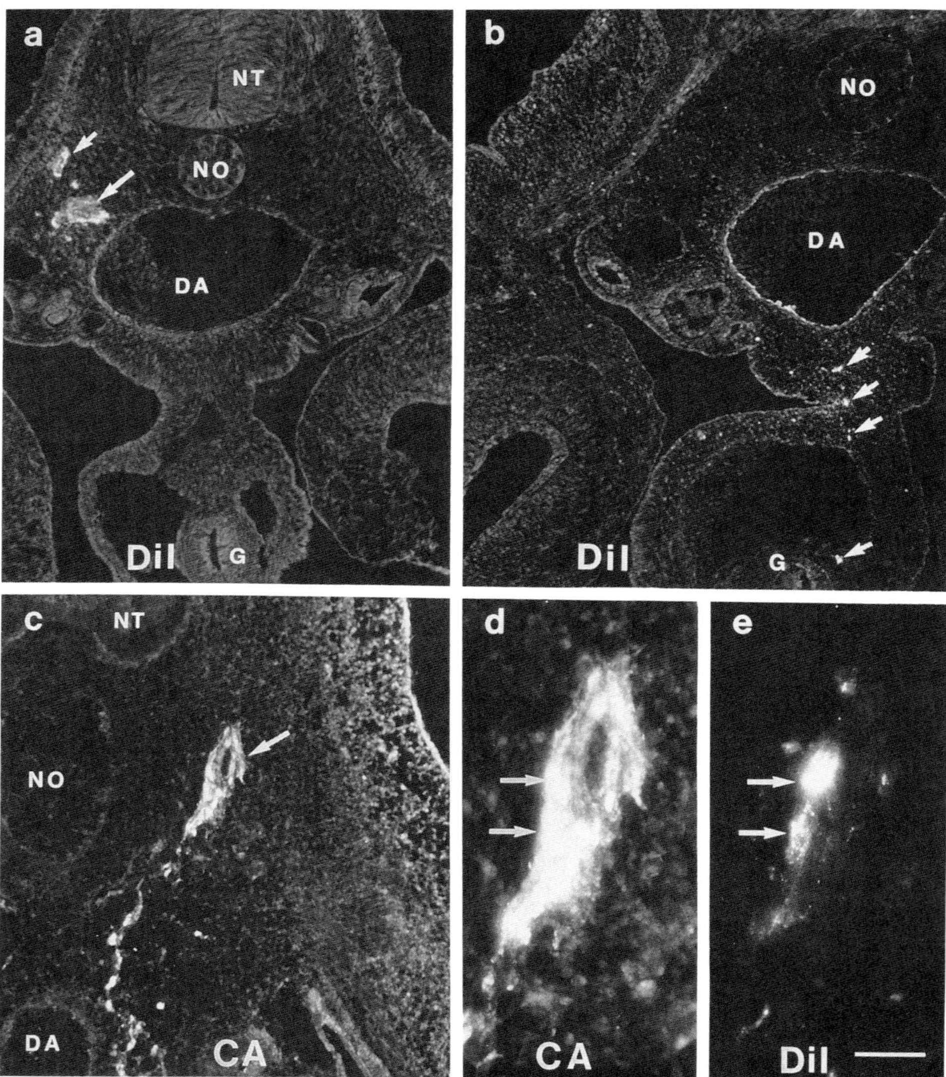

Figure 8. Transverse sections through chick embryos after injection of DiI-labeled quail ciliary ganglion cells. Embryos were fixed with an aldehyde mixture resulting in catecholamine (CA) fluorescence. a. Embryo 1 day after injection of 8-day ciliary ganglion cells into somites at the forelimb level; DiI-labeled cell aggregates (*arrows*) near the injection site were clearly visible in the sclerotome lateral to the notochord and dorsal aorta. b. Embryo 2 days after injection of 8-day ciliary ganglion cells into somites at the forelimb level; DiI-labeled cells (*arrows*) have moved below the dorsal aorta into the dorsal mesentery as far ventral as the gut. c. Embryo 2 days after injection of 6-day ciliary ganglion cells just

VIII. Conclusions Regarding Mechanisms of Cell-Type Segregation in the Neural Crest

An idea of how cell lineage segregation may occur in the vertebrate neural crest can be inferred from the collective data described in this chapter. Accumulating evidence suggests that the majority of premigratory and early migrating neural crest cells are multipotent in their developmental potential, both in the trunk and in the head. The potential derivatives arising from these multipotent precursors in the head and trunk are similar but not completely overlapping. Although the neural crest precursors in the trunk can give rise to pigment cells, neurons, and nonneuronal cells, trunk neural crest cells never form cartilage. On the other hand, a single cranial neural crest cell can give rise to cartilage and neurons. These multipotent progenitors are likely to be distributed uniformly at their respective axial levels. Intermingled with these multipotent cells may be minority populations that are more restricted in developmental potential. These "restricted" or "predetermined" progenitors appear to be most prevalent in rostral regions of the embryo (LeDouarin and Teillet, 1974).

Either during late stages of migration or in the vicinity of their final destinations, the multipotent precursors become committed to neural-crest-derived sublineages such as the sympathoadrenal lineage. The choice of sublineage, as well as the commitment to a single cell fate in a lineage, may be in part stochastic, but also appears to be influenced by signals present in the external environment. One exogenous factor is timing—the time at which a cell leaves the neural tube may limit its potential sites of localization (Serbedzija *et al.*, 1989). Another influence is dictated by molecules present in the local environment. These regionally restricted "growth factors" may affect proliferation, differentiation, or survival factors of appropriate neural-crest-derived cells. Other factors may be required for maintenance of the differentiated state, for example, the choice of neurotransmitter in some neural-crest-derived neurons. Although some factors that affect neural crest cell

---

caudal to forelimb level; catecholamine histofluorescence (violet filter) shows adrenergic cells forming a definitive sympathetic ganglion (*arrow*) and extending in a row ventrally toward the developing adrenal gland. d. Higher magnification of sympathetic ganglion show in c; arrows point to cells with catecholamine that are also labeled with DiI as shown in e. e. Note that the DiI-labeled cells include one that is weakly labeled and one that is small and brightly labeled; a larger bright cell just above the small brightly labeled one contains very little catecholamine. Bar: 100 μm (a–c); 40 μm (d, e). DA, dorsal aorta; G, gut; NO, notochord; NT, neural tube. (Reprinted from Sechrist *et al.*, 1990, with permission.)

development have been identified, little is known about their region-specific distribution in the embryo. Some or many of these may be associated with extracellular matrix molecules in defined regions of the embryo and may be produced by selected tissues surrounding sites of neural crest cell localizations.

One proposed mechanism of cell type diversification in the neural crest is by "neuropoiesis," in which a multipotent neural crest stem cell gives rise to a committed progenitor sublineage that finally differentiates into one of several related phenotypes (Anderson, 1989). This model is based on the principles of cell-type segregation in the hematopoietic system. In contrast to the permanently renewing hematopoietic stem cell, the proposed neural crest stem cell is short-lived. This hypothesis makes some testable predictions that deserve further exploration. In addition to cell lineage, other determinants, such as a neural crest cell's position and its pathway of migration, are likely to influence its differentiation.

The neural crest is a particularly intriguing system because of the diversity of cell types arising from a precursor population that appears to be relatively homogeneous. New techniques have recently become available to study the question of neural crest cell lineage. These include clonal analysis *in vitro* and *in vivo*, the production of immortalized neural crest cell lines, immunoablation and cell sorting of neural crest cells and their derivatives, and improved cell markers for identification of differentiated phenotypes. Such approaches promise to give new insights into the mechanisms of cell type selection in this unique population.

Acknowledgments

Parts of this work were supported by United States Public Health Services grant HD-25138.

References

Anderson, D. J. (1989). The neural crest cell lineage problems: Neuropoiesis? *Neuron* **3**, 1–12.
Anderson, D. J., and Axel, R. (1986). A bipotential neuroendocrine precursor whose choice of cell fate is determined by NGF and glucocorticoids. *Cell* **47**, 1079–1090.
Barald, K. (1982). Monoclonal antibodies to embryonic neurons. Cell-specific markers for chick ciliary ganglion. *In* "Neuronal Development" (N. C. Spitzer, ed.), pp. 101–119. New York: Plenum.

Barald, K. (1988a). Monoclonal antibodies made to chick mesencephalic neural crest cells and to ciliary ganglion neurons identify a common antigen on the neurons and a neural crest subpopulation. *J. Neurosci. Res.* **21,** 107–118.

Barald, K. (1988b). Antigen recognized by monoclonal antibodies to mesencephalic neural crest and to ciliary ganglion neurons is involved in the high-affinity choline uptake mechanism in the cells. *J. Neurosci. Res.* **21,** 119–134.

Barbu, M., Ziller, C., Rong, P. M., and LeDouarin, N. M. (1986). Heterogeneity in migrating neural crest cells revealed by a monoclonal antibody. *J. Neurosci.* **6,** 2215–2225.

Barde, Y.-A. (1989). Trophic factors and neuronal survival. *Neuron* **2,** 1525–1534.

Baroffio, A., Dupin, E., and LeDouarin, N. M. (1991). Common precursors for neural and mesecto-dermal derivatives in the cephalic neural crest. Development 112: 301–306.

Baroffio, A., Dupin, E., and LeDouarin, N. M. (1988). Clone-forming ability and differentiation potential of migratory neural crest cells. *Proc. Natl. Acad. Sci. U.S.A.* **85,** 5325–5329.

Birren, S. J., and Anderson, D. J. (1990). A v-*myc*-immortalized sympathoadrenal progenitor cell line in which neuronal differentiation is initiated by FGF but not NGF. *Neuron* **4,** 189–201.

Bronner-Fraser, M. E., and Cohen, A. M. (1980). The neural crest: What can it tell us about cell migration and determination? *In* "Current Topics in Developmental Biology," vol. 15, pp. 1–25. (R. K. Hunt, Ed.) New York: Academic Press.

Bronner-Fraser, M. E., Sieber-Blum, M., and Cohen, A. M. (1980). Clonal analysis of the avian neural crest: Migration and maturation of mixed neural crest clones injected into host chicken embryos. *J. Comp. Neurol.* **193,** 423–434.

Bronner-Fraser, M., and Fraser, S. (1988). Cell lineage analysis shows multipotentiality of some avian neural crest cells. *Nature (London)* **335(8),** 161–164.

Bronner-Fraser, M., and Fraser, S. (1989). Developmental potential of avian trunk neural crest cells *in situ. Neuron* **3(6),** 755–766.

Carr, V. McM. and Simpson, S. B. (1978). Proliferative and degenerative events in the early development of chick dorsal root ganglia. I. Normal development. *J. Comp. Neurol.* **182,** 727–740.

Ciment, G., and Weston, J. A. (1982). Early appearance in neural crest and crest-derived cells of an antigenic determinant present in avian neurons. *Dev. Biol.* **93,** 355–367.

Ciment, G., and Weston, J. A. (1985). Segregation of developmental abilities in neural-crest-derived cells: Identification of partially restricted intermediate cell types in the branchial arches of avian embryos. *Dev. Biol.* **111,** 73–83.

Claude, P., Parada, I. M., Gordon, K. A., D'Armore, P. A., and Wagner, J. A. (1988). Acidic fibroblast growth factor stimulates adrenal chromaffin cells to proliferate and to extend neurites, but is not a long-term survival factor. *Neuron* **1,** 783–790.

Cohen, A. M. (1972). Factors directing the expression of sympathetic nerve traits in cells of neural crest origin. *J. Exp. Zool.* **179,** 167–182.

Cohen, A. M. (1977). Independent expression of the adrenergic phenotype by neural crest *in vitro. Proc. Natl. Acad. Sci. U.S.A.* **74,** 2899–2903.

Cohen, A. M., and Konigsberg, I. R. (1975). A clonal approach to the problem of neural crest determination. *Dev. Biol.* **46,** 262–280.

Cowell, L., and Weston, J. A. (1970). An analysis of melanogenesis in cultured chick embryo spinal ganglia. *Dev. Biol.* **22,** 670–697.

Coulombe, J. N., and Bronner-Fraser, M. E. (1986). Cholinergic neurones acquire adrenergic neurotransmitters when transplanted into an embryo. *Nature (London)* **324,** 569–572.

Davies, A. M., Thoenen, H. and Barde, Y. A. (1986). The response of chick sensory neurons to brain-derived neurotrophic factor *J. Neurosci.* **6(7),** 1897–1904.

DiCiccio-Bloom, E., and Black, I. B. (1988). Insulin growth factors regulate the mitotic cycle in cultured rat sympathetic neurons. *Proc. Natl. Acad. Sci. U.S.A.* **85,** 4066–4070.

Doupe, A. J., Landis, S. C., and Patterson, P. H. (1985a). Environmental influences in the development of neural crest derivatives: Glucocorticoids, growth factors, and chromaffin cell plasticity. *J. Neurosci.* **5,** 2119–2142.

Doupe, A. J., Landis, S. C., and Patterson, P. H. (1985b). Small intensely fluorescent cells in culture: Role of glucocorticoids and growth factors in their development and interconversions with other neural crest derivatives. *J. Neurosci.* **5,** 2143–2160.

Dupin, E. (1984). Cell division in the ciliary ganglion of quail embryos *in situ* and after back transplantation into the neural crest migration pathways of chick embryos *Dev. Biol.* **105,** 288–299.

Ernsberger, U., Sendtner, M., and Rohrer, H. (1989). Proliferation and differentiation of embryonic chick sympathetic neurons: Effects of ciliary neurotrophic factor. *Neuron* **2,** 1275–1284.

Fraser, S. E., and Bronner-Fraser, M. (1991). Migrating neural crest cells in the trunk of the avian embryo are multipotent. *Development* **112,** 913–920.

Fukada, K. (1985). Purification and partial characterization of a cholinergic neuronal differentiation factor. *Proc. Natl. Acad. Sci. U.S.A.* **82,** 8795–8799.

Gimlich, R. L., and Braun, J. (1986). Improved fluorescent compounds for tracing cell lineage. *Dev. Biol.* **109,** 509–514.

Girdlestone, J., and Weston, J. A. (1985). Identification of early neuronal subpopulations in avian neural crest cell cultures. *Dev. Biol.* **109,** 274–287.

Hamburger, V., and Levi-Montalcini, R. (1949). Proliferation, differentiation and degeneration in the spinal ganglia of the chick embryo under normal and experimental conditions. *J. Exp. Zool.* **111,** 457–501.

Hofer, M. M., and Barde, Y. A. (1988). Brain-derived neurotrophic factor prevents neuronal death *in vivo. Nature (London)* **331,** 261–262.

Hörstadius, S. (1950). The Neural Crest: Its Properties and Derivatives in the Light of Experimental Research. New York: Oxford University Press.

Holt, C., Bertsch, T. W., Ellis, H. M., and Harris, W. A. (1988). Cellular determination in the *Xenopus* retina is independent of lineage and birth date. *Neuron* **1,** 15–26.

Howard, M., and Bronner-Fraser, M. (1985). The influence of neural tube derived factors on differentiation of neural crest cells *in vitro.* Histochemical study on the appearance of adrenergic cells. *J. Neurosci.* **5,** 3302–3309.

Howard, M., and Bronner-Fraser, M. (1986). Neural tube derived factors influence the differentiation of neural crest cell *in vitro:* Effects on activity of neurotransmitter biosynthetic enzymes. *Dev. Biol.* **117,** 45–54.

Jerdan, J. A., Varner, M. M., Greenberg, J. H., Horn, V. J., and Martin, G. R. (1985). Isolation and characterization of a factor from calf serum that promotes the pigmentation of embryonic and transformed melanocytes. *J. Cell Biol.* **100,** 1493–1498.

Kalcheim, C., and LeDouarin, N. M. (1986). Requirement of a neural tube signal for the differentiation of neural crest cells into dorsal root ganglia. *Dev. Biol.* **116,** 451–466.

Kalcheim, C., Barde, Y.-A., Thoenen, H., and LeDouarin, N. M. (1987). *In vivo* effect of brain-derived neurotrophic factor on the survival of developing dorsal root ganglion cells. *EMBO J.* **6,** 2871–2873.

Landis, S. C., and Patterson, P. H. (1981). Neural crest cell lineages. *Trend Neurosci.* **4,** 172–175.

Landis, S. C., and Keefe, D. (1983). Evidence for neurotransmitter plasticity *in vivo:* Developmental changes in properties of cholinergic sympathetic neurons. *Dev. Biol.* **98,** 349–372.

LeDouarin, N. M. (1982). "The Neural Crest." New York: Cambridge University Press.

LeDouarin, N. M. (1986). Cell line segregation during peripheral nervous system ontogeny. *Science* **231,** 1515–1522.

LeDouarin, N. M., and Teillet, M. A. (1973). The migration of neural crest cells to the wall of the digestive tract in avian embryo. *J. Embryol. Exp. Morph.* **30,** 31–48.

LeDouarin, N. M., and Teillet, M. A. (1974). Experimental analysis of the migration and differentiation of neuroblasts of the autonomic nervous system and of neuroectodermal mesenchymal derivatives, using a biological cell marking technique. *Dev. Biol.* **41,** 162–184.

LeDouarin, N. M., Renaud, D., Teillet, M. A., and LeDouarin, G. (1975). Cholinergic differentiation of presumptive adrenergic neuroblasts in interspecific chimeras after heterotropic transplantations. *Proc. Natl. Acad. Sci. U.S.A.* **72,** 728–732.

LeDouarin, N. M., Teillet, M. A., Ziller, C., and Smith, J. (1978). Adrenergic differentiation of cells of the cholinergic ciliary and Remak ganglia in avian embryo after *in vivo* transplantation. *Proc. Natl. Acad. Sci. U.S.A.* **75,** 2030–2034.

LeLievre, C. S., Schweizer, G. G., Ziller, C. M., and LeDouarin, N. M. (1980). Restrictions of developmental capabilities in neural crest cell derivatives as tested by *in vivo* transplantation experiments. *Dev. Biol.* **77,** 362–378.

Lemke, G. E., and Brockes, J. P. (1984). Identification and purification of glial growth factor. *J. Neurosci.* **4,** 75–83.

Levi-Montalcini, R. (1982). Developmental neurobiology and the natural history of nerve growth factor. *Ann. Rev. Neurosci.* **5,** 341–362.

Lumsden, A. G. S. (1989). Multipotent cells in the avian neural crest. *Trends Neurosci.* **12,** 81–83.

Maxwell, G. D. (1976). Cell cycle changes during neural crest cell differentiation *in vitro. Dev. Biol.* **49,** 66–79.

Maxwell, G. D., and Forbes, M. E. (1987). Exogenous basement membrane-like matrix stimulates adrenergic development in avian neural crest cultures. *Development* **101,** 767–776.

Maxwell, G. D., Forbes, M. E., and Christie, D. S. (1988). Analysis of the developmental and cellular subsets present in the neural crest using cell sorting and cell culture. *Neuron* **1,** 557–568.

Maxwell, G. D., and Forbes, M. E. (1990). The phenotypic response of cultured quail trunk neural crest cells to a reconstituted basement membrane-like matrix is specific. *Dev. Biol.* **141,** 233–237.

Nichols, D. H., and Weston, J. A. (1977). Melanogenesis in cultures of peripheral nervous tissue. I. The origin and prospective fate of cells giving rise to melanocytes. *Dev. Biol.* **60,** 226–237.

Noden, D. M. (1975). An analysis of the migratory behavior of avian cephalic neural crest cells. *Dev. Biol.* **42,** 106–130.

Norr, S. C. (1973). *In vitro* analysis of sympathetic neuron differentiation from chick neural crest cells. *Dev. Biol.* **34,** 16–38.

Patterson, P. H. (1978). Environmental determination of autonomic neurotransmitter functions. *Ann. Rev. Neurosci.* **1,** 1–17.

Payette, R. F., Bennett, G. S., and Gershon, M. D. (1984). Neurofilament expression in vagal neural crest-derived precursors of enteric neurons. *Dev. Biol.* **105,** 273–287.

Perris, R., von Boxberg, Y., and Löfberg, J. (1988). Local embryonic matrices determine region-specific phenotypes in neural crest cells. *Science* **241,** 86–89.

Potter, D. D., Landis, S. C., Matsumoto, S. G., and Furshpan, E. J. (1983). Synaptic functions in rat sympathetic neurons in microcultures. II. Adrenergic/cholinergic dual status and plasticity. *J. Neurosci.* **6,** 1080–1090.

Ratner, N., Bunge, R. P., and Glaser, L. (1985). A neuronal cell surface heparan sulfate proteoglycan is required for dorsal root ganglion neuron stimulation of Schwann cell proliferation. *J. Cell Biol.* **101,** 744–754.

Ratner, N., Hong, D., Lieberman, M. A., Bunge, R. P., and Glaser, L. (1988). The neuronal cell-surface molecule mitogenic for Schwann cells is a heparin-binding protein. *Proc. Natl. Acad. Sci. U.S.A.* **85,** 6992–6996.

Rickmann, M., Fawcett, J. W., and Keynes, R. J. (1985). The migration of neural crest cells and the growth of motor axons through the rostral half of the chick somite. *J. Exp. Morph. Embryol.* **90**, 437.

Rohrer, H., Henke-Fahle, S., El-Sharkawy, T., Jux, H. D., and Thoenen, H. (1985). Progenitor cells from embryonic chick dorsal root ganglia differentiate *in vitro* to neurons: Biochemical and electrophysiological evidence. *EMBO J* **4**, 1709–1714.

Sanes, J. R., Rubenstein, J. L. R., and Nicholas, J.-F. (1986). Use of a recombinant retrovirus to study postimplantation lineage in mouse embryos. *EMBO J* **5**, 3133–3142.

Satoh, M., and Ide, H. (1987). Melanocyte-stimulating hormone affects melanogenic differentiation of quail neural crest cells *in vitro*. *Dev. Biol.* **119**, 579–586.

Schotzinger, R. J., and Landis, S. C. (1988). Cholinergic phenotype developed by noradrenergic sympathetic neurons after innervation of a novel cholinergic target *in vivo*. *Nature (London)* **335**, 637–639.

Sechrist, J., Coulombe, J., and Bronner-Fraser, M. (1989). Combined vital dye labeling and catecholamine histofluorescence of transplanted ciliary ganglion cells. *J. Neural Transplantation* 1(3,4): 113–128.

Serbedzija, G., Bronner-Fraser, M., and Fraser, S. E. (1989). Vital dye analysis of the timing and pathways of avian trunk neural crest cell migration. *Development* **106**, 806–816.

Serbedzija, G., Fraser, S. E., and Bronner-Fraser, M. (1990). Pathways of trunk neural crest cell migration in the mouse embryo revealed by vital dye analysis. *Development* **108**, 605–612.

Serbedzija, G., Fraser, S. E., and Bronner-Fraser, M. (1991). Pathways of sacral neural crest cell migration in the chick and the mouse. *Development* **111**, 857–866.

Sieber-Blum, M. (1989). Commitment of neural crest cells to the sensory neuron lineage. *Science* **243**, 1608–1611.

Sieber-Blum, M., and Cohen, A. M. (1980). Clonal analysis of quail neural crest cells: They are pluripotent and differentiate *in vitro* in the absence of non-crest cells. *Dev. Biol.* **80**, 96–106.

Smith, J., Cochard, Ph., and LeDouarin, N. M. (1977). Development of choline acetyltransferase activities in enteric ganglia derived from presumptive adrenergic and cholinergic levels of the neural crest. *Cell Diff.* **6**, 199–216.

Stemple, D. L., Maganthappa, N. K., and Anderson, D. J. (1988). Basic FGF induces neuronal differentiation, cell division, and NGF dependence in chromaffin cells: A sequence of events in sympathetic development. *Neuron* **1**, 517–525.

Stern, C. D., Artinger, K. B., and Bronner-Fraser, M. (1991). Tissue interactions affecting the migration and differentiation of neural crest cells in the trunk of the avian embryo. *Development* (in press).

Teillet, M.-A., and LeDouarin, N. M. (1983). Consequences of neural tube and notochord excision on the development of the peripheral nervous system in the chick embryo. *Dev. Biol.* **98**, 192–211.

Tucker, G. C., Aoyama, H., Lipinski, M., Tursz, T. and Thiery, J. P. (1984). Identical reactivity of monoclonal antibodies HNF-1 and NC-1: Conservation in vertebrates on cells derived from the neural primordium and on some leukocytes. *Cell Diff.* **14**, 223–230.

Turner, D. L., and Cepko, C. L. (1987). A common progenitor for neurons and glia persists in rat retina late in development. *Nature (London)* **328**, 131–136.

Vogel, K. S., and Weston, J. A. (1988). A subpopulation of cultured avian neural crest cells has transient neurogenic potential. *Neuron* **1**, 569–577.

Vogel, K. S., and Weston, J. A. (1990a). The sympathoadrenal lineage in avian embryos. I. Adrenal chromaffin cells lose neuronal traits during embryogenesis. *Dev. Biol.* **139**, 1–12.

Vogel, K. S., and Weston, J. A. (1990b). The sympathoadrenal lineage in avian embryos. II. Effects of glucocorticoids on cultured neural crest cells. *Dev. Biol.* **139**, 13–23.

Weisblat, D. A., Sawyer, R. T., and Stent, G. S. (1978). Cell lineage analysis by intracellular injection of a tracer enzyme. *Science* **202,** 1295–1298.

Weston, J. A., and Butler, S. L. (1966). Temporal factors affecting the localization of neural crest cells in chick embryos. *Dev. Biol.* **14,** 246–266.

Wetts, R., and Fraser, S. E. (1988). Multipotent precursor cells can give rise to all major cell types of the frog retina. *Science* **239,** 1142–1145.

Yamamori, T., Fukada, K., Aebersold, R., Korsching, S., Fann, M.-J., and Patterson, P. H. (1989). The cholinergic neuronal differentation factor from heart cells is identical to leukemia inhibitory factor. *Science* **246,** 1412–1416.

Ziller, C., Dupin, E., Brazeau, P., Paulin, D., and LeDouarin, N. M. (1983). Early segregation of a neural precursor cell line in neural crest as revealed by culture in a chemically defined medium. *Cell* **32,** 627–638.

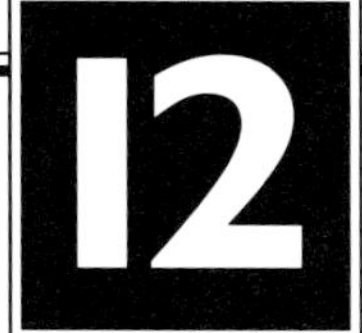

The Determination of Neuronal Identity
in the Mammalian Cerebral Cortex

Susan K. McConnell

Department of Biological Sciences
Stanford University
Stanford, California

I. Introduction

The generation of neuronal diversity in the nervous system stands as one of the most complex problems in developmental biology. The last decade has seen significant progress in our ability to explore these issues. Recently several advances have been made in weeding out the influences of intrinsic and extrinsic determinants of neuronal identity in the mammalian cerebral cortex, the seat of our highest perceptual abilities and cognitive functions. The cortex has long been considered an interesting and important area of the brain in its own right, and its development has garnered the scrutiny of such early pioneers of developmental neurobiology as Ramon y Cajal (1911). Over the past decade it also has become clear that the cortex presents an experimentally manipulable system in which basic questions concerning the mechanisms of neurogenesis and cell migration in development can be addressed: several of its features (shared with other layered structures, such as the retina and tectum) greatly simplify the study of basic developmental processes. The most important of these features is that cell types are highly organized, in both the radial and tangential domains of the cortex, into layers and columns, respectively. This organizational scheme results in a system in which the laminar position of a neuron is strongly correlated with its phenotype, as defined by its physiological properties, morphology, and axonal connections. The further finding that neurons in the different cortical layers are generated at distinct times during development has enabled us to begin to ask at what stage of development young neurons become committed to adopting their normal fates, and what influences act on the cell during its differentiation along particular developmental pathways.

In this chapter I will describe some of the initial efforts that have been made to understand the timing and mechanisms of neuronal determination in the developing mammalian central nervous system. One of the prerequisites of such an effort is that one is somehow able to predict the normal fate of an undifferentiated cell. The correlation found in the developing cortex between the birthday of a given neuron and its ultimate laminar fate has provided us with such a tool. Through a combination of cell lineage tracing experiments and transplantation experiments designed to challenge cells to change their normal fates, it is becoming apparent that cortical neurons are derived from a multipotent precursor cell. This cell appears to interact with its local environment around the time of mitosis to generate a committed neuron, one capable of migrating into the correct layer of cortex and forming axonal projections that are typical of its birthday.

II. Organization and Development of the Mammalian Cerebral Cortex

The cerebral cortex consists of the rind of neurons that covers the two cerebral hemispheres of the brain, and contains of many hundreds of thousands of neurons with a multitude of phenotypes and projection patterns. The neocortex is parcelled out into many functionally distinct areas that process different types of sensory inputs, perform associational tasks, or coordinate motor outputs. The cortical region about which we know the most is the primary visual cortex, also known as area 17 or visual area 1 (V1), the organization of which was explored initially through the groundbreaking studies of Hubel and Wiesel in the early 1960s (c.f., Hubel and Wiesel, 1962). Their and subsequent studies of the adult organization of the visual cortex have laid down an essential framework in which studies of the development of cortical neurons have been generated.

A. Organization of the Adult Cerebral Cortex

The first and central feature of cortical organization is immediately noticeable even on simple inspection of a section through the cortex, that is, that the cortex is organized into layers of neurons, with each layer defined by the density and morphology of its constituent cells. Neurons in each cortical layer tend to share several features with one another. First, they tend to have similar physiological properties. For example, in the visual cortex, "simple" cells predominate in the layers that receive direct thalamic input (layers 4 and 6) and layer 5 contains large numbers of "special complex" neurons (Hubel and Wiesel, 1962; LeVay and Gilbert, 1976; Gilbert, 1977; LeVay *et al.*, 1987). Second, neurons in a layer tend to share common morphological properties, although this is not a hard and fast rule. The middle layer, layer 4, is populated by a population of stellate-shaped neurons (Lund, 1973; Lund *et al.*, 1979) that are derived from cells that are initially pyramidal in shape early in development (Peinado and Katz, 1990). Projection neurons in the remaining cortical layers are pyramidal in form, but the characteristics of their particular dendritic morphologies vary from layer to layer. For example, as shown in Fig. 1, the apical dendrites of layer 6 corticothalamic neurons reach only into layer 4, but those of layer 5 corticotectal cells extend all the way into layer 1 (Lund, 1973; Gilbert and Wiesel, 1979; Lund *et al.*, 1979; Gilbert, 1983; Martin and Whitteridge, 1984). Presumably these differences reflect the manner in which these neurons gather and integrate presynaptic inputs along their dendritic trees. Finally, neurons in each cortical layer tend to share similar patterns of local and long-distance axonal connections. As a general rule for primary sensory areas, upper-layer neurons send their axons to other cortical areas, whereas deep-layer neurons project to subcortical targets (Gilbert and Kelly, 1975; Lund *et al.*, 1975; LeVay and Sherk, 1981; Katz *et al.*, 1984; Symonds and Rosenquist, 1984; McConnell and LeVay, 1986; McConnell, 1988a).

Figure 1 also provides a summary of the axonal targets of several classes of projection neurons in the mammalian visual cortex. The particular cells on which we have focused our own experiments are the corticothalamic neurons of layer 6, which constitute about half the total population of layer 6 neurons (Gilbert and Kelly, 1975; McConnell, 1988a), and the association neurons of the upper cortical layer 2/3, which sends axons to higher visual cortical areas such as areas 18 and 19 (Gilbert and Kelly, 1975; Lund *et al.*, 1975; Symonds and Rosenquist, 1984; McConnell and LeVay, 1986; McConnell, 1988a). It is interesting to note that the local intrinsic axonal projections of cortical neurons also vary by layer; these patterns may underlie the sequential processing of visual information from layer to layer (Fig. 1; Lund and Boothe, 1975; Gilbert and Wiesel, 1979; Gilbert, 1983; Katz *et al.*, 1984; Martin and Whitteridge, 1984; Katz, 1987). Layer 4 neurons, which receive the bulk of the primary thalamic input, project axons directly upward into cortical layer 2/3. The layer 2/3 cells send axon collaterals locally in layer 2/3 and down into layer 5. Layer 5 neurons project in turn to layer 6 (as well as sending a minor projection back into layer 2/3), and the layer 6 neurons provide a feedback input to layer 4, thus completing the circuit.

These studies of the normal organization of the adult visual cortex have revealed that, despite the overwhelmingly large numbers of cells in the cortex,

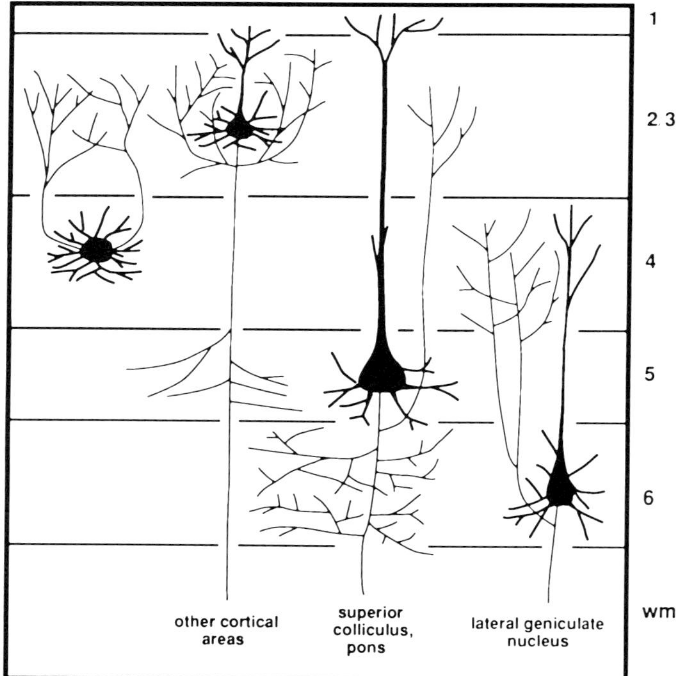

Figure 1. Local and long-distance axonal targets of the major classes of projection neurons in the primary visual cortex. Note that the many classes of inhibitory interneurons of the cortex are not shown. Abbreviations: wm, white matter. (Adapted from Gilbert and Wiesel, 1985.)

they can be broken down into a more manageable number of cell types as defined by the neuron's physiological properties, morphology, and pattern of axonal projections. What's more, these different types of neurons are neatly stacked one on top of another and segregated into separate layers. The final characteristic of the neocortex that makes studies of its development tractable is its columnar organization: roughly each millimeter of cortex contains all the cellular machinery required to analyze visual information from a small region of the visual world (Hubel and Wiesel, 1962). These columnar units are then reiterated to cover the whole visual field. The reiteration of a relatively small number of basic cell types somewhat compensates for the drawback in developmental studies that the cerebral cortex does not contain individually identifiable neurons, as are found in simple animals such as the nematode (Sulston and Horvitz, 1977) or simpler systems such as the spinal cord of zebrafish (see Chapter 14). Instead, the cortex presents a system in which a relatively small number of cell types is segregated into different layers, and each unit is repeated many times.

B. Early Development: Neurogenesis and Migration

Both the neurons and the glial cells of the developing neocortex are generated from a dense region of proliferating cells that lines the lateral ventricle of the brain (Fig. 2). This region is called the ventricular zone early in embryonic life (Boulder Committee, 1970). It contains a pseudostratified columnar epithelium of cells that cycle in a characteristic series of cellular movements (Sidman *et al.*, 1959; Fujita, 1963). Figure 3 shows that, in G1 of the cell cycle, cell nuclei occupy the middle of the ventricular zone. Nuclei move upward to the top of the zone (away from the ventricular surface) with the initiation of DNA synthesis in S phase of the cell cycle. As cells complete DNA replication and enter G2, their nuclei descend to the ventricular surface, where they proceed through mitosis to generate two daughters, each of which now re-enters G1 of the cell cycle. If one or both daughters then decide to leave the cell cycle and become forever postmitotic—the mechanisms by which this decision is regulated are entirely unclear—the cell is faced with the challenge of translocating its cell body out into the region called the cortical plate, which will become the layered cerebral cortex of the adult animal (Fig. 2). Migration in the cortex is accomplished with the aid of a special class of glial cells, the radial glia, which form a striking palisade of fibers extending from the ventricular to the pial surface of the brain (Rakic, 1971a,b, 1978, 1985, 1990; Rakic *et al.*, 1974). Young neurons associate intimately with radial glial cells during their migration, as they travel through the cell-sparse intermediate zone (which is also populated by both incoming and outgoing axons) and into

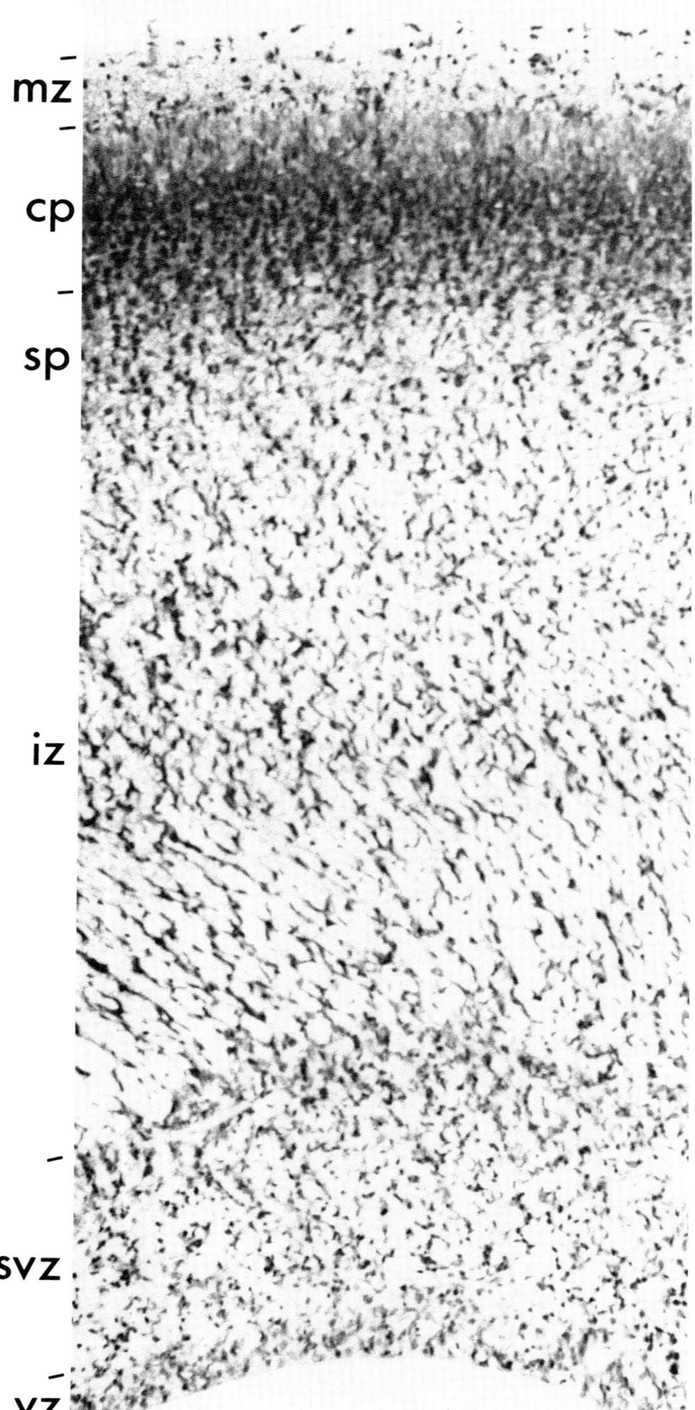
mz
cp
sp
iz
svz
vz

the cortical plate (Fig. 2). The elegant experiments of Hatten and co-workers (Hatten, 1990; Hatten and Mason, 1990) have demonstrated that the radial glial cells can support neuronal migration *in vitro*, and that neurons express a cell-surface molecule (or molecules) called astrotactin that both mediates the attachment of neurons to glia and is essential for the translocation of neuronal cell bodies along the radial fibers. In normal development, young neurons migrate out to the top of the cortical plate, where it borders the marginal zone or future layer 1; here cells detach from the radial glial fibers and subsequently complete their differentiation of dendrites and local and long-distance axonal projections (reviewed in McConnell, 1988b).

The time at which young neurons are generated can be marked by the simple technique of pulse-labeling with [³H]thymidine. If an animal is injected with [³H]thymidine, cells in S phase of the cell cycle incorporate the label during DNA replication. Because the [³H]thymidine is quickly metabolized, the label is available for only a short period of time, ranging from 10 min to 1 hr or so (Nowakowski and Rakic, 1974; Hickey *et al.*, 1983). Progenitor cells

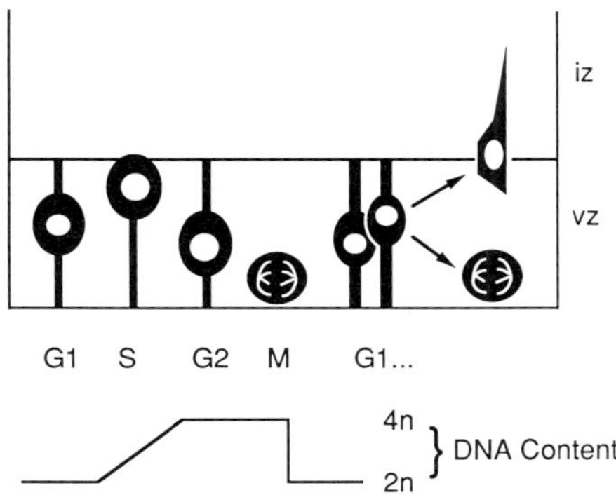

Figure 3. Summary of cell cycle progression in the embryonic ventricular zone. Cells in G1 have diploid DNA content. They translocate their nuclei to the top of the ventricular zone when they enter S phase and initiate DNA replication. In G2 (cells with doubled DNA content), nuclei move downward toward the ventricular surface, where they complete mitosis (M). Upon dividing, DNA contents are halved to diploid levels; one or both daughter cells may then become postmitotic and migrate radially toward the cortical plate. Lineage tracing experiments suggest that the predominant mode of cell division in the ventricular zone is asymmetric, that is, one daughter cell commonly reenters the cell cycle. Abbreviations: vz, ventricular zone; iz, intermediate zone. (Reproduced from McConnell and Kaznowski, 1991, with permission, copyright 1991 by the AAS.)

Figure 2. Organization of the developing cerebral wall in a neonatal ferret. Abbreviations: vz, ventricular zone; svz, subventricular zone; iz, intermediate zone; sp, subplate; cp, cortical plate; mz, marginal zone. The total thickness of the cerebral wall is about 1 mm.

then complete mitosis to produce two labeled daughters; however, any cell that becomes forever postmitotic at that point will remain heavily labeled with [^{3}H]thymidine, whereas any cell that re-enters the cell cycle will incorporate cold thymidine and progressively dilute out the label. These [^{3}H]thymidine "birthdating" studies of the developing cerebral cortex have revealed that, with one important set of exceptions, the cortical layers are generated in an inside-first, outside-last gradient of development (Angevine and Sidman, 1961; Rakic, 1974; Luskin and Shatz, 1985a). The first neurons to be born constitute the exception: these earliest-generated neurons leave the ventricular zone to reside in a single layer near the pial surface of the brain called the primordial plexiform layer or preplate (Marin-Padilla, 1971; Luskin and Shatz, 1985b). These neurons are subsequently split into two layers by the formation of the cortical plate. The upper layer is called the marginal zone and will become layer 1 of the adult animal. The deeper layer, or subplate (so called because it sits beneath the cortical plate), constitutes an extremely interesting population of transient neurons: the vast majority of these cells disappears in a wave of programmed cell death early in postnatal life (for review, see Shatz *et al.*, 1990). The genesis of cortical layers 2–6 follows and is characterized by an extremely orderly procession of cell birth, migration, and differentiation. The cells of the deepest layer, layer 6, are the earliest to become postmitotic and migrate out, inserting themselves between the nascent marginal zone and subplate neurons. With time, the cells of the more superficial layers are generated; the neurons of each layer migrate out to the top of the cortical plate, so the very last cells to be born and migrate are the neurons found in the uppermost layer of the cortical plate, layer 2.

III. Mechanisms of Neuronal Determination

This remarkable correlation between the time at which a neuron is generated and its ultimate fate (as defined by its laminar position and the related traits of cell morphology, physiology, and connections) raises several hypotheses about how cell fates might be determined. Any viable mechanism must account for the orderly production of neurons that are destined for distinct layers at different times during development. In general, there are two possible mechanisms that might contribute to the sculpting of different neuronal phenotypes. The first mechanism is that a cell might inherit some restriction of developmental potential from its parent or ancestor, in other words, cell fates are determined by patterns of cell lineage. In the cortex, one can imagine two possible variations on this theme. One variation on this mechanism is that separate pools of progenitor cell populations might sequentially give rise to neurons of the different cortical layers: different layers could conceivably be derived from different precursors that produce their progeny in a series of waves during development. If this were the case, one would predict that lineage studies would show that neurons in a particular layer are clonally related to neurons in that same layer, but not to neurons in other layers. Another variation on the lineage theme is that a common precursor generates the cells of all or several cortical layers, but does so by a preformed plan in which the postmitotic neuron generated in the first mitotic division becomes a layer-6 neuron, the second a layer-5 neuron, the third a layer-4 cell, and so on. In this scheme, the precursor is multifated (in the sense that it produces daughters that adopt a variety of fates) but it produces these different neurons according to a preset intrinsic "clock." The prediction generated by this hypothesis is that lineage studies would reveal that neurons in different layers are clonally related, and would show consistent patterns of clonal relatedness from column to column and animal to animal. Such invariability would be observed if the "clock" operated over a fixed sequence of mitotic divisions. One could also imagine, however, a determinative clock that runs on real time, in which any variability in the length of the mitotic cycle (between precursors or from cycle to cycle) would produce some variability in the laminar composition of individual clones. Thus variability in the composition of clones from animal to animal would not definitively rule out a role for cell lineage in fate determination.

The second possible mechanism by which cortical cell fates might be determined is one in which cortical precursors are truly multipotent, that is, that precursors have not gone through a lineage-based restriction of their developmental potential, but are naive with respect to the fates of their daughters. Thus, cell fates would be determined through interactions of these cells with their local microenvironment. In this scheme, the environment would provide an instructive influence on the progenitor or the newly generated neuron, and would actively signal the production of specific neuronal phenotypes at different times during neurogenesis. It is important to note that this model is consistent with finding either invariable or variable patterns of cell lineages. The former possibility is somewhat counterintuitive—that lineage studies might reveal apparently inherited restrictions of cell fate, but that lineage *per se* might not provide the mechanism that determines cell fate. The best example of this paradox has been found in studies of the nematode *C. elegans.* Observations of the early development of individual identifiable cells in the worm have revealed that patterns of cell lineage are, for the most part, completely reproducible from animal to animal (Sulston and Horvitz, 1977). These findings led several authors to the premature conclusion that lineage-based inheritance provides the mechanisms by which cell fates are determined in this simple creature. However, cell ablation experiments in several systems provided startling evidence that cell–cell interactions play a crucial and determinative role in the induction of specific cell phenotypes; the role of lineage is to put the cell in the right place at the right time for these interactions to occur (Greenwald, 1989). These and other studies have provided two important lessons for developmental biologists. First, clonally related cells need not be identical for lineage to play an important role in fate determination. In the nematode, cells as different as a neuron and a muscle cell can be derived from a common precursor. This precursor may be described as both multifated (since the fates of its two daughters differ) and committed (since, in many such cases, cell fates are intrinsically determined). The second lesson is that lineage studies alone provide insufficient information to distinguish between intrinsic and extrinsic influences on the determination of cell fate. To make this distinction, one needs to challenge the cell to change its normal fate—experiments that are accomplished by changing the local environment of the cell by ablating or mutating its neighbors, or by transplanting the cell into a foreign environment.

A. Tracing Cell Lineages

The genetic engineering of retroviral vectors as lineage tracers has revolutionized the study of early cortical development. For the first time it has become possible to directly test several hypotheses that have addressed the predicted lineal relationships and patterns of migration of cortical neurons (Rakic, 1978, 1989). Retroviral vectors provide a means of stably introducing foreign genes into dividing progenitor cells, so the progeny of these cells will reliably inherit and express the foreign gene (Sanes *et al.*, 1986; Turner and Cepko, 1987). Expression of this gene (usually the *lac Z* gene from *E. coli*, from which the enzyme β-galactosidase is derived) then serves as a marker for identifying clonally related cells at various times after the retrovirus has been injected into the developing nervous system.

Lineage studies of the developing cortex from several laboratories have provided evidence that clones commonly span more than one layer, and can even span all the cortical layers (Luskin *et al.*, 1988; Price and Thurlow, 1988; Walsh and Cepko, 1988; Austin and Cepko, 1990). This evidence suggests that cortical progenitor cells are multifated in the sense that they can give rise to cells that lie in several cortical layers. An important and fascinating exception to this general conclusion has apparently been found by Parnavelas *et al.* (1990), who asked whether projection neurons and interneurons share a common or separate precursor. Electron microscopy of β-galactosidase-labeled neurons revealed that most clones contained either pyramidal neurons or nonpyramidal neurons, but not both. These data suggest that two separate sets of neuronal progenitors, one for projection neurons and one for interneurons, may coexist in the ventricular zone.

Lineage studies also have shown that there can be wide variability in the specific laminar patterns of cells from clone to clone. In other words, lineage appears to be largely indeterminate in predicting the laminar fate of a neuron. This finding lends credence to the possibility that cell–cell or other environmental interactions play a central role in the determination of cell fates during cortical development, but makes no predictions about when or where such interactions might take place.

B. Transplantation Experiments

In classical developmental biology, cells are said to be committed to their normal fates if they continue to develop in a cell-autonomous manner following changes to their local environment, changes that can be generated by a variety of methods including cell ablation, mutation, or transplantation (Stent, 1985). We have chosen to take this type of manipulative approach to exploring the determination of neuronal fates in the developing cerebral cortex. In the cortex of higher mammals, such as cat, ferret, and primate, there is a powerful correlation between the birthdate of a neuron and its eventual laminar position (Rakic, 1974; Luskin and Shatz, 1985a; McConnell, 1988a,b; Jackson *et al.*, 1989). In the ferret, for example, the majority of neurons generated on embryonic day (E) 29 will migrate out to form deep-layer (subplate and layer 6) neurons (Fig. 4A), whereas neurons generated roughly 2 wk later on postnatal day (P) 1, will come to reside in the upper cortical layers 2 and 3 (Fig. 4B). One way of asking whether and when young neurons become committed to their normal laminar fates is to transplant cells into an older or younger brain in which the host cohort of neurons is migrating into a position quite different from that typical of cells being generated in the donor environment. Such experiments can address the question of whether progenitor cells at different ages are fully capable of producing any laminar phenotype, or whether the competence of precursors to generate specific layers changes over time. One can also ask whether newly generated neurons are committed to sitting in the layer typical of their birthday prior to the time that they initiate migration, or whether these young neurons are naive with respect to their eventual fates and are instructed by cues from the local microenvironment to adopt the position and connections typical of the new environment.

These transplantation experiments presented a significant technical challenge: in order to study the influences that might shape cell fates, it is

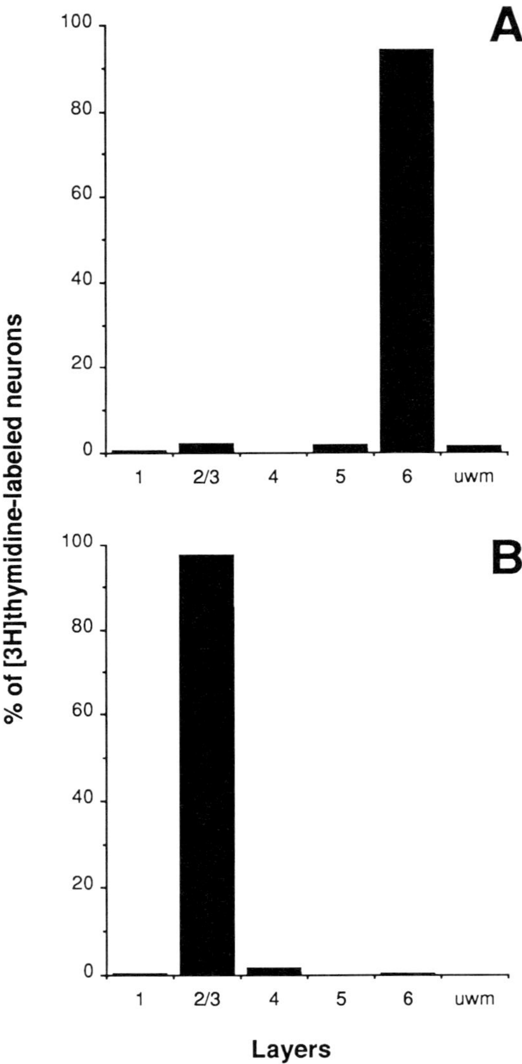

Figure 4. Laminar positions of neurons generated on (A) E29 or (B) P1 in the ferret visual cortex. Animals were injected with [³H]thymidine on the day indicated; their brains were processed for autoradiography in adulthood. The laminar distributions of heavily labeled neurons generated on these two days are nonoverlapping. It is worth noting that when animals injected on E29 are examined at younger (neonatal) ages, in addition to labeled layer-6 cells, substantial numbers of labeled subplate neurons are found (not shown). Presumably these cells disappear during postnatal life by cell death (Shatz *et al.*, 1991). Abbreviations: uwm, underlying white matter (the adult remnant of the embryonic subplate zone). [Fig. 4B is reproduced with permission from McConnell (1988a) *Journal of Neuroscience* **8**, 945–974.]

important to introduce young neurons into a brain in which they are fully subject to any environmental cues that might direct or permit normal development. Thus, in the ideal transplantation experiment, young neurons would migrate out into a foreign brain along host radial glial fibers and, in the host cortical plate, choose the layer in which to lie and which axonal connections to form. An initial set of "isochronic" transplantation experiments demonstrated the feasibility of this approach: presumptive upper-layer cortical neurons from a P1 ferret donor were prelabeled with [³H]thymidine, removed from the ventricular zone prior to migration, dissociated into a single-cell suspension, then transplanted back into the ventricular region of a neonatal host (see Fig. 5). These labeled neurons migrated out normally into the cortical plate of the host animal, where they assumed positions in layer 2/3 and formed axonal projections to visual association areas, just as they would normally (see Fig. 7A; McConnell, 1985, 1988a).

These experiments set the stage for performing the more interesting "heterochronic" transplants, in which presumptive deep-layer neurons are challenged to change their normal fates after transplantation into an older

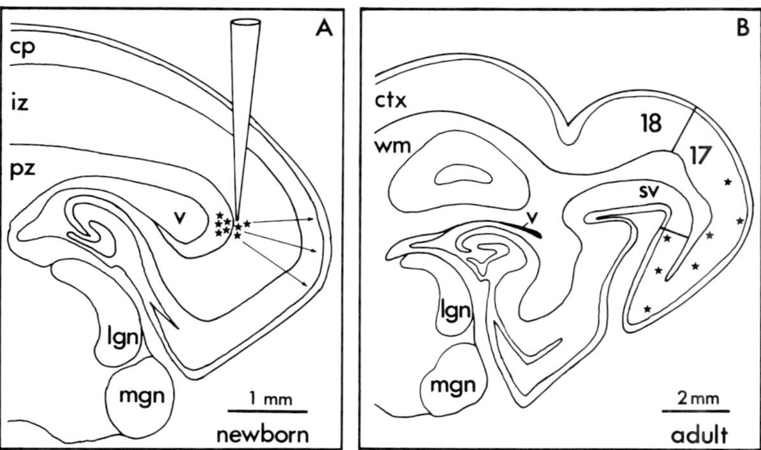

Figure 5. Methods for cell transplantation. A. Reconstruction of a neonatal host ferret brain, showing the pipette containing dissociated cells injecting cells (*stars*) into or near the host ventricular zone. Sagittal view, posterior to the right. The goal of the experiment is for transplanted cells to migrate radially (*arrows*) into areas of the host cortical plate that will differentiate into the visual cortex in the adult. B. The positions of transplanted neurons in the adult host brain can be determined by looking for cells heavily labeled with [³H]thymidine (*stars*). Abbreviations: v, lateral ventricle; pz, proliferative zone; iz, intermediate zone; cp, cortical plate; lgn, lateral geniculate nucleus; mgn, medial geniculate nucleus; wm, white matter; ctx, cortex; 17, primary visual cortex (area 17); 18, area 18; sv, splenial visual area. [Reproduced with permission from McConnell (1988a) *Journal of Neurosciece* **8**, 945–974.]

host environment (McConnell, 1988a; McConnell and Kaznowski, 1990, 1991). In these studies, donor ferrets were injected with [³H]thymidine either on E29 (when subplate and layer 6 cells are generated) or on E31/32 (layers 5 and 6). After various time intervals, which will be described more fully subsequently, the donor cerebrum was removed, dissociated, and the resulting cell suspension injected into the ventricular region of a newborn host ferret, in which the current cohort of newly generated neurons was destined for the upper layers 2/3. The two possible outcomes of such an experiment are summarized in Fig. 6. If the transplanted neurons are committed to the fates typical of their birthday, they should migrate out along host radial glia, recognize the deep cortical layers as their normal positions, and develop the subcortical projections appropriate for those layers. If, however, these cells are multipotent and the local environment has a determinative influence on their development, one would expect the cells to migrate out along with host neurons to the upper cortical layers and there develop the cortical connections appropriate for neurons generated in early postnatal life.

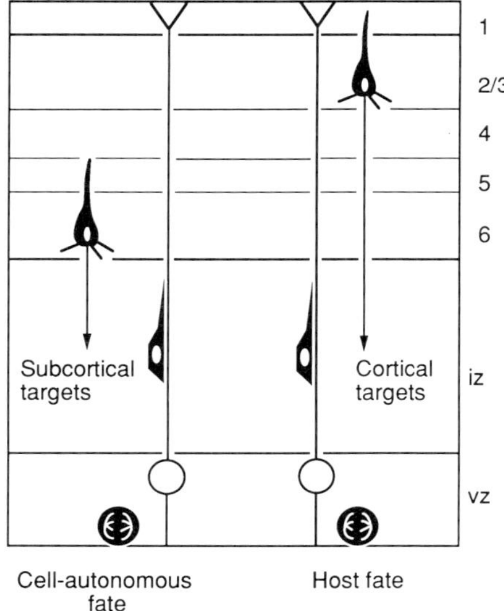

Figure 6. Two possible outcomes of heterochronic transplantation. (*Left*) Neurons committed to their normal fates at the time of transplantation should migrate to the deep cortical layers and form subcortical axonal projections. (*Right*) If environmental signals determine cellular identities, transplanted neurons should adopt the host fate by migrating to layer 2/3 and extending axons to cortical targets. Abbreviations: vz, ventricular zone; iz, intermediate zone. (Reproduced from McConnell and Kaznowski, 1991, with permission, copyright 1991 by the AAS.)

Results from the first series of heterochronic transplants, which are summarized in Fig. 7B (McConnell, 1988a, 1989), did not provide a clear answer to the question of when cells become committed to their normal laminar fates. We found about half of the transplanted neurons that migrated into the cortex in the deep cortical layers, positions typical of their birthday (cells were labeled on E31/32); the remaining half were found in layer 2/3, the position typical of the host environment. Strikingly, a majority of thymidine-labeled cells failed to migrate at all, remaining clustered near the lateral ventricle at the site into which they were injected (not shown). Despite the lack of a uniform choice made by transplanted cells, these results suggested for the first time the possibility that at least some young cortical neurons—those that ended up in the deep layers—were committed to their normal fates prior to their migration out into the cortical plate. In support of this conclusion, many of the transplanted neurons in layer 6 were shown to send axons to the lateral geniculate nucleus of the thalamus, an axonal target unique to the deep layers (McConnell, 1988a). However, the results of these first experiments also presented the possibility that some neurons (those that migrated to layer 2/3) were multipotent and could change their normal fate on transplantation to a new environment. The obvious question is, why didn't all the cells behave the same way in the transplantation assay? Our laboratory has been addressing this question over the last few years; we have found that the reason for the variability in laminar choices has to do with the interval of time between [^{3}H]thymidine labeling and transplantation, in other words, with the position of a cell in the cell cycle at the time of transplantation.

Our first hypothesis, which was laid out by McConnell (1989), was that the site of a precursor cell's final mitotic division plays an important role in determining cell fate. In the original transplants, we noticed that although the heavily labeled neurons could be found in either the deep or superficial layers, lightly labeled cells were always in the upper layers (McConnell, 1989). Of course, a cell that is lightly labeled with [^{3}H]thymidine must have re-entered the mitotic cycle after the initial [^{3}H]thymidine injection and completed an additional round of cell division (thereby diluting the label) before migrating out into the cortex. Because of the timing of the original experiments, these cells must have gone through that second mitotic cycle in the new environment—and all these cells changed their normal fates. This observation led to the hypothesis that the environment in which a cell divides determines its final fate. It predicts that if presumptive deep-layer neurons are allowed to divide in their original embryonic environment, and are then transplanted just prior to initiating migration, these cells should demonstrate a powerful commitment to their normal fate.

We tested this hypothesis directly by labeling E29 deep-layer progenitors with [^{3}H]thymidine, then waiting for 24 hr before removing the cells from the

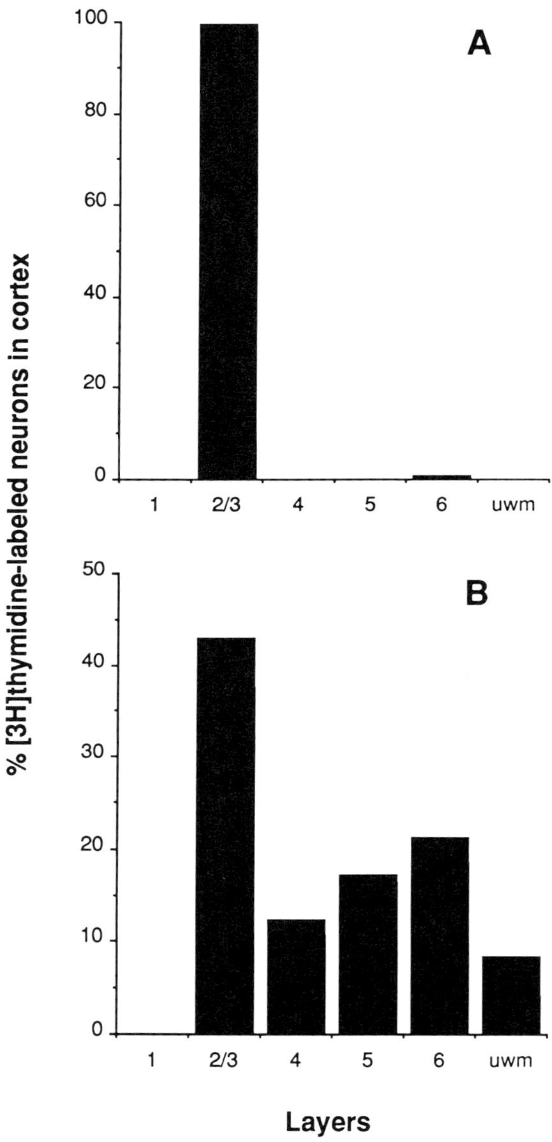

Figure 7. The distributions of heavily labeled neurons in the visual cortex of host brains following (A) isochronic transplantation of presumptive upper-layer neurons into a neonatal host (in which layer 2/3 neurons are being generated) and (B) heterochronic transplantation of cells labeled on E31 or E32 (presumptive deep-layer neurons) into a newborn host brain. A. In isochronic controls (n=383), neurons generated on P1 migrate normally into layer 2/3, their normal laminar position. About 97% of all labeled cells migrated into the visual cortex (not shown). B. In heterochronic transplants (n=273), E31 or E32 donors received four injections of [³H]thymidine spaced 1 hr apart, and were transplanted 1 hr after the last injection into newborn hosts. In contrast to isochronic controls, only about 20% of

donor brain for transplantation into an older environment. This 24-hr time interval between labeling and transplantation allowed progenitor cells that incorporated [³H]thymidine in S phase ample time to complete mitosis in their original environment (see Fig. 3). Thus heavily labeled neurons recovered in the host brain are cells that were newly postmitotic at the time of transplantation. In these experiments, the great majority of heavily labeled neurons that migrated into the host cortex were found in the deep cortical layers, positions appropriate for their birthday (Fig. 8D; McConnell and Kaznowski, 1990, 1991). These results provide strong support for our suggestion that the laminar fate of a cortical neuron is determined by the time that cell is born, in other words, that cortical neurons are committed to adopting a laminar position appropriate for their birthday by the time they initiate their migration to the cortical plate. Somehow this commitment results in a neuron that is capable of recognizing that position as it migrates and terminating its journey when it reaches that position. These results also imply that the termination of migration is an active process. The radial glia do not merely act as a conveyor belt that dumps out all young neurons at the top of the cortical plate; instead, neurons are capable of making active choices about the cells with which to group.

The next issue we considered was whether there was a time in the development of a given neuron at which it or its precursor was multipotent. In other words, is there an instructive role for the environment in the generation of specific neuronal phenotypes at different times during development? The alternative is that E29 progenitor cells are preprogrammed to produce only layer-6 and subplate cells at this age by employing some kind of intrinsic determinative "clock." To ask whether E29 progenitors are committed to producing deep-layer neurons, we performed another variation of the transplant assay. This time E29 progenitors were labeled with [³H]thymidine during a short period *in vitro*, and were immediately transplanted into a neonatal host brain. Thus, in this paradigm, the precursors themselves were transplanted while still in S phase of the cell cycle (see Fig. 3), and would therefore have to complete the rest of the cycle in the older host environment. Strikingly, the vast majority of heavily labeled cortical neurons that were derived from these precursors and migrated out into the host cortex switched their normal fates after transplantation; they were found in the layer appro-

---

heavily labeled cells migrated into the visual cortex (not shown). Shown is the laminar distribution of those cells that did migrate. This distribution was bimodal: about half the cells that migrated to the cortex apparently changed their normal fates and migrated to the upper layers 2/3; the other half of the cells were found in their cell-autonomous position in the deep layers, mainly in layers 5 and 6 (positions typical for their birthday). Abbreviations: uwm, underlying white matter (the adult remnant of the embryonic subplate zone). [Reproduced with permission from McConnell (1988a) *Journal of Neurosciece* **8,** 945–974.]

priate for host neurons: layer 2/3 (Fig. 8A). This result implies that the precursors of deep-layer neurons are truly multipotent, as suggested by the cell lineage studies. They are capable of producing either deep-layer or upper-layer neurons, depending on the environment in which they divide. [An important caveat here is that we do not know yet whether the axonal connections of these transplanted neurons in the upper layers are typical of the new environment. It remains a possibility that, like neurons in the *reeler* mouse (a mutation that perturbs the normal lamination of the cortex; Caviness, 1976, 1982; Dräger, 1981; Lemmon and Pearlman, 1981), neurons may maintain axonal connections appropriate for their birthday although they lie in ectopic laminar positions.]

The question now arises, who makes the decision to be a deep-layer neuron, the newly generated neuron itself (just after its final mitotic division) or the progenitor cell (at some point prior to mitosis)? We have recently addressed this issue using two separate techniques: transplantation assays similar to those already described, and flow cytometry to ascertain the DNA content of labeled cells as they progress through the cell cycle.

First, a series of transplantation experiments was performed to try to pinpoint the timing of neuronal commitment. The experiments described earlier show that cells become committed at some time between 0 and 24 hr after being labeled with [3H]thymidine. It is worth making the point here that the [3H]thymidine labeling provides a fortunate additional benefit: cortical progenitors cycle asynchronously, yet only cells in the process of DNA replication incorporate [3H]thymidine. Thus thymidine labeling provides a means of looking at a subpopulation of progenitor cells that are in rough synchrony by virtue of having been in S phase at the time of the injection. We asked when these cells become committed to making deep-layer neurons by labeling donor animals with [3H]thymidine at time 0, then waiting various intervals of time (2 hr, 4 hr, 8 hr, etc.) to allow the cells to progress through the cycle before removing and transplanting them. The results of these experiments are shown in Fig. 8B,C. By only 4 hr after [3H]thymidine labeling, cells are committed to a deep-layer fate. [This finding coincides perfectly with the results of the first set of heterochronic transplants in which cells assumed a bimodal distribution (Fig. 7B). In those experiments, cells were given four [3H]thymidine injections over 4 hr and were then removed and transplanted; the bimodal distribution correlates with the more recent finding that cells at time 0 are uncommitted, whereas cells at 4 hr are committed.]

If cells transplanted at 4 hr after [3H]thymidine labeling are committed to a deep-layer phenotype, who makes this decision—the progenitor cell itself or the newly generated cortical neuron just after mitosis? We could answer this question if we knew the DNA content of [3H]thymidine-labeled cells 4 hr after labeling. The following section maps out the strategy for addressing this issue,

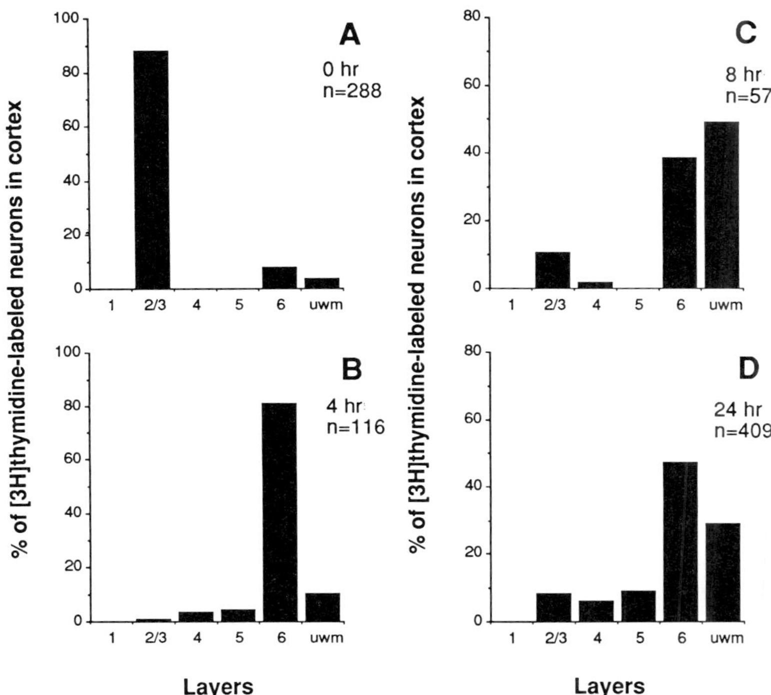

Figure 8. Histograms of the laminar positions of heavily labeled neurons that were labeled with [³H]thymidine on E29, and were removed and transplanted into newborn hosts at four different times after labeling: (A) 0 hr; (B) 4 hr; (C) 8 hr; (D) 24 hr. Cells transplanted immediately after thymidine labeling are multipotent, but at later times have undergone a commitment to a deep-layer fate. The fraction of neurons found in the subplate rather than in layer 6 (uwm) in B–D is variable, but both of these layers constitute normal destinations of neurons generated on E29. The variability between experiments might be explained by small variations in dating the gestational age of the donors (± 1 day), which would affect the fraction of subplate neurons being generated. Furthermore, because subplate neurons go through a substantial period of cell death in the first few months of postnatal life, differences in the time of sacrifice of host animals could affect the fraction of subplate neurons recovered. Abbreviations: uwm, underlying white matter (the adult remnant of the embryonic subplate zone). (Reproduced from McConnell and Kaznowski, 1991, with permission, copyright 1991 by the AAS.)

and provides evidence that the cortical progenitor cell makes the commitment to generating a deep-layer neuron prior to mitosis.

C. Cell Cycle Kinetics

Figure 3 provides a reminder of how progenitor cells progress through the cell cycle and how their DNA content varies with different stages. Cells in

G1 have normal diploid DNA contents. During S phase, through the process of DNA replication, they gradually increase this level, so in G2 and just prior to mitosis the cells have doubled their DNA content. If one knew that the DNA content of cells labeled with [³H]thymidine at 4 hr after the pulse (i.e., committed cells) was the normal diploid level, then one would conclude that commitment was likely to occur sometime at or after the cell's final mitotic division, when DNA contents have been halved by cell division. If, however, labeled cells at 4 hr had intermediate or doubled DNA contents, then one would conclude that the progenitor cell itself makes a commitment to the fate of its daughter.

The [³H]thymidine label is not a very useful marker for directly determining the DNA content of a subset of cycling cells; however, the thymidine analog 5-bromo-2′-deoxyuridine (BrdU) is quite useful in this regard. Antibodies to BrdU can be used to fluorescently tag those cells that are in S phase at the time of a BrdU pulse; this fluorescence makes these cells detectable by a fluorescence-activated cell sorter (FACS). The dye propidium iodide (PI), which is incorporated into chromatin and fluoresces in a manner proportional to the DNA content of the cell, is used in conjunction with BrdU to follow the progression of BrdU-labeled cells through the cell cycle with time after labeling (Hoy *et al.*, 1987). In these experiments, animals are injected with BrdU *in vivo* and the cortex is removed and dissociated into a single-cell suspension, as in the transplantation experiments, at different time points after the injection. At this point, however, the cells are fixed, immunoreacted with antibodies to BrdU, stained with PI, and passed through the FACS. The FACS determines both the BrdU fluorescence and PI staining of each cell, then generates a two-dimensional histogram of BrdU fluorescence vs. DNA content for the whole population (McConnell and Kaznowski, 1991). BrdU-labeled cells (cells with high BrdU fluorescence; Fig. 9A) that are fixed immediately after incorporating BrdU are primarily in S phase of the cell cycle, just as one would expect. Their DNA contents are intermediate between those of the unlabeled cells in G1 and G2/M (Fig. 9A). With increasing time after the pulse,

Figure 9. Contour plots of BrdU fluorescence and PI fluorescence (DNA content) derived from flow cytometry of cells obtained at four different times after labeling on E29 with BrdU. A. 0 hr: Cells that are not labeled with BrdU (bottom half of graph) have predominantly diploid and doubled DNA contents, as would be expected, since BrdU is only incorporated into DNA during S phase (see Fig. 3). BrdU-labeled cells (top half of plot) are in S phase, with intermediate DNA contents. With increasing time after the BrdU pulse, labeled cells in the top halves of each plot progress through the cell cycle; their shifting DNA contents reflect this progression. B. 6 hr: Many BrdU-labeled cells in the top half of the plot have completed S phase, with DNA contents that have shifted to the G2/M level. C. 12 hr: As labeled cells complete mitosis, their DNA contents appear on the left of the plot at diploid levels (above unlabeled G1 cells). D. 24 hr: A few BrdU-labeled cells have re-entered S phase, with intermediate DNA contents. (Reproduced from McConnell and Kaznowski, 1991, with permission, copyright 1991 by the AAS.)

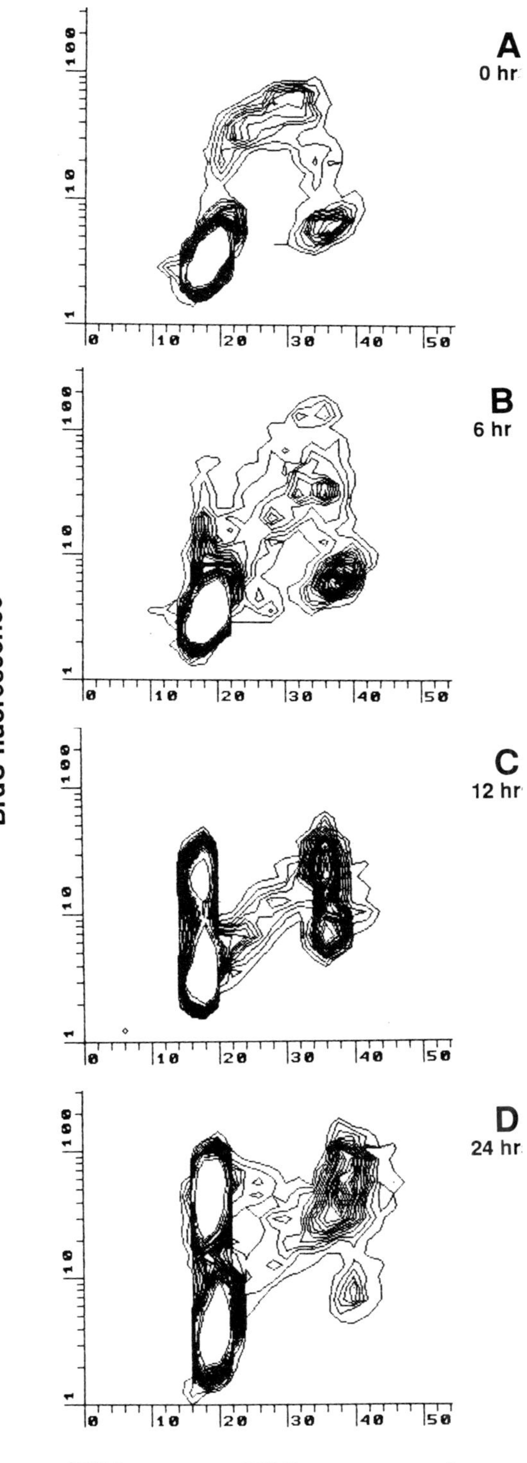

A
0 hr
B
6 hr
C
12 hr
D
24 hr
BrdU fluorescence
DNA content (PI fluorescence)

however, the DNA contents of labeled cells shift to the right of the histogram. These cells have completed S phase and are in G2 prior to mitosis (Fig. 9B). With time, as these cells divide and thereby halve their DNA contents, a large number of labeled cells gradually appears in the left-hand side of the plot, above the unlabeled G1 cells (Fig. 9C).

The progression of labeled cells through the cell cycle can be quantified by determining the fraction of BrdU-labeled cells in each of three areas of the plots: those in S phase, in G2/M, and in G1 (McConnell and Kaznowski, 1991). The results of these determinations are shown in Fig. 10. Just as expected, the percentage of labeled cells in S phase is quite high at first (Fig. 10A), then falls with time as the labeled cells complete replication and enter G2/M (Fig. 10B). The number of labeled cells in G1 subsequently begins to increase as the first of these cells completes a mitotic division to achieve diploid DNA contents (Fig. 10C).

Returning to the question of who makes the commitment to a deep-layer fate, the progenitor or its daughter, the relevant time point to examine in Fig. 10 is 4 hr. The flow cytometry data demonstrate that at 4 hours after BrdU labeling, some cells have left S-phase and entered G2/M, but very, very few cells have completed a mitotic division. This result strongly suggests that the cell making the commitment to a deep-layer fate is in fact the progenitor cell, prior to mitosis, probably at around the S to G2 transition (McConnell and Kaznowski, 1991).

This result is somewhat surprising, perhaps because it seems difficult to envision the cellular mechanisms required to instruct a precursor cell about the fate of its daughter; we don't even understand the rules by which the daughter decides whether to become postmitotic or to reenter the cell cycle.

Figure 10. The percentages of BrdU-labeled cells in three stages of the cell cycle—S, G2/M, and G1—as determined by their DNA contents, measured at a variety of times after BrdU labeling on E29. The percentages were obtained from histograms like those in Fig. 9. Each point represents the average from two samples of cells obtained from one litter of E29 ferret fetuses; points with error bars represent the average of two samples from each of two litters (error bars ± S.D.). A quadstat data analysis program was used to first determine the total number of BrdU-labeled cells in each contour plot (Fig. 9) by positioning a horizontal line in the valley separating the upper (BrdU-labeled) and lower (unlabeled) halves of each plot. A vertical line was then moved into position to distinguish cells on the far right (with G2/M DNA contents) from those with intermediate or diploid DNA contents. Another vertical line was then drawn to separate cells at the far left of each plot G1 cells) from S-phase cells with intermediate contents. The percentages of BrdU-labeled cells in each of these three phases were calculated. The number of labeled cells in S phase (Fig. 10A) should theoretically be 100% at time 0; however, the methods used have underestimated this fraction since early S-phase cells have DNA contents that overlap with G1 cells, and the DNA contents of late S-phase cells overlap with G2/M cells. Thus the fraction of labeled cells in S phase is an underestimate of the actual percentage; however, such an underestimation should not affect the overall kinetics of cell movement between the various phases. (Reproduced from McConnell and Kaznowski, 1991, with permission, copyright 1991 by the AAS.)

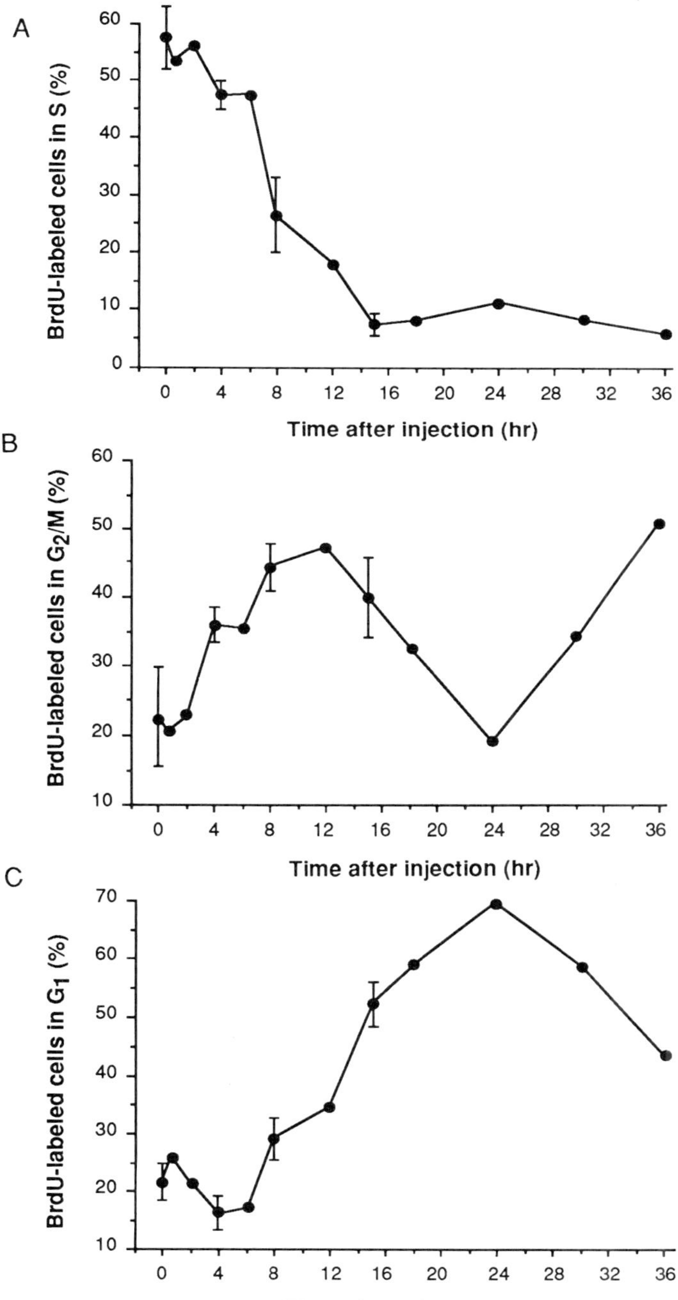
A
BrdU-labeled cells in S (%)
60
50
40
30
20
10
0
0 4 8 12 16 20 24 28 32 36
Time after injection (hr)

B
BrdU-labeled cells in G$_2$/M (%)
60
50
40
30
20
10
0 4 8 12 16 20 24 28 32 36
Time after injection (hr)

C
BrdU-labeled cells in G$_1$ (%)
70
60
50
40
30
20
10
0 4 8 12 16 20 24 28 32 36
Time after injection (hr)

One thing seems clear: if a daughter resulting from a cell division becomes a precursor itself—in other words, if the division is asymmetric, with one daughter migrating away to become a deep-layer neuron and the other re-initiating S phase—the cell that continues to cycle must somehow "forget" the commitment undergone by its parent. We believe this must be the case, because lightly labeled cells in the transplantation experiments, which have gone through an additional round of synthesis and division in the new, host environment, adopt the fate typical of host neurons (McConnell, 1989). These data thus provide a glimpse of what may be a complex series of regulatory decisions tied to progression through the cell cycle, in which a multipotent precursor cell is influenced by its environment midway through the cell cycle to produce a neuronal phenotype appropriate for that stage in gestation. If a neuron produced by that division leaves the cell cycle to become forever postmitotic and migrate out into the cortical plate, it appears to be equipped with the information it needs to home to its correct laminar position and form axonal projections typical of its birthday. If, however, a daughter cell re-enters the cycle and divides again, it presumably either never inherits or forgets the information acquired by its mother, to encounter afresh the signals provided by the environment in which it divides. Interestingly, a similar scheme has been encountered in the leech central nervous system, in which the o/p progenitor cell makes a stepwise series of commitments in producing cells of the "O" lineage (Shankland and Weisblat, 1984).

The timing of commitment in early cortical progenitors, which occurs late in S phase or at the S-to-G2 transition, is an interesting time in molecular terms. Ultimately it seems that changes in cell commitment must involve the regulation of the set of a cell's potentially activatable genes against those genes that are either repressed or inaccessible for activation or expression. One possible mechanism of regulation is at the level of chromatin configuration: changes in DNAase-hypersensitive sites or DNA methylation can affect the expression of different genes (Weintraub, 1985; Vandenbergh et al., 1989). Several authors have speculated that alterations in chromatin configuration may be enhanced by DNA replication (Brown, 1984; Weintraub, 1985; Wolffe and Brown, 1986), although others have shown that replication is not required for such changes to occur (Blau, 1989). It will be interesting to determine, in this context, whether the commitment of cortical progenitors to producing deep-layer neurons is dependent on the cell completing replication, or whether it occurs independent of DNA synthesis. One way to test this would be to block replication with an inhibitor of DNA polymerase, such as aphidicolin (Ikegami et al., 1978), during the 4-hr time period in which cells normally make a commitment to a deep-layer fate. If the completion of replication is an essential feature of commitment, the cells should be frozen in time with respect to fate determination and retain their multipotence. If, however, the process is independent of replication, perhaps involving changes on the cell surface or in second messenger systems, then one might expect the precursors to commit to making deep-layer cells even in the absence of DNA synthesis.

D. Unanswered Questions

These experiments have left a host of other issues unaddressed or unanswered. The first and most obvious among them is, what is the nature of the environmental cue that induces the production of deep- or upper-layer neurons? Indeed, at this point it is not even clear whether there is a "default" pathway for the production of specific cell types, as has been suggested for the developing retina (see Chapter 13 for review), or whether an active signal is required for the production of each neuronal phenotype. Progress in this realm could be achieved if one could study the development of different laminar phenotypes *in vitro*, a goal that necessitates the development of layer-specific markers or antibodies to distinguish different cell types in a dish.

A second issue concerns the competence of progenitor cells to produce cells of different layers as time passes during development. All the transplantation experiments described have employed early embryonic precursors, cells that will normally give rise to neurons in several layers. However, late in development comes a time at which the only neurons that remain to be produced are neurons of the upper layer 2/3. Do the late progenitors of these cells retain the capacity to produce deep-layer neurons, or has their competence to do so been lost over time in development? One way of addressing this question would be to transplant late precursor cells into embryonic hosts in which deep-layer neurons are being generated.

Finally, one outcome of commitment is that the young, postmitotic neuron is able to recognize its correct laminar position as it migrates out into a foreign cortical plate. Several lines of experiments have suggested that layer formation in the cortex involves an active process of cell recognition, conceivably mediated by specific adhesion between neurons of similar birthdays. The first line of evidence is derived from reaggregation cultures of cortical neurons: dissociated cortical neurons will reaggregate and form histotypically organized structures in rotating cultures (DeLong, 1970; DeLong and Sidman, 1970). The second line of evidence is from similar reaggregation experiments in which neurons were birthdated prior to dissociation: early-generated neurons, normally destined for the deep cortical layers, appear to associate preferentially with like neurons in these cultures (Krushel and van der Kooy, 1987). Because both sets of experiments were performed in long-term cultures, it is impossible to determine whether selective adhesion is the mechanism by which similar neurons associate with one another. It is of course an interesting possibility that one of the results of cell commitment is that deep-layer neurons express a layer-specific cell-surface molecule (or combination of molecules) that confers on the cell the ability to "home" to the correct layer.

IV. Axon Outgrowth in the Developing Cerebral Cortex

Once in its correct laminar position, the young cortical neuron is still faced with the monumental tasks of growing its axon to the correct target region and receiving appropriate synaptic inputs. These problems are complicated by the fact that not only do neurons have to make layer-specific sets of connections, but their connections must also be appropriate for the cortical area in which the neuron lies. We have considered so far only the radial dimension of cortical organization, in which layers form. However, orthogonal to this axis the cortex is also subdivided in the tangential domain into anatomically and functionally distinct areas that are responsible for processing information from different sensory modalities and for relaying motor output information to a variety of subcortical and spinal targets. Thus, the visual cortex receives incoming thalamic information from the visual thalamus, and relays this information to other visual areas, back to the lateral geniculate nucleus, and to subcortical areas such as the superior colliculus that are involved in the motor control of eye and head movements. The somatosensory cortex, in contrast, receives inputs from the ventrolateral and ventrobasal thalamus and sends descending projections both back to these areas and down into the spinal cord. The development of these area-specific patterns of axonal projections has been a major focus of work in the development of the cerebral cortex. Unlike a cell's laminar identity, which seems to be determined early in the cell's life history prior to its migration out into the cortex, the regional identity of neocortical neurons appears to be relatively plastic in early development. The determination of this identity may involve interactions between these cells and a unique class of cells found during development, the subplate neurons.

A. Regional Variations across the Cerebral Cortex

Two lines of thought have been developed with respect to the origins of regional diversity in the developing cerebral cortex. The first, laid out most forcefully by Rakic (1989), posits that regional differences in cortical areas are predetermined in the ventricular zone, which contains a "protomap" of the eventual layout of all the areas. An alternative view is that the ventricular zone, and even the postmitotic neuron, is initially naive with respect to area-specific identity, and that this identity is achieved through a gradual epigenetic process of interactions between cortical neurons, their afferents, and other environmental influences. Indeed, evidence for both views has been obtained. It is likely that the development of different areas in the cortex will involve an interplay between both mechanisms.

In favor of an early parcelling of cortical regions is the finding of molecular heterogeneity in the ventricular zone at times at which neurogenesis is in full swing. The strongest example of this comes from Levitt and co-workers, who have characterized the cell-surface glycoprotein LAMP (limbic-associated membrane protein), expressed specifically in limbic cortical regions of the rat (Levitt, 1984; Horton and Levitt, 1988). The limbic cortex is a phylogenetically old cortical region, also called mesocortex, and can be easily distinguished from evolutionarily newer neocortical regions. To test whether differences between limbic and neocortex are set up early in development, Barbe and Levitt (1990, 1991) transplanted small pieces of embryonic limbic cortex into ectopic neocortical locations. Their experiments demonstrate that presumptive limbic cortex from E17 rat fetuses retains many features of its original limbic phenotype, such as LAMP expression, in the novel position (Barbe and Levitt, 1991). Transplanted neurons also attract some of the afferent inputs of normal limbic cortex, and develop efferent connections that are at least partially correct for their donor origin (Barbe and Levitt, 1990). When the limbic regions are transplanted at E12, however, transplanted cells fail to express LAMP, suggesting that, at very early times in neurogenesis, prior to the production of most of the neurons of this region, some developmental plasticity is still retained (Barbe and Levitt, 1991). These experiments suggest that differences between such different cortical regions as the phylogenetically old limbic mesocortex and the evolutionarily newer neocortex may emerge relatively early in development, when neurogenesis is still occurring. However, similar experiments designed to explore the development of regional differences *among* neocortical regions (discussed next) have suggested that area-specific patterns of connections are likely to emerge much later in development.

I. EXUBERANT PROJECTIONS IN DEVELOPMENT

One of the first clues that differences among neocortical areas might emerge gradually during development came from studies of growing cortical axons. In particular, the finding that cortical neurons often extend axons "exuberantly" to multiple targets early in development, only to later retract inappropriate axons, suggested the possibility that neurons express regional differences relatively late in development. The best-studied example is of layer 5 neurons throughout the neocortex. In the adult rodent, layer 5 cells in the caudal, visual regions of the cortex project axons primarily to the superior colliculus and the rostral pons; more rostral layer 5 neurons, in contrast, project heavily to the spinal cord and to the caudal pons, among other targets. In early development, however, layer 5 neurons throughout the cortex extend axons to "inappropriate" targets (with respect to their region of origin): neurons in the visual cortex, for example, initially extend axons into the spinal cord and later retract these axons as they form their permanent connections with the tectum and pons (Stanfield *et al.*, 1982; Stanfield and O'Leary, 1985a; O'Leary and Stanfield, 1985). One way to think about these early projections is that they are mistakes of axon targeting that result from flawed outgrowth. A compelling alternative is the possibility that layer 5 neurons throughout the cortex employ a common program of development that directs axonogenesis to many or all the possible targets of layer 5 cells; region-specific differences only emerge subsequent to the bulk of axon outgrowth as the cells acquire a discrete areal identity.

2. TRANSPLANTATION STUDIES OF THE DETERMINATION OF CORTICAL AREAS

To test whether cortical neurons are committed to developing the cytoarchitectonic features and axonal connections typical of their region of origin, an elegant series of transplantation experiments have been performed in developing rats (Stanfield and O'Leary, 1985b; Schlagger and O'Leary, 1988; O'Leary and Stanfield, 1989). In these experiments, small pieces of cortex from the visual/occipital region of E16 rats were transplanted into more rostral regions such as motor or somatosensory cortex of neonatal hosts; the converse transplants of motor into occipital cortex were also done. Visual cortical neurons, which would normally retract their exuberantly projecting axon down the spinal cord, retained this projection following transplantation into more rostral cortical areas, in which spinal axons are normally maintained. This result demonstrates that the pattern of target selection by layer 5 neurons in visual cortex is not preprogrammed or intrinsically determined; in this sense, visual cortex can become motor cortex under appropriate environmental circumstances. Likewise, motor cortex transplanted to the visual region developed subcortical axonal projections typical of visual cortex.

To test whether layer 5 neurons are unique in displaying this developmental plasticity, pieces of embryonic occipital cortex have been transplanted into the somatosensory region of neonatal hosts (Schlagger and O'Leary, 1988). The somatosensory cortex of the normal rat is characterized by a beautiful cytoarchitectonic feature called the barrel fields, regions of layer 4 in which the whisker barrels are represented physiologically and in which the cells of layer 4 actually differentiate in barrel-like arrays, visible using either a simple Nissl stain or other markers including lectins and antibodies to cytotactin (Steindler *et al.*, 1989). When visual cortex is transplanted into the somatosensory region, the transplanted cortex not only develops projections typical of its new locale, but it also develops barrel fields in register with those of the host brain (Schlagger and O'Leary, 1990). This result indicates that the differentiation of the cortex appears to be completely normal for the new location, in inputs, cytoarchitectonic features, and efferent connections.

These transplantation experiments indicate that neocortical areas appear to have an equivalent developmental potential at E17, when many of the neurons that will constitute the adult cortex already have been generated. These experiments argue that the layout of different neocortical areas is not strictly determined in the ventricular zone, but is achieved through a series of interactions between cortical neurons and their neighbors, their afferent inputs, or their long-distance targets, by mechanisms that remain quite unknown.

B. Subplate Neurons: Pioneer Neurons of the Developing CNS?

The studies reviewed here suggest the possibility that some kind of epigenetic process, involving interactions between neurons, their inputs, and their targets, may be involved in the parcelling of the cortex into distinct areas. Possible players in this epigenetic process are the subplate neurons, a special class of transient neurons that are among the first postmitotic cells of the developing cerebral wall and are uniquely situated to play a role in the parcelling of the cortex into different areas (Shatz *et al.*, 1990). Several lines of evidence have demonstrated that subplate cells are indeed neurons: they express the neuron-specific marker microtubule-associated protein 2 (MAP-2), as well as several neuropeptides (Chun *et al.*, 1987; Wahle and Meyer, 1987; Chun and Shatz, 1989a,b; Antonini and Shatz, 1990). Subplate cells receive synaptic inputs, both morphologically (Chun *et al.*, 1987) and physiologically (Friauf *et al.*, 1990); they fire action potentials (Friauf *et al.*, 1990) and make both long-distance and local axonal projections (Marin-Padilla, 1971; Chun *et al.*, 1987; Wahle and Meyer, 1987; Valverde and Valverde, 1988; McConnell *et al.*, 1989; Antonini and Shatz, 1990). The most interesting feature of subplate neurons is that the vast majority of these cells disappears during postnatal life in a wave of cell death (Luskin and Shatz, 1985b; Valverde and Valverde, 1987; Chun and Shatz, 1989; Woo *et al.*, 1990). One of the questions that has puzzled us and others since subplate neurons were first described is, why does the brain go to all the trouble of making subplate neurons, only to wipe them out later in life?

One clue about a possible function of subplate neurons was obtained through a study of the development of the long-distance subcortical projections from the cortex. Much to our surprise, experiments in which axons are studied with the tracer DiI revealed the presence of a substantial projection of axons that enter the internal capsule and descend into the thalamus at very early stages of fetal life, prior to the generation of the permanent subcortical projection neurons of the cortex (McConnell *et al.*, 1989). One obvious possibility is that subplate neurons, which are already postmitotic at these early times, might be responsible for forming the first descending axons. We tested this by using DiI as a retrograde tracer and labeling the cells of origin of this pathway from the internal capsule, the gateway between the thalamus and the cortex. Figure 11 shows that a substantial population of cells could be labeled and identified as subplate neurons, based on their position and early presence in the cortical preplate (McConnell *et al.*, 1989).

These results raised the possibility that subplate neurons may act as early pioneer neurons in the development of descending cortical projections. Pioneer neurons were originally described in invertebrates, and are defined as the first neurons to extend axons toward long-distance targets when the distances between neurons and those targets are at a minimum (Bate, 1976; Bentley and Keshishian, 1982; Bastiani *et al.*, 1985). In these systems, the pioneer axons are subsequently followed by later-growing axons; there is evidence in a few cases that follower axons require the presence of the early pioneers to find their appropriate targets (Klose and Bentley, 1989; Bastiani *et al.*, 1985). In the cat and ferret, subplate neurons project into the thalamus and superior colliculus, targets of adult deep-layer neurons in layers 6 and 5, respectively (McConnell *et al.*, 1989). We have thus been curious to know whether the axons of deep-layer cortical neurons depend on the pioneering subplate axons to grow toward or innervate long-distance subcortical targets.

I. FORMATION OF DESCENDING PROJECTIONS

We considered first whether the descending axons of deep-layer neurons grow at roughly the same time as, or much later than, the axons of subplate neurons, and second whether these axons might actually fasciculate with the axons of subplate neurons. The answer to the first question seems clear: the

Figure 11. Subplate neurons retrogradely labeled with DiI from the internal capsule on E30. these labeled neurons pioneer the earliest axon pathway from the cortex into the thalamus (McConnell *et al.*, 1989). The axons of subplate neurons run in the intermediate zone, just above the ventricular zone.

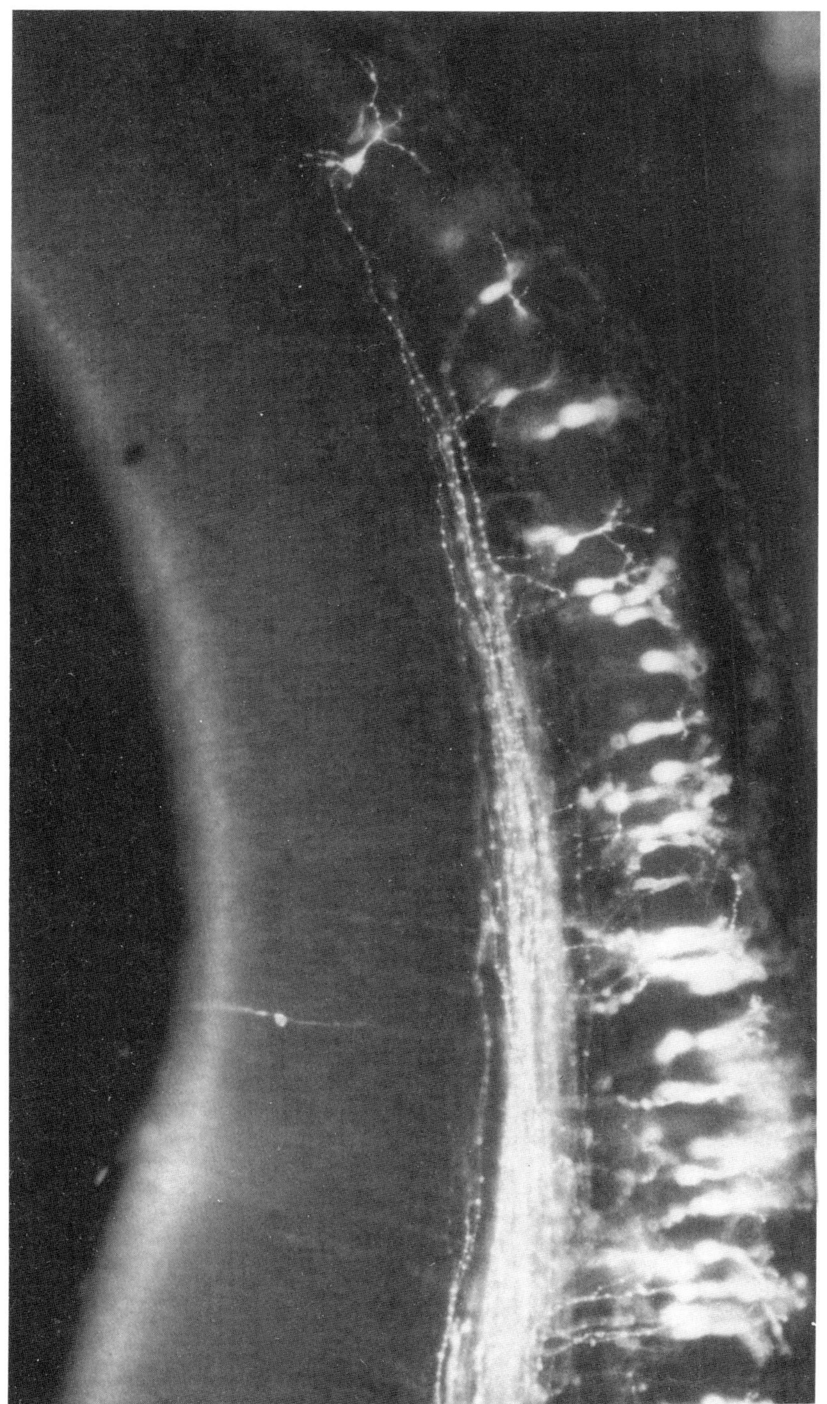

axons of deep-layer neurons develop significantly later than do the axons of subplate neurons. This can be demonstrated by placing small crystals of DiI superficially in the cortical plate so not to mark subplate cells. Descending axons labeled by these superficial injections appear to grow out with a significant lag, traversing the distance from visual cortex to thalamus over a period of weeks (not surprising, since this distance is ever-increasing with the growth of the whole brain); axons finally invade the lateral geniculate nucleus (LGN) of the thalamus at about E56 in the cat (McConnell and Shatz, 1988; unpublished observations).

It turns out that the second question (of fasciculation) has been particularly difficult to address. The axons of subcortical projection neurons appear to elongate primarily along the upper surface of the ventricular zone, deep within the intermediate zone. We are not yet sure exactly where subplate axons run, although it is likely that they are located primarily in the middle region of the intermediate zone, perhaps intermingled with the ascending axons of thalamic neurons (see subsequent text). It seems somewhat unlikely that cortical and subplate axons are physically intermingled in the intermediate zone and, therefore, unlikely that they fasciculate with one another. We have, however, found a striking difference in the complexity of the growth cones of subplate and cortical neurons. Early-growing axons, likely to belong to subplate cells, terminate in very large and complex growth cones with many filopodia at all points along the corticothalamic pathway. In contrast, later-growing subcortical axons have very simple clublike growth cones with few or no filopodia (Kim *et al.*, 1991). Several studies in other systems have suggested that the morphology of growth cones is correlated with the complexity of choices or decisions they face: growth cones become more complex at "choice points" along an axon pathway, where an axon must make a decision among several possible growth pathways (Tosney and Landmesser, 1985; Bovolenta and Mason, 1987; Holt, 1989). The growth cones of leading axons are typically more complex than the growth cones of axons that fasciculate along behind them (LoPresti *et al.*, 1973). If one draws a parallel between the developing cortex and these other systems, the differences observed in growth cone complexity suggest that late-growing axons face fewer decisions than do earlier axons, consistent with the possibility that subplate axons pioneer an initial pathway that cortical axons then later simply follow.

The most direct test of the subplate pioneer hypothesis would be to selectively ablate subplate neurons early in development, prior to the outgrowth of deep-layer cortical axons, and study the effects of removing this early pathway on axonal outgrowth of later-growing cells. It is indeed possible to selectively ablate subplate neurons in fetal life, using the neurotoxin kainic acid (Chun and Shatz, 1988; Ghosh *et al.*, 1990). In such experiments, layer-6 neurons in visual cortex, which normally project to the lateral geniculate nucleus of the thalamus, can no longer be retrogradely labeled from this target, implying that, in the absence of subplate neurons, these cells can no longer find or recognize their appropriate thalamic target (Ghosh *et al.*, 1990; see Fig. 12B). We are still in the process of trying to ascertain whether the deep-layer cortical axons can pathfind normally to the thalamus but fail to innervate the correct nucleus, or whether axogenesis is so abnormal that the axons never even reach the vicinity of their target. These two results would imply very different roles for subplate neurons in cortical axogenesis. The former would imply that subplate axons are not needed for pathfinding along the subcortical projection toward and through the internal capsule, but that subplate neurons play a role in defining the identity of cortical or thalamic areas as visual (as opposed to other modalities). The latter would imply that subplate axons play a role in physically defining the corticothalamic pathway itself, and that cortical axons rely on following this pathway during develop-ment (either by directly fasciculating onto subplate axons or by following other cues that are somehow defined by or dependent on the presence of subplate axons).

2. THALAMOCORTICAL TARGET RECOGNITION

The pathway between the cortex and the thalamus is, of course, a two-way street. In addition to the descending axons just discussed, axons from the thalamus course upward through the internal capsule to diverge and in-nervate appropriate cortical targets. Indirect evidence has long suggested that subplate neurons might be involved in thalamocortical axogenesis and target recognition: In higher mammals such as cat and primate, thalamic axons grow into the cortical white matter prior to the generation of their ultimate post-synaptic targets, the neurons of cortical layer 4 (Rakic, 1983; Shatz and Luskin, 1986; Shatz *et al.*, 1988, 1990). The thalamic axons growing from the cat's LGN, for example, arrive in the vicinity of the visual cortex on and after E35; layer-4 neurons are only beginning to be generated at that time and take an additional week or so to migrate out into their final positions, which they do by about E55 (Shatz and Luskin, 1986; Shatz *et al.*, 1988, 1990). During this 2–3-wk period, LGN axons accumulate in the subplate region below the cortical plate, and finally grow into the cortical plate itself beginning around E50–56, concomitant with the arrival of the layer-4 neurons in their final positions. The findings that subplate neurons receive synapses on their cell bodies (Chun *et al.*, 1987) and can be driven to fire monosynaptic action potentials on stimulation of the optic radiations (Friauf *et al.*, 1990) have supported the hypothesis that subplate neurons act as transient synaptic targets of the waiting geniculocortical axons (reviewed in Shatz *et al.*, 1990). We were therefore interested to examine the possible roles that subplate neurons might play in determining the pattern of innervation between thalamic axons and their cortical targets.

To this end, subplate neurons were selectively ablated with injections of kainic acid on E38–E42, when LGN axons are accumulating beneath the cortical plate. The effect of this ablation on the axons was examined at a variety of times after the ablation by placing small crystals of DiI into the LGN. Geniculocortical axons displayed a striking change in their behavior following ablation of subplate neurons. The first effect of subplate ablation is that the cortical plate in effect sits directly on top of the optic radiations containing LGN axons, since the intervening subplate region has collapsed. However, despite their apparently easy access to the cortical plate, LGN axons do not invade the visual cortex prematurely. Instead, they continue to grow past the visual cortex altogether, into regions of white matter below cortical areas that never contain LGN axons in normal animals (Ghosh *et al.*, 1990). Even in postnatal life, when geniculocortical axons are normally branching in cortical layer 4 (Fig. 12A), LGN axons in the subplate-ablated animals fail to innervate the visual cortex (Fig. 12B). We do not know yet whether these axons eventually invade, or form synaptic contacts with, other normally nonvisual cortical regions.

These results suggest that the cortical plate itself does not have sufficient information to attract the ingrowth of normal afferent connections *in vivo*, and that somehow subplate neurons stand as a crucial link in the process of matching the different thalamic inputs to their appropriate cortical targets. Several control experiments have been performed that suggest that these effects on LGN axonogenesis are specific to the disappearance of the subplate neurons (Ghosh *et al.*, 1990). First, MAP-2 immunohistochemistry and Nissl staining reveal that subplate neurons are missing in the area of the lesion, whereas the cortical plate remains intact. Second, radial glial fibers in the area of the lesion can be labeled with DiI and are unaffected by kainic acid. Third, the migration of layer-4 neurons, the ultimate targets of LGN axons in normal animals, continues normally in the absence of the subplate. Fourth, immunohistochemistry using antibodies to vimentin and GFAP reveal no abnormalities in the glia underlying the cortical plate. Finally, A. Ghosh and C. J. Shatz (unpublished results) have shown that similar results can also be obtained for subplate ablations beneath other neocortical areas such as auditory cortex, which is normally innervated by the medial geniculate nucleus (MGN). These experiments raise the interesting possibility that subplate neurons serve as intermediaries in parcelling out the cortex into functionally distinct areas. The fact that subplate neurons form axonal projections into the overlying cortical plate (Marin-Padilla, 1971; Wahle and Meyer, 1987; Chun and Shatz, 1989a; Friauf *et al.*, 1990) provides a possible conduit for communication between subplate cells, waiting axons, and their eventual targets in the cortical plate.

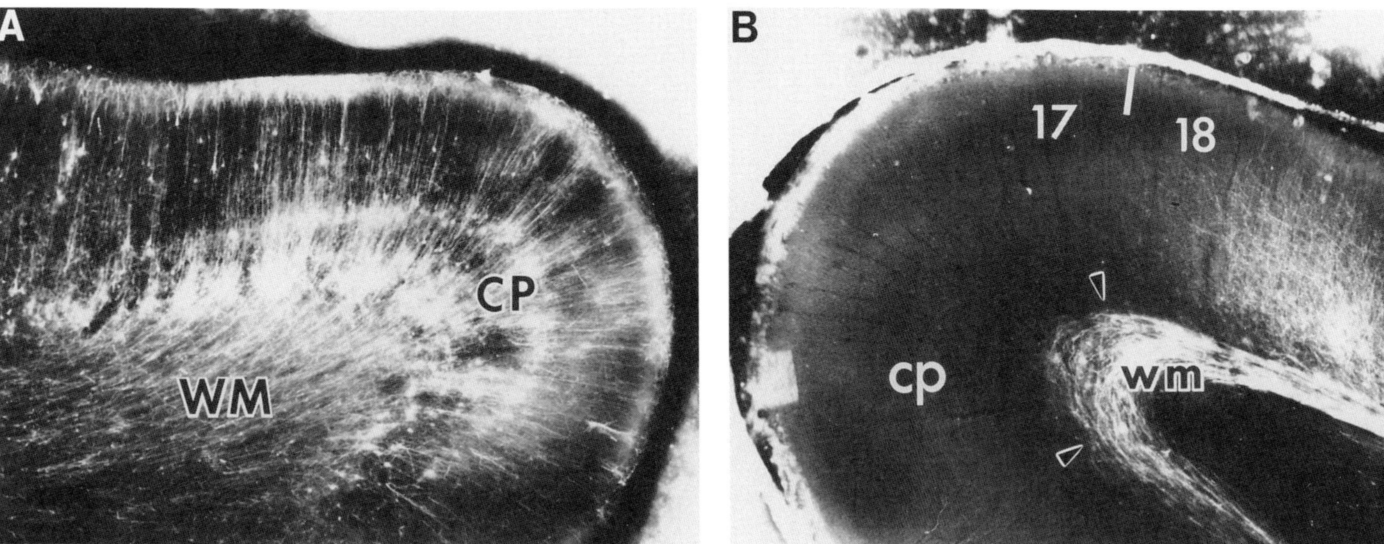

Figure 12. A. Axons from the LGN have innervated layer 4 of the visual cortex by P2 in normal cat brains. Seen here is a combination of anterograde and retrograde labeling following an injection of DiI into the LGN of a fixed P2 brain. This coronal section shows an abundance of anterogradely labeled LGN axons that enter the cortex from the white matter (wm) and branch extensively in layer 4. Retrograde labeling is seen in the deep cortical layers (the neurons of which project axons to subcortical targets). B. Abnormal development of LGN axons observed at P5, following a kainic acid ablation of subplate neurons on E42. Kainic acid was injected into the subplate underlying the primary visual cortex on E42, and fetuses were allowed to grow to P5. At this time, DiI was placed in the LGN to reveal the axons of LGN neurons. LGN axons (*arrowheads*) have failed to recognize and innervate the primary visual cortex, and instead have grown past their normal target into regions of the cerebral hemispheres not normally occupied by LGN axons. Note that some LGN axons have entered cortical area 18, a normal target; the subplate neurons below area 18 were not destroyed by the kainic acid injection. Note also the absence of retrograde labeling in layer 6, consistent with the hypothesis that the pioneering axons of subplate neurons are required for the axons of layer 6 cells to find their normal thalamic targets. Bar: 750 μm. Abbreviations: wm, white matter; cp, cortical plate; 17, area 17; 18, area 18. [Reproduced with permission from Ghosh *et al.* (1990) *Nature* **347**, 179–181; copyright © 1990, Macmillan Magazines Ltd.]

V. Summary

The experiments described in this chapter point to a process of progressive determination of neuronal fates in the developing cortex. These decisions collectively employ a variety of mechanisms, including lineage-based restrictions of cell fates, commitments to a laminar phenotype at roughly the time a cell is born, and a progressive and epigenetic process by which the neocortex is parcelled out into functionally distinct areas. Transplantation studies of presumptive limbic and neocortex suggests that differences between these broad regions may be laid out early in development during neurogenesis. In the neocortex, retroviral lineage studies have demonstrated that early cortical progenitors normally generate neurons destined for several different layers, yet recent studies suggest that separate lineages may produce projection neurons and interneurons. Transplantation experiments in which thymidine-labeled progenitor cells have been injected into older host brains have shown that commitment to a laminar position in the cortex occurs prior to a neuron's migration away from the ventricular zone into the cortex. The progeny of precursor cells transplanted in S phase of the cell cycle, however, alter their fate in the novel environment, suggesting that environmental cues play an instructive role in the progressive generation of specific neuronal phenotypes over time in development. Regional differences in patterns of connectivity between cortical areas emerge late in development: layer-5 neurons in the rodent go through a common program of exuberant axon outgrowth followed by selective retraction of axons in a pattern appropriate for the tangential position of the neuron. Transplantation experiments suggest that different neocortical regions are developmentally equivalent, even after many neurons have become postmitotic. Less is known about the nature of environmental cues responsible for these commitments and decisions, but recent evidence suggests that one of the epigenetic steps in the parcelling of the neocortex may involve interactions with the specialized subplate region, whose neurons seem to mediate the establishment of normal connections between the cortex and other regions of the brain.

Acknowledgments

I thank Marty Shankland and Carla Shatz for their thoughtful comments on the manuscript. The author's work is supported by grants from the NIH (EY08411), the Pew Scholars Program, Searle Scholars/The Chicago Community Trust, and a Clare Boothe Luce professorship.

References

Angevine, J. B., Jr., and Sidman, R. L. (1961). Autoradiographic study of cell migration during histogenesis of cerebral cortex in the mouse. *Nature (London)* **192,** 766–768.

Antonini, A., and Shatz, C. J. (1990). Relationship between putative transmitter phenotype and connectivity of subplate neurons during cerebral cortical development. *Eur. J. Neurosci.* **2,** 744–761.

Austin, C. P., and Cepko, C. L. (1990). Cellular migration patterns in the developing mouse cerebral cortex. *Development* **110,** 713–732.

Barbe, M. F., and Levitt, P. (1990). Connectivity of fetal limbic cortex transplanted into nonlimbic cortex. *Soc. Neurosci. Abstr.* **16,** 1151.

Barbe, M. F., and Levitt, P. (1991). The early commitment of fetal neurons to limbic cortex. *J. Neurosci.* **11,** 519–533.

Bastiani, M. J., Doe, C. Q., Helfand, S. L., and Goodman, C. S. (1985). Neuronal specificity and growth cone guidance in grasshopper and *Drosophila* embryos. *Trends Neurosci.* **8,** 257–266.

Bate, C. M. (1976). Pioneer neurones in an insect embryo. *Nature (London)* **260,** 54–56.

Bentley, D., and Keshishian, H. (1982). Pathfinding by peripheral pioneer neurons in grasshoppers. *Science* **218,** 1082–1087.

Blau, H. M. (1989). How fixed is the differentiated state? *Trends Genet.* **5,** 268–272.

Boulder Committee (1970). Embryonic vertebrate central nervous system: Revised terminology. *Anat. Rec.* **166,** 257–262.

Bovolenta, P., and Mason, C. (1987). Growth cone morphology varies with position in the developing mouse visual pathway from retina to first targets. *J. Neurosci.* **7,** 1447–1460.

Brown, D. D. (1984). The role of stable complexes that repress and activate eucaryotic genes. *Cell* **37,** 359–365.

Caviness, V. S., Jr. (1976). Patterns of cell and fiber distribution in the neocortex of the reeler mutant mouse. *J. Comp. Neurol.* **170,** 435–448.

Caviness, V. S., Jr. (1982). Neocortical histogenesis in normal and reeler mice: A developmental study based on [³H]thymidine autoradiography. *Dev. Brain Res.* **4,** 293–302.

Chun, J. J. M., Nakamura, M. J., and Shatz, C. J. (1987). Transient cells of the developing mammalian telencephalon are peptide-immunoreactive neurons. *Nature (London)* **325,** 617–620.

Chun, J. J. M., and Shatz, C. J. (1988). Redistribution of synaptic vesicle antigens is correlated with the disappearance of a transient synaptic zone in the developing cerebral cortex. *Neuron* **1,** 297–310.

Chun, J. J. M., and Shatz, C. J. (1989a). The earliest-generated neurons of the cat cerebral cortex: Characterization by MAP2 and neurotransmitter immunohistochemistry during fetal life. *J. Neurosci.* **9,** 1648–1667.

Chun, J. J. M., and Shatz, C. J. (1989b). Interstitial cells of the adult neocortical white matter are the remnant of the early generated subplate neuron population. *J. Comp. Neurol.* **282,** 555–569.

DeLong, G. R. (1970). Histogenesis of fetal mouse isocortex and hippocampus in reaggregating cell cultures. *Dev. Biol.* **22,** 563–583.

DeLong, G. R., and Sidman, R. L. (1970). Alignment defect of reaggregating cells in cultures of developing brains of reeler mutant mice. *Dev. Biol.* **22,** 584–600.

Dräger, U. C. (1981). Observations on the organization of the visual cortex in the reeler mouse. *J. Comp. Neurol.* **201,** 555–570.

Friauf, E., McConnell, S. K., and Shatz, C. J. (1990). Functional circuits in the subplate during fetal and early postnatal development of cat visual cortex. *J. Neurosci.* **10**, 2601–2613.

Fujita, S. (1963). Analysis of neuron differentiation in the central nervous system by tritiated thymidine autoradiography. *J. Comp. Neurol.* **122**, 311–328.

Ghosh, A., Antonini, A., McConnell, S. K., and Shatz, C. J. (1990). Requirement for subplate neurons in the formation of thalamocortical connections. *Nature (London)* **347**, 179–181.

Gilbert, C. D. (1977). Laminar differences in receptive field properties of cells in cat primary visual cortex. *J. Physiol. (London)* **268**, 391–421.

Gilbert, C. D. (1983). Microcircuitry of the visual cortex. *Ann. Rev. Neurosci.* **6**, 217–247.

Gilbert, C. D., and Kelly, J. P. (1975). The projections of cells in different layers of the cat's visual cortex. *J. Comp. Neurol.* **163**, 81–106.

Gilbert, C. D., and Wiesel, T. N. (1979). Morphology and intracortical projections of functionally characterized neurones in the cat visual cortex. *Nature (London)* **280**, 120–125.

Gilbert, C. D., and Wiesel, T. N. (1985). Intrinsic connectivity and receptive field properties in visual cortex. *Vision Res.* **25**, 365–374.

Greenwald, I. (1989). Cell–cell interactions that specify certain cell fates in *C. elegans* development. *Trends Genet.* **5**, 237–241.

Hatten, M. E. (1990). Riding the glial monorail: A common mechanism for glial-guided neuronal migration in different regions of the developing mammalian brain. *Trends Neurosci.* **13**, 179–184.

Hatten, M. E., and Mason, C. A. (1990). Mechanisms of glial-guided neuronal migration *in vivo* and *in vitro*. *Experientia* **46**, 907–916.

Hickey, T. L., Whikehart, D. R., Jackson, C. A., Hitchcock, P. F., and Peduzzi, J. D. (1983). Tritiated thymidine experiments in the cat: A description of techniques and experiments to describe the time-course of radioactive thymidine availability. *J. Neurosci. Meth.* **8**, 139–147.

Holt, C. E. (1989). A single-cell analysis of early retinal ganglion cell differentiation in *Xenopus*: From soma to axon tip. *J. Neurosci.* **9**, 3123–3145.

Horton, H. L., and Levitt, P. (1988). A unique membrane protein is expressed on early developing limbic system axons and cortical targets. *J. Neurosci.* **8**, 4653–4744.

Hoy, C. A., Rice, G. C., Kovacs, M., and Schimke, R. T. (1987). Over-replication of DNA in S phase Chinese hamster ovary cells after DNA synthesis inhibition. *J. Biol. Chem.* **262**, 11927–11934.

Hubel, D. H., and Wiesel, T. N. (1962). Receptive fields, binocular interaction and functional architecture in the cat's visual cortex. *J. Physiol. (London)* **160**, 106–154.

Ikegami, S., Taguchi, T., Ohashi, M., Oguro, M., Nagano, H., and Mano, Y. (1978). Aphidicolin presents mitotic cell division be interfering with the activity of DNA polymerase-α. *Nature (London)* **275**, 258–260.

Jackson, C. A., Peduzzi, J. D., and Hickey, T. L. (1989). Visual cortex development in the ferret. I. Genesis and migration of visual cortical neurons. *J. Neurosci.* **9**, 1242–1253.

Katz, L. C. (1987). Local circuitry of identified projection neurons in cat visual cortex brain slices. *J. Neurosci.* **7**, 1223–1249.

Katz, L. C., Burkhalter, A., and Dreyer, W. J. (1984). Fluorescent latex microspheres as a retrograde neuronal marker for *in vivo* and *in vitro* studies of visual cortex. *Nature (London)* **310**, 498–500.

Kim, G. J., Shatz, C. J., and McConnell, S. K. (1991). Morphology of pioneer and follower growth cones in the developing cerebral cortex. *J. Neurobiol.* **22**, 629–642.

Klose, M., and Bentley, D. (1989). Transient pioneer neurons are essential for formation of an embryonic peripheral nerve. *Science* **245**, 982–983.

Krushel, L. A., and van der Kooy, D. (1987). Selective *in vitro* reassociation of early vs. late postmitotic neurons from the rat forebrain. *Soc. Neurosci. Abstr.* **13**, 1114.

Lemmon, V., and Pearlman, A. L. (1981). Does laminar position determine the receptive field properties of cortical neurons? A study of corticotectal cells in area 17 of the normal mouse and the reeler mutant. *J. Neurosci.* **1,** 83–93.

LeVay, S., and Gilbert, C. D. (1976). Laminar patterns of geniculocortical projection in the cat. *Brain Res.* **113,** 1–19.

LeVay, S., and Sherk, H. (1981). The visual claustrum of the cat. I. Structure and connections. *J. Neurosci.* **1,** 956–980.

LeVay, S., McConnell, S. K., and Luskin, M. B. (1987). Functional organization of primary visual cortex in the mink (*Mustela vision*) and a comparison with the cat. *J. Comp. Neurol.* **257,** 422–441.

Levitt, P. (1984). A monoclonal antibody to limbic system neurons. *Science* **223,** 299–301.

LoPresti, V., Macagno, E. R., and Levinthal, C. (1973). Structure and development of neuronal connection in isogenic organisms: Cellular interactions in the development of the optic lamina of daphnia. *Proc. Natl. Acad. Sci. U.S.A.* **70,** 433–437.

Lund, J. S. (1973). Organization of neurons in the visual cortex, area 17, of the monkey (*Macaca mulatta*). *J. Comp. Neurol.* **147,** 455–496.

Lund, J. S., and Boothe, R. G. (1975). Interlaminar connections and pyramidal neuron organization in the visual cortex, area 17, of the macaque monkey. *J. Comp. Neurol.* **159,** 305–334.

Lund, J. S., Lund, R. D., Hendrickson, A. E., Bunt, A. H., and Fuchs, A. F. (1975). The origin of efferent pathways from the primary visual cortex, area 17, of the macaque monkey as shown by retrograde transport of horseradish peroxidase. *J. Comp. Neurol.* **164,** 287–304.

Lund, J. S., Henry, G. H., MacQueen, C. L., and Harvey, A. R. (1979). Anatomical organization of the primary visual cortex (area 17) of the cat. A comparison with area 17 of the macaque monkey. *J. Comp. Neurol.* **184,** 599–618.

Luskin, M. B., and Shatz, C. J. (1985a). Studies of the earliest generated cells of the cat's visual cortex: Cogeneration of subplate and marginal zones. *J. Neurosci.* **5,** 1062–1075.

Luskin, M. B., and Shatz, C. J. (1985b). Neurogenesis of the cat's primary visual cortex. *J. Comp. Neurol.* **242,** 611–631.

Luskin, M. B., Pearlman, A. L., and Sanes, J. R. (1988). Cell lineage in the cerebral cortex of the mouse studied *in vivo* and *in vitro* with a recombinant retrovirus. *Neuron* **1,** 635–647.

McConnell, S. K. (1985). Migration and differentiation of cerebral cortical neurons after transplantation into the brains of ferrets. *Science* **229,** 1268–1271.

McConnell, S. K. (1988a). Fates of visual cortical neurons in the ferret after isochronic and heterochronic transplantation. *J. Neurosci.* **8,** 945–974.

McConnell, S. K. (1988b). Development and decision-making in the mammalian cerebral cortex. *Brain Res. Rev.* **13,** 1–23.

McConnell, S. K. (1989). The determination of neuronal fate in the cerebral cortex. *Trends Neurosci.* **12,** 342–349.

McConnell, S. K., and LeVay, S. (1986). Anatomical organization of the visual system of the mink (*Mustela vision*). *J. Comp. Neurol.* **250,** 109–132.

McConnell, S. K., and Shatz, C. J. (1988). Prenatal development of axonal projections from the cat's visual cortex. *Soc. Neurosci. Abstr.* **14,** 743.

McConnell, S. K., Ghosh, A., and Shatz, C. J. (1989). Subplate neurons pioneer the first axon pathway from the cerebral cortex. *Science* **245,** 278–281.

McConnell, S. K., and Kaznowski, C. E. (1990). Laminar commitment occurs prior to migration in the developing cerebral cortex. *Soc. Neurosci. Abstr.* **16,** 1272.

McConnell, S. K., and Kaznowski, C. E. (1991). Cell cycle dependence of laminar determination in developing cerebral cortex. *Science* **254,** 282–285.

Marin-Padilla, M. (1971). Early prenatal ontogenesis of the cerebral cortex (neocortex) of the cat (*Felis domestica*). A Golgi study. I. The primordial neocortical organization. *Z. Anat. Entwicklungsgesch.* **134**, 117–145.

Martin, K. A. C., and Whitteridge, D. (1984). Form, function and intracortical projections of spiny neurones in the striate visual cortex of the cat. *J. Physiol. (London)* **353**, 463–504.

Nowakowski, R. S., and Rakic, P. (1974). Clearance rate of exogenous [^{3}H]thymidine from the plasma of pregnant rhesus monkeys. *Cell Tissue Kinet.* **7**, 189–194.

O'Leary, D. D. M., and Stanfield, B. B. (1985). Occipital cortical neurons with transient pyramidal axons extend and maintain collaterals to subcortical but not intracortical targets. *Brain Res.* **336**, 326–333.

O'Leary, D. D. M., and Stanfield, B. B. (1989). Selective elimination of axons extended by developing cortical neurons is dependent on regional locale. *J. Neurosci.* **9**, 2230–2246.

Parnavelas, J. G., Barfield, J. A., and Luskin, M. B. (1990). Lineage relationships of pyramidal and nonpyramidal neurons in the rat cerebral cortex. *Soc. Neurosci. Abstr.* **16**, 1272.

Peinado, A., and Katz, L. C. (1990). Development of cortical spiny stellate cells: Retraction of a transient apical dendrite. *Soc. Neurosci. Abstr.* **16**, 1127.

Price, J., and Thurlow, L. (1988). Cell lineage in the rat cerebral cortex: A study using retroviral-mediated gene transfer. *Development* **104**, 473–482.

Rakic, P. (1971a). Neuron–glia relationship during graunule cell migration in developing cerebellar cortex. A golgi and electronmicroscopic study in *Macacus rhesus. J. Comp. Neurol.* **141**, 283–312.

Rakic, P. (1971b). Guidance of neurons migrating to the fetal monkey neocortex. *Brain Res.* **33**, 471–476.

Rakic, P. (1974). Neurons in the rhesus monkey visual cortex: Systematic relationship between time of origin and eventual disposition. *Science* **183**, 425–427.

Rakic, P. (1978). Neuronal migration and contact guidance in the primate telencephalon. *Postgrad. Med. J.* **54**, 25–40.

Rakic, P. (1985). Contact regulation of neuronal migration. *In* "The Cell in Contact: Adhesions and Junctions as Morphogenetic Determinants" (G. M. Edelman and J.-P. Thiery, eds.), pp. 67–91. Cambridge: Neurosciences Research Foundation.

Rakic, P. (1989). Specification of cerebral cortical areas. *Science* **241**, 170–176.

Rakic, P. (1990). Principles of neural cell migration. *Experientia* **46**, 882–891.

Rakic, P. (1974). Neurons in the rhesus monkey visual cortex: Systematic relationship between time of origin and eventual disposition. *Science* **183**, 425–427.

Rakic, P. (1983). Geniculo-cortical connections in primates: normal and experimentally latered development. In *Molecular and Cellular Interactions Underlying Higher Brain Functions* (Changeux, J.-P., Glowinski, J., Imbert, M., and Bloom, F. E., eds.), pp. 393–404. New York: Elsevier Science Publishers, B. V.

Rakic, P. (1989). Specification of cerebral cortical areas. *Science* **241**, 170–176.

Ramon y Cajal, S. (1911). "Histologie du système nerveux de l'homme et des vertèbrès" Vol. 2, pp. 847–861. Paris: Maloine.

Sanes, J. R., Rubenstein, J. L. R., and Nicolas, J.-F. (1986). Use of a recombinant retrovirus to study post-implantation cell lineage in mouse embryos. *EMBO J.* **5**, 3133–3142.

Schlagger, B. L., and O'Leary, D. D. M. (1988). Embryonic rat neocortex transplanted homotopically into newborn neocortex develops area appropriate features. *Soc. Neurosci. Abstr.* **15**, 1050.

Schlagger, B. L., and O'Leary, D. D. M. (1990). Glycoconjugate boundaries outline barrels that form in visual cortex transplanted to the barrelfield of SI cortex. *Soc. Neurosci. Abstr.* **16**, 631.

Shankland, M., and Weisblat, D. A. (1984). Stepwise commitment of blast cell fates during the positional specification of the O and P cell lines in the leech embryo. *Dev. Biol.* **106,** 326–342.

Shatz, C. J., and Luskin, M. B. (1986). The relationship between the geniculocortical afferents and their cortical target cells during the development of the cat's primary visual cortex. *J. Neurosci.* **6,** 3655–3668.

Shatz, C. J., Chun, J. M., and Luskin, M. B. (1988). The role of the subplate in the development of the mammalian telencephalon. *In* "Cerebral Cortex" (A. Peters and E. G. Jones, eds.), Vol. 7, pp. 35–57. New York: Plenum Press.

Shatz, C. J., Ghosh, A., McConnell, S. K., Allendoerfer, K. L., Friauf, E., and Antonini, A. (1990). Pioneer neurons and target selection in cerebral cortical development. *Cold Spring Harbor Symp. Quant. Biol.* **55,** 469–480.

Sidman, R. L., Miale, I. L., and Feder, N. (1959). Cell proliferation and migration in the primitive ependymal zone: An autoradiographic study of histogenesis in the nervous system. *Exp. Neurol.* **1,** 322–333.

Stanfield, B. B., O'Leary, D. D. M., and Fricks, C. (1982). Selective collateral elimination in early postnatal development restricts cortical distribution of rat pyramidal tract neurons. *Nature (London)* **298,** 371–373.

Stanfield, B. B., and O'Leary, D. D. M. (1985a). The transient corticospinal projection from the occipital cortex during the postnatal development of the rat. *J. Comp. Neurol.* **238,** 236–248.

Stanfield, B. B., and O'Leary, D. D. M. (1985b). Fetal occipital cortical neurones transplanted to the rostral cortex can extend and maintain a pyramidal tract axon. *Nature (London)* **313,** 135–137.

Stanfield, B. B., O'Leary, D. D. M., and Fricks, C. (1982). Selective collateral elimination in early postnatal development restricts cortical distribution of rat pyramidal tract neurons. *Nature (London)* **298,** 371–373.

Steindler, D. A., Faissner, A., and Schachner, M. (1989). Brain "cordones:" Transient boundaries of glia and adhesion molecules that define developing functional units. *Comm. Dev. Neurobiol.* **1,** 29–60.

Stent, G. S. (1985). The role of cell lineage in development. *Phil. Trans. R. Soc. London (B.)* **312,** 3–19.

Sulston, J. E., and Horvitz, H. R. (1977). Postembryonic cell lineages of the nematode *Caenorhabditis elegans. Dev. Biol.* **56,** 110–156.

Symonds, L. L., and Rosenquist, A. C. (1984). Laminar origins of visual corticocortical connections in the cat. *J. Comp. Neurol.* **229,** 39–47.

Tosney, K. W., and Landmesser, L. T. (1985). Growth cone morphology and trajectory in the lumbosacral region of the chick embryo. *J. Neurosci.* **5,** 2345–2358.

Turner, D. L., and Cepko, C. L. (1987). Cell lineage in the rat retina: A common progenitor for neurons and glia persists late in development. *Nature (London)* **328,** 131–136.

Valverde, F., and Facal-Valverde, M. V. (1987). Transitory population of cells in the temporal cortex of kittens. *Dev. Brain Res.* **32,** 283–288.

Valverde, F., and Facal-Valverde, M. V. (1988). Postnatal development of interstitial (subplate) cells in the white matter of the temporal cortex of kittens: a correlated Golgi and electron microscopic study. *J. Comp. Neurol.* **269,** 168–192.

Vandenbergh, D. J., Wuenschell, C. W., Mori, N., and Anderson, D. J. (1989). Chromatin structure as a molecular marker of cell lineage and developmental potential in neural crest-derived chromaffin cells. *Neuron* **3,** 507–518.

Wahle, P., and Meyer, G. (1987). Morphology and quantitative changes of transient NPY-ir neuronal populations during early postnatal development of the cat visual cortex. *J. Comp. Neurol.* **161,** 165–192.

Walsh, C., and Cepko, C. L. (1988). Clonally related cortical cells show several migration patterns. *Science* **241,** 1342–1345.

Weintraub, H. (1985). Assembly and propagation of repressed and derepressed chromosomal states. *Cell* **42,** 705–711.

Wolffe, A. P., and Brown, D. D. (1986). DNA replication *in vitro* erases a *Xenopus* 5S gene transcription complex. *Cell* **47,** 217–227.

Woo, T. U., Beale, J. M., and Finlay, B. L. (1990). Dual fate of subplate neurons in the rodent. *Soc. Neurosci. Abstr.* **16,** 836.

Generation of Neuronal Diversity in the Vertebrate Retina

Thomas A. Reh
Department of Biological Structure
University of Washington
Seattle, Washington

I. Introduction
II. Embryology of the Eye
III. Sensory Retinal Histogenesis
    A. Progenitor Cells in the Retinal Germinal Neuroepithelium Are Multipotent at All Stages of Development
    B. Progenitor Cells Are Progressively Restricted in Their Prospective Fate during Retinal Neurogenesis *in Vivo*
    C. Progenitor Cells Are Progressively Restricted in Their Prospective Fate during Retinal Neurogenesis *in Vitro*
IV. Mechanisms of Cell Determination in the Sensory Retina
    A. Do Intrinsic or Microenvironmental Interactions Determine the Phenotype of a Differentiating Retinal Cell?
    B. Is Neurogenesis Unidirectional?
    C. Is There a Default Phenotype for the Retinal Neuroepithelial Cell?
    D. When Does a Neuroepithelial Cell Make a Commitment?
    E. To What Extent Are Determination and Differentiation Separable Events?
V. Conclusions
    References

I. Introduction

The development of the eye has long fascinated embryologists. The ease of identification of ocular phenotypes after embryological manipulation is likely to be part of the explanation for the inordinate amount of attention this structure has received; however, in addition, the number of different tissue types that must coordinate their differentiation for the appropriate organo-genesis of the eye has no doubt contributed to its interest. The degree to which inductive interactions are important to eye development is highlighted by the fact that our current concepts of embryonic induction arose initially through Spemann's studies of lens formation. In addition, the retina has been the subject of a considerable number of developmental studies, since it is easily isolated from the rest of the central nervous system (CNS). Also, the various cell types that make up the retina have well characterized morphology, electrophysiology, and biochemistry. Since this structure arises from a ger-minal neuroepithelium continuous with that of the neural tube, the principles of neural development that control the formation of the retina are likely to be the same as those that control the rest of the central nervous system. In this chapter, I will describe briefly some of the early embryology of the eye, to show the degree to which the determination and differentiation of the eye-forming cells appears to be dependent on interactions with other tissues. Then I will discuss recent experiments that have demonstrated that the same types of interactions are likely to be important in the determination of the phenotypes of various classes of neurons in the retina.

II. Embryology of the Eye

During eye development, as during the development of other areas of the embryo, there appears to be a progressive restriction in the potential fates that cells can adopt (von Baer, 1828). The possibility that the commitment to a particular cell fate might arise as a direct consequence of a cell's history led several investigators to analyze the lineages of blastomeres in the frog and fish. Using injections of fluorescent dyes or peroxidase tracers, the lineages of ocular tissues, along with the cells in the rest of the animal, have been determined for two vertebrate species. These studies have found that many different blastomeres have the potential to give rise to ocular tissues. Although there is some regularity in *Xenopus,* and at the 32-cell-stage only four blas-tomeres are likely to contribute to the retina (Moody, 1987), virtually every blastomere participates in the formation of the eye in a zebrafish at the same stage (Streisinger *et al.,* 1989). In general, tissue specific lineages are first observed at gastrulation; prior to this stage, it appears that the tissue con-tribution of a particular blastomere is largely indeterminate (Kimmel and Warga, 1986;1987;1988).

At gastrulation it also first becomes possible to identify by the methods of traditional embryology the cells that will ultimately give rise to the eye. Several different types of studies have been carried out over almost 100 years to determine the position of the eye-forming cells in the embryo and assay their state of commitment. It is beyond the scope of this chapter to review this literature in detail. (For an excellent review of the earlier literature, see Lopashov and Stroeva, 1964.) However, at the risk of oversimplification, I will summarize the overall conclusions of these studies. Although most of this work has been done in amphibians, studies in chick embryos indicate a very similar developmental process (Clarke, 1936; Rawles, 1936; Coulombre and Coulombre, 1965; Hilfer *et al.*, 1981). The types of studies that have attempted to identify and localize the presumptive eye primordia at various stages of development can be classified as follows: (1) vital dye labeling of neural plate cells; (2) excision of regions of the neural plate and folds; (3) transplantation of neural plate or fold cells; and (4) rearrangement or rotation of presumptive eye primordia in the neural plate. These experiments have been done on urodeles and anurans at various stages, from late gastrula to neural fold.

One major conclusion of the studies in amphibian embryos is that induction of the eye primordia from ectoderm occurs during gastrulation, as a consequence of general neural induction by the invaginating archenteron roof (Spemann, 1938). By transplantation of the eye primordia from the ectoderm of various stages of urodele embryos (early gastrula to neurula) to an ectopic location on a later staged host embryo, Mangold (1929) found that the youngest transplant that produced definitive eye tissue was a *"Triton alpestris* gastrula with a medium-sized yolk plug" (quoted from Alderman, 1935). The probability that an eye will form from a transplant increases with the age of the donor so by neurulation, eyes are reliably produced. These transplantation experiments have been confirmed by explantation of the same tissue to balanced salt solution and culture as fragments (von Woellwarth, 1952). Table 1 summarizes these results. Complete or fragmentary eyes were present in up to 45% of the cases in which the presumptive eye-forming neural ectoderm was explanted from embryos at blastopore closure.

The second general conclusion that can be drawn from the embryological experiments in the amphibian is that a well-defined region of anterior neural plate is normally responsible for generating the eye (Fig. 1). In addition to excision or transplantation experiments, several investigators have used vital dye mapping methods to establish the position of the eye primordia at neural plate stages (Manchot, 1929; Woerdeman, 1929; Jacobson, 1959; Eagleson and Harris, 1990). Although all these studies are in general agreement on this issue, controversies have arisen over the years about exactly where the eye-forming cells are positioned in the neural plate. For example, Spemann (1938) claimed that the eye primordia are located medially, on the basis of excision experiments, whereas Adelman (1929, 1930), using a very similar experimental design, found that the lateral third of the anterior neural plate must be removed instead to inhibit eye formation. Some of the differences in experimental results can probably be attributed to minor variations among

TABLE I

Change in Frequency of Appearance of Eyes and Their Number during Explantation of Anterior Neural Plate Section with Neural Crests and Adjacent Ectoderm in *Triturus alpestris*[a]

Stage of experiment	Undifferentiated ectoderm	Neural structures	Nasal placodes		Eyes (%)				
						Cyclopia		Synoph-thalmia	Two separated eyes
			Single	Paired	Fragments	Complete	Incomplete		
Late gastrula	73	15	4	–	4	4	–	–	–
Blastopore closure	30	65	45	–	5	45	10	–	–
Neural groove appearance	–	100	95	–	–	57	24	19	–
Neural plate appearance	–	100	90	–	–	38	20	29	–
Early neurula	–	100	100	–	–	20	32	48	–
Middle neurula	–	100	100	–	–	18	27	55	–
Late neurula	–	100	40	–	–	–	10	60	30
Neural tube closure	–	100	–	–	–	–	–	–	100

[a]Reprinted from von Woellwarth, 1952.

species and to differences in technique; however, a relatively recent study by Brun (1981) reinvestigated the issue with excision experiments and time lapse recordings and found that the cells that will ultimately give rise to the eye move rapidly across the surface of the neural plate as the folds are forming. (Fig. 1 shows the position of the eye primordia at three stages of neural plate development, as described by Brun, 1981.) Thus, much of the inconsistency in the earlier reports may have been caused by the fact that the embryologist attempting to remove the eye primordia for transplantation is faced with a moving target.

Transplantation experiments have also been used to determine the state of commitment of the eye primordia at neurula stages in amphibians. As noted earlier, transplantation of presumptive eye-forming cells from embryos as early as late gastrula stages results in the development of eye tissue in a percentage of the cases. At neural plate stages, this commitment appears to be largely complete, since transplantation of anterior neural plate cells, either with (Spemann, 1938) or without (Adelman, 1929, 1930; Alderman, 1935) under-lying mesoderm (or "substrate") will develop into complete eyes in ectopic locations. Figure 2 (E,F,G) schematically demonstrates these experiments and their typical (>50% of cases) result. On the other hand, several experiments in which the neural plate has been rotated have been interpreted as evidence that the commitment of the neural plate cells is still labile at the neural plate stage. When a piece of neural plate was rotated, either with or without the underlying mesoderm, Alderman (1935) found "the material which would go

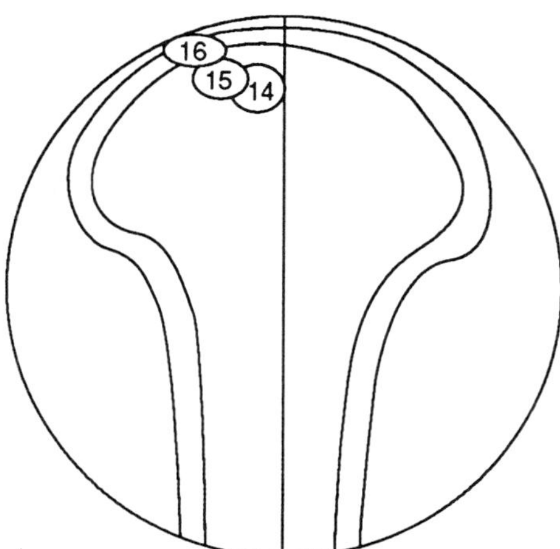

Figure 1. Location of the eye primordia at three successive neural plate stages (14, 15, 16) in a *Xenopus* embryo, showing the movement of these cells across the surface of the neural plate. Adapted from Brun (1981).

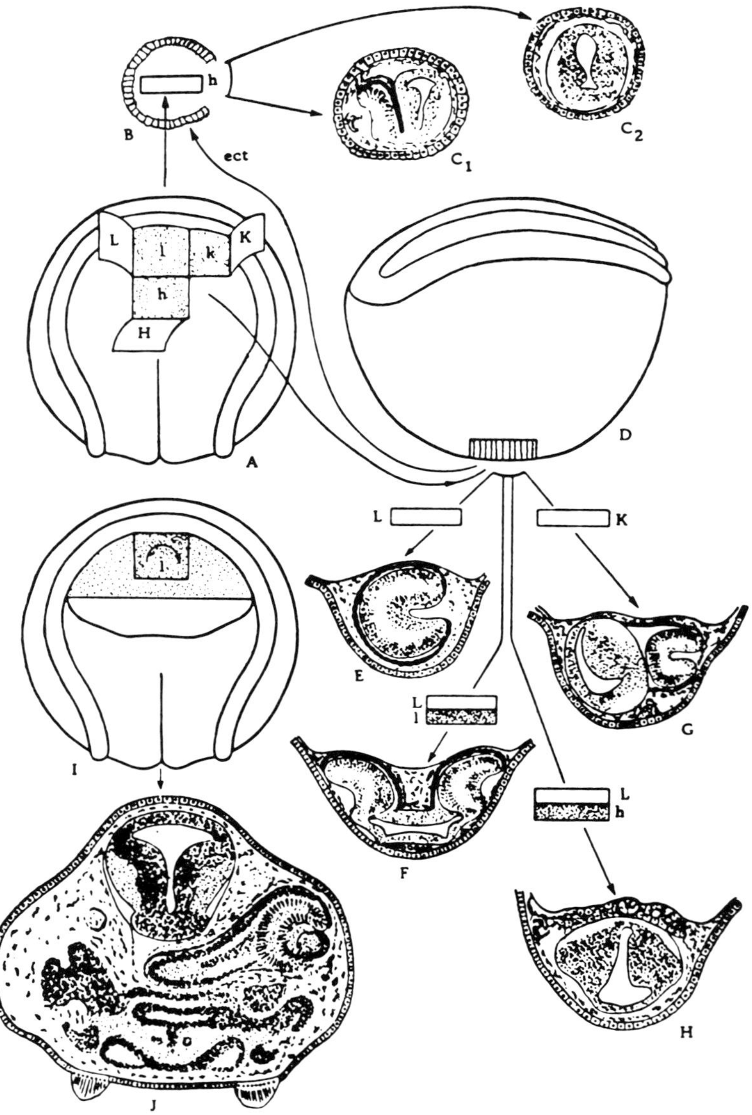

Figure 2. Schematic representation of the various experimental transplantation paradigms used to study the location and state of commitment of eye-forming cells in amphibian embryos. A neural plate staged embryo (A) is shown with the neuroectoderm peeled away (L, H, K) to show the underlying mesoderm (l, h, k). Pieces of mesoderm, cultured with "indifferent" ectoderm (B), produce primarily brain tissue (C_1, C_2). Grafts of neuroectoderm from eye primordial regions of the neural plate (L, K) transplanted to ectopic locations in other embryos produce eyes (E, G); however, when eye primorida are combined with mesoderm from a region of neural plate that normally produces hindbrain (h), eyes fail to develop in the graft (H). (Reproduced from Lopashov and Stroeva, 1964, with permission.)

to form eye, now forms brain. Material which left in place would form brain, under these circumstances forms eye." Additional experiments further suggest that the commitment of these cells to generate only ocular phenotypes is not yet fixed; several of these different experimental paradigms are shown along with the typical result in Fig. 2. In one of these experiments—shown schematically as the "L" and "h" combination—pieces of the anterior neural plate ("L") that normally produce eyes (when transplanted to a neutral site on another embryo) can be induced to generate more posterior neural structures when co-transplanted with pieces of mesoderm ("h") from more posterior regions of the embryo (Alderman, 1935; Takaya, 1955).

Although the molecular mechanisms responsible for the commitment to the ocular phenotype are not known, one speculation is that position-determining genes are stably expressed only through consistent expression in both the mesoderm and the adjacent ectoderm. Normally by neurula stages of development, these genes are coordinately expressed in both of these tissues at a particular axial position; therefore, when the ectoderm is isolated or transplanted to a "neutral" location, such as the ventral surface of the embryo, the eye positional signals in the neuroectoderm remain active and eyes develop. However, when the eye ectoderm is co-cultured or co-transplanted with mesoderm that is expressing positional genes from a different axial location, the ectoderm now begins to express the positional genes of the mesoderm and neural structures other than eyes develop from the cells. The positional genes important in specifying the ocular phenotype may be related to the homeobox genes that appear to play a role in determining axial position in more caudal regions of the embryo. The expression of *Pax2* (Nornes *et al.,* 1990) and *Hox*7.1 (Hill *et al.,* 1989) have been described in developing retina.

By the time the optic vesicles form, however, the cells are apparently restricted to develop into ocular phenotypes exclusively. The anterior part of the optic vesicle normally forms the neural retina, whereas the posterior part of this anlage gives rise to the retinal pigmented epithelium. Once again it appears that this commitment is not immediately fixed since, under experimental conditions, there is a period of development during which the fates of these two issues can be reversed. Most of these experiments, again, have used amphibian embryos; if the optic cup is transplanted in such a manner that the posterior cell layer (presumptive pigment epithelium) is adjacent to the ectoderm or the otic vesicle (shown in Fig. 3), fully differentiated retina, albeit inverted in orientation, will form from this layer (Detwiler and van Dyke, 1953, 1954). The length of this labile period varies with species and reaches its extreme in urodeles, in which neural retinal precursors can develop from well-differentiated pigmented epithelial cells in mature animals, following retinal removal or degeneration (Stone, 1950a,b, 1960; Lopashov and Sologub, 1972; Reyer, 1977; Okada, 1980; Reh and Nagy, 1987; Reh *et al.,* 1987). In the chick embryo there appears to be a definite period during which the pig-

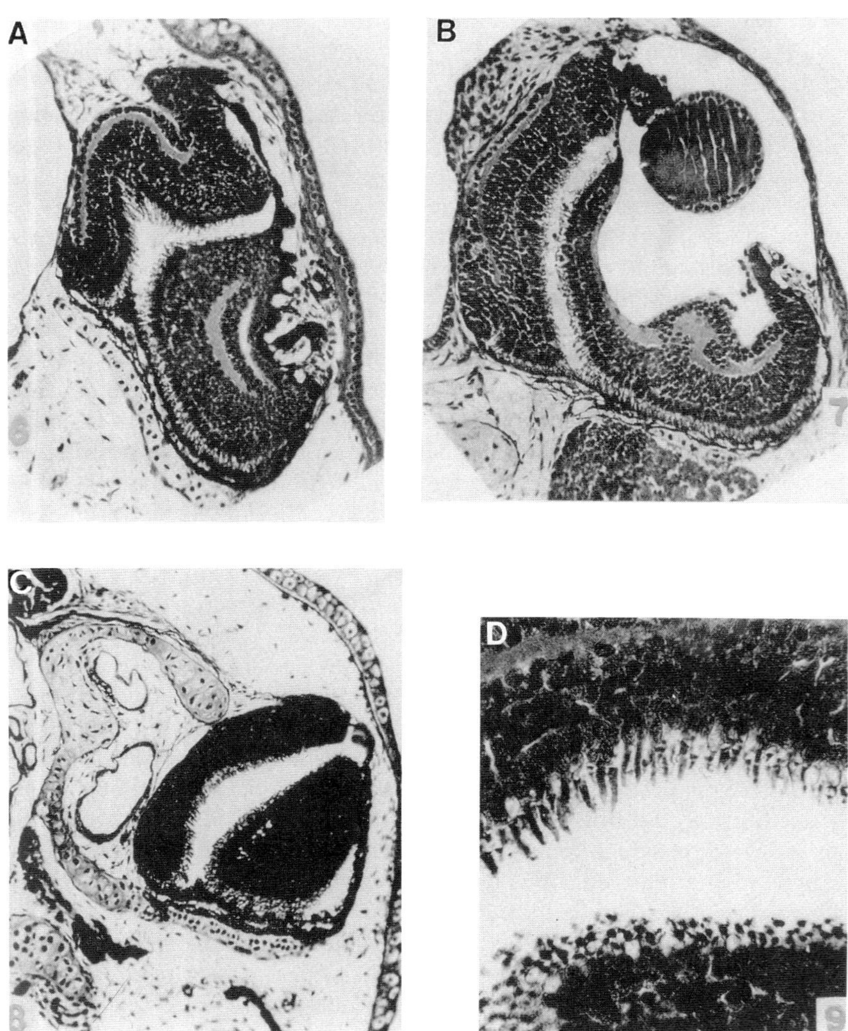

Figure 3. Neural retina "induced" from the pigment epithelium following transplantation to the otic vesicle region in *Amblystoma punctatum* embryos. A, B, C. Three examples in which the retina derived from the pigment epithelium is to the left, whereas the normal retina is to the right. D. Higher magnification of the photoreceptor outer segments in the induced retina. (A, B: 80×; C: 56×; D: 224×) (Reproduced from Detwiler and van Dyke, 1953, with permission.)

mented epithelial cells can be induced to form sensory retinal progenitors and, ultimately, retinal neurons (Coulombre and Coulombre, 1965; Park and Hollenberg, 1989). Several types of experiments, including transplantation or explant culture of the eye primordia and examination of regeneration after retinal removal, have led to the conclusion that "the capacity of prospective tapetal tissue to form sensory retina . . . is retained at least through the 36-somite stage" (Alexander, 1937; Gayer, 1942; Orts-Llorca and Genis-Galvez, 1960; Coulombre and Coulombre, 1965), 3–4 days of incubation.

In summary, the development of the eye is clearly a complex process that is likely to involve several different inductive interactions. The ability to form ocular tissues apparently does not reside in a particular set of blastomeres in blastula-stage embryos and, in the case of the zebrafish embryo, the eye can receive a contribution from virtually every blastomere. However, during gastrulation, a set of neuroectoderm cells acquires the ability to form eye tissue when cultured in isolation or in ectopic locations in the embryo. In the zebrafish gastrula, there may be as few as 40 cells (out of several thousand) that become committed to generate the pigmented epithelium (Streisenger *et al.,* 1989). This commitment to presumptive eye primordia is thought to be the result of a position-dependent inductive interaction via the underlying mesoderm. Recent studies have proposed that concentration gradients of peptide growth factors may be responsible for the induction of various CNS structures, including the eyes (Godsave *et al.,* 1988; Kimmelman *et al.,* 1988; Rosa *et al.,* 1988; Sokol *et al.,* 1990). The commitment of these cells to the exclusive generation of ocular tissue appears to remain labile throughout neurula stages. If the position of the eye primordium is changed with respect to the underlying mesoderm, the fate of these cells may be changed. Their commitment to ocular phenotypes appears to be fixed, however, once the eye vesicles have formed, although both the anterior and posterior walls of the optic vesicle have the ability to generate either sensory or pigmented retina. Ultimately, this plasticity is also lost in most species, although pigment epithelial cells from urodele amphibians retain the capacity to generate retinal neuronal progenitors throughout the animal's life.

III. Sensory Retinal Histogenesis

A. Progenitor Cells in the Retinal Germinal Neuroepithelium Are Multipotent at All Stages of Development

The next stage of retinal development is characterized by the generation of the various neuronal and glial cell classes. Under normal conditions, the precursor cells of the sensory germinal neuroepithelium give rise to all the classes of neurons found in the retina, as well as the Müller glial cells. Retinal astrocytes are not produced by the retinal germinal neuroepithelium, but migrate into the retina via the optic nerve (Watanabe and Raff, 1988). Due to its relatively simple laminar organization, and the distinct morphological features of the various cell classes found in the retina, several recent studies examining the lineal relationships among the neurons and glia of the CNS have focused on the retina as a model system. Using either retroviral infection in rodent retina at various stages of retinal development (Turner and Cepko, 1988; Turner *et al.*, 1990) or dye injections of individual progenitor cells in both embryonic and larval frogs (Holt *et al.*, 1988; Wetts and Fraser, 1988; Wetts *et al.*, 1989), several investigators have shown that retinal neurons and glia have indeterminate lineages; the clones of infected or injected neuroepithelial cells can vary in number from one to hundreds of cells, and are composed of many different neuronal and glial phenotypes. In addition to demonstrating the lack of a clear pattern in the lineages of the various retinal cell classes, these studies also suggest that the neuroepithelial cells are multipotent. This interpretation relies on the following assumptions: (1) cell death in clones is minimal (or at least equal among the retinal cell classes); (2) the neuroepithelial cells at any given stage of development are a homogeneous population; and, at least for the retroviral infection studies, (3) the reporter gene is expressed in all cells of a clone. Although these assumptions are generally held to be valid, it will be important to demonstrate that an isolated neuroepithelial cell can generate multiple neuronal phenotypes *in vitro,* where these assumptions can be directly tested.

In this context, the two-cell clones resulting from retroviral infection or dye injection are particularly informative, since they are likely to be the products of the final mitotic division of a neuroepithelial cell. In the frog, in which the development of the central retina is very rapid, any combination of retinal cell classes can arise in these two-cell clones. However, in the rat, although the neuroepithelial cells appear to be capable of generating all the combinations of retinal phenotypes, at any given time in the development of the retina certain combinations are more likely than others. For example, when retroviral infections are made in postnatal rats, clones with only two cells, which presumably represent the terminal mitosis of a neuroepithelial cell, can consist of any combination of bipolar, Müller, or rod photoreceptor cells; however, two-cell clones that consist of any of these aforementioned cell classes and a cone photoreceptor, horizontal cell, or ganglion cell were not observed (Turner and Cepko, 1988). This is almost certainly because different retinal cell classes are generated at different times during development (see subsequent text), a phenomenon present throughout the CNS. This apparent restriction of the neuroepithelial cells to generate only a subset of the range of retinal phenotypes can be explained in two ways: (1) The progenitor cell has changed during the course of development, either by some intrinsic mechanism or by some influence from its local environment; (2) The neuroepithelial cells from all stages of development are identical, but are continuously restricted in their potential through interactions with their local environment. As noted earlier, the cells of the pigment epithelium initially arise from a similar region of the neural plate as the sensory retina; even after the pigment epithelium has formed, these cells retain the capacity to revert to neuroepithelial cells. However, over a relatively short period of development they become restricted (by factors in their local environment) to the pigmented phenotype. If an analogous mechanism exists for the neuroepithelial cells, we could predict that there is also a progressive restriction in their potential that comes about through interactions with the differentiating cells in their immediate environment.

B. Progenitor Cells Are Progressively Restricted in Their Prospective Fate during Retinal Neurogenesis *in Vivo*

The [^{3}H]thymidine birthdating experiments of Sidman (1961) first suggested that cells of the germinal neuroepithelium might undergo progressive changes with development. From these early studies, it was clear that germinal neuroepithelial cells generated different types of retinal cells during particular periods of neurogenesis. Birthdating studies in other areas of the CNS soon demonstrated that a similar phenomenon occurred in diverse CNS regions (see Jacobson, 1978, for review). In the mouse retina, Sidman found that ganglion cells, horizontal cells, and amacrine cells were the first cell classes to be generated in the retina, whereas most bipolar cells and photoreceptors became postmitotic postnatally. Since these initial studies, a large number of further experiments using a wide variety of different species, has essentially confirmed the early work, and extended the idea of defined birthdates for particular cell classes in the retina (Hollyfield, 1968; Kohn, 1974; Blanks and Bok, 1977; Hinds and Hinds, 1978, 1979; Carter-Dawson and LaVail, 1979; Young, 1985; Rappaport *et al.,* 1987, 1988; Zimmerman *et al.,* 1988; see also Holt *et al.,* 1988). More detailed analysis has shown that, in a general class of cells, particular subclasses may have different schedules of production. For example, in the cat retina, the alpha and beta ganglion cells have distinct periods of generation (Walsh *et al.,* 1983; Walsh and Polley, 1985); in addition, the A- and B-type horizontal cells are likely to have separable birthdates as well (Zimmerman *et al.,* 1988). The periods of generation of the two classes of photoreceptors—the rods and the cones—are also distinct; cone production precedes rod histogenesis by a considerable degree

(Carter-Dawson and LaVail, 1979). Thus, although there is considerable overlap in the timing of production of the different cell classes in the retina of most species, the period of development over which a given cell class is produced is very well defined in a particular species (Fig. 4).

C. Progenitor Cells Are Progressively Restricted in Their Prospective Fate during Retinal Neurogenesis *in Vitro*

Additional evidence for a developmental change in the potential range of retinal cell phenotypes capable of being generated by the neuroepithelial cells comes from recent *in vitro* studies in the rat and the chick. As in the classical embryological experiments described earlier, the status of determination of a given cell is assayed operationally by isolating the cell from other neighboring cells and examining the phenotypes that are generated in isolation. This kind of experiment assumes that the cells in question have the ability to survive and differentiate their normal phenotypic characteristics under the isolation protocol used in the experiment. Although there are some important caveats to these assumptions (see subsequent text), in general the process of dissociation and low density cell culture inhibits the mitotic activity of retinal neuroepithelial cells (Reh and Kljavin, 1989) so these cells will differentiate into identifiable neuronal phenotypes. In the experiments with rat retinal cells, the phenotypes that dissociated neuro-

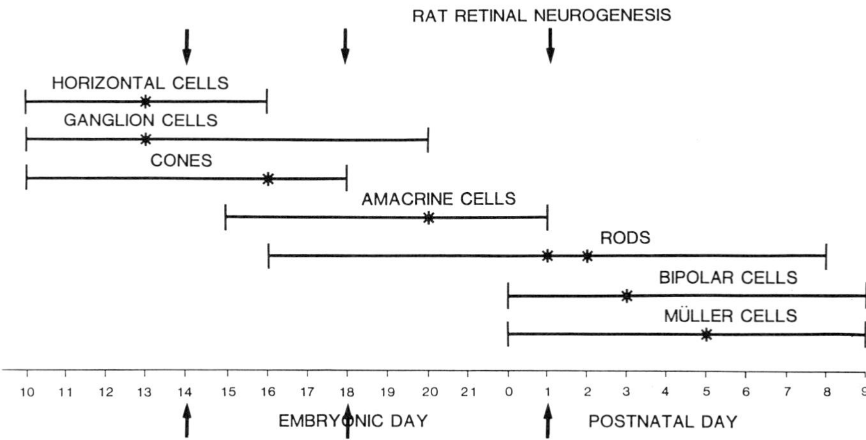

Figure 4. Chart of [³H]thymidine birthdating studies by LaVail (unpublished observations) showing the range of cell birthdates of the various cell classes in the rat retina. The asterisk denotes the day at which the greatest number of cells of a particular type become postmitotic, the bars indicate the range over which that cell type becomes postmitotic.

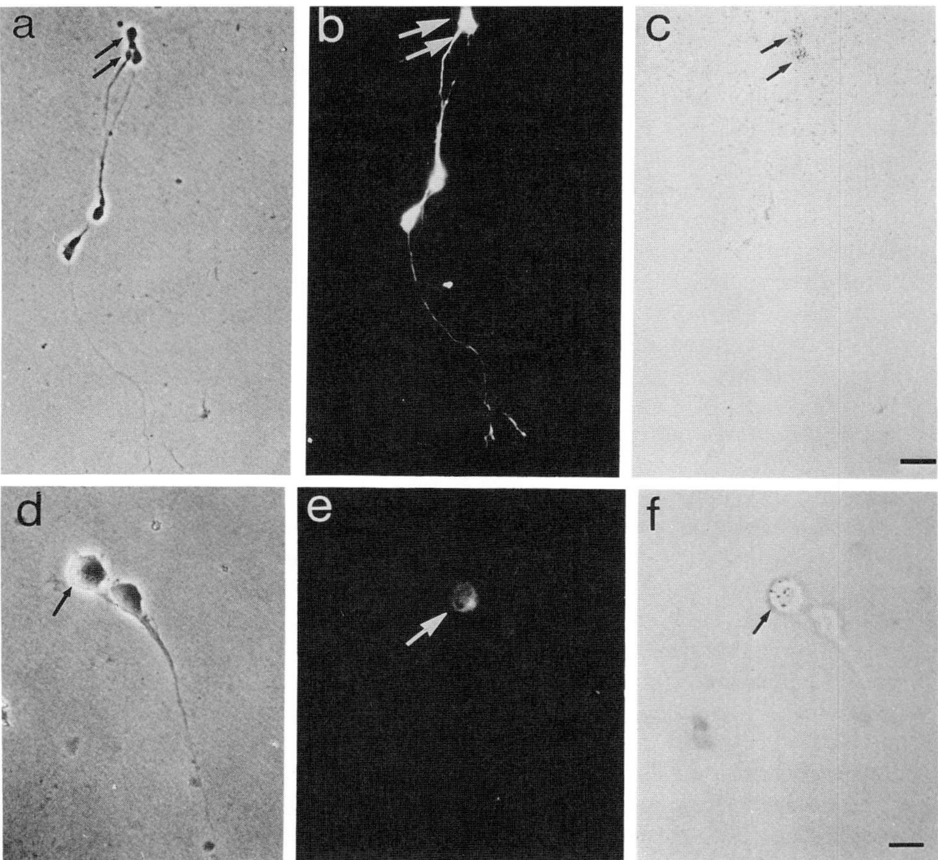

Figure 5. Ganglion cells derived from E14 retina after 4 days in culture. a–c. Corresponding phase, fluorescent, and bright field micrographs of the same field of cells labeled with B-50 antibodies. d–f. Corresponding phase, fluorescent, and bright field micrographs of the same two cells labeled with a monoclonal antibody to neurofilament. Several of the immunoreactive cells are also labeled with [³H]thymidine, as shown by the silver grain over their nuclei (*arrows*), indicating that they were in the S phase of the cell cycle within 6 hr of dissociation. Bars: 19 μm (a–c); 13 μm (d–f).

epithelial cells expressed in culture were determined by labeling the mitotically active cells in the retina with [³H]thymidine prior to dissociation and subsequently identifying the phenotypes of the thymidine-labeled cells after several days *in vitro* with a variety of cell-class-specific antibodies. When the retinas are cultured from early embryonic stages (E14), a large percentage of the germinal neuroepithelial cells differentiate into ganglion cells (Figs. 5,6b), whereas rod photoreceptors are only found in cultures when the cells are dissociated from postnatal animals (Reh and Kljavin, 1989). In addition, no double-labeled ganglion cells were found in the postnatal cultures, indicating that the late-stage neuroepithelial cells no longer differentiate into retinal ganglion cells (Fig. 6b). We therefore concluded that germinal neuroepithelial cells that are prematurely induced to differentiate by dissociation are limited in their differentiation to the types of neurons that were being generated at the time of dissociation.

In the chick, a similar type of experiment results primarily in the differentiation of "photoreceptor" cells from early-stage retinas (Fig. 6), whereas "multipolar neurons" predominate in cultures from later-stage animals (Adler and Hatlee, 1989). The results in the chick have been interpreted as evidence that photoreceptors are the "default" phenotype (see subsequent text). The data from retinal dissociation experiments in rodents and chicks would seem to be contradictory; however, the disparities can be explained by differences in the cellular composition of the retina. In the birthdating studies reviewed earlier, cones, horizontal cells, and ganglion cells are generated early in retinal development, whereas rods, bipolar cells, and Müller glia come later in the sequence of generation of the different retinal cell types. Since the predominant photoreceptor in the chick retina is the cone, and these cells are among the first to become postmitotic during development, chick retinal neuroepithelial cells, induced to differentiate by dissociation, would be expected to differentiate into cones with increasing frequency as the age of the animal *decreases*. Alternatively, since the predominant photoreceptor in the rat retina is the later-developing rod, the percentages of photoreceptors should increase with *increasing* developmental age. Both of these studies indicate that the stage of retinal development at which a neuroepithelial cell differentiates determines the range of cell types that it can become. Neuroepithelial cells isolated from early stages of retinal development and prematurely induced to differentiate will become those cell types normally generated during this period; whereas the progenitor cells isolated from later stages of retinal development will differentiate into those retinal cell types normally generated late in development.

These studies indicate that the probability that any given cell type is generated by a particular cell division changes progressively with development. Postmitotic daughter cells from cell divisions early in retinal development are most likely to give rise to ganglion cells, cone photoreceptors, or horizontal cells, whereas those cells that become postmitotic during the final stages of retinal development are most likely to be committed to becoming rod photoreceptors, bipolar cells, or Müller glia. Is this shift in the developmental potential of the neuroepithelial cells due to an intrinsic or internal clock mechanism that keeps track of the number of prior cell divisions, or is the change in the probability of generation of particular phenotypes due to interactions with previously generated cells and

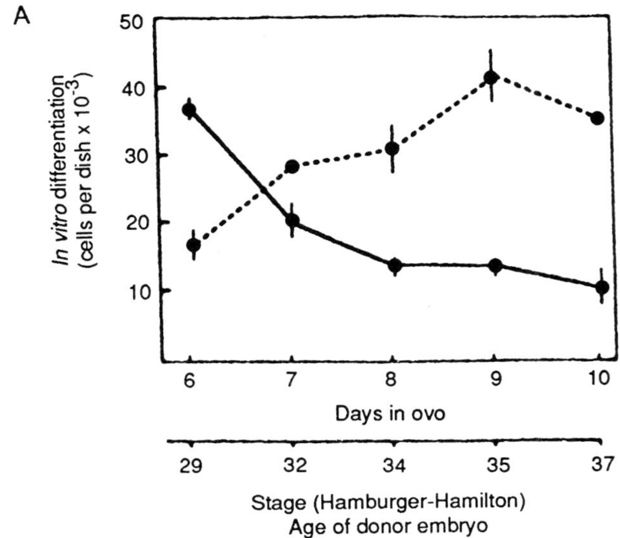

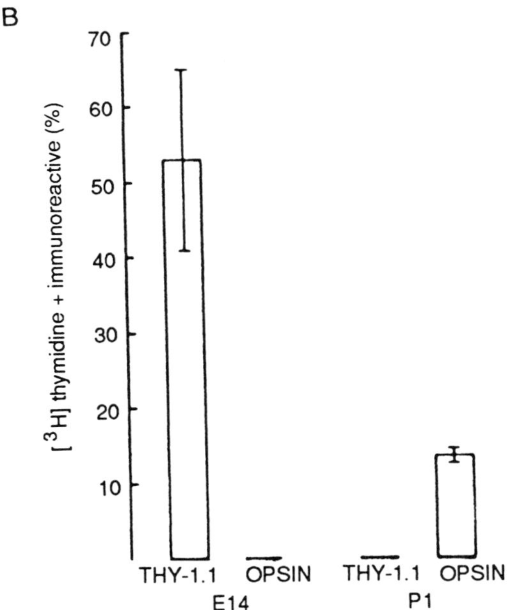

Figure 6. A. Percentage of chick retinal cells differentiating into either multipolar neurons (—) or photoreceptors (---), when dissociated and cultured at various embryonic stages. (Reproduced from Adler and Hatlee, 1989, with permission.) B. Percentages of [3H]thymidine-labeled cells that express either thy-1.1 or opsin 2–6 days after dissociation. Bars represent means and SE of the percentage of double-labeled cells from three experiments. Six fields from three coverslips were counted in each experiment. (Reproduced from Reh and Kljavin, 1989, with permission.)

factors in their local microenvironment? Although this is the central question to be addressed in the rest of this chapter, several additional questions are also relevant. First, is the progressive change in the potential of neuroepithelial cells an irreversible process? In other words, does a neuroepithelial cell from a late stage of retinal development retain the capacity to generate retinal cells of all phenotypes, or are these cells now restricted to producing only those cell types normally generated late in retinal histogenesis, regardless of the surrounding microenvironment? Second, if the phenotype of retinal neurons and glia is determined by interactions between the dividing neuroepithelial cells and previously generated differentiating neuroblasts, what is the phenotype of the first cells to differentiate, that is, what is the default condition. Third, are the processes of determination or commitment to a particular phenotype, and differentiation of particular aspects of that phenotype (such as cell-specific antigen expression), under the control of separate factors, or do all characteristics of a particular phenotype develop by a cell-autonomous program once the cell has been committed to a particular type? Finally, are retinal neurons committed to a particular phenotype at their terminal mitotic division; or is the neuronal phenotype plastic for several days after their final mitosis?

IV. Mechanisms of Cell Determination in the Sensory Retina

A. Do Intrinsic or Microenvironmental Interactions Determine the Phenotype of a Differentiating Retinal Cell?

Experiments in both mammals and nonmammalian vertebrates, using both cell cultures and *in vivo* lesion studies of developing retina, indicate that the choice of phenotype by the multipotent retinal precursor cells can be influenced by neighboring cells. For some time it has been known that the retina is capable of a considerable amount of regeneration following retinal damage in embryos of amphibians (see Reyer, 1977, for review), chicks (Coulombre and Coulombre, 1965; Park and Hollenberg, 1989), and mammals (Rugh and Wolff, 1955a,b). Although these studies did not assay the various phenotypes of the cells that constituted such regenerated retinas, their overall histology and size was approximately normal. This indicates that the cells of the retinal germinal neuroepithelium are capable of producing many more cells than they normally would in response to damage. This is in contrast to some other areas of the CNS, for which it has been argued from chimeric studies that the germinal neuroepithelial cells are somehow intrinsically programmed to generate particular numbers and types of neurons as early as neural plate stages (for review, see Williams and Herrup, 1988; see also Cowan and Finger, 1982).

Neurotoxin experiments in the developing fish and frog retinas have provided more direct evidence that the choice of neuronal phenotypes, as well as overall cell number, is regulated by interactions with previously differentiating neurons. Relatively selective neuronal destruction can be experimentally induced in the developing retinas of larval frogs and adult fish. In both of these animals, the central retina has fully differentiated and functions normally, yet a small zone of neuroepithelial cells at the peripheral margin of the retina continues to generate new neurons and glia. When the neurotoxin 6-hydroxy dopamine (6-OHDA) is injected intravitreally in larval frogs or fish of various ages, the dopamineragic amacrine cells in the mature regions of retina are destroyed within a few days. However, since new cell production continues at the retinal margin in these species, it is possible to assess whether the loss of this particular cell type in the differentiated retina will have any effect on the types of new cells produced by the mitotically active marginal precursor cells. Negishi and his collaborators (Negishi *et al.*, 1982, 1985, 1987) examined the distribution of monoaminergic cells after neurotoxic lesions in the goldfish retina, using formaldehyde-induced monoaminergic fluorescence. They reported an increase in the density of the dopaminergic amacrine in the newly generated peripheral retina in those animals that had received 6-OHDA injections several weeks earlier. In similar experiments with the frog, *Rana pipiens,* using immunohistochemical labeling for several types of amacrine cells, the generation of new cells at the retinal margin is influenced by the neurotoxin lesion in a highly specific manner: after the destruction of the mature dopaminergic amacrine cells, there is a specific increase in the production of new dopaminergic amacrines, but not of the other amacrine cell classes (those containing serotonin or substance P) that were examined (Reh and Tully, 1986).

Similar lesion experiments with the neurotoxin kainic acid (KA) further support the idea that the retinal precursor cells at the retinal margin will specifically increase their production of new cells of the types that are destroyed (Reh, 1987). KA causes degeneration in the inner nuclear layer (INL) and ganglion cell layer (GCL) of several vertebrate species, including the frog (Erlich and Morgan, 1980; Hampton *et al.*, 1981; Ingham and Morgan, 1983; Reh, 1987). In the *Rana* tadpole, intraocular injections of KA resulted in a 52% decline in the cell density of the INL, a 37% decline in the density of the GCL and no significant change in the density of cells in the outer nuclear layer (ONL) (Reh, 1987). In the 3 wk after KA administration, the tadpoles were injected with [^{3}H]thymidine to detect any changes in the number and laminar distribution of newly generated cells in the lesioned eyes as compared with the controls. In animals that received the [^{3}H]thymidine injection more than 1 wk after the KA lesion, there was a large increase in the number of new neurons generated in the treated retina over the uninjected eye. Moreover, the INL which had sustained the greatest cell loss as a result of the KA treatment, showed the greatest increase over control in the number of new cells, with the other layers receiving proportionally less (Table 2).

These results provide evidence for some type of negative feedback control of neuronal production, at the marginal proliferative zone, by the specific channeling of precursor differentiation into certain pathways in a density-dependent manner. On the basis of these results, we proposed the following model (Reh and Tully, 1986). Mitotically active neuroepithelial cells are exposed to a complex microenvironment produced by dividing cells, postmitotic migrating immature neurons, and some differentiated neurons. The first cells to differentiate do so as a result of some interactions with the developing ocular extracellular matrix and other ocular tissues (Reh, 1989a). These first differentiating cells produce some type of signal that inhibits further differentiation of cells of this particular phenotype. As each new cell type is then generated in the sequence, it also provides a specific feedback inhibition of further production. This kind of mechanism would not rigidly determine the phenotype of a given daughter from a neuroepithelial cell division, but the balance of signals present in the cell's local microenviron-

TABLE 2
Cells in Retinal Layers after Kainic Acid Treatment

	Retinal ganglion cell layer (%)	Inner nuclear layer (%)	Outer nuclear layer (%)
Degenerating cells in layers, 1 day after KA (n=4)	10.3±4.5	23.3±8.7	<1
Change in cell density 2–6 weeks after KA (n=16)	−37.6±3.8	−52.3±4.2	−5.8±2.9
Change in [^{3}H]thymidine-labeled cells/layer: KA/control (<1 wk)(n=5)	−2.1±19	−9±12	−10±20
Change in [^{3}H]thymidine-labeled cells/layer: KA/control (>1 wk) (n=5)	+15.2±2.7	+22.2±2.4	+1.6±3

ment at any given time would predispose a cell to differentiate along a particular path. In this model, when a given cell class is experimentally reduced, as in the experiments just described, the inhibitory signals for that cell type are also lost and the germinal neuroepithelial progenitor cells will, therefore, be more likely to differentiate into that cell type. Although the molecular nature of these interactions has not been defined, our results in the larval frog retina indicated that the distance over which the signals could regulate cell phenotype were restricted to the area of mature retina immediately adjacent to the developing marginal neuroepithelium. It is possible that the differentiating neuro- and glioblasts can only influence those neuroepithelial cells that they directly contact, either through cell-surface interactions, short-range diffusible signals, or gap junctional coupling.

It is important to emphasize that this model does not require that the proliferating neuroepithelial cells undergo a particular *number* of cell divisions to become competent to generate those phenotypes normally generated late in development, but that the *sequence* of generation of different cell types is critical, since an early differentiating cell class restricts the phenotypic choice of the remaining neuroepithelial cells. A recent study by Harris and Hartenstine (1991) dissociated the process of cell division from phenotypic commitment; various retinal cell phenotypes develop in *Xenopus* embryos in which cell division is blocked with aphidicolin and hydroxyurea prior to the birthdates of any retinal neurons.

In order to more directly test whether the developing microenvironment has the potential to influence the choice of phenotype of neuroepithelial cells, as well as to develop assay systems for the ultimate identification of these factors, several *in vitro* experimental paradigms have recently been employed. The basic experimental design has been to label the cells from one developmental age, using either [³H]thymidine, 5-bromo-2′-deoxyuridine (BrdU), or a species-specific antibody, and to co-culture the labeled cells with unlabeled cells from a different developmental stage. These heterochronic co-culture experiments have concentrated on the late developing rod photoreceptor, using cultures of either dissociated cells or aggregates. For the dissociated cell culture experiment, early embryonic cells from E14 rat embryos were labeled for 6 hr with [³H]thymidine prior to dissociation, and co-cultured with unlabeled cells from various postnatal ages. After 6–10 days in culture, the cells were fixed, processed for opsin immunoreactivity to identify the rods in the cultures, and autoradiographed to identify the E14 cells. These cultures were then examined for the presence of [³H]thymidine-labeled cells that had differentiated into rod photoreceptors, which are found after this period *in vitro* when E14 cells are cultured alone. In this study, there were many examples of cells with both labels in the co-cultures of E14 and the early postnatal retinal cells, while only a few double-labeled cells were present in the co-cultures of E14 and retinal cells from animals older than postnatal day 8 (Reh, 1989b). Similar results also have been obtained recently by Watanabe and Raff (1990) using reaggregate cultures in which E15 and P1 retinal cells have been combined, after labeling the E15 cells with BrdU and the rod photoreceptors with a monoclonal antibody against opsin. They also find that the postnatal environment has an influence on the number of rods that differentiate from the E15 cells; approximately 40 times more E15 cells differentiate into rods in the co-cultures than would normally develop in the aggregates during the same period in culture.

Chimeric co-cultures and transplant experiments have also extended this conclusion. Several species-specific monoclonal antibodies have been raised against mouse neurons and glia; since these antibodies do not recognize a similar epitope on rat cells, they can be used to identify the mouse cells in chimeric cultures or transplant studies (Lagenauer *et al.*, 1984; Lund *et al.*, 1985). We have recently used such chimeric heterochronic cultures, as well as *in vivo* intraretinal grafts, for our studies of retinal cell determination. Our preliminary results are shown in Figs. 7–9. The results obtained with the chimeric cultures so far confirm those observed in the previous heterochronic studies. When E14 mouse cells are cultured with 100-fold excess postnatal rat cells, we found that a much higher percentage of the embryonic cells expressed the rod phenotype than in E14 mouse cells cultured alone or with E14 rat cells after the same period *in vitro* (Fig. 7,8). Similarly, in our initial transplant experiments, we found that a high percentage of the E14 mouse neuroepithelial cells grafted into postnatal rat retina differentiated into rods after 3 days; this is several days prior to the normal appearance of rods in the mouse retina.

These results, considered together, extend the previously described neurotoxin lesion studies, and provide strong support for the hypothesis that the developing microenvironment can influence the determination or differentiation of the multipotent progenitors that generate the neurons and intrinsic glia of the developing retina. These interactions are likely to occur normally over a restricted range, both spatially and temporally, since the types of neurons generated at any particular time during histogenesis vary from central to peripheral retina.

B. Is Neurogenesis Unidirectional?

As described earlier, several lines of evidence led to the proposal that the fate of the progeny of retinal neuroepithelial cells depends on the composition of their immediate environment. In addition to the apparent spatial restriction of these phenotype-determining cues, there is evidence that these

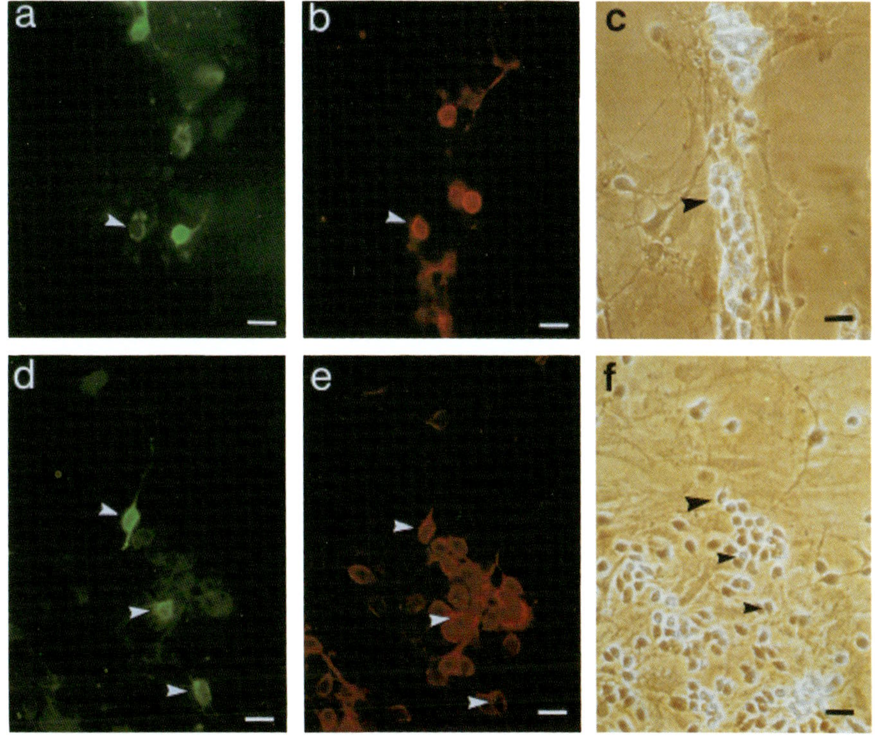

FIGURE 7. Chimeric cultures of rat and mouse retinal cells. a–f. E14 mouse retinal cells were cocultured with a 10-fold excess of P3 rat retinal cells for 6 days, fixed, and labeled with M6 to reveal all mouse neurons (b, e) and Rho4D2 (anti-opsin) to show the rods in the culture (a, d). Arrows point to the same cells in the fluorescent and phase micrographs. Bar: 13 μm (a, b); 19 μm (c).

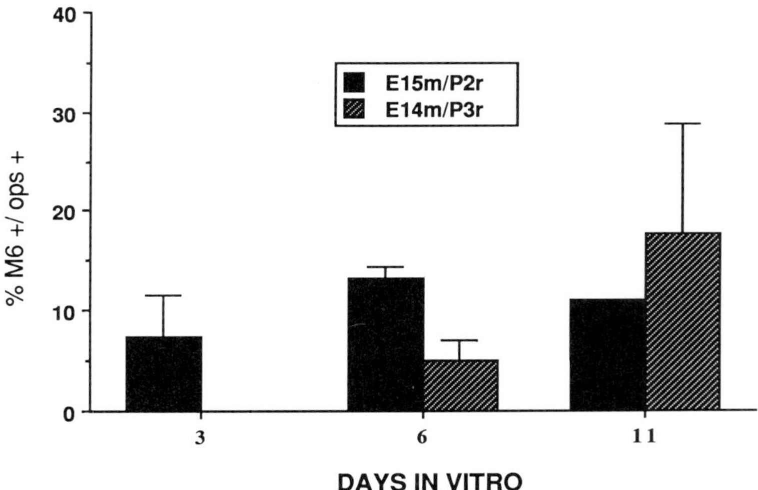

Figure 8. Summary graph of heterochronic chimeric coculture experiments. The percentage of M6 + (E14 or E15) mouse neurons that also expresses opsin immunoreactivity is graphed after 3, 6, or 11 days in coculture with either P2 or P3 rat retinal cells. When E14 or E15 mouse retinal cells are cultured alone or with E14 or E15 rat retinal cells, no opsin-positive cells are observed after this period in culture. The fact that up to 20% of the E14/15 mouse neurons become rods when cocultured with postnatal retinal cells indicates that the environment in which a cell develops can influence the phenotype into which it will differentiate.

environmental determinants are restricted temporally during retinal developmental as well. The earlier cited birthdating studies in mammals have demonstrated that the various cell classes of retinal cells are generated in a sequential manner. Lesion experiments of developing mammalian retinas suggest that neuroepithelial cells may only be able to respond to a particular range of phenotypic determination signals at any given point in their development.

A large number of X-irradiation studies have shown that the most sensitive cell populations in the CNS are the newly postmitotic migrating neuroblasts; the proliferating neuroepithelial cells are surprisingly resistant (reviewed in Hicks and D'Amato, 1978). In the cerebral cortex, such irradiation experiments typically result in a "scrambled cortex," in which it is not possible to reliably sort out the locus of the damage or the process of repair. However, the simpler structure of the retina permits a more straightforward interpretation of this type of experiment. In a series of studies, Rugh and Wolff (1955a,b) analyzed mice, both acutely and chronically, after exposure to several different doses of X rays during the early stages of embryonic development. Within a few hours of irradiation of E12.5 or E13.5 embryos, with 150–300 rad, there is massive destruction of the newly migrated cells in the retinal ganglion cell

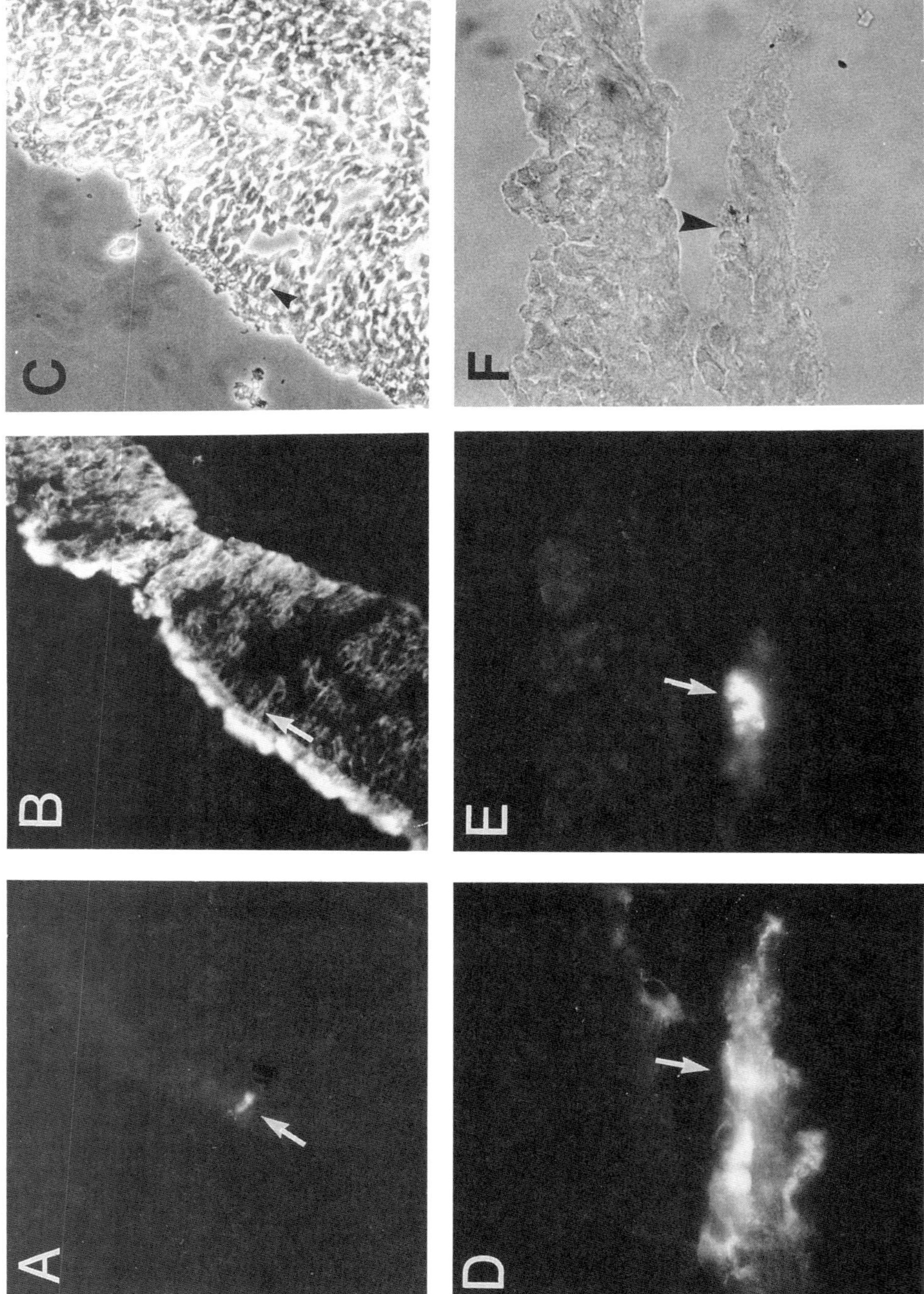

layer; virtually the entire ganglion cell layer undergoes phagocytosis by 24 hr. However, by birth, little to no residual damage is apparent in the majority of retinas. The retinal ganglion cell layer appears to have been completely replaced. In addition, the other retinal layers have a normal histological appearance; although the eyes of irradiated animals are somewhat smaller than those of controls, as is the whole animal, the retinas are appropriately proportioned. The repair of the damaged retinas comes about as a result of an increase in the overall level of proliferation of the progenitor cells, and specifically in a relative increase in the proportion of new cells committed to the earlier retinal phenotypes that had been destroyed by the X irradiation. Thus, early lesions of the retina will apparently lead to considerable replacement of the types of cells that are lost, so the final proportions of cells in the retina approximate those in the normal retina. In addition, since the histological composition of the mature retina was grossly normal in these cases, it is likely that a specific overproduction of the deleted cell types (e.g., retinal ganglion cells) must have occurred.

In contrast with these X-irradiation studies, a more recent experiment (Beazley *et al.*, 1987) has examined the effects of ganglion cell destruction in postnatal rats (after ganglion cell genesis is completed) on the further histogenesis of the retina. Following the destruction of the majority of the retinal ganglion cells, by neonatal optic nerve section, the overall number of mitotic figures in the retina does not change, and the ganglion cells are not replaced, although histogenesis of other cell types is ongoing in the retina (Beazley *et al.*, 1987). A further experiment that also demonstrates a lack in the germinal neuroepithelial cells to replace earlier generated cell classes used kainic-acid-mediated destruction of horizontal cells in the postnatal rabbit retina (Messersmith and Redburn, 1990). Although cell proliferation continued after the kainic acid treatment, and a considerable number of rod photoreceptor cells were generated, the horizontal cells were not replaced.

Since fetal destruction of ganglion cells results in their replacement, whereas postnatal destruction of this same cell type has no apparent effect on the subsequent retinal histogenesis, it appears that lesions to a particular cell class will result in the regeneration of that cell type only during the period in which that cell class is being generated. These lesion studies imply that the

---

Figure 9. Heterochronic chimeric transplantation experiments. E14 mouse retinal cells (M6$^+$) were dissociated and injected into the subretinal space of postnatal day 3 rat pups. After 3 days, the retinas were fixed and double labeled for M6 to reveal transplanted cells (A, D) and for Rho4D2 to demonstrate rods (B, E). Many examples of double-labeled cells were observed (*arrows*); when single E14 mouse neurons were found in the outer nuclear layer (A–C), they were frequently found to also express opsin. These results also support the conclusion that the microenvironment influences the choice of commitment.

environmental cues that regulate the differentiation of retinal ganglion cells or horizontal cells are restricted to (or only "readable" in) a particular window of time. However, it is also possible that there is a progressive restriction in the potential phenotypes capable of being produced by the progenitor cells during development. Heterochronic transplants should discriminate between these possibilities.

C. Is There a Default Phenotype for the Retinal Neuroepithelial Cell?

There is evidence from several developing systems that cells have ground states or default conditions when deprived of necessary cellular interactions (see, for example Chapter 1). Adler and Hatlee (1989) have suggested that the photoreceptor cell is the default condition of the retinal neuroepithelial cell, since the percentage of cells that differentiate into photoreceptors increases with decreasing stage of dissociation. As noted previously, another interpretation of this finding is that the neuroepithelial cells, prematurely induced to differentiate by the dissociation, will differentiate into the types of neurons that were being generated at the time of dissociation, that is, cone photoreceptors are generated early in retinal development in all species examined.

Evidence against the notion that photoreceptor cells are a default phenotype comes from the *in vitro* studies of the rat retina just described. In the rat, the percentage of photoreceptors that develops in dissociated culture decreases with decreasing developmental stage. Since the predominant photoreceptor cell class in the rat is the rod, this result would appear to at least rule out this class of photoreceptor as a potential candidate for the ground state of retinal neuroepithelial cells. What about the possibility that cone photoreceptors are the default condition? The [³H]thymidine birthdating data from both chicks and rodents indicate that cones are one of the fist cell types that are produced during development (see previous text), consistent with the possibility that cones are the default condition; however, retinal histogenesis is somewhat compressed in these species, so the technical limitations on birthdating analysis preclude definitive determination of the first cell type. The examination of a species in which the histogenesis is more extended would be more appropriate to determine the first cell type generated by neuroepithelial cells, when there are presumably no other previously produced retinal neurons to influence their choice of phenotype. The monkey retina provides such an extended developmental sequence (LaVail *et al.,* 1991, 1987; Curcio and Hendrickson, 1990); it appears that, in this species, the cone photoreceptor is not one of the first cell types generated; instead, the first cells to become postmitotic in the retina are committed to become horizontal cells and ganglion cells. Therefore, when the first neuroepithelial cells undergo their final mitotic division, and there are no other types of postmitotic neurons or glia around to influence their choice of phenotype, the neuroepithelial cells do not differentiate into either rod or cone photoreceptor cells.

Is there likely to be a single default phenotype? Of the various classes of retinal cells in the retina, the two that are generated first are the ganglion cells and the horizontal cells. Even in the monkey, there is no detectable distinction between the onset of generation in these two cell types (Rappaport *et al.*, 1987). Therefore, it is likely that one, or both, of these two cell types is the first cell generated in the retina; this is certainly consistent with the *in vitro* results of rat retinal cultures (see previous text) in which a large percentage of the neuroepithelial cells differentiates as ganglion cells (Reh and Kljavin, 1989). Recent results obtained with chimeric co-cultures support this possibility. When 10–50 E11 mouse retinal cells are plated onto confluent monolayers of rat retinal neurons, a wide variety of different retinal phenotypes are generated; however, when these same mouse cells are plated onto confluent monolayers of rat cerebral cortical neurons, virtually all of the mouse cells differentiate into large multipolar neurons with a highly branched dendritic arborization and a single axonal process. These results support the possibility that either ganglion cells, horizontal cells, or both types of neurons are the default phenotype in the mammalian retina.

D. When Does a Neuroepithelial Cell Make a Commitment?

Several authors have suggested that a cell becomes committed to differentiating into a particular type of neuron at or near the final mitotic division. Support for this idea is based on several lines of evidence. First, serial section analysis of developing mouse retina has shown that cells begin to show characteristic features of their morphology within hours of their terminal mitosis, prior to their migration to their final destinations (Hinds and Hinds, 1978). Second, immunohistochemical studies of the developing retina have shown that newly generated retinal ganglion cells begin to express proteins specific to these cells while still at the ventricular margin of the retina, again prior to any migration (Bennett and DiLullo, 1985; McLoon and Barnes, 1989). Third, since the neuroepithelial cells can give rise to any two retinal cell types generated at the time of their final mitotic division (see previous text), it does not appear that commitment to a particular phenotype occurs prior to their terminal mitosis. Thus, it does not seem likely that there are committed progenitor cells in the mammalian or frog retina, as are found in the hematopoietic system. However, although such a committed retinal progenitor cell does not appear to be present during embryogenesis, several studies of the postembryonic goldfish retina provide evidence for a progenitor cell that appears to only give rise to rod photoreceptor cells (Johns and Fernald, 1981). The rod progenitor cell, as it is called, continues to generate new rods throughout the life of the goldfish and, in so doing, maintains a constant density of rods in the retina as the eye enlarges. Although this appears to be an exception to the hypothesis that commitment to a particular phenotype occurs at the final mitotic division, recent studies of retinal regeneration following neurotoxic damage in this species suggests that these cells can revert to a multipotent state and give rise to all retinal cell classes (Raymond *et al.*, 1988). Therefore, the rod progenitor may represent a multipotent neuroepithelial cell that is extremely restricted by its normal environment in the postembryonic fish to generate only rods, and no other retinal cell type; however, when released from this environmental constraint by retinal damage, it will then produce all retinal phenotypes.

The *in vitro* study by Adler and Hatlee (1989) has also addressed the issue of when commitment takes place during retinal histogenesis; specifically, they tested whether the fate of retinal neuroblasts, generated (postmitotic) prior to embryonic day 5, could be changed if they were isolated from other retinal cells by low density culturing, either 1 or 3 days after their terminal mitosis. They found that 70% of the postmitotic cells became photoreceptors when cultured on ED 6 (>1 day after their birthdate), whereas 35% of the cells became photoreceptors when cultured on ED 8 (>3 days after their birthdate). The authors interpreted this result as suggesting that commitment to a particular phenotype does not occur at the final mitosis, but is made several days later, after the neuroblast cells have migrated to their final positions in the retina. This interpretation is obviously at variance with the studies on the appearance of cell-specific traits prior to migration cited earlier. Although it is possible that chick photoreceptor cells are an exception to the notion that neuronal phenotype is determined at the terminal mitosis of a neuroepithelial cell, this result could also be explained by the possibility that, for some cell types, cell survival in culture depends on how long after their birthdate the cells are dissociated (see subsequent text).

E. To What Extent Are Determination and Differentiation Separable Events?

Since much of the information concerning the development of the different cell types in the retina is derived from *in vitro* studies, it is essential to address the possibility that the factors necessary for the expression of a particular phenotype may not be present in the culture dish, even though the progenitor cells have become committed to that cell type. To what extent are the processes of determination, or commitment to a particular phenotype, and the differentiation of particular characteristics of that phenotype, under separate regulatory factors, either *in vitro* or during normal development? Obviously, this is both an important theoretical point, as well as a critical factor in the interpretation of the cell culture studies just reviewed.

The differentiation of retinal cells in tissue culture has been the subject of many studies. These studies have taken advantage of the fact that the retina is composed of well-defined cell classes that have characteristic morphology and antigenic properties that are expressed *in vitro.* For example, retinal ganglion cells express the highest levels of several neuron-specific proteins, both *in vivo* and *in vitro,* for example, the neurofilament proteins, thy 1.1 and GAP-43 (Shaw and Weber, 1983; Barnstable and Drager, 1984; McCaffrey *et al.,* 1984; Reh and Kljavin, 1989). In addition, the morphology of these cells in culture is reminiscent of that observed *in vivo,* with a single long axonal process and several shorter dendritic neurites (Reh and Kljavin, 1989). Similarly, other cultured retinal cells display substantial similarities to their *in vivo* counterparts. Chick photoreceptors are among the most striking examples of cell autonomy in the development of their normal morphology and pattern of antigenic expression of any of the retinal cell types yet examined; even characteristic outer segments and oil droplets are expressed (Adler *et al.,* 1985; Adler, 1986). Bipolar cells express the pcd5 antigen (Madl *et al.,* 1990; Oberdick *et al.,* 1990) and also show a bipolar morphology in cell cultures (personal observations), Müller cells are either flat or elongated in culture and are immunoreactive for both vimentin and cellular retinaldehyde binding protein (Deleeuw *et al.,* 1990), and amacrine cells develop immunoreactivity for a variety of antigens in culture (Akagawa and Barnstable, 1986; Politi *et al.,* 1988).

Although many of the normal aspects of any particular cell phenotype appear to develop in cell cultures, some of these normal phenotypic characteristics show only rudimentary development or fail to differentiate at all in the cultures. For example, in the case of rat rod photoreceptors, typical outer segments, with morphological evidence of disc formation, will not develop *in vitro* (Araki *et al.,* 1987; Politi *et al.,* 1988; Reh and Kljavin, 1989; Kljavin and Reh, 1990). In addition, the overall development of the retina in low density cultures appears to be substantially slower than that observed *in vivo* or in high density or aggregate cultures (see subsequent text). Finally, the culture conditions, such as the presence or absence of serum in the culture media, can influence the differentiation of particular aspects of a cell's phenotype (see, for example, Politi *et al.,* 1988). All these considerations are important in evaluating the studies of determination of particular cell phenotypes using the tissue culture models currently available. Moreover, several additional considerations are important in interpretation of the available tissue culture data. There is likely to be substantial cell loss during the process of tissue dissociation and culture of retinal neurons from any age of animal. Retinal cell cultures from particular ages appear to be more vulnerable to cell death, possibly due to changes in the trophic dependence of particular cell classes at different periods in their development (McCaffery *et al.*, 1984). Although this would appear to be more of a problem in low-density serum-free conditions, the amount of cell loss in retinal organ or reaggregate cultures may also be substantial, but this is more difficult to assess, since cell loss is accompanied by continued proliferation.

Several other reports have examined retinal histogenesis in organ or reaggregate cultures. Barnstable *et al.*, (1988; Sparrow *et al.*, 1990) put E13 rat retinas in organ culture, after removing the lens and the RPE. After 2 wk the retinas developed into the three normal layers and some opsin-positive cells with bipolar morphology were present that approximate those observed *in vivo;* however, the number or percentage of rods was much lower than that normally observed at P5, the equivalent *in vivo* age. Taylor and Reh (1990) cultured retinas from both pre- and postnatal rats and showed that neurogenesis continues at approximately normal rates for at least the first 3 days *in vitro;* in addition, several types of neurons differentiate in these cultures. Probably the best *in vitro* development of the retina has been reported by Caffe *et al.*, (1990), in which the pigment epithelium (RPE) is kept adjacent to the retina, and both tissues are sandwiched between a nitrocellulose membrane and a polyamide gauze grid on a shaker platform. These retinas continued their morphological development in a manner strikingly similar to that observed *in vivo* and at approximately normal rates; they even showed extension of photoreceptor outer segments from the rods. Reaggregate cultures, in either chick or rat, also have shown a degree of retinal development that most closely approximates that observed *in vivo,* for a variety of different aspects of retinal structure. The early studies of chick reaggregate cultures have demonstrated the ability of the constituent cells to organize into normal cellular layers and to exhibit some degree of continued neurogenesis, particularly if the RPE was included (Vollmer and Layer, 1986). More recently, Watanabe and Raff (1990) have described reaggregate pellet cultures in which the genesis of rod photoreceptors continues at a rate that closely approximates normal histogenesis of this cell type.

In addition, these studies indicate that several of the retinal cell types will develop many of their normal phenotypic characteristics in culture; some cell types appear to develop much of their normal phenotype in a cell-autonomous fashion (e.g., chick photoreceptors and rat ganglion cells) whereas other cell classes appear to require interactions with other retinal cells to develop appropriately (e.g., rat rod photoreceptors). The latter cell types more closely approximate their normal *in vivo* development as the cell density in the cultures is increased.

What about the relationship between determination and differentiation *in vivo*? As discussed earlier, retinal ganglion cells begin to express both morphological and immunohistochemical aspects of their differentiated phenotype almost immediately after their terminal mitosis (Hinds and Hinds, 1974; McLoon and Barnes, 1989). In addition, for several of the other cell classes, it appears that some of their morphological features develop prior to their migration. However, some of the antigens present in a particular cell class may not be expressed at detectable levels, although the cell may be committed to differentiation along a particular path. The rod photoreceptor cell provides a good example of this phenomenon. Figure 10 shows a running total of the birthdates of rods in the rat retina, from [³H]thymidine data (from M. LaVail, unpublished observations) plotted with a similar total of opsin-immunoreactive cells at the same ages. It is clear from the figure that there is a substantial delay between when a rod becomes committed to this particular phenotype

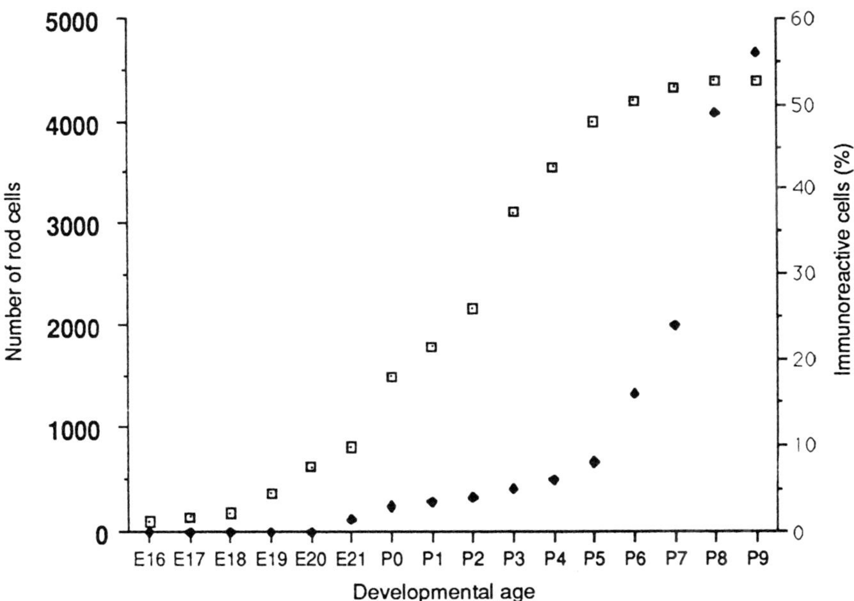

Figure 10. Graph of the total number of cells committed to become rods (□) as a function of developmental age (from [³H]thymidine data), along with the percentage of cells expressing immunoreactivity (◆), following dissociation and labeling with Rho4D2, also expressed as a function of age. The graph shows that there is a substantial delay between the birthdate of a rod and the time at which it begins to express opsin.

and when it expresses immunoreactivity for opsin. This suggests that either the expression of opsin to detectable levels requires several days after commitment, although it proceeds autonomously, or additional cellular interactions are necessary for the expression of opsin that are independent of the commitment to the rod phenotype.

V. Conclusions

The determination and differentiation of the various cell phenotypes present in the mature eye is clearly an extremely complex process, involving many levels of cellular interactions. However, although inductive interactions have been postulated to be important in eye development for almost 100 years, only very recently has any progress been made in defining the molecular basis for these interactions. Many of the questions raised in this chapter are only likely to be answered when more is known about the molecules that are involved in the various developmental decisions. There are clear analogies with other systems that may help identify the important molecular determinants. For example, in the formation of the *Drosophila* peripheral nervous system, the entire sense organ seems to be determined prior to the commitment of cells to the various phenotypes in it (Ghysen and Dambly-Chaudière, 1989; see also Chapter 8), much as the entire vertebrate eye appears to be determined prior to the commitment of cells to either a particular cell type (such as pigmented epithelial or neural) or a particular class of neurons. Also, the determination of the various cell classes in the *Drosophila* eye seems to occur by a cascade of cellular interactions, much like that proposed for the vertebrate retina, and several of the genes involved in these determination events in the fly have been identified in the past few years (see Chapter 7). If the analogy can be carried through to the molecular level, we will develop a much more thorough understanding of the generation of cellular diversity in the vertebrate retina.

References

Adelmann, H. B. (1929). Experimental studies on the development of the eye. II. The eye-forming potencies of the median portions of the urodelan neural plate (*Triton taeniatus* and *Amblystoma punctatum*). *J. Exp. Zool.* **54**, 219–317.

Adelmann, H. B. (1930). Experimental studies on the development of the eye. III. The effect of substrate on the heterotropic development of median and lateral strips of the anterior end of the neural plate of *Amblystoma. J. Exp. Zool.* **57**, 223–281.

Adler, R. (1986). Developmental predetermination of the structural and molecular polarization of photoreceptor cells. *Dev. Biol.* **117**, 520–527.

Adler, R., Jerdan, J., and Hewitt, A. T. (1985). Responses of cultured neural retinal cells to substratum-bound laminin and other extracellular matrix molecules. *Dev. Biol.* **112**, 100–114.

Adler, R., and Hatlee, M. (1989). Plasticity and differentiation of embryonic retinal cells after terminal mitosis. *Science* **243**, 391–393.

Akagawa, K., and Barnstable, C. J. (1986). Identification and characterization of cell types in monolayer cultures of rat retina using monoclonal antibodies. *Brain Res.* **383**, 110–120.

Alderman, A. L. (1935). The determination of the eye in the anuran, *Hyla regilla. J. Exp. Zool.* **70**, 205–232.

Alexander, L. E. (1937). An experimental study of the role of optic cup and overlying ectoderm in lens formation in the chick embryo. *J. Exp. Zool.* **75**, 41–73.

Araki, M., Iida, Y., Taketami, S., Watanabe, M., Ohta, K., and Saito, J. (1987). Characterization of photoreceptor cell differentiation in the rat retinal cell culture. *Dev. Biol.* **124**, 239–247.

Barnstable, C. J., and Drager, U. C. (1984). Thy-1 antigen: A ganglion cell specific marker in rodent retina. *Neurosci.* **11**, 847–855.

Barnstable, C. J., Blum, A. S., Devoto, S. H., Hicks, D., Morabito, M. A., Sparrow, J. R., and Triesman, J. E. (1988). Cell differentiation and pattern formation in the developing mammalian retina. *Neurosci. Res.* **8**, 527–541.

Beazley, L. D., Perry, V. H., Baker, B., and Darby, J. E. (1987). An investigation into the role of ganglion cells in the regulation of division and death of other retinal cells. *Dev. Brain Res.* **33**, 169–184.

Bennett, G. S., and DiLullo, C. (1985). Transient expression of a neurofilament protein by replicating neuroepithelial cells of the embryonic chick brain. *Dev. Biol.* **107**, 107–127.

Blanks, J. C., and Bok, D. (1977). An autoradiographic analysis of postnatal cell proliferation in the normal and degenerative mouse retina. *J. Comp. Neurol.* **145**, 317–328.

Brun, R. B. (1981). The movement of the prospective eye vesicles from the neural plate into the neural fold in *Amblystoma mexicanum* and *Xenopus laevis. Dev. Biol.* **88**, 192–199.

Caffe, A. R., Jansen, H., and Sanyal, S. (1990). Histogenesis of retina from newborn mouse in organ culture over the postnatal period. *Int. Cong. Eye Res. Abstr.* **9**, 52.

Carter-Dawson, L. D., and LaVail, M. M. (1979). Rods and cones in the mouse retina. II. Autoradiographic analysis of cell generation using tritiated thymidine. *J. Comp. Neurol.* **188**, 263–272.

Clarke, L. F. (1936). Regional differences in eye-forming capacity of the early chick blastoderm as studied in chorio-allantoic grafts. *Physiol Zool.* **9**, 102–128.

Coulombre, J. L., and Coulombre, A. J. (1965). Regeneration of neural retina from the pigmented epithelium in the chick embryo. *Dev. Biol.* **12**, 79–92.

Cowan, W. M., and Finger, T. E. (1982). Regenerating and regulation in the developing central nervous system. *In* "Neuronal Development" (N. C. Spitzer, ed.), pp. 377–415. New York: Plenum Press.

Curcio, C. A., and Hendrickson, A. E. (1991). Organization and development of the primate photoreceptor mosaic. *Prog. Retinal Res.* Vol 10 (N. Osborne and J. Chader, eds.) pp. 89–120. Oxford: Pegamon Press.

Deleeuw, A. M., Gaur, V. P, Saari, J. C., and Milam, A. H. (1990). Immunolocalization of cellular retina, retinaldehyde, and retinoic acid-binding proteins in rat retina during pre- and postnatal development. *J. Neurocytol.* **19**, 253–264.

Detwiler, S. R., and van Dyke, R. H. (1953). The induction of the neural retina from the pigment epithelial layer of the eye. *J. Exp. Zool.* **122,** 367–383.

Detwiler, S. R., and van Dyke, R. H. (1954). Further experimental observations on retinal inductions. *J. Exp. Zool.* **126,** 135–155.

Dorris, F. (1938). Differentiation of the chick eye *in vitro. J. Exp. Zool.* **78,** 385–415.

Eagleson, G. W., and Harris, W. A. (1990). Mapping of the presumptive brain regions in the neural plate of *Xenopus laevis. J. Neurobiol.* **21(3),** 427–440.

Erlich, O., and Morgan, I. G. (1980). Kainic acid lesions in chick retina amacrine cells. *Neurosci. Lett.* **17,** 43–48.

Gayer, K. (1942). A study of coloboma and other abnormalities in transplants of eye primordia from normal and creeper chick embryos. *J. Exp. Zool.* **89,** 103–145.

Ghysen, A., and Dambly-Chaudière C. (1990). Early events in the development of the *Drosophila* peripheral nervous system. *J. Physiol. (Paris)* **84,** 11–20.

Godsave, S. F., Isaacs, H. V., and Slack, J. M. W. (1988). Mesoderm-inducing factors: A small class of molecules. *Development* **102,** 55–566.

Hampton, C. K., Garcia, C., and Redburn, D. A. (1981). Localization of kainic acid sensitive cells in the mammalian retina. *J. Neurosci. Res.* **6,** 99–111.

Harris, W. A., and Hartenstein, V. (1991). Neuronal determination without cell division in *Xenopus* embryos. *Neuron* **6,** 499–515.

Hicks, S. P., and D'Amato, C. J. (1978). Effects of ionizing radiation on developing brain and behavior. *In* "Studies on the Development of Behavior and the Nervous System," pp. 35–72. New York: Academic Press.

Hilfer, S. R., Brady, R. C., and Yang, J. W. (1981). Intracellular and extracellular changes during early ocular development in the chick embryo. *In* "Ocular Size and Shape. Regulation during Development" (S. R. Hilfer and J. B. Sheffield, eds.), pp. 45–78. New York: Springer-Verlag.

Hill, R. E., Jones, P. F., Rees, A. R., Sime, C. M., Justice, M. J., Copeland, N. G., Jenkins, N. A., Graham, E., and Davidson, D. R. (1989). A new family of mouse homeobox containing genes: molecular structure and developmental expression of Hox 7.1. *Genes and Development* **3,** 26–37.

Hinds, J. W., and Hinds, P. L. (1974). Early ganglion cell differentiation in the mouse retina: An electron microscopic analysis utilizing serial sections. *Dev. Biol.* **37,** 381–416.

Hinds, J. W., and Hinds, P. L. (1978). Early development of amacrine cells in the mouse retina: An electron microscopic, serial section analysis. *J. Comp. Neurol.* **179,** 277–300.

Hinds, J. W., and Hinds, P. L. (1979). Differentiation of photoreceptors and horizontal cells in the embryonic mouse retina: An electron microscopic, serial section analysis. *J. Comp. Neurol.* **187,** 495–512.

Hollyfield, J. G. (1968). Differential addition of cells to the retina in *Rana pipiens* tadpoles. *Dev. Biol.* **18,** 163–179.

Holt, C. W., Bertsch, T. W., Ellis, H. M., and Harris, W. A. (1988). Cellular determination in the *Xenopus* retina is independent of lineage and birthdate. *Neuron* **1,** 15–26.

Ingham, C. A., and Morgan, I. G. (1983). Dose-dependent effects of intravitreal kainic acid on specific cell types in chicken retina. *Neurosci.* **9,** 151–181.

Jacobson, C. O. (1959). The localization of the presumptive cerebral regions in the neural plate of the *Axolotl* larva. *J. Embryol. Exp. Morph.* **7,** 1–21.

Jacobson, M. (1978). "Developmental Neurobiology." New York: Plenum Press.

Johns, P. R., and Fernald, R. D. (1981). Genesis of rods in teleost fish retina. *Nature (London)* **293,** 141–142.

Kahn, A. J. (1974). An autoradiographic analysis of the time of appearance of neurons in the developing chick neural retina. *Dev. Biol.* **38,** 30–40.

Kimmelman, D., Abraham, J. A., Haaparanta, T., Palishi, T. M., and Kirschner, M. W. (1988). The presence of fibroblast growth factor in the frog egg: Its role as a natural mesoderm inducer. *Science* **242**, 1053–1056.

Kimmel, C. B., and Warga, R. M. (1986). Tissue-specific cell lineages originate in the gastrula of the zebrafish. *Science* **231**, 365–368.

Kimmel, C. B., and Warga, R. M. (1987). Indeterminate cell lineage of the zebrafish embryo. *Dev. Biol.* **124**, 269–280.

Kimmel, C. B., and Warga, R. M. (1988). Cell lineage and developmental potential of cells in the zebrafish embryo. *Trends Genet.* **4**, 68–73.

Kljavin, I. J., and Reh, T. A. (1991). Müller cells are a preferred substrate for *in vitro* neurite extension by rod photoreceptors. *J. Neurosci.* (in press).

Lagenaur, R. D., Fushili, S., and Schachner, M. (1984). Monoclonal antibody M6 blocks neurite extension in cultured mouse cerebellar neurons. *Soc. Neurosci. Abs.* **11**, 223.

LaVail, M. M., Rapaport, D. H., and Rakic, P. (1991). Cytogenesis in the monkey retina. *J. Comp. Neurol.* **309**, 86–114.

Lopashov, G. V., and Stroeva, O. G. (1964). "Development of the Eye. Experimental Studies" (translated by B. Meytar). Jerusalem:S. Monson.

Lopashov, G. V., and Sologub, A. A. (1972). Artificial metaplasia of pigmented epithelium into retina in tadpoles and adult frogs. *J. Embryol. Exp. Morph.* **28**, 521–546.

Lund, R. D., Change, F. L. F., Hankin, M. H., and Lagenaur, C. F. (1985). Use of a species-specific antibody for demonstrating mouse neurons transplanted to rat brains. *Neurosci. Lett.* **61**, 221–226.

McCaffrey, C. A., Raju, T. R., and Bennett, M. R. (1984). Effects of cultured astroglia on the survival of neonatal rat retina ganglion cells *in vitro. Dev. Biol.* **104**, 441–448.

McLoon, S. C., and Barnes, R. B. (1989). Early differentiation of retinal ganglion cells: An axonal protein expressed by premigratory and migrating retinal ganglion cells. *J. Neurosci.* **9**, 1424–1432.

Madl, J. E., Nordquist, D. T., Orr, H. T., and Beitz, A. J. (1990). Expression of the protein encoded by the cDNA clone PCD5 is restricted to cerebellar Purkinje cells and retinal bipolar cells. *J. Cell Biol.* (in press).

Manchot, E. (1929). Abgrenzung des Augenmaterials und anderer Teilbezirke in der Medullarplatte; die Teilbewegungen während der Auffaltung (Farbmarkierungsversuche an Keimen von Urodelen). *Roux's Arch. Entw.-Mech.* **116**, 689–708.

Mangold, O. (1929). Experimente zue Analyse der Determinatin und Induktion der Medullarplatte. *Roux's Arch. Entw. Mech.* **117**, 586–696.

Messersmith, E. K., and Redburn, D. A. (1990). Kainic acid lesioning alters development of the outer plexiform layer in neonatal rabbit retina. *Int. J. Dev. Neurosci.* (in press).

Metcalf, D. (1989). The molecular control of cell division, differentiation commitment and maturation of haemopoietic cells. *Nature (London)* **339**, 27–30.

Moody, S. A. (1987). Fates of the blastomeres of the 32-cell-stage *Xenopus* embryo. *Dev. Biol.* **122**, 300–319.

Negishi, K., Teranishi, T., and Kato, S. (1982). New dopaminergic and idoleamine-accumulating cells in the growth zone of goldfish retinas after neurotoxic destruction. *Science* **216**, 747–749.

Negishi, K., Teranishi, T., and Kato, S. (1985). Growth rate of a peripheral annulus defined by neurotoxic destruction in the goldfish retina. *Dev. Brain Res.* **20**, 291–295.

Negishi, K., Teranishi, T., Kato, S., and Nakamura, Y. (1987). Paradoxical induction of dopaminergic cells following intravitreal injection of high doses of 6-hydroxydopamine in juvenile carp retina. *Dev. Brain Res.* **33**, 76–79.

Nornes, H. O., Dressler, G. R., Knapik, E. W., Deutsch, V. and Gruss, P. (1990). Spatially and temporally restricted expression of Pax2 during murine neurogenesis. *Development* **109**, 797–809.

Oberdick, J., Smeyne, R. J., Mann, J. R., Zackson, S., and Morgan, J. I. (1990). A promoter that drives transgene expression in cerebellar Purkinje and retinal bipolar neurons. *Science* **248**, 223–226.

Okada, T. S. (1980). Cellular metaplasia or transdifferentiation as a model for retinal cell differentiation. *In* "Current Topics in Developmental Biology" (S. Denis-Donini and G. Augusti-Tocco, eds.), pp. 349–380. New York: Academic Press.

Orts-Llorca, F., and Genis-Galvez, J. M. (1960). Experimental production of retinal septa in the chick embryo. Differentiation of pigment epithelium into neural retina. *Acta Anat.* **42**, 31–70.

Park, C. M., and Hollenberg, M. J. (1989). Basic fibroblast growth factor induces retinal regeneration *in vivo. Dev. Biol.* **134**, 201–205.

Politi, L. E., Lehar, M., and Adler, R. (1988). Development of neonatal mouse retinal neurons and photoreceptors in low density cell culture. *Invest. Ophthalm. Vis. Sci.* **29**, 534–543.

Rawles, M. E. (1936). A study in the localization of organ-forming areas in the chick blastoderm of the head-process stage. *J. Exp. Zool.* **72**, 271–315.

Raymond, P. A., Reifler, M. J., and Rivlin, P. K. (1988). Regeneration of goldfish retina: Rod precursors are a likely source of regenerated cells. *J. Neurobiol.* **19**, 431–464.

Reh, T. A. (1987). Cell-specific regulation of neuronal production in the larval frog retina. *J. Neurosci.* **7**, 3317–3324.

Reh, T. A. (1989a). Regulation of neuronal production in the vertebrate retina. *In* "Development of the Vertebrate Retina" (B. Finlay and D. Senglaub, eds.), pp. 43–67. New York: Plenum Publishing.

Reh, T. A. (1989b). Environmental cues influence differentiation of rat retinal germinal neuroepithelial cells. *Soc. Neurosci. Abstr.* **15**, 96.

Reh, T. A., and Tully, T. (1986). Regulation of tyrosine hydroxylase-containing amacrine cell number in larval from retina. *Dev. Biol.* **114**, 463–469.

Reh, T. A., and Nagy, T. (1987). A possible role for the vascular membrane in retinal regeneration in *Rana catesbienna* tadpoles. *Dev. Biol.* **122**, 471–482.

Reh, T. A., Redshaw, J. D., and Bisby, M. A. (1987). Axons of the pyramidal tract do not increase their transport of growth-associated proteins after axotomy. *Mol. Brain Res.* **2**, 1–6.

Reh, T. A., and Kljavin, I. J. (1989). Age of differentiation determines rat retinal germinal cell phenotype: Induction of differentiation by dissociation. *J. Neurosci.* **9**, 4179–4189.

Reyer, R. W. (1977). The visual system in vertebrates. *In* "The Amphibian Eye: Development and Regeneration" (F. Crescitelli, ed.), pp. 309–390. Berlin: Springer-Verlag.

Rosa, F., Roberts, A. B., Danielpour, D., Dart, L. L., Sporn, M. B., and Dawid, I. B. (1988). Mesoderm induction in amphibians: The role of TGF-β2-like factors. *Science* **239**, 783–785.

Rugh, R. (1962). "Experimental embryology: Techniques and procedures." Minneapolis: Burgess.

Rugh, R., and Wolff, J. (1955a). Reparation of the fetal eye following radiation insult. *Arch. Ophthalm.* **54**, 351–359.

Rugh, R., and Wolff, J. (1955b). Resilience of the fetal eye following radiation insult. *Proc. Soc. Exp. Biol. Med.* **89**, 248–253.

Shaw, G., and Weber, K. (1983). The structure and development of the rat retina: An immunofluorescence microscopical study using antibodies specific for intermediate filament proteins. *J. Cell Biol.* **30**, 219–232.

Sidman, R. L. (1961). Histogenesis of mouse retina studied with [^{3}H]thymidine. *In* "The Structure of the Eye" (G. Smelser, Ed.), pp. 487–506. New York: Academic Press.

Sokol, S., Wong, G. G., and Melton, D. A. (1990). A mouse macrophage factor induces head structures and organizes a body axis in *Xenopus. Science* **249**, 561–564.

Sparrow, J. R., Hicks, D., and Barnstable, C. J. (1990). Cell commitment and differentiation in explants of embryonic rat neural retina. Comparison with the developmental potential of dissociated retina. *Dev. Brain Res.* **51**, 69–84.

Spemann, H. (1938). "Embryonic Development and Induction." New Haven, Connecticut: Yale University Press.

Stone, L. S. (1950a). Neural retina degeneration following regeneration by surviving retinal pigment cells in grafted adult salamander eyes. *Anat. Rec.* **106**, 89–109.

Stone, L. S. (1950b). The role of retinal pigment cells in regenerating neural retinae of adult salamander eyes. *J. Exp. Zool.* **113**, 9–31.

Stone, L. S. (1960a). Regeneration of the lens, iris and neural retina in a vertebrate eye. *Yale J. Biol. Med.* **32**, 464–473.

Streisinger, G., Coale, F., Taggart, C., and Grunwald, D. J. (1989). Clonal origins of cells in the pigmented retina of the zebrafish eye. *Dev. Biol.* **131**, 60–69.

Takaya, H. (1955). Formation of the brain from the prospective spinal cord of amphibian embryos. *Proc. Japan Acad.* **31**, 360–356.

Taylor, M., and Reh, T. A. (1990). Induction of differentiation of rat retinal, germinal, neuroepithelial cells by dbcAMP. *J. Neurobiol.* **21**, 470–481.

Turner, D. L. and Cepko, C. L. (1988). A common progenitor for neurons and glia persists in rat retina late in development. *Nature (London)* **328**, 131–136.

Turner, D. L., Snyder, E. Y., and Cepko, C. L. (1990). Lineage-independent determination of cell type in the embryonic mouse retina. *Neuron* **4**, 833–845.

Vollmer, G., and Layer, P. G. (1986). An *in vitro* model of proliferation and differentiation of the chick retina: Coaggregates of retinal and pigment epithelial cells. *J. Neurosci.* **6**, 1885–1896.

von Baer, K. E. (1828). "Über Entwicklungsgeschichte der Thiere." Königsberg.

von Woellwarth, C. (1952). Die Induktionsstufen des Gehirns. *Arch. Entw.-Mech.* **145**, 582–668.

Walsh, C., Polley, E. H., Hickey, T. L., and Guillery, R. W. (1983). Generation of cat retinal ganglion cells in relation to central pathways. *Nature (London)* **302**, 611–614.

Walsh, C., and Polley, E. H. (1985). The topography of ganglion cell production in the cat's retina. *J. Neurosci.* **5**, 751–750.

Watanabe, T., and Raff, M. C. (1988). Retinal astrocytes are immigrants from the optic nerve. *Nature (London)* **332**, 834–837.

Watanabe, T., and Raff, M. C. (1990). Rod photoreceptor development *in vitro*: Intrinsic properties of proliferating neuroepithelial cells change as development proceeds in the rat retina. *Neuron* **2**, 461–467.

Wetts, R., and Fraser, S. E. (1988). Multipotent precursors can give rise to all major cell types of the frog retina. *Science* **239**, 1142–1145.

Wetts, R., Serbedzija, G. N., and Fraser, S. E. (1989). Cell lineage analysis reveals multipotent precursors in the ciliary margin of the frog retina. *Dev. Biol.* **136**, 254–263.

Williams, R. W., and Herrup, K. (1988). The control of neuron number. *Ann. Rev. Neurosci.* **11**, 423–453.

Woerdeman, W. W. (1929). Experimentelle Untersuchungen über Lage und Bau der augenbildenden Bezirke in der Medullarplatte dem *Axolotl. Arch. Entw.-Mech.* **116**, 220–241.

Young, R. W. (1985). Cell proliferation during postnatal development of the retina in the mouse. *Dev. Brain Res.* **21**, 229–239.

Zimmerman, R. P., Polley, E. H., and Fortney, R. L. (1988). Cell birthdays and rate of differentiation of ganglion and horizontal cells of the developing cat's retina. *J. Comp. Neurol.* **274**, 77–90.

Development of Motoneuronal
Identity in the Zebrafish

Judith S. Eisen
Institute of Neuroscience
University of Oregon
Eugene, Oregon

I. Introduction

One of the most striking features of the nervous system is the high degree of structural and biochemical diversity among neurons. Even in organisms with a relatively small number of neurons, these cells show a remarkable

DETERMINANTS OF NEURONAL IDENTITY

469

variety in their differentiated features such as shape, synaptic connectivity, neurotransmitters, and distribution of ion channels and receptors. The factors that contribute to neuronal differentiation are not well understood, but both intrinsic cellular properties and extrinsic interactive events are likely to be important. One of the fundamental issues in developmental neuroscience is understanding how neurons acquire their characteristic differentiated properties.

My colleagues and I have been addressing this question by studying the development of a small set of identified neurons in the embryonic zebrafish. The zebrafish embryo is ideal for cellular studies of neuronal development for several reasons: (1) Early in development the nervous system has a relatively small number of postmitotic neurons, many of which can be recognized as unique individuals. (2) The embryo is nearly transparent; thus, we can visualize developing neurons and their progenitors and study these cells *in situ* through the first several days of embryonic development. (3) The embryo develops relatively rapidly; thus, it is possible to follow the entire course of development of the same identified neuron from birth through the outgrowth of processes and formation of synaptic connections.

We have devoted much of our attention to a specific set of motoneurons because each cell in this set can be recognized as a unique individual. We find that, under normal conditions, each identified motoneuron undergoes a stereotyped pattern of development. To dissect the factors that contribute to the proper development of these cells, we have used techniques such as single-cell ablation and transplantation. In addition, we have taken advantage of the pioneering work of George Streisinger (Streisinger *et al.*, 1981) and have begun to use a mutational approach to study motoneuronal development in this "simple" vertebrate. In this chapter I will focus primarily on work that addresses the question of how a cell becomes a particular primary motoneuron.

II. Early Patterning of the Embryo

A. The Embryonic Cell Lineage Is Indeterminate

Like the eggs of other fish (Balinsky, 1970), zebrafish eggs undergo meroblastic cleavage, resulting in a cap of blastomeres positioned on the animal hemisphere of a large uncleaved yolk cell. Because yolk granules are segregated into the yolk cell, the blastomeres are nearly transparent, making it possible to follow their early division patterns *in situ*. The first few cell divisions are regular and result in a stereotyped pattern of blastomeres (Kimmel and Law, 1985a), raising the possibility that the zebrafish embryo might arise from a determinate cell lineage, as do the nematode *Caenorhabditis elegans* (Sulston *et al.*, 1983) and leeches (Weisblat *et al.*, 1984). To learn whether the zebrafish lineage was determinate, Kimmel and Warga (1986) labeled single blastomeres with nontoxic fluorescent dyes and followed the lineages of the marked cells and the movements of their progeny in living embryos. They found that blastomeres arising from the same pattern of cell divisions in different embryos gave rise to progeny with different fates and located in different positions, showing that the lineage of the zebrafish embryo is indeterminate (Kimmel and Warga, 1987).

B. Tissue-Level Restrictions Occur during Gastrulation

Although the zebrafish embryo has an indeterminate cell lineage, restrictions occur during embryogenesis that limit the tissues to which an individual cell normally contributes progeny. The first restriction occurs relatively early, at about the midblastula stage, and segregates cells that contribute to an extraembryonic tissue from those that contribute to the embryo proper (Kimmel and Law, 1985b). Restrictions in embryonic lineages occur later, during gastrulation; single cells from this stage typically contribute progeny to only a single tissue (Kimmel and Warga, 1986; Kimmel *et al.*, 1990). Learning whether these tissue-level restrictions occur because cells have become committed to produce only a specific type of progeny will require challenging the cells with a novel environment by transplanting them to new positions in the embryo. If transplanted cells develop in accordance with their new positions, they were not committed to a particular fate, although they may always express this fate under the conditions they normally encounter in an unmanipulated embryo.

III. Differentiation of the Nervous System

A. Different Types of Neurons Arise from Different Embryonic Locations

Kimmel *et al.* (1990) followed the lineages of cells marked during the late blastula stage, and constructed a fate map for the zebrafish embryo that shows the correspondence between the position of a cell at the onset of gastrulation and the phenotypes of that cell's progeny later in development (Fig. 1). Based on these studies, they found that cells that give rise to the nervous system are located in specific regions of the fate map. Moreover, at the onset of gastrulation there is a direct correspondence between the location of cells that are in a position to contribute progeny to the nervous system and the region of the nervous system that their progeny will populate. For example, forebrain structures arise from a more anterior position than do hindbrain structures, and spinal motoneurons arise from a more dorsal position than do spinal sensory neurons. However, because of the extensive rearrangements that take place during gastrulation, it is not possible to predict which cells will be the progenitors of specific neurons, or even of specific types of neurons. For example, spinal interneurons and motoneurons may arise from the same ancestral cell (Kimmel *et al.*, 1990).

B. Neurons That Arise at Different Times Have Characteristic Features

Zebrafish neurons fall into distinct classes that may subserve different functions in the developing embryo. Neurons of one class, called "primary"

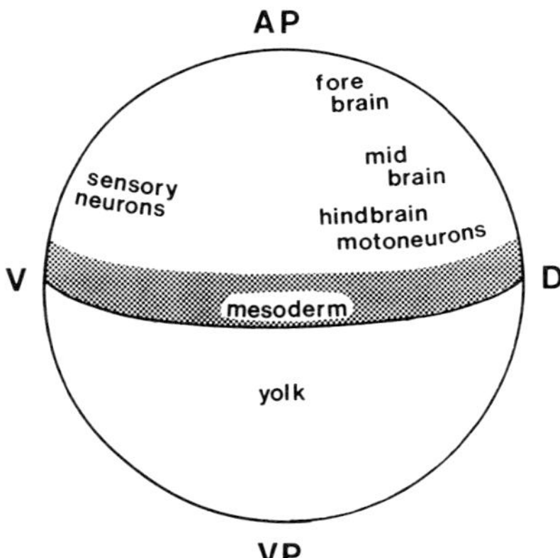

Figure 1. Zebrafish fate map at the beginning of gastrulation. The cells of the embryo constitute the upper region in the drawing; they are situated on the uncleaved yolk cell. Neurons of specific types arise from progenitors located in the regions indicated. The stippled region indicates progenitors of mesoderm-derived tissues; progenitors of endoderm-derived tissues are not illustrated here. They are most likely to be located ventral to the mesodermal progenitors. Abbreviations: AP, animal pole; VP, vegetal pole; D, dorsal (indicates the future dorsal side of the embryo); V, ventral (indicates the future ventral side of the embryo). (Adapted and redrawn from Kimmel *et al.*, 1990.)

neurons (see Kimmel and Westerfield, 1990), are distinguished from neurons that arise later by their characteristic early development, large soma sizes, and small numbers. Primary neurons become postmitotic during gastrulation or shortly thereafter (Mendelson, 1986; Myers *et al.*, 1986) and include cells of different functional modalities. Primary neurons are the first to extend growth cones; their axons establish the first nerve pathways in the embryo and form a simple scaffold (Chitnis and Kuwada, 1990; Wilson *et al.*, 1990), that may be important for proper extension of the growth cones of later-developing neurons (Kuwada, 1986; Pike *et al.*, 1989). Within a few hours of sprouting growth cones, primary sensory neurons, primary interneurons, and primary motoneurons begin to establish the synaptic connections that will form the first functional circuitry that is probably responsible for generating early swimming behavior (see Kahn and Roberts, 1982). Perhaps because they are crucial for establishing the early functional circuitry as well as for providing the axonal pathways that may help guide the growth cones of later-developing neurons, at least some aspects of the development of zebrafish primary neurons may be regulated by a different set of mechanisms than those used by later-developing zebrafish neurons or by neurons in other vertebrates (see Liu and Westerfield, 1990).

In addition to the morphological and developmental criteria by which they can be distinguished, primary neurons can also be distinguished from later-arising neurons because they have different patterns of gene expression. In embryos homozygous for the neural degeneration mutation *ned-1(b39)* (Grunwald *et al.*, 1988), the nervous system begins to develop normally and embryos exhibit normal early behaviors, suggesting that the primary neurons establish functional circuitry. However, during the second day of development, later-arising neurons of all functional classes begin to degenerate, while all primary neurons remain viable. This observation suggests that there may be fundamental differences between the primary neurons and neurons that arise later.

C. Many Primary Neurons Can Be Individually Identified

The small number, large size, and characteristic axonal trajectories of the primary neurons have allowed many of these cells to be identified as unique individuals by explicit morphological, and in some cases physiological, criteria. The most famous identified neuron of vertebrates is the Mauthner cell found in fish and amphibia (see Faber and Korn, 1978). This cell is present as a single bilateral pair of homologs whose somata are located in the hindbrain and whose axons decussate and extend caudally in the spinal cord. Although the

Mauthner cell was probably the first identified neuron, it has often been assumed that such cells are peculiar to invertebrates. However, recent work from larval and adult zebrafish has shown that many neurons can be individually identified, including specific motoneurons (Myers, 1985; Westerfield *et al.*, 1986) and interneurons (Kuwada *et al.*, 1990) in the spinal cord and interneurons in the hindbrain (Metcalfe *et al.*, 1986). Figure 2 shows a synopsis of some of the identified neurons of the zebrafish spinal cord.

To learn how individual neurons acquire their identities during development of the zebrafish, we have focused on the primary motoneurons. The following sections describe the criteria by which these cells can be uniquely identified and summarize our current understanding of the events involved in determination of primary motoneuron identity.

IV. Criteria for Identification of Primary Motoneurons

A. Segmental Arrangement of Primary Motoneuronal Somata

All vertebrate embryos develop segmented mesodermal structures called somites that give rise to segmented axial musculature and bone. The segmented musculature is innervated by a segmental pattern of motor and sensory nerves. In zebrafish, the segmental motor nerves are initially formed by the axons of the primary motoneurons; at later stages the axons of later-developing secondary motoneurons contribute to these nerves as well (Myers, 1985; Westerfield *et al.*, 1986). Although the motor nerves are segmentally arranged during some stages in all vertebrates, motoneurons in most verte-

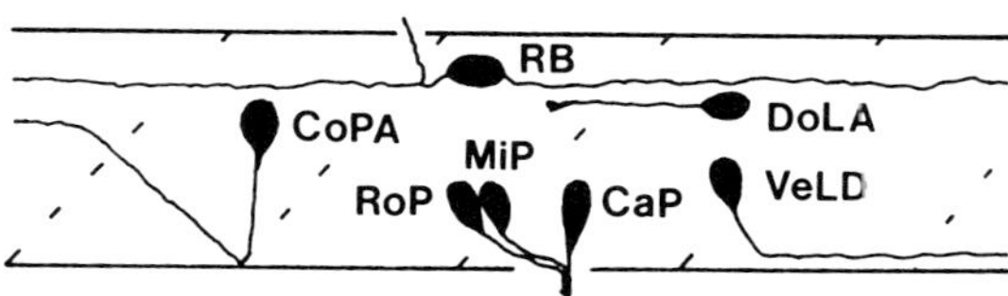

Figure 2. Phenotypes of some of the identified primary neurons in the spinal cord of the embryonic zebrafish. The CaP, MiP, and RoP primary motoneurons and VeLD primary interneuron are segmentally distributed so one set of these cells is present on each side of every trunk spinal segment; in some segments there may be two VeLDs on one or both sides. The CoPA and DoLA primary interneurons and Rohon Beard (RB) primary sensory neurons do not appear to be segmentally distributed. (Adapted and redrawn from Kuwada *et al.*, 1990.)

brate spinal cords are not obviously organized in a segmental arrangement. However, at least in some cases, the motoneurons may initially be segmentally arranged, but this arrangement is later lost, in part because of morphogenetic changes during development (see Westerfield and Eisen, 1985). In zebrafish, the somata of the primary motoneurons retain an obvious segmental organization into adulthood, although it is not yet clear whether the somata of secondary motoneurons are also segmentally organized.

B. Adults

Every trunk muscle segment of the adult zebrafish is innervated by three primary motoneurons whose somata are arranged in bilaterally paired clusters (Westerfield *et al.*, 1986). Several criteria can be used to identify each primary motoneuron uniquely. (1) Because the somata of zebrafish primary motoneurons remain in register with the muscle segments innervated by their axons, each primary motoneuron soma is located on the right or left side of a particular spinal segment defined by the muscle segment it innervates. For example, the primary motoneurons on the right side of segment 7 (R7) innervate the seventh muscle segment on the right side of the fish. (2) On both sides of every spinal segment, each primary motoneuron has a specific soma position. CaP, the *ca*udal *p*rimary, has the most caudally located soma. RoP, the *ro*stral *p*rimary, has the most rostrally located soma. MiP, the *mi*ddle *p*rimary, has a soma between the CaP and RoP somata. (3) Each primary motoneuron has an axonal projection in a discrete region of its muscle segment and innervates muscle fibers exclusively in that region (Fig. 3a). CaP extends its axon along a ventral pathway and innervates muscle fibers in the ventral third of the ipsilateral muscle segment, RoP extends its axon along a ventrolateral pathway and innervates fibers in the middle third of the ipsilateral muscle segment, and MiP extends its axon along a dorsal pathway and innervates fibers in the dorsal third of the ipsilateral muscle segment.

C. Larvae

In larval zebrafish, as in adults, soma position correlates with the region of muscle innervated by an individual primary motoneuron. Myers (1985) labeled motoneurons by retrograde transport of horseradish peroxidase (HRP) and observed that the somata of both primary and secondary motoneurons in the CaP and RoP positions could be labeled by lesions made in the ventral muscle. However, only somata in the MiP position were labeled by lesions made in the dorsal muscle. Thus, only cells in the MiP position have

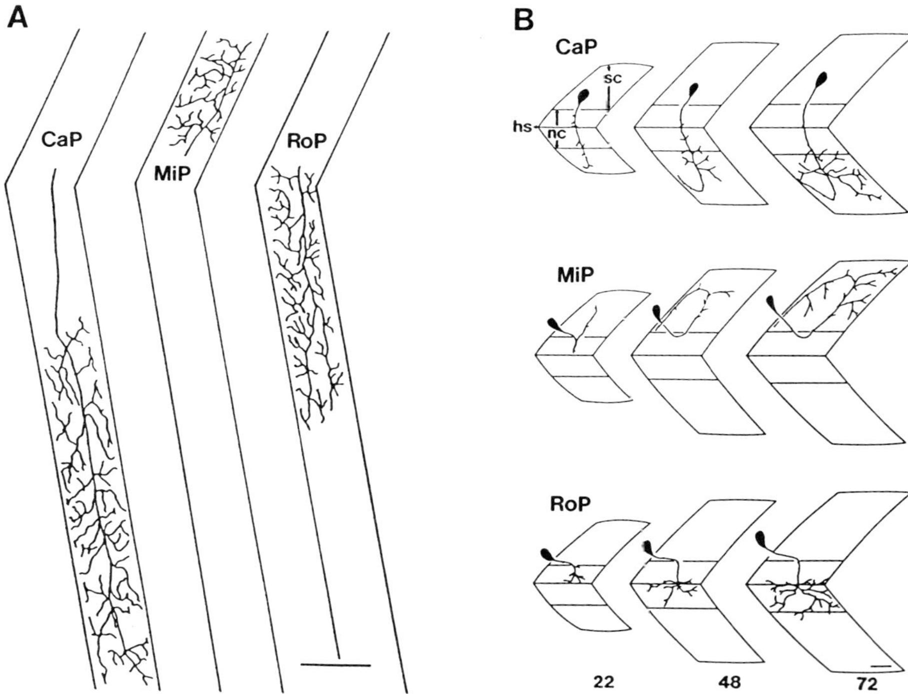

Figure 3. Each primary motoneuron can be identified by its soma position, axonal arbor, and pattern of outgrowth. A. Adults. Outlines of three muscle segments from an adult zebrafish, each with the axon of a single identified primary motoneuron. Each primary motoneuron innervates an exclusive muscle territory in its own muscle segment. CaP innervates the ventral third of the muscle segment, MiP innervates the dorsal third of the muscle segment, and RoP innervates the middle third of the muscle segment. Bar: 1 mm. [Redrawn from Westerfield *et al.* (1986) by permission of the *Journal of Neuroscience.*] B. Embryos. Outgrowth of CaP, MiP, and RoP at three stages of development (times are given in hours postfertilization at 28.5°C). Cells were labeled with DiI, and axonal outgrowth monitored using low-light-level video microscopy. Abbreviations: sc, spinal cord; nc, notochord; hs, horizontal septum. Bar: 20 μm. See text, Eisen *et al.* (1986, 1989), and Pike and Eisen (1990) for a complete description of the stereotyped pattern of axonal outgrowth. [Reprinted from Pike and Eisen (1990), by permission of the *Journal of Neuroscience.*]

dorsal axons, whereas cells in the CaP and RoP positions have ventral axons. The same results have recently been obtained in late stage embryos by retrograde labeling with DiI (Liu and Westerfield, 1990; S. Pike, personal communication) as well as by labeling individual primary motoneurons anterogradely by intracellular injection of fluorescent dyes or DiI (J. Eisen, S. Pike, and E. Melancon, unpublished observations).

D. Embryos

Primary motoneurons can be identified in embryonic zebrafish by their individual patterns of axonal outgrowth (Fig. 3b). To learn how these cells developed their individual morphologies and innervation patterns, we followed the development of labeled motoneurons in living embryos (Eisen *et al.*, 1986; Myers *et al.*, 1986). We found that the growth cones of the identified primary motoneurons extended only to the regions of muscle appropriate for their adult functions. Not only do these neurons extend their growth cones directly to their functionally appropriate targets, but the primary motoneurons that innervate each muscle segment initiate axonal outgrowth in a stereotyped sequence in which CaP precedes MiP, and MiP precedes RoP. The MiP and RoP growth cones initially extend caudally in the spinal cord, reorienting and extending into the periphery when they encounter CaP. The CaP growth cone pioneers a common pathway to a "choice point" at which the horizontal septum separating the dorsal and ventral muscle of each embryonic muscle segment, or myotome will form. The MiP and RoP growth cones follow the CaP axon along the common pathway to the horizontal septum choice point. At the choice point, the growth cones of all three motoneurons pause; then each growth cone selects a separate cell-specific pathway along which to extend. The result of cell-specific pathway extension is that each growth cone arrives at the region of the myotome containing appropriate muscle fiber targets.

The arrangement of primary motoneurons seen in embryonic and larval zebrafish is the same as that seen in adults, with one possible exception. In some segments of embryonic zebrafish there is a fourth primary motoneuron (Eisen *et al.*, 1990); because this cell is variably present we have called it VaP (*va*riable *p*rimary; Fig. 4). The VaP soma is adjacent to the CaP soma, and early in development the two cells cannot be distinguished. However, the VaP growth cone does not extend ventrally from the horizontal septum choice point. Instead, most (probably more than 85%) VaPs die without projecting to specific muscle fibers. The VaPs that do not die arborize in the region between the MiP and RoP arbors. These cells persist into larval de-

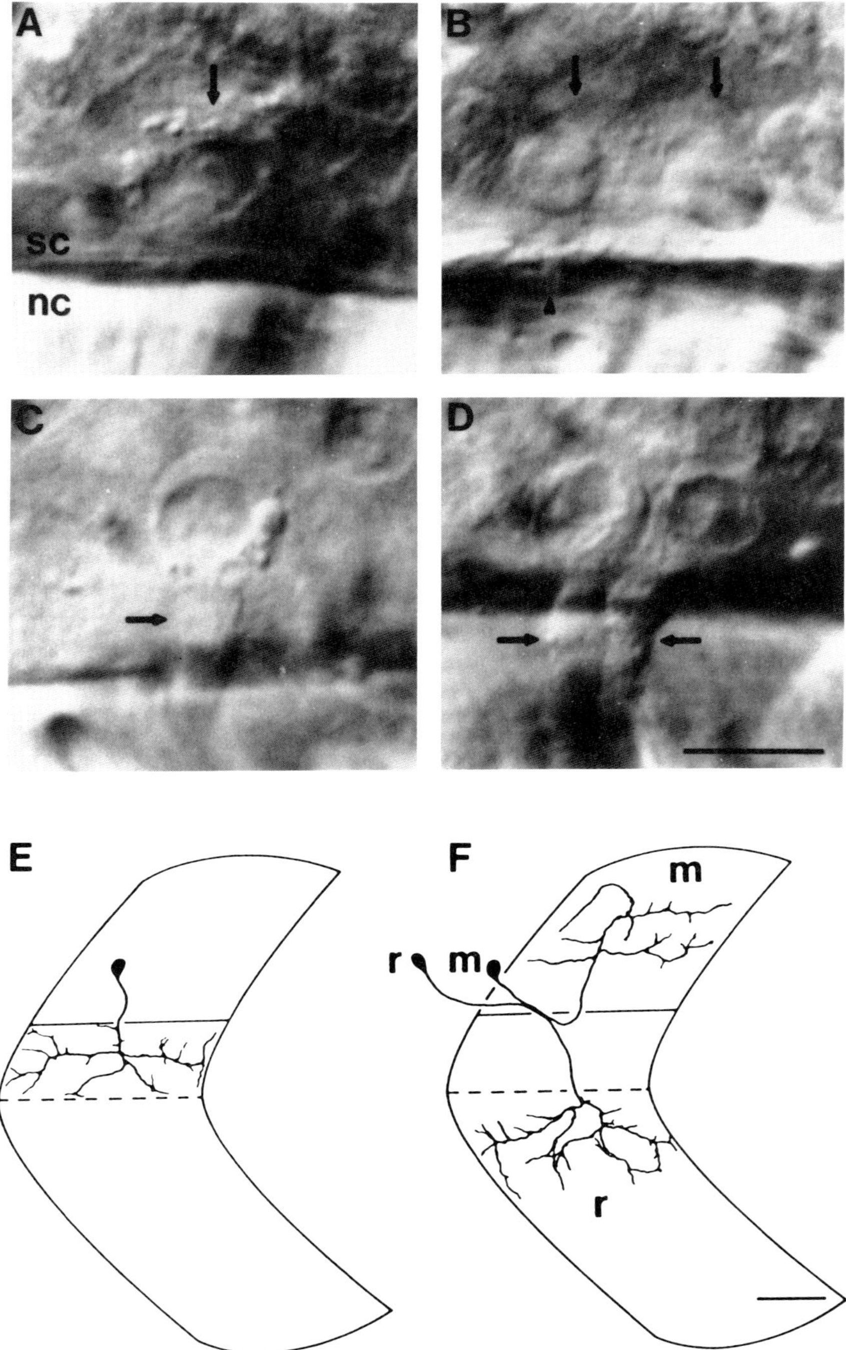

velopment (3-day), but we have not yet determined whether they are present in adults.

V. Development of Primary Motoneuronal Identity

A. Environmental Influences on Pathfinding

1. EXTRACELLULAR MATRIX MOLECULES MAY CONTRIBUTE TO THE SEGMENTAL PATTERN OF PRIMARY MOTONEURON AXONS

Extracellular matrix molecules have been suggested as possible guidance cues for growth cones during axonal pathfinding (Rogers *et al.*, 1983). Frost and Westerfield (1986) examined the distribution of several extracellular matrix glycoproteins in embryonic zebrafish and found that the regions traversed by the primary motoneuronal growth cones showed laminin-like immunoreactivity whereas the regions avoided by the primary motoneuronal growth cones, such as the myotomal borders, showed fibronectin-like immunoreactivity. This observation suggests that the distribution of a fibronectin-like molecule may contribute to the segmental pattern of the motor axons by determining where they cannot grow (see Patterson, 1988; Walter *et al.*, 1990).

2. TARGET MUSCLE MAY BE REQUIRED FOR PROPER PATHFINDING

Interactions between motoneurons and the muscles they innervate are likely to be important for formation of normal motoneuron axonal pathways (Lewis *et al.*, 1981; Tosney, 1987). We used a mutational approach to investigate whether target muscle affected axonal development of zebrafish

Figure 4. Location and development of VaP. VaP is present in about half of the trunk spinal hemisegments. A,C. Nomarksi photomicrographs of hemisegments in which VaP is not present. A. CaP (*arrow*) before axogenesis. C. CaP after axogenesis; the arrow in C is pointing to the CaP growth cone. B,D. Nomarski photomicrographs of hemisegments in which both CaP and VaP are present; at this stage it is not possible to tell which cell is which. B. Arrows point to the somata; one of the cells already has begun to elaborate a growth cone (*arrowhead*). D. Both cells have growth cones (*arrows*). E. An 89-hr VaP labeled with DiI. This cell arborized in a region between the arbors of the 87-hr MiP (m) and RoP (r) shown in F. Bar: 10 μm. [Reprinted from Eisen *et al.* (1990), by permission of the *Journal of Neuroscience.*]

primary motoneurons (Eisen and Pike, 1991). We examined the development of primary motoneurons in zebrafish embryos homozygous for the *spt-1(b104)* mutation, nicknamed "spadetail" (Kimmel *et al.*, 1989). In mutants, cells normally fated to make trunk muscle migrate improperly during gastrulation; these cells enter the tail rudiment and develop fates in accordance with their new positions. This leaves the trunk depleted of muscle cells. By transplanting cells between mutant and wild-type embryos during gastrulation, Ho and Kane (1990) showed that the *spt-1* mutation acts cell autonomously in the progenitors of trunk muscle cells by affecting their ability to undergo specific migratory movements. They also showed that the progenitors of other mesoderm-derived trunk structures, such as the notochord, are unaffected, as are the gastrulation movements of prospective neuroectoderm. Thus, the direct action of the mutation appears to be restricted to the precursors of segmented mesoderm of the trunk.

In mutant embryos, the pattern of primary motoneuronal somata is disrupted, probably because of abnormal early interactions with developing segmented mesoderm (Eisen and Pike, 1991). In addition, although at least some primary motoneurons extend growth cones out of the spinal cord, they form axons that are morphologically aberrant (Eisen and Pike, 1991). The aberrant morphology of primary motoneuron axons in spadetail embryos might arise in two very different ways: the mutation could act directly to alter some intrinsic feature of the primary motoneurons or it could be the result of an alteration in some feature of their environment that is critical for proper pathfinding, for example, the presence of target muscle, its surrounding organized extracellular matrix, or other cells in the somites. To learn whether the mutation acts directly on motoneuronal pathfinding or is due to environmental changes related to the loss of target muscle cells, we performed a genetic mosaic analysis by transplanting individual primary motoneurons between mutant and wild-type embryos (Fig. 5). Donor embryos were labeled with fluorescent lineage-tracer dye at the single-cell stage so the entire donor embryo contained the dye; primary motoneuronal somata were transplanted from labeled donors to unlabeled hosts. These experiments revealed that wild-type primary motoneurons transplanted to *spt-1* hosts had an aberrant morphology, whereas *spt-1* primary motoneurons transplanted to wild-type hosts had a wild-type morphology. Thus, the mutation did not appear to affect the motoneurons directly, suggesting that their abnormal development was environmentally imposed, perhaps by the loss of their target muscles. To test this idea directly, we deprived somites of wild-type embryos of target muscle by removing precursor cells at a stage before primary motoneurons had undergone axonogenesis. We found that wild-type primary motoneurons in muscle-deprived regions resembled *spt-1* primary motoneurons. This result is consistent with the idea that the aberrant morphology of *spt-1* primary

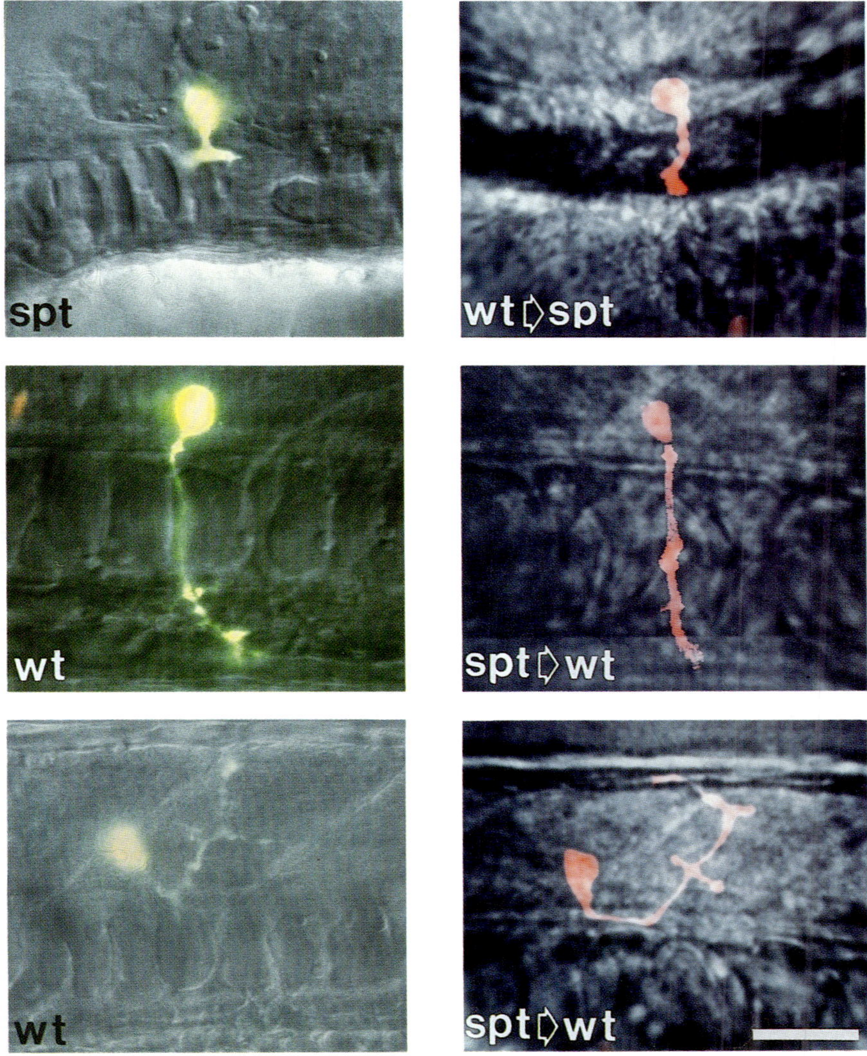

FIGURE 5. The *spt-1* mutation alters pathfinding by the primary motoneurons. *(Left)* Combined Nomarksi and fluorescence photomicrographs of native primary motoneurons labeled by intracellular iontophoresis of lucifer yellow. The upper photograph shows a motoneuron in a mutant embryo, the middle photograph shows a CaP motoneuron in a wild-type embryo, and the bottom photograph shows a MiP motoneuron in a wild-type embryo. *(Right)* Image-processed photomicrographs of single primary motoneurons transplanted between *spt-1* and wild-type embryos. The upper photograph shows that wild-type motoneurons transplanted to *spt-1* hosts have a mutant phenotype. The middle and bottom photographs show that *spt-1* motoneurons transplanted to wild-type hosts have a wild-type phenotype. Bar: 30 μm. Adapted from Eisen and Pike (1991) with the permission of *Cell Press*.

motoneurons was due to environmental changes resulting from lack of target muscle, and suggests that the muscle provides something that primary motoneurons require for proper development.

3. TARGET ACTIVITY IS NOT NECESSARY FOR PROPER PATHFINDING OR ARBORIZATION

Interactions between motoneurons and their targets based on target activity are thought to be important for the formation of proper synaptic connections (Purves and Lichtman, 1985). Westerfield and his colleagues investigated the role of activity in pathfinding and synapse formation by zebrafish primary motoneurons by blocking muscle activity pharmacologically and genetically. Liu and Westerfield (1990) allowed embryos to develop under conditions in which sodium channels or acetylcholine receptors were blocked, and found that pathfinding, synaptogenesis, and the pattern of muscle innervation by the primary motoneurons were normal. Westerfield *et al.* (1990) examined pathfinding in embryos homozygous for the nicotinic acetylcholine receptor mutation *nic-1(b107)*. Because these embryos do not respond to cholinergic agonists and labeling of their muscles cannot be detected by α-bungarotoxin or monoclonal antibodies to acetylcholine receptor subunits, they probably lack functional acetylcholine receptors. Despite the absence of functional acetylcholine receptors, motoneurons in mutant embryos undergo proper pathfinding. Morphologically normal neuromuscular junctions were also observed by electron microscopy. These two sets of results suggest that transmitter-evoked muscular activity is not important for proper pathfinding or synapse formation by zebrafish primary motoneurons.

Although target activity appears unnecessary for proper pathfinding, it is still possible that primary motoneurons might compete for innervation of particular muscle fibers. Liu and Westerfield (1990) directly observed branching by CaP and RoP; they found that both primary motoneurons make branches on muscle fibers in the vicinity of the horizontal septum choice point. These muscle fibers are in an inappropriate territory for CaP innervation and the branches are later retracted. The time course of retraction is consistent with a model in which primary motoneurons compete for innervation of these muscle fibers. To test whether retraction is actually caused by competition, Liu and Westerfield removed potential competition by ablating RoP with a laser microbeam focused onto the cell soma. When potential competition was removed in this way, CaP still withdrew the inappropriate branches, suggesting that CaP and RoP were not competing for innervation of these muscle fibers. Thus, in this situation, competition appears unimportant in determining the muscle fibers that individual motoneurons innervate.

B. Interactions among Primary Motoneurons

Because the growth cones of the primary motoneurons reach their targets by a process of directed pathfinding, it is tempting to speculate that these cells may have individual identities even prior to axonogenesis. This hypothesis predicts that, by the time of axonogenesis each primary motoneuron would have become committed to develop in a characteristic way that differed from the other primary motoneurons in its own segment. Commitment might involve activation of an intrinsic program that caused the cell to develop a specific morphology, as has been described for regenerating neurons of the leech (Acklin and Nicholls, 1988). Alternatively, it might involve expression of a set of receptors that recognized particular extrinsic cues that would provide guidance information to the navigating growth cone. Of course these possibilities are not mutually exclusive and they could be combined with other possibilities not considered here. By transplanting identified primary motoneurons to novel locations, it should be possible to learn whether the growth cones of particular primary motoneurons show specific recognition for their own region of the myotome. Preliminary results support the idea that, even when the primary motoneurons are in ectopic locations, their growth cones recognize the appropriate cell-specific pathways. The growth cones of CaP motoneurons transplanted to the choice point region at which the cell-specific primary motoneuronal pathways diverge appear to extend specifically along the CaP pathway, whereas the growth cones of MiPs transplanted to the same position appear to extend specifically along the MiP pathway (C. Gatchalian, personal communication). These results suggest that the pathways followed by the growth cones of the different primary motoneurons may differ in some way that the growth cones recognize.

Another possibility is that, although the primary motoneurons have different morphologies and innervate different muscle regions, they are all equivalent and achieve their individual characteristics by interactions in which they compete for pathways leading to specific target regions. Such interactions could be based on timing, so the growth cone of a later-developing primary motoneuron is excluded from extending along a pathway occupied by the axon of an earlier-developing primary motoneuron. This hypothesis makes a specific prediction: in segments in which VaP is not present, the first primary motoneuron to extend an axon will select the CaP pathway, the second one will select the MiP pathway, and the third one will select the RoP pathway. Thus, in the absence of CaP, the MiP growth cone should extend into CaP territory rather than MiP territory, and in the absence of both CaP and MiP, the RoP growth cone should extend into CaP territory.

To test this idea, we ablated primary motoneurons by focusing a laser microbeam onto their somata prior to axonogenesis (Eisen *et al.*, 1989, 1990; Pike and Eisen, 1990). We found that, even when we ablated all but one primary motoneuron on one side of a spinal segment, that cell always extended its axon along the cell-specific pathway it would have chosen if the other primary motoneurons were still present. Thus, competitive interactions among the primary motoneurons are unlikely to be important in pathway choice, suggesting that pathway choice is governed by other factors.

Although CaP, MiP, and RoP appear to develop their individual morphologies and undergo proper pathfinding independent of one another, this may not be the case for VaP. Early in their development, CaP and VaP are often so similar in their appearance and time-course of axonal outgrowth that they cannot be distinguished (Fig. 4). This observation suggested that the two cells might be equivalent (Eisen *et al.*, 1990) and that perhaps interactions between the two cells resulted in only one of them developing the CaP morphology. Interactions among specific sibling neurons in grasshoppers (Kuwada and Goodman, 1985) and between particular contralateral homologs in the leech (Macagno and Stewart, 1987; Martindale and Shankland, 1990) have been shown to be involved in determining which cell of the pair adopts a specific fate.

To test whether the development of the CaP and VaP phenotypes depended on interactions between the two cells, we ablated one of the two cells prior to axogenesis. Our rationale was that if these cells competed to become CaP, then removal of one of them would force the remaining cell to become CaP. However, our initial results did not support this hypothesis. When we examined the ablated segments several hours after the ablation, half of the remaining cells had a CaP phenotype, having axons that extended to the ventral edge of the ventral muscle, and half of them had a VaP phenotype, having axons that had not extended beyond the horizontal septum choice point. However, when we examined ablated segments at later stages, we observed cells with a phenotype intermediate between those of VaP and CaP (J. Eisen, unpublished observations). The interpretation of this result is that, after pausing at the horizontal septum choice point, the growth cones of these cells resumed extension. These observations suggest that CaP and VaP may initially be equivalent cells that compete for innervation of the CaP muscle territory.

More recently, this issue was examined further by transplanting presumptive CaPs/VaPs to new locations (J. Eisen, unpublished observations). When a segment was created with three primary motoneurons in the CaP/VaP position by transplanting an additional cell into that segment (either a CaP or a VaP; it is not possible to tell at this stage which fate the cell would have adopted if it had not been moved), only one of the cells became a CaP. Which cell becomes CaP seems to depend on which cell extends its growth cone first. Thus, when the native motoneurons have already extended growth cones before the third cell is transplanted into the segment, a native primary motoneuron becomes CaP and the transplanted cell becomes VaP. However, if

the cell is transplanted into a segment in which the native primary motoneurons have not yet extended growth cones, then the transplanted cell and
the native ones appear to have equal probabilities of becoming CaP. In any
case, *only one* cell became CaP; when that cell was one that was transplanted
into the segment, then the growth cones of both of the native motoneurons
in the segment did not extend ventrally from the horizontal septum choice
point, at least as late as they have been examined. The current interpretation
of this result is that there is some kind of interaction among primary motoneurons in the CaP/VaP position, so when one of them adopts the CaP fate,
the others cannot. This interaction could be directly among the primary
motoneurons, or it could be between the primary motoneurons and other
cells; one possibility that we are currently investigating is that the CaP axonal
pathway can only be occupied by the axon of a single primary motoneuron.

This issue has also been examined by transplanting presumptive CaP/VaPs
to segments in which the native primary motoneurons have been removed. In
this case, all the surviving transplanted cells adopt the CaP phenotype. Although the possibility that the VaPs specifically do not survive cannot be ruled
out, this seems unlikely. In the most extreme cases, transplantation of both
CaP and VaP from a single segment into adjacent segments lacking native
primary motoneurons result in both transplanted cells adopting the CaP
phenotype.

As a whole, these experiments show that both CaP and VaP have the
potential to become CaP, and they suggest that the VaP phenotype arises
because of interactions. It is possible that when one cell extends an axon
ventrally from the choice point it becomes CaP, suppressing axonal extension
along that pathway by the other cell, which then becomes VaP. Our results are
also consistent with the idea that there may be earlier interactions between
these cells, perhaps occurring before axonogenesis, that influence which cell
adopts the CaP phenotype and which cell adopts the VaP phenotype. However, we cannot rule out the possibility that ablating one cell of the CaP/VaP
pair sometimes causes the remaining cell to develop more slowly than its
homologs in adjacent segments. Why VaPs appear to be present in only about
half the trunk segments of any given embryo is still unresolved.

C. The Role of Position in Determining Primary Motoneuron Identity

I. PRIMARY MOTONEURON PROGENITORS APPEAR TO BE MULTIPOTENT

Using lineage analysis, Kimmel and Warga (1986) found that divisions of
neuronal precursors occurring just before the neural tube forms often give
rise to two cells on opposite sides of the midline, although this is not always

the case. In some cases, this division is the final one and generates two cells that are bilateral homologs. For example, a progenitor cell may produce CaPs on the left and right sides of the same segment. However, just as the early division pattern of the embryo is not invariant, the pattern of cells produced by a primary motoneuron progenitor is not invariant (C.B. Kimmel, personal communication). Thus, the sibling of a CaP is not necessarily another CaP, and in some cases it may not be another primary motoneuron (C.B. Kimmel and R.M. Warga, personal communication).

These observations suggest that, even at the time of the final mitosis, progenitors that may produce primary motoneurons are not committed to do so, although they may already have some limitations on the types of progeny they can produce. Thus, the progenitors of the primary motoneurons appear to be multipotent. The idea that vertebrate neuronal precursors are multipotent has received considerable support from lineage-tracing studies that suggest the presence of a population of multipotent precursor cells in several regions of the vertebrate CNS, including the retina (Turner and Cepko, 1987; Holt *et al.*, 1988; Wetts and Fraser, 1988; see Chapter 13), cerebral cortex (Luskin *et al.*, 1988; Price and Thurlow, 1988; Walsh and Cepko, 1988), optic tectum (Gray *et al.*, 1988), spinal cord (Hartenstein, 1989; Leber *et al.*, 1990), and neural crest (see Chapter 11). To demonstrate rigorously that primary motoneuronal progenitors are multipotent would require learning whether they are a homogeneous population of cells, whether specific primary motoneuronal progenitors always produce the same progeny, and whether the fates of the progeny can be altered in response to different environments. If neuronal progenitors are not committed to produce specific progeny, then it seems likely that some environmental influence, perhaps the position the cell occupies during or after its final division, determines what its progeny will become.

2. THE DEVELOPMENTAL POTENTIAL OF PRIMARY NEURONS APPEARS TO BE RESTRICTED

Since the progenitors of primary motoneurons appear to be multipotent, is seems reasonable to ask whether postmitotic neurons arising from these progenitors are also multipotent, or whether their potential to develop as other neuronal types is restricted. To examine this issue, primary motoneurons and primary interneurons were transplanted to new spinal cord locations and their subsequent development examined. Cells were transplanted prior to axonogenesis; following the transplant, it was determined whether they developed fates appropriate for their sites of origin or fates appropriate for their new positions.

Primary motoneurons were taken from the CaP or MiP position and placed in the positions of CaP, MiP, and RoP motoneurons as well as in the position of VeLD primary interneurons. All the surviving cells developed a motoneuronal morphology, that is, all extended peripheral axons along pathways normally followed by the axons of primary motoneurons (Fig. 6a; see also Eisen, 1991). This result argues that, by the time these cells were moved, they were already committed to become primary motoneurons. Preliminary results suggest that these cells retain features of primary motoneurons, for

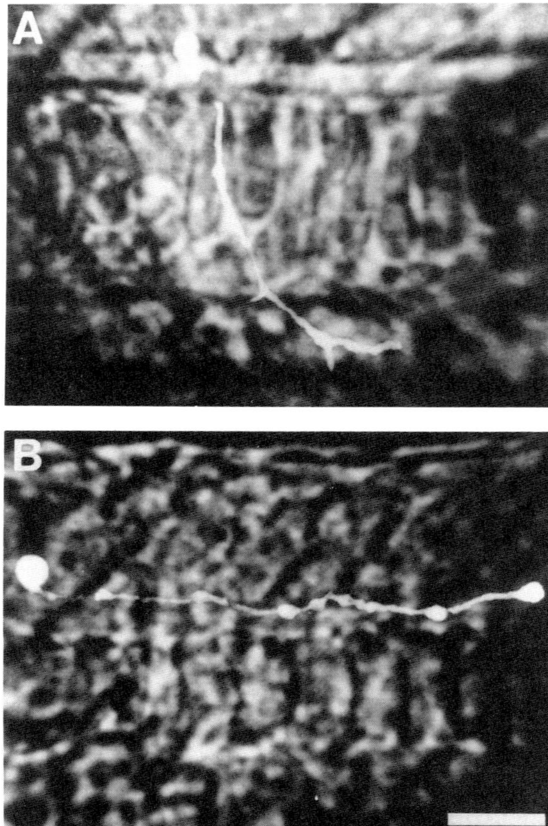

Figure 6. Functional class commitment of postmitotic primary neurons. The results of transplantation experiments argue that, even before axogenesis, cells are already committed to be neurons of a particular functional class. A. Image-processed photomicrograph of a cell from the CaP position of a labeled donor embryo transplanted to an unlabeled host about 2 hr before axogenesis. This cell developed as a normal CaP. [Adapted from Eisen (1991) with permission of *Science*; copyright © 1991 by the AAAS.] B. Image-processed photomicrograph of a cell transplanted from the VeLD position of a labeled donor to an unlabeled host about 2 hr before axogenesis. This cell developed as a normal VeLD. Bar: 25 μm.

example, extending axons along normal primary motoneuronal pathways even when they are challenged further by transplantation outside of the spinal cord into the space between the notochord or spinal cord and the overlying muscle (Gatchalian and Eisen, 1990). This finding strengthens the idea that by this stage these cells are committed to becoming primary motoneurons and that they are, therefore, restricted in their potential to develop as other cell types.

To learn whether other cell types were also committed by this stage, VeLD primary interneurons were transplanted to primary motoneuronal positions in the spinal cord. VeLD interneurons transplanted to the position of CaP, MiP, or RoP motoneurons extended axons caudally in the spinal cord (Fig. 6b), as do normal VeLDs, arguing that these cells were committed to become primary interneurons by the time they were moved.

These transplantation experiments suggest that, although primary motoneurons and primary interneurons may arise from uncommitted progenitors, cells arising from the final mitosis are committed to the class of neurons they will become before axonogenesis. It seems likely that commitment occurs after the cells become postmitotic, although this has not been demonstrated directly. What causes these cells to become committed and how soon after the final mitosis does it happen? If position is actually the determining factor, then cell-type commitment may not occur until the progeny have "settled" in some particular position. Based on this hypothesis, I would predict that, if cells were transplanted very soon after they became postmitotic, they might be able to develop appropriately for their new soma positions. However, even at early times cells may have made commitments based on their positions and migration patterns, so their developmental options are limited, despite the fact that they are not committed to specific fates. Alternatively, there might be a "default" developmental pathway taken by all cells in the ventral spinal cord that have early birthdays, if they do not receive some position-dependent signal that prompts them to begin to differentiate as primary motoneurons.

3. DETERMINATION OF PRIMARY MOTONEURONS MAY INVOLVE SEVERAL STEPS

Primary motoneurons transplanted to new spinal cord locations extend axons along normal motoneuronal pathways, even when they are transplanted several hours before axonogenesis. Thus, these cells appear to be committed to develop as primary motoneurons. Since each identified primary motoneuron has a characteristic morphology, a detailed analysis of the soma position and axonal trajectory of each transplanted primary motoneuron should reveal whether these cells are committed to extend their axons along specific pathways and to innervate particular muscle territories. Cells moved to new positions that develop axonal trajectories appropriate for their *original* soma positions would be considered committed, whereas cells that develop axonal trajectories appropriate for their *new* soma positions would be considered uncommitted (Eisen, 1991).

Examination of the morphologies of transplanted motoneurons revealed that the cells fell into several different categories. Cells transplanted *homotopically*, from the CaP position to the CaP position or from the MiP position to the MiP position, developed normal morphologies appropriate for their soma positions. However, cells transplanted *heterotopically*, from the CaP position to the MiP position or from the MiP position to the CaP position, developed in three different ways. These three classes of cells are described in the following paragraphs.

The first class of cells included motoneurons transplanted 1–3 hr before axonogenesis. The cells in this group developed axonal trajectories that were appropriate for their original soma positions. By the definition of commitment set forth earlier, these cells could be considered committed, at least with respect to their axonal trajectories. However, these cells did something quite surprising that made it difficult to evaluate whether their axonal trajectories actually were committed. After they were transplanted, the somata of these cells moved from their new positions to positions that corresponded to their original positions; examples of two of these cells are shown in Fig. 7a,b. Since the somata did not stay in the new positions in which they were placed, the axonal trajectories of these cells were appropriate for both their new soma positions and their original soma positions. Thus, it is not certain that these cells were committed.

Figure 7. Commitment of primary motoneuronal axonal trajectories. Primary motoneurons transplanted before axogenesis develop in three different ways. Many cells transplanted 1–3 hrs before axogenesis did not remain where they were placed, but moved to a position equivalent to their site of origin. A,B. Image-processed photomicrographs of cells transplanted from the CaP position to the MiP position and from the MiP position to the CaP position, respectively. The somata of both cells returned to their original positions and both cells developed morphologies appropriate for their sites of origin. The inset in A shows the position of the cell right after transplantation. Cells transplanted about 1 hr before axogenesis developed axonal trajectories appropriate for their sites of origin. C,D. Image-processed photomicrographs of cells transplanted from the CaP position to the MiP position and from the MiP position to the RoP position, respectively. Both cells extended axons along the pathways appropriate for their original soma positions. Cells transplanted 2–3 hrs before axogenesis developed axonal trajectories appropriate for their new soma positions. E,F. Image-processed photomicrographs of cells transplanted from the CaP position to the MiP position and from the MiP position to the CaP position, respectively. Both cells extended axons along the pathways appropriate for their new soma positions. Bar: 25 μm. [Adapted from Eisen (1991) with permission of *Science*; copyright © 1991 by the AAAS.]

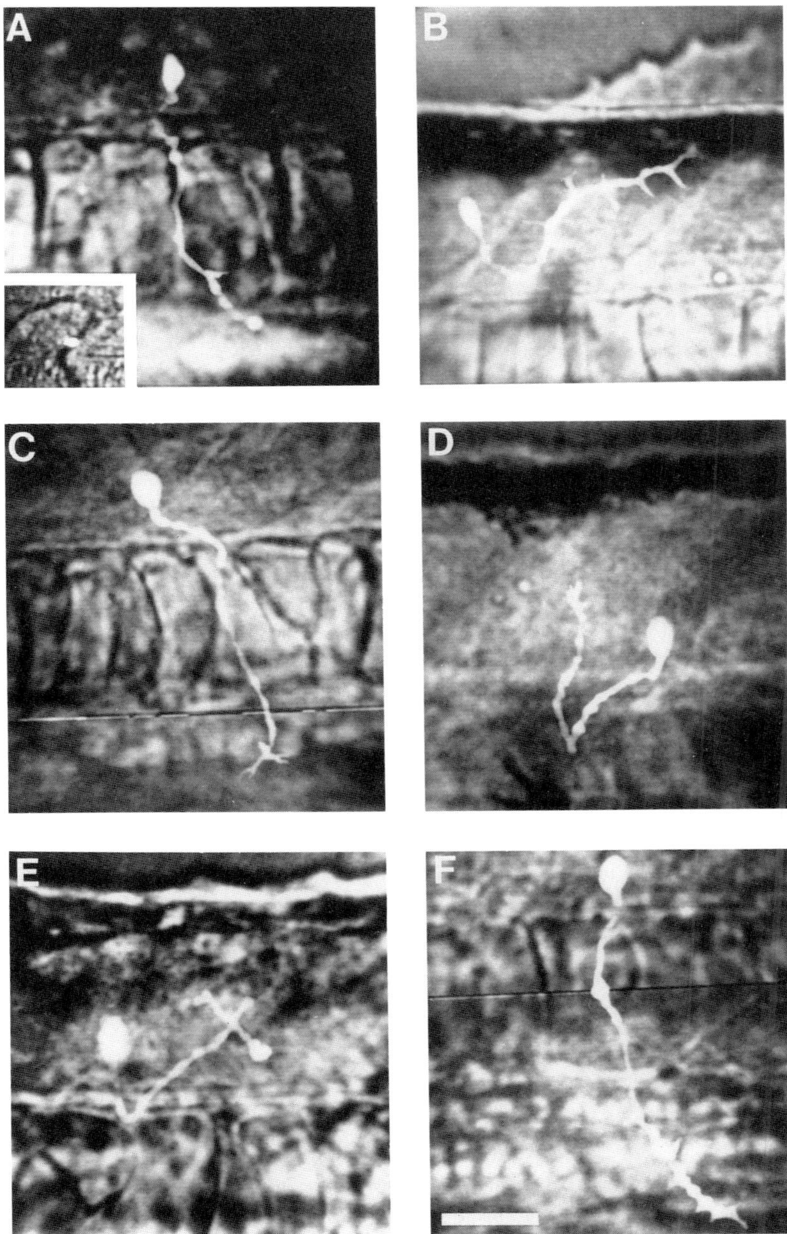

The second class of cells was composed of motoneurons transplanted about 1 hr before axonogenesis. These cells developed novel morphologies in which their axonal trajectories were appropriate for their original soma positions, but not for their new soma positions (Fig. 7c,d). Since the somata of all these cells remained in their new positions, the axonal trajectories of these cells were deemed committed by the time the cells were transplanted. This idea is strengthened by preliminary results (C. Gatchalian, personal communication) that, even when these cells are transplanted to the region of the horizontal septum choice point, they seem to extend axons along primary motoneuronal pathways appropriate for their sites of origin.

The third class of cells included motoneurons transplanted 2–3 hr before axonogenesis. These cells developed axonal trajectories appropriate for their new soma positions, but not for their original soma positions (Fig. 7e,f). Again, the somata of all these cells remained in their new positions; thus, the axonal trajectories of these cells were uncommitted at the time the cells were transplanted.

These results suggest that the process by which primary motoneurons become committed to express their individual identities may involve several steps. These cells appear to be committed as primary motoneurons before they are committed to express particular axonal trajectories, suggesting that initially all the primary motoneurons may be equivalent. Primary motoneurons whose somata are in different locations develop different axonal trajectories, suggesting that local cues in the vicinity of the soma may influence expression of particular motoneuronal phenotypes. Before they are committed, these cells can respond to a new set of cues by developing an axonal trajectory appropriate for a new position. A short time later, after they are committed, these cells can no longer respond to a new set of cues, and they develop the axonal trajectories appropriate for their original positions. Thus, each cell develops an individual identity, with the possible exception that CaP and VaP may remain equivalent. It is interesting that we have never observed either native or transplanted primary motoneurons to extend axons along multiple cell-specific pathways. This observation suggests that axonal pathway selection may involve a switch in which recognition of one pathway prevents recognition of other pathways.

A surprising finding in this study was that, after they were transplanted to new positions, the somata of many primary motoneurons moved back to their original positions. Whether these cells were committed or not is somewhat difficult to say, since a committed cell must, by definition, express its original fate in a novel position. However, these results suggest that these cells may recognize and respond to local positional cues; this ability might be a reflection of the cells having undergone an earlier commitment that occurs before commitment to express a particular axonal trajectory.

VI. Conclusions

Our results suggest that, in the zebrafish embryo, primary motoneurons become committed to develop their individual morphologies before axonogenesis. The commitment process can be considered to involve at least two steps, since cells seem to be committed to become primary motoneurons before they are committed to develop specific axonal trajectories. Once their axonal trajectories become committed, their growth cones retain the ability to recognize the appropriate cell-specific axonal pathways, even when the cells are transplanted to ectopic locations outside the spinal cord. This is consistent with the idea that identity is established and maintained independent of retrograde information from the growth cone. At this time, morphology has been our only assay for motoneuronal identity; ideally, we would like to have molecular markers for the different cell types. The ability of the growth cones of specific primary motoneurons to recognize particular pathways suggests at least one molecular distinction among different motoneurons: the expression of specific receptors for pathway cues localized to the different pathways. We hope to identify additional molecular differences between specific primary motoneurons and, thus, to learn more about the basis of neuronal identity.

Several lines of evidence suggest that soma position may be a major determinant of cellular identity and, thus, of primary motoneuronal growth cone pathway selection. First, the primary motoneuronal somata have stereotyped positions; second, soma position correlates with axonal trajectory; and third, motoneurons transplanted to new positions after their axonal trajectories are committed extend growth cones along pathways appropriate for their *original* soma positions. Position also appears to be important in determining neuronal identity in other species. In the *Drosophila* retina, position is correlated with cell fate, consistent with the idea that cell fate may be influenced by a position-dependent process (see Chapter 7). One photoreceptor, called R8, is specified first. R8 cells arise in a precise pattern in which they are equidistant from one another, suggesting that their initial specification may involve competition in which specified R8 cells inhibit neighboring cells from becoming R8 (Baker *et al.*, 1990). Other photoreceptors are specified later by a cascade of interactions (Karpilow *et al.*, 1989; Banerjee and Zipursky, 1990). In the grasshopper CNS (Doe and Goodman, 1985), a position-dependent process appears to determine which cell will enlarge to become a neuroblast; this cell then inhibits its neighbors from becoming neuroblasts. In amphibians, a position-dependent process may determine which cell will become the Mauthner neuron; the Mauthner neuron in turn appears to inhibit neighboring cells from adopting this fate (Stefanelli, 1951; Schlenoff and Model, 1985;

see Kimmel and Eaton, 1976). Perhaps in zebrafish the primary motoneurons arise by a similar position-dependent process. This idea is consistent with the cell lineage data. If it is the case, then early removal of a primary motoneuron should lead to its replacement by another cell, as just described for amphibian Mauthner cells and grasshopper neuroblasts.

Primary motoneurons whose somata are in different positions extend growth cones along different cell-specific pathways and do not seem to compete for those pathways or for innervation of their cell-specific muscle territories. Again, these observations are consistent with a role for soma position in determining axonal trajectory. Further, primary motoneurons whose somata are located in similar positions, such as CaP and VaP, do appear to compete for an axonal trajectory. The basis of this competition is currently unknown, but it will be interesting to learn whether it is similar to the competition seen between leech neurons (Martindale and Shankland, 1990) or between motoneurons in other vertebrates.

We have begun using a mutational approach to examine features of the zebrafish embryo that might provide the signals involved in determining the identities of the primary motoneurons or in promoting proper pathfinding. Analysis of embryos homozygous for three different embryonic lethal mutations has begun to shed light on these processes. Embryos homozygous for the *cyc-1(b16)* mutation lack a differentiated floor plate of the CNS (Hatta *et al.*, 1991). In avian embryos lacking a floor plate, adjacent motoneurons appear to be absent (Hirano *et al.*, 1991). In contrast, primary motoneurons are present and appear to have a normal morphology in *cyc-1* mutants (Eisen, 1991), suggesting that the floor plate is not a unique source of positional cues that influence the identities of the primary motoneurons. However, the putative positional cues could be provided by a combination of sources that includes the floor plate. Embryos homozygous for the *spt-1* mutation have primary motoneurons with stunted axons (Eisen and Pike, 1991). Transplantation of primary motoneurons between wild-type and mutant embryos suggests that the mutation affects the motoneurons indirectly, by altering the amount of muscle in the somites, implying that muscle cells are important for proper motoneuronal differentiation. Embryos homozygous for the *nic-1* mutation lack functional acetylcholine receptors (Westerfield *et al.*, 1990). In these embryos, the morphology of the primary motoneurons is normal, suggesting that neuromuscular activity does not influence motoneuronal development.

It seems likely that ordered spatiotemporal patterns of gene expression are involved in the acquisition of the individual identities of the primary motoneurons. Recent work in murine embryos (Gaunt *et al.*, 1988; Wilkinson *et al.*, 1989; Kessel and Gruss, 1990) as well as in the zebrafish (see Molven *et al.*, 1990) has revealed an intriguing pattern of expression of homeobox-containing genes along the body axis. In the mouse hindbrain, specific genes are expressed in particular segments, and other genes are expressed in overlapping segmental patterns. It is tempting to speculate that the products of these or other genes, which are likely to be transcriptional regulators, could be involved in providing positional cues to the somata of the developing primary motoneurons. However, even if such genes are involved, it will still require a great deal of work to understand how their expression could regulate the development and morphologies of individual neurons.

Acknowledgments

It is a pleasure to thank Charles Kimmel, Monte Westerfield, Christine Gatchalian, Sue Pike, Peter O'Day, Marty Shankland, and Eduardo Macagno for criticism of earlier drafts of this manuscript, Sean Poston for photography, and Pat Edwards for typing. Work in my laboratory has been supported by the NIH, NSF, American Heart Association, Procter and Gamble Company, and a Searle Scholar Award.

References

Acklin, S. E., and Nicholls, J. G. (1988). Reduplication of specific branching patterns expressed in the CNS of the leech by isolated identified neurons in culture. *Soc. Neurosci. Abstr.* **14,** 596.

Baker, N. E., Mlodzik, M., and Rubin, G. M. (1990). Spacing differentiation in the developing *Drosophila* eye: A fibrinogen-related lateral inhibitor encoded by *scabrous. Science* **250,** 1370–1377.

Balinsky, B. I. (1970). "An introduction to embryology." Philadelphia: Saunders.

Banerjee, U., and Zipursky, S. L. (1990). The role of cell–cell interaction in the development of the *Drosophila* visual system. *Neuron* **4,** 177–187.

Chitnis, A. B., and Kuwada, J. Y. (1990). Axonogenesis in the brain of zebrafish embryos. *J. Neurosci.* **10,** 1892–1905.

Doe, C. Q., and Goodman, C. S. (1985). Early events in insect neurogenesis II. The role of cell interactions and cell lineage in the determination of neuronal precursor cells. *Devel. Biol.* **111,** 206–219.

Easter, S. S., Jr., and Taylor, J. S. H. (1989). The development of the *Xenopus* retinofugal pathway: Optic fibers join a pre-existing tract. *Development* **107,** 553–573.

Eisen, J. S. (1991). Determination of primary motoneuron identity in developing zebrafish embryos. *Science* **252,** 569–572.

Eisen, J. S., Myers, P. Z., and Westerfield, M. (1986). Pathway selection by growth cones of identified motoneurons in live zebrafish embryos. *Nature (London)* **320,** 269–271.

Eisen, J. S., Pike, S. H., and Debu, B. (1989). The growth cones of identified motoneurons in embryonic zebrafish select appropriate pathways in the absence of specific cellular interactions. *Neuron* **2,** 1097–1104.

Eisen, J. S., Pike, S. H., and Romancier, B. (1990). An identified neuron with variable fates in embryonic zebrafish. *J. Neurosci.* **10,** 34–43.

Eisen, J. S., and Pike, S. H. (1991). The *spt-1* mutation alters the segmental arrangement and axonal development of identified neurons in the spinal cord of the embryonic zebrafish. *Neuron* **6,** 767–776.

Faber, D. S., and Korn, H. (1978). "Neurobiology of the Mauthner cell." New York: Raven Press.

Frost, D., and Westerfield, M. (1986). Axon outgrowth of embryonic zebrafish neurons is promoted by laminin and inhibited by fibronectin. *Soc. Neurosci. Abstr.* **12,** 1114.

Gatchalian, C. L., and Eisen, J. S. (1990). Growth cones of ectopic motoneurons select normal pathways in embryonic zebrafish. *Soc. Neurosci. Abstr.* **16,** 624.

Gaunt, S. J., Sharpe, P. T., and Duboule, D. (1988). Spatially restricted domains of homeogene transcripts in mouse embryos: Relation to a segmented body plan. *Development* **104** *Suppl,* 159–179.

Gray, G. E., Glover, J. C., Majors, J., and Sanes, J. R. (1988). Radial arrangement of clonally related cells in the chicken optic tectum: Lineage analysis with a recombinant retrovirus. *Proc. Natl. Acad. Sci. U.S.A.* **85,** 7356–7360.

Grunwald, D. J., Kimmel, C. B., Westerfield, M., Walker, C., and Streisinger, G. (1988). A neural degeneration mutation that spares primary neurons in the zebrafish. *Dev. Biol.* **126,** 115–128.

Hanneman, E., Trevarrow, B., Metcalfe, W. K., Kimmel, C. B., and Westerfield, M. (1988). Segmental pattern of development of the hindbrain and spinal cord of the zebrafish embryo. *Development* **103,** 49–58.

Hanneman, E., and Westerfield, M. (1989). Early expression of acetylcholinesterase activity in functionally distinct neurons of the zebrafish. *J. Comp. Neurol.* **284,** 350–361.

Hartenstein, V. (1989). Early neurogenesis in *Xenopus*: The spatio-temporal pattern of proliferation and cell lineages in the embryonic spinal cord. *Neuron* **3,** 399–411.

Hatta, K., Kimmel, C. B., Ho, R. K., and Walker, C. (1991). The cyclops mutation blocks specification of the floor plate of the zebrafish central nervous system. *Nature (London)* **350,** 339–341.

Hirano, S., Fuse, S., and Sohal, G. S. (1991). The effect of the floor plate on pattern and polarity in the developing central nervous system. *Science* **251,** 310–313.

Ho, R. K., and Kane, D. A. (1990). Cell-autonomous action of zebrafish *spt-1* mutation in specific mesodermal precursors. *Nature (London)* **348,** 728–730.

Holt, C. E., Bertsch, T. W., Ellis, H. M., and Harris, W. A. (1988). Cellular determination in the *Xenopus* retina is independent of lineage and birth date. *Neuron* **1,** 15–26.

Kahn, J. A., and Roberts, A. (1982). Experiments on the central pattern generator for swimming in amphibian embryos. *Phil. Trans. R. Soc. Lond. B.* **296,** 229–243.

Karpilow, J., Kolodkin, A., Bork, T., and Venkatesh, T. (1989). Neuronal development in the *Drosophila* compound eye: *rap* gene function is required in photoreceptor cell R8 for ommatidial pattern formation. *Genes Devel.* **3,** 1834–1844.

Kessel, M., and Gruss, P. (1990). Murine developmental control genes. *Science* **249,** 374–379.

Kimmel, C. B., and Eaton, R. C. (1976). Development of the Mauthner Cell. *In* "Simpler Networks and Behavior" (J. C. Fentress, ed.), pp. 186–202. Sunderland, Massachusetts: Sinauer Assoc.

Kimmel, C. B., and Law, R. D. (1985a). Cell lineage of zebrafish blastomeres. I. Cleavage pattern and cytoplasmic bridges between cells. *Dev. Biol.* **108,** 78–85.

Kimmel, C. B., and Law, R. D. (1985b). Cell lineage of zebrafish blastomeres. II. Formation of the yolk syncytial layer. *Dev. Biol.* **108,** 86–93.

Kimmel, C. B., and Warga, R. M. (1986). Tissue-specific cell lineages originate in the gastrula of the zebrafish. *Science* **231,** 365–368.

Kimmel, C. B., and Warga, R. M. (1987). Indeterminate cell lineage of the zebrafish embryo. *Dev. Biol.* **124,** 269–280.

Kimmel, C. B., Kane, D. A., Walker, C., Warga, R. M., and Rothman, M. B. (1989). A mutation that changes cell movement and cell fate in the zebrafish embryo. *Nature (London)* **337,** 358–362.

Kimmel, C. B., Warga, R. M., and Schilling, T. F. (1990). Origin and organization of the zebrafish fate map. *Development* **108,** 581–594.

Kimmel, C. B., and Westerfield, M. (1990). Primary neurons of the zebrafish. *In* "Signals and Sense: Local and Global Order in Perceptual Maps" (G. M. Edelman, W. E. Gall, and W. M. Cowan, eds.), pp. 561–588. New York: John Wiley & Sons.

Kuwada, J. Y. (1986). Cell recognition by neuronal growth cones in a simple vertebrate embryo. *Science* **233,** 740–746.

Kuwada, J. Y., and Goodman, C. S. (1985). Neuronal determination during embryonic development of the grasshopper nervous system. *Dev. Biol.* **110,** 114–126.

Kuwada, J. Y., Bernhardt, R. R., and Chitnis, A. B. (1990). Pathfinding by identified growth cone in the spinal cord of zebrafish embryos. *J. Neurosci.* **10,** 1299–1308.

Lance-Jones, C., and Landmesser, L. (1981). Pathway selection by embryonic chick motoneurons in an experimentally altered environment. *Proc. R. Soc. Lond. B.* **214,** 19–52.

Leber, S. M., Breedlove, S. M., and Sanes, J. R. (1990). Lineage, arrangement, and death of clonally related motoneurons in chick spinal cord. *J. Neurosci.* **10,** 2451–2462.

Lewis, J., Chevallier, A., Kieny, M., and Wolpert, L. (1981). Muscle nerve branches do not develop in chick wings devoid of muscle. *J. Embryol. Exp. Morphol.* **64,** 211–232.

Liu, D. W., and Westerfield, M. (1990). The formation of terminal fields in the absence of competitive interactions among primary motoneurons in the zebrafish. *J. Neurosci.* **10,** 3947–3959.

Luskin, M. B., Pearlman, A. L., and Sanes, J. R. (1988). Cell lineage in the cerebral cortex of the mouse studied *in vivo* and *in vitro* with a recombinant retrovirus. *Neuron* **1,** 635–647.

Macagno, E. R., and Stewart, R. R. (1987). Cell death during gangliogenesis in the leech: Competition leading to the death of PMS neurons has both random and nonrandom components. *J. Neurosci.* **7,** 1911–1918.

Martindale, M. Q., and Shandland, M. (1990). Neuronal competition determines the spatial pattern of neuropeptide expression by identified neurons of the leech. *Dev. Biol.* **139,** 210–226.

Mendelson, B. (1986). Development of reticulospinal neurons of the zebrafish. I. Time of origin. *J. Comp. Neurol.* **251,** 160–171.

Metcalfe, W. K., Mendelson, B., and Kimmel, C. B. (1986). Segmental homologies among reticulospinal neurons in the hindbrain of the zebrafish larva. *J. Comp. Neurol.* **251,** 147–159.

Molven, A., Wright, C. V. E., BreMiller, R., De Robertis, E. M., and Kimmel, C. B. (1990). Expression of a homeobox gene product in normal and mutant zebrafish embryos: Evolution of the tetrapod body plan. *Development* **109,** 279–288.

Myers, P. Z. (1985). Spinal motoneurons of the larval zebrafish. *J. Comp. Neurol.* **236,** 555–561.

Myers, P. Z., Eisen, J. S., and Westerfield, M. (1986). Development and axonal outgrowth of identified motoneurons in the zebrafish. *J. Neurosci.* **6,** 2278–2289.

Patterson, P. H. (1988). On the importance of being inhibited, or saying no to growth cones. *Neuron* **1,** 263–267.

Pike, S. H., Brandenburg, E. F., and Eisen, J. S. (1989). Extension of motoneuronal growth cones is disrupted by the absence of pre-existing axonal pathways. *Soc. Neurosci. Abstr.* **15,** 1262.

Pike, S. H., and Eisen, J. S. (1990). Interactions between identified motoneurons in embryonic zebrafish are not required for normal motoneuron development. *J. Neurosci.* **10,** 44–49.

Price, J., and Thurlow, L. (1988). Cell lineage in the rat cerebral cortex: a study using retroviral-mediated gene transfer. *Development* **104**, 473–482.

Purves, D., and Lichtman, J. W. (1985). "Principles of Neural Development." Sunderland, Massachusetts: Sinauer Assoc.

Rogers, S. L., Letourneau, P. C., Palm, S. L., McCarthy, J., and Furcht, L. T. (1983). Neurite extension by peripheral and central nervous system neurons in response to substratum-bound fibronectin and laminin. *Dev. Biol.* **98**, 212–220.

Schlenoff, D. H., and Model, P. G. (1985). The amphibian Mauthner cell is determined during very early neurulation. *Soc. Neurosci. Abstr.* **11**, 1062.

Stefanelli, A. (1951). The Mauthnerian apparatus in the ichthyopsida; Its nature and function and correlated problems of neurohistogenesis. *Q. Rev. Biol.* **26**, 17–34.

Streisinger, G., Walker, C., Dower, N., Knauber, D., and Singer, F. (1981). Production of clones of homozygous diploid zebra fish (*Brachydanio rerio*). *Nature (London)* **291**, 293–296.

Sulston, J. E., Schierenberg, E., White, J. G., and Thomas, J. N. (1983). The embryonic lineages of the nematode *Caenorhabditis elegans. Dev. Biol.* **100**, 64–119.

Tosney, K. W. (1987). Proximal tissues and patterned neurite outgrowth at the lumbosacral level of the chick embryo: Deletion of the dermamyotome. *Dev. Biol.* **122**, 540–558.

Trevarrow, B., Marks, D. L., and Kimmel, C. B. (1990). Organization of hindbrain segments in the zebrafish embryo. *Neuron* **4**, 669–679.

Turner, D. L., and Cepko, C. L. (1987). A common progenitor for neurons and glia persists in rat retina late in development. *Nature (London)* **328**, 131–136.

Walsh, C., and Cepko, C. L. (1988). Clonally related cortical cells show several migration patterns. *Science* **241**, 1342–1346.

Walter, J., Allsopp, T. E., and Bonhoeffer, R. (1990). A common denominator of growth cone guidance and collapse? *Trends Neurosci.* **13**, 447–452.

Weisblat, D. A., Kim, S. Y., and Stent, G. S. (1984). Embryonic origins of cells in the leech *Helobdella triserialis. Dev. Biol.* **104**, 65–85.

Westerfield, M., and Eisen, J. S. (1985). The growth of primary motor axons in *Xenopus* embryos. *Dev. Biol.* **109**, 96–101.

Westerfield, M., McMurray, J., and Eisen, J. S. (1986). Identified motoneurons and their innervation of axial muscles in the zebrafish. *J. Neurosci.* **6**, 2267–2277.

Westerfield, M., Kimmel, C. B., Walker, C., and Liu, D. W. (1990). Pathfinding and synapse formation in a zebrafish mutant lacking acetylcholine receptors. *Neuron* **4**, 867–874.

Wetts, R., and Fraser, S. E. (1988). Multipotent precursors can give rise to all major cell types of the frog retina. *Science* **239**, 1142–1145.

Wilkinson, D. G., Bhatt, S., Cook, M., Boncinelli, E., and Krumlauf, R. (1989). Segmental expression of Hox-2 homeobox-containing genes in the developing mouse hindbrain. *Nature* **341**, 405–409.

Wilson, S. W., Ross, L. S., Parrett, T., and Easter, S. S., Jr. (1990). The development of a simple scaffold of axon tracts in the brain of the embryonic zebrafish, *Brachydanio rerio. Development* **108**, 121–145.

Cellular and Molecular Mechanisms Determining Neurotransmitter Phenotypes in Sympathetic Neurons

Story C. Landis
Department of Neurosciences
Case Western Reserve University
School of Medicine
Cleveland, Ohio

I. Introduction

During development, neurons make many important decisions that define their phenotype. These decisions are the consequences of a complex interplay between the lineage history of particular neurons and a variety of environmental factors. Clearly, the normal function of the mature nervous system depends on the appropriateness of the decisions. One such decision is which neurotransmitter(s) to use. Although numerous descriptions exist of the developmental onset of transmitter properties in particular

DETERMINANTS OF NEURONAL IDENTITY

497

neuron populations, the cellular and molecular mechanisms that determine neurotransmitter phenotype remain largely unexplored. This may reflect, in part, an implicit assumption that the developmental mechanisms that are responsible for determining neuron class will specify a transmitter function as well. Many examples, however, now exist of diversity of transmitter and neuropeptide expression in a single class of neuron. For example, although most sympathetic neurons synthesize and release norepinephrine, a minority uses acetylcholine. Further, in addition to a small molecule or classical transmitter, many sympathetic neurons contain one or more neuropeptides. One striking exception to the general lack of information concerning neurotransmitter specification is our understanding of the regulation of transmitter choice by sympathetic neurons. This chapter summarizes present knowledge of the developmental mechanisms that determine transmitter choice, focusing on the determination of cholinergic sympathetic neurons.

II. Neurotransmitter Phenotypes of Sympathetic Neurons

By far the greatest proportion of principal sympathetic neurons in paravertebral ganglia is noradrenergic. Most investigators estimate that they account for over 95% of the neurons in the paravertebral ganglia and they innervate a host of autonomic targets. A small proportion of principal neurons is cholinergic. Evidence for their existence has come primarily from the identification and characterization of sympathetic postganglionic projections that exhibit cholinergic, rather than adrenergic, pharmacology. Two such systems have been identified. One of these, the innervation of eccrine sweat glands, has been well characterized. A second system, incompletely characterized, is responsible for sympathetic vasodilation in the limb of carnivores (Uvnas, 1966), but does not appear to exist in rodents (Yardley and Hilton, 1987). Histochemical and biochemical, as well as pharmacological, evidence exists for the presence of cholinergic neurons in sympathetic ganglia. Histochemical studies have disclosed a small number of sympathetic neurons that do not contain detectable levels of catecholamines (see, for example, Hamberger *et al.*, 1963; Yamauchi and Lever, 1971; Yamauchi *et al.*, 1973). Single neurons dissected from lumbar ganglia have been found to contain high levels of choline acetyltransferase (ChAT) activity (Buckley *et al.*, 1967), suggesting that the neurons that are not catecholaminergic are cholinergic.

It is now clear that sympathetic neurons, like many of other classes of neurons, contain one or more neuropeptides in addition to either acetylcholine or norepinephrine. Although the roles that neuropeptides play in neurotransmission have not been defined in many instances, the general assumption is that they act as co-transmitters or neuromodulators (Hokfelt *et al.*, 1980; Lundberg *et al.*, 1980, 1982b; Lundberg and Hokfelt, 1986). Many noradrenergic sympathetic neurons in the paravertebral ganglia contain neuropeptide Y (NPY); estimates range from 50% in the rat to 65% in the cat (Lundberg *et al.*, 1982a,b, 1983; Jarvi *et al.*, 1986). Similarly, many noradrenergic neurons contain immunoreactivity (IR) for galanin (Lindh *et al.*, 1989); a subset of the galanin neurons, however, lack NPY. In guinea pig, somatostatin-like immunoreactivity is also present in a small proportion of noradrenergic neurons (Hokfelt *et al.*, 1977), as is Leu-enkephalin (Schultzberg *et al.*, 1979; P. Henion and S. Landis, unpublished observations). The extent to which NPY, somatostatin, and Leu-enkephalin are colocalized is unclear. Immunoreactivity for vasoactive intestinal peptide (VIP) is normally present in neurons that are not noradrenergic and therefore are presumed to be cholinergic (Lundberg *et al.*, 1979, 1980, 1982a; Lindh *et al.*, 1989). A subset of the VIP-immunoreactive neurons in rat and cat contains immunoreactivity to calcitonin-gene-related peptide (CGRP; Landis and Fredieu, 1986; Lindh *et al.*, 1989). Although there appear to be similarities in the general principles that govern peptide expression in sympathetic neurons of different species, it is evident that there are differences. For example, substance P (SP) is colocalized with CGRP and VIP in some neurons in the cat but not in the rat (Landis and Fredieu, 1986; Lindh *et al.*, 1989). The extent to which there are interspecies differences among cat, rat, and guinea pig must still be defined.

The notion that has emerged from mapping studies of neuropeptides is that their distribution reflects chemical coding of functional pathways (Lundberg *et al.*, 1982; Morris and Gibbins, 1989). There are a number of correlations between the presence of a neuropeptide and innervation of particular target tissues. For example, NPY is present in the sympathetic innervation of the vasculature, the iris, the pineal gland, and the heart, but is absent from the innervation of glandular parenchyma (Lundberg *et al.*, 1982; Lindh *et al.*, 1989). Similarly, neurons that contain VIP and CGRP project to sweat glands (Lundberg *et al.*, 1979, 1982a; Landis and Fredieu, 1986; Landis *et al.*, 1988; Lindh *et al.*, 1989). The developmental mechanisms that give rise to this specificity have not been explored yet in detail.

III. A System for Studying Cholinergic Sympathetic Neurons: Sweat Gland Innervation

When we began our studies, the best-characterized cholinergic sympathetic neurons were those that innervate eccrine sweat glands in the footpads of the cat. In the 1890s, Langley described a sympathetic outflow from the stellate and lower lumbar ganglia to the front and hind footpads that caused sweat secretion (Langley, 1891, 1894; Patton, 1948). A surprising finding was that this response was cholinergic and not adrenergic in its pharmacology; muscarinic agonists elicited sweating and adrenergic did not, whereas muscarinic antagonists blocked nerve-stimulation-induced sweating and adrenergic antagonists did not (Langley, 1922; Foster and Weiner, 1970). Further evidence for the secretion of acetylcholine from these sympathetic fibers was obtained when the presence of acetylcholine was demonstrated in the venous effluent from footpads following nerve stimulation (Dale and Feldberg, 1934). The terminals around the sweat glands stain strongly for acetylcholinesterase (AChE) (Sjoqvist, 1963; Lundberg *et al.*, 1980) and some neurons present in the stellate and 6th lumbar ganglia, which provide innervation to the sweat glands in the front and hind feet, are intensely AChE-positive (Sjoqvist, 1963; Lundberg *et al.*, 1979). Lundberg and colleagues have demonstrated that sweat gland innervation in the cat contains VIP, CGRP, and SP (Lundberg *et al.*, 1979; Lindh *et al.*, 1989) and suggested that, in this system, acetylcholine stimulates sweat secretion and the neuropeptides serve to increase local blood flow. In cats and other laboratory animals, sweat secretion does not appear to serve a thermoregulatory function since it can be elicited most effectively by mechanical rather than thermal stimuli; instead, sweating has been hypothesized to keep the hairless skin maximally flexible and sensitive (Janig *et al.*, 1983).

Rats, like cats, have sweat glands concentrated in the pads of their feet (Ring and Randall, 1947). In the adult rat, the hind footpads contain 30–40 individual glands. Each gland contains a single tightly coiled secretory tubule connected to the surface by a duct, a capillary network, fat cells, and mast cells. Secretory and myoepithelial cells constitute tubule wall. Their basal surfaces contact a thick basement membrane that is surrounded by an incomplete sheath of fibrocytes. A plexus of intensely AChE-positive fibers enmeshes the secretory tubule. Ultrastructural examination of the innervation reveals bundles of 8–12 axons, partially ensheathed by Schwann cells and equidistant from the coiled secretory tubule and the capillaries (Landis and Keefe, 1983). The axonal varicosities contain small clear synaptic vesicles and larger dense-core vesicles, and lack membrane specializations. Thus, like certain other autonomic junctions, the axons are separated from the target secretory and myoepithelial cells by an intervening basement membrane as well as by fibrocyte processes.

Several lines of evidence indicate that sweat gland innervation is cholinergic and sympathetic in the rat as well as in the cat. Transmission is functionally cholinergic; sweating evoked by nerve stimulation is blocked by local injections of atropine, a muscarinic antagonist, and treatment with cholinergic agonists elicits sweat secretion (Hayashi and Nakagawa, 1963; Stevens and

Landis 1987). Recent studies to characterize the muscarinic receptors present on the sweat glands have demonstrated that they are the M_2 glandular pharmacological subtype and the m3 molecular subtype (Grant *et al.*, 1991). Homogenates of footpad tissue contain high levels of ChAT activity, gland-containing tissue pieces synthesize acetylcholine from choline and store it, and ChAT immunoreactivity is present in nerve terminals in the glands (Leblanc and Landis, 1986). Finally, no catecholamines are detectable in the sweat gland innervation of adult rats following glyoxylic acid fluorescence or permanganate fixation and ultrastructural examination. In contrast, the sympathetic innervation of arterioles and arteries in the connective tissue trabeculae between the glands, or deep in the pads, contains catecholamine fluorescence and small granular vesicles (SGV) following permanganate fixation.

The sweat gland innervation also contains immunoreactivity for several neuropeptides. VIP- and peptide HI (PHI)-containing fibers are coextensive with the terminal plexus revealed by a monoclonal antibody that recognizes a synaptic vesicle antigen (Yodlowski *et al.*, 1984; Landis *et al.*, 1988). The coexpression of VIP and PHI is not surprising, since they are produced from a common precursor (Itoh *et al.*, 1983; Nishizawa *et al.*, 1985). In addition, the sweat gland innervation contains immunoreactivity for CGRP (Landis and Fredieu, 1986), a neuropeptide previously described in cholinergic motoneurons as well as in sensory neurons (Rosenfeld *et al.*, 1983; Lee *et al.*, 1985; Takami *et al.*, 1985). Unlike in the cat, however, substance P is not evident. Since sweat secretion is blocked by atropine (Stevens and Landis, 1987), the role of the neuropeptides in rat sweat gland function is unclear.

Retrograde tracing studies provide evidence that the innervation of rat sweat glands is sympathetic in origin. Following injection of fluorescent tracers into front and hind footpads, labeled neurons are present in the stellate and lower lumbar paravertebral sympathetic ganglia, respectively (R. Siegel and S. Landis, unpublished observations). Since many of the retrogradely labeled neurons display VIP-IR, which in the footpads is restricted to sweat gland innervation, these double-labeled cells give rise to the sweat gland innervation. The retrogradely labeled neurons exhibit a distinctive pattern of peptide immunoreactivity; both VIP-IR and CGRP-IR are distributed in the perinuclear Golgi region.

IV. Developmental History of Sympathetic Neurons

The neural crest cells that will give rise to sympathetic neurons receive an adrenergic signal from their environment early in development. The nature of this signal appears to involve interactions between the migrating crest cells and tissues along their migratory pathway or at the site of ganglion formation, particularly somitic mesenchyme, ventral neural tube, and notochord (Cohen, 1972; Norr, 1973; Teillet *et al.*, 1978; Howard and Bronner-Fraser, 1985, 1986). Sympathetic precursors do not express noradrenergic properties until after they aggregate at the site of the future ganglia. In rat and mouse, catecholamine fluorescence as well as catecholamine synthetic enzymes become detectable in the sympathetic neuroblasts as they coalesce into ganglia (DeChamplain *et al.*, 1970; Cochard *et al.*, 1979; Teitelman *et al.*, 1979). Before sympathetic precursors undergo a final mitosis to become neurons, they have acquired a number of neuronal properties including tyrosine hydroxylase (TH) and neurofilament immunoreactivities, catecholamine fluorescence, and neuronal surface markers (Rothman *et al.*, 1978, 1980; Anderson and Axel, 1986; Rohrer and Thoenen, 1987). The early acquisition of neuronal traits by sympathoblasts contrasts with the expression of neuronal phenotype by other derivatives of the neural crest only after a terminal mitosis (Rohrer and Thoenen, 1987). The developmental mechanisms responsible for the early neuronal differentiation of sympathetic precursors and the consequences of such early differentiation for subsequent development must still be defined. As sympathetic neurons are born, they extend axons and dendrites and become innervated by preganglionic fibers (Rubin, 1985a,b,c). At birth in the rat, virtually all sympathetic neurons are generated and exhibit catecholamine histofluorescence (Eranko, 1972; Hendry, 1977). In contrast to our detailed knowledge of the development of catecholaminergic properties in mammalian sympathetic neurons, relatively little is known about the onset of neuropeptidergic properties and their regulation.

A. Sweat Gland Innervation Changes Its Transmitter Properties

The sweat glands and their sympathetic innervation develop in concert postnatally in the rat (Landis and Keefe, 1983). At birth, numerous invaginations are evident in the epidermis of the hind footpads. During the first 10 days, these extend to form long straight tubules. At 10 days, the tubules begin to coil and connective tissue elements encapsulate the developing glands. By 2 wk, many glands possess differentiated myoepithelial and secretory cells. At 21 days, the glands appear morphologically mature and many secrete in response to nerve stimulation (Stevens and Landis, 1987). Axons, visualized using a monoclonal antibody that recognizes a synaptic vesicle antigen, first become associated with the developing sweat glands at 4 days postnatal. As the gland primordia enlarge and mature, the associated axonal plexus increases. It is of interest that one of the first signs of differentiation in the developing glands is the appearance of mRNA for muscarinic receptors and ligand binding sites (Grant and Landis, 1991). Since these receptors appear in the absence of sympathetic innervation, it appears that their expression is not regulated by neuron–target interactions.

The neurotransmitter properties initially expressed by the developing sweat gland innervation are strikingly different from those expressed by the mature innervation (Fig. 1; Landis and Keefe, 1983; Leblanc and Landis, 1986; Stevens and Landis, 1987; Landis *et al.*, 1988). When axons first contact the developing glands during early postnatal development, they exhibit only catecholaminergic markers. These include intense catecholamine histofluorescence, immunoreactivity for the catecholamine synthetic enzymes TH and dopamine β-hydroxylase (DBH), and small granular vesicles after permanganate fixation. In contrast, mature cholinergic and peptidergic markers are undetectable: ChAT activity, AChE, and VIP and CGRP immunoreactivities are absent (Landis and Keefe, 1983; Leblanc and Landis, 1986; Landis *et al.*, 1988). It is of interest that we did not find any evidence in the developing innervation for the expression of the several neuropeptides that have been colocalized with catecholaminergic properties in sympathetic neurons; NPY, somatostatin, SP, and Leu- and Met-enkephalin were not detectable at any age.

The neurotransmitter properties that characterize the mature innervation appear during the second and third postnatal weeks. AChE staining is first detectable between 7 and 10 days, VIP-IR at 10 days, and ChAT activity at postnatal day 11. Sweat secretion in response to nerve stimulation is first evident in a small proportion of glands at 14 days and, as in the adult, is muscarinic cholinergic in pharmacology (Stevens and Landis, 1987). CGRP-IR, the last property to appear, becomes detectable between days 14 and 21. The relatively close correspondence in the appearance of ChAT, AChE, and VIP raises the possibility that these properties are coordinately regulated during development. CGRP, however, may be independently regulated. It is important to point out that in these studies, however, the appearance of the several markers has been assayed only in the axonal plexus, which may not reflect the onset of expression in the cell body. Clarification of this issue will require developmental studies of the cell bodies of origin of the gland innervation. As the gland innervation acquires cholinergic and peptidergic markers, detectable stores of catecholamines disappear and immunoreactivity for the catecholamine synthetic enzymes TH and DBH decreases.

Several lines of evidence indicate that the changes in transmitter properties observed in the development of sweat gland innervation take place in a single population of fibers rather than as the loss of an early-arriving noradrenergic population and its replacement by a late-arriving population of cholinergic fibers. First, ultrastructural studies of the developing innervation, after fixation with potassium permanganate to localize vesicular stores of norepinephrine, provide evidence for the presence of a single population of axons

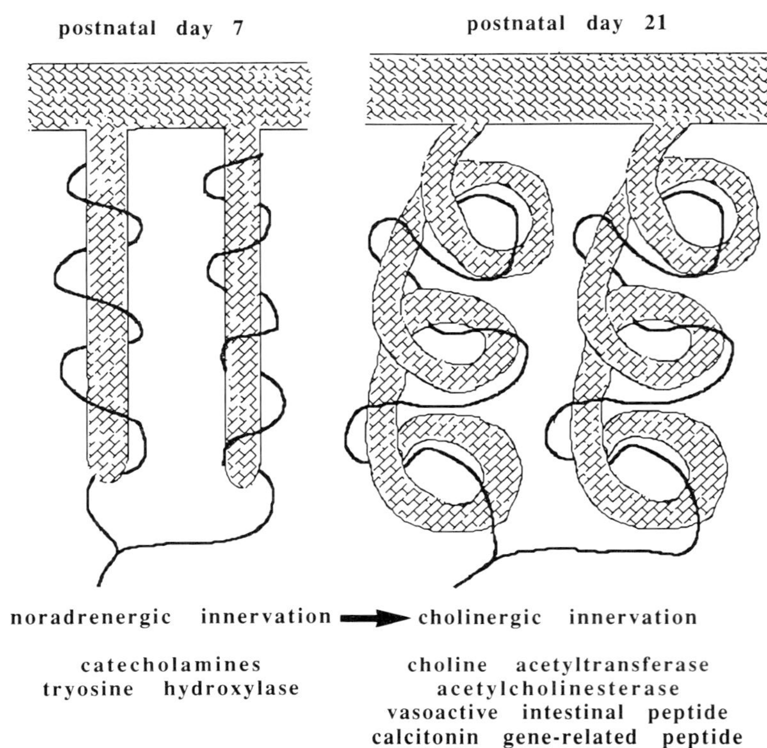

Figure 1. During normal postnatal development, the sweat glands and their sympathetic innervation undergo major morphogenetic and neurochemical changes. At postnatal day 7, the presumptive glands consist of epidermal invaginations which have not yet begun to coil, and which do not contain either secretory or myoepithelial cells. The sympathetic axons that are associated with the developing glands at this age contain catecholamines and immunoreactivity for their synthetic enzymes. By postnatal day 21, the glands have grown extensively, formed secretory coils and contain both secretory and myoepithelial cells. During this same period, the innervation has changed from noradrenergic to cholinergic and peptidergic; catecholamine fluorescence disappears while cholinergic and peptidergic markers appear.

whose cytochemical properties change with time (Landis and Keefe, 1983). There was no evidence for two populations of terminals, one of which was noradrenergic and contained many SGVs and the other of which was cholinergic and contained only clear synaptic vesicles. A second line of evidence comes from examination of the mature innervation for the expression of noradrenergic properties. If the sweat gland innervation is initially noradrenergic and becomes cholinergic, then the mature and functionally cholinergic innervation might continue to express catecholaminergic properties. We found that the innervation does, in fact, possess low but detectable levels of immunoreactivity for TH and DBH (Landis *et al.*, 1988). In addition, the high-affinity catecholamine uptake system is present; incubation of sweat-gland-containing tissue pieces with exogenous catecholamine reveals a catecholamine histofluorescent plexus (Landis and Keefe, 1983). These several catecholaminergic properties appear to be expressed at significantly lower levels in the mature innervation than in the developing innervation or the noradrenergic sympathetic innervation of adjacent blood vessels. It is obvious that the weight that can be attached to this argument is related to the extent to which the expression of catecholaminergic properties is restricted to functionally noradrenergic neurons. Although there are a number of instances in which immunoreactivity for one or both catecholamine synthetic enzymes is evident in nonadrenergic neurons (Grzanna and Coyle, 1978; Landis *et al.*, 1987; Baetge *et al.*, 1990), this is the only example to date in which all three properties are present.

A final line of evidence comes from studies using 6-hydroxydopamine (6-OHDA) and guanethidine. These adrenergic neurotoxins are taken up selectively by catecholaminergic neurons and, when administered to neonatal rats, cause the destruction of peripheral noradrenergic cell bodies and nerve terminals (Eranko and Eranko, 1971; Finch *et al.*, 1973). In using the adrenergic neurotoxins, we reasoned that if the developing sweat gland innervation was initially noradrenergic and became cholinergic, then treatment of newborn rats with 6-OHDA or guanethidine would eliminate the sweat gland innervation whereas treatment of adults should not (Yodlowski *et al.*, 1984). If, however, the glands were innervated by two populations of axons, an adrenergic one that was later lost and a cholinergic one that was retained, then neither neonatal nor adult treatment with 6-OHDA or guanethidine should eliminate the sweat gland fibers. Following treatment of neonatal rats with either 6-OHDA or guanethidine, no AChE, VIP-IR, ChAT, or characteristic sympathetic varicosities are present in the glands. In contrast, treatment of adult rats with the identical dose of 6-OHDA had no effect on AChE, VIP, or ultrastructure of the sweat gland innervation whereas noradrenergic sympathetic fibers disappeared from the iris, salivary glands, and blood vessels in the footpads. These results indicate that the mature cholinergic and peptidergic innervation is derived from the initial catecholaminergic innervation. It is of interest that the sweat glands that had been sympathetically denervated did not remain uninnervated. Sensory fibers containing SP and/or CGRP and possessing a characteristic ultrastructure grew into and formed a plexus in the sweat glands. They did not, however, acquire any of the neurotransmitter-related properties that characterize the mature sympathetic innervation.

It seemed likely that the elimination of the developing sweat gland innervation by 6-OHDA was a consequence of nerve growth factor (NGF) deprivation. We examined directly the question of whether the cholinergic sympathetic neurons that innervate sweat glands, like their noradrenergic counterparts that innervate other peripheral tissues, require NGF during development (Landis *et al.*, 1985). Neonatal rats were treated with an antiserum generated against NGF and their sweat glands were examined 3 wk later. We found that AChE and VIP were absent. Further, when the glands were examined with the electron microscope, no axons or nerve terminals, sympathetic or sensory in morphology, were evident. The failure of sensory sprouting in the anti-NGF-treated animals indicates that the neurons that grew into the sympathetically denervated sweat glands are NGF-responsive and suggests that NGF produced by the target may have been responsible for their ingrowth following chemical sympathectomy. These observations indicate that the elaboration of the sweat gland plexus is NGF dependent and suggest that at least one population of cholinergic sympathetic neurons is NGF dependent. Since, during development, these neurons closely resemble noradrenergic sympathetic neurons, it is perhaps not surprising that they require NGF.

It will be of interest to determine whether this developmental history is common to all cholinergic sympathetic neurons. Although at present no other cholinergic sympathetic systems have been identified in the rat, the presence of catecholamine-negative and ChAT-immunoreactive neurons in sympathetic ganglia that do not innervate footpads makes it clear that other cholinergic sympathetic neurons exist. Evidence consistent with a similar switch in a second cholinergic system has been obtained in developing piglets. Swine, like cats and dogs (Uvnas, 1966), have a well-characterized cholinergic sympathetic vasodilation of femoral circulation. When the development of this system is examined, noradrenergically mediated vasoconstriction is evident early in postnatal development but cholinergic vasodilation is not apparent until approximately 1 mo, despite the early appearance of muscarinic receptors in the vasculature (Buckley *et al.*, 1981). The late onset of cholinergic function is most easily explained if the neurons responsible are initially noradrenergic.

B. Target Dependence of Changes in Neurotransmitter Phenotype

Although in principle the alterations in neurotransmitter-related properties that occur in the sweat gland innervation could be intrinsically determined, the studies of sympathetic neurons developing in cell culture that will be described next suggest that environmental cues specify transmitter properties in this system. In addition to the neurotransmitter repertoire that these sympathetic neurons express, the sweat gland neurons are distinguished by their target. Thus, the sweat glands themselves present a reasonable source for a transmitter specifying signal. In an initial series of experiments, the normal developmental interaction between the glands and the neurons that innervate them was disrupted by a single dose of 6-OHDA on postnatal day 2 (Stevens and Landis, 1988). As a consequence, the arrival of the innervation in the target tissue was delayed (most likely because of chemical axotomy by the adrenergic neurotoxin), as was the normal decline in endogenous catecholamines and the appearance of cholinergic function. These findings are consistent with a target role but do not provide direct evidence.

In a second series of experiments, neonatal superior cervical ganglia (SCG) were transplanted to the anterior chamber of the eye with either sweat glands (a cholinergic sympathetic target) or pineal gland (an adrenergic sympathetic target) (Stevens and Landis, 1990). After 4 wk, the neurons were examined for the target-appropriate expression of transmitter systems. In the SCG/sweat gland co-transplants, the surviving neurons lost catecholamine fluorescence and consistently acquired ChAT-IR. In contrast, surviving neurons in the SCG/pineal co-transplants maintained catecholamine fluorescence and inconsistently acquired ChAT-IR. Most interesting was the finding that peptide expression was also target-appropriate; many neurons co-transplanted with sweat glands contained VIP whereas neurons co-transplanted with pineal gland contained NPY, the peptide normally present in the sympathetic innervation of the pineal gland (Schon *et al.*, 1985). Since virtually no SCG neurons contained NPY whereas many SCG neurons contained NPY-IR at the time that the transplantation was done, the co-transplanted sweat glands appear to have suppressed NPY expression and induced VIP. Thus, in these experiments, several aspects of neuronal phenotype, catecholamine fluorescence and neuropeptide immunoreactivity, were expressed in a target-appropriate fashion. Because only a small number of neurons survived transplantation, the issue of selective survival complicates interpretation of these results. However, since developing cholinergic sympathetic neurons *in vivo* as well as *in vitro* are NGF-dependent (Landis *et al.*, 1985), it seems unlikely that the observed differences in transmitter phenotype result from the survival of subpopulations of neurons.

The role of sweat glands in inducing the observed change in neurotransmitter-related properties has been tested directly in two cross-innervation studies (Fig. 2). In the first series of experiments, we determined whether sweat glands are required to induce the changes normally observed in transmitter phenotype by replacing sweat gland primordia in early postnatal rats with parotid gland, a target that receives noradrenergic sympathetic innervation (Norberg and Olson, 1965; Hand, 1972). Since catecholaminergic properties appear in sympathetic precursors as the ganglia coalesce and, therefore, before target innervation (DeChamplain *et al.*, 1970; Cochard *et al.*, 1979), the parotid gland does not appear to instruct the neurons that innervate it to express a noradrenergic phenotype but promotes the maintenance and maturation of noradrenergic properties that have been previously induced. The innervation of the transplanted parotid gland retains intense catecholamine fluorescence and fails to develop ChAT activity. Thus, the presence of the sweat gland is required for the normal loss of catecholamines and induction of cholinergic function (Schotzinger and Landis, 1990a).

A second set of experiments was performed to determine whether sweat glands could induce changes in neurotransmitter phenotype in neurons that normally would not innervate them. We took advantage of the topographical segregation of cholinergic and noradrenergic sympathetic targets in rat skin. Hairy skin normally receives noradrenergic sympathetic innervation, particularly of piloerectors and blood vessels, but not cholinergic sympathetic innervation (Schotzinger and Landis, 1990b). In contrast, the sweat-gland-containing glabrous skin of the footpads receives cholinergic sympathetic innervation. By transplanting sweat-gland-containing skin to the lateral thorax of early postnatal inbred Lewis rats, we forced the sympathetic neurons that innervate noradrenergic targets in the hairy skin to innervate sweat glands instead. Since piloerectors and their innervation, like sweat glands, develop postnatally, these transplantation studies involved the *de novo* growth of sympathetic fibers rather than regeneration. Further, the transplanted glands are innervated by middle thoracic ganglia that do not normally provide innervation to sweat glands.

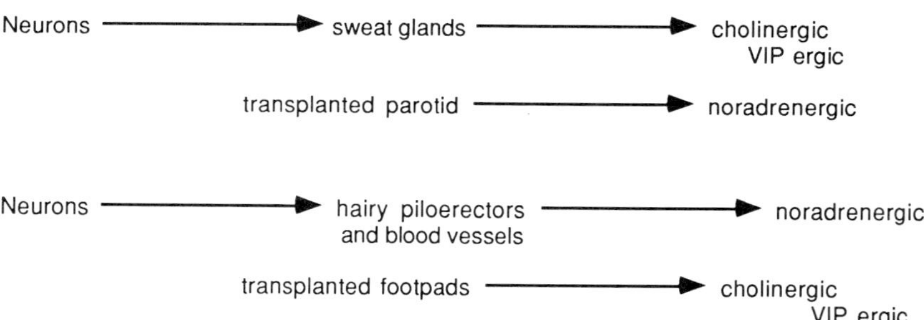

Figure 2. The results of several transplantation studies to examine the role of the target in inducing alterations in neurotransmitter phenotype are diagramed above. When neurons that ordinarily innervate sweat glands, a target of cholinergic sympathetic neurons, innervate parotid glands instead, they fail to develop their normal phenotype; catecholamines are maintained and cholinergic and peptidergic properties do not appear. In the converse experiment, when neurons that ordinarily innervate piloerectors and blood vessels in the hairy skin are induced to innervate sweat glands instead they lose their noradrenergic properties and acquire cholinergic and peptidergic function. These studies indicate that the target can retrogradely specify the neurotransmitter properties of the neurons which innervate it.

The innervation of the transplanted sweat glands exhibited neurotransmitter-related properties appropriate for the novel target rather than for normal hairy-skin targets (Schotzinger and Landis, 1988). Although catecholamine-containing fibers formed an intensely fluorescent plexus in the transplanted glands by 3 wk, at 6 wk only occasional faintly fluorescent fibers were present. AChE, ChAT activity, and VIP were initially absent but appeared in the innervation of the transplanted glands between 3 and 6 wk. These changes reflect a specific target influence, since replacing hairy skin with hairy skin does not elicit them. Treatment of the rats with 6-OHDA before transplantation to eliminate catecholaminergic sympathetic fibers prevents both the ingrowth of catecholaminergic fluorescent fibers and the development of ChAT, AChE, and VIP immunoreactivity. Thus, the observed changes occur in sympathetic fibers. It is of interest that, although in each of the experimental paradigms employed—delayed innervation, anterior chamber transplantation, and skin transplantation—all the sympathetic neurons lose catecholamines and acquire cholinergic function, only a subset appears to become immunoreactive for VIP. The reason for this difference is unclear.

In summary, these experiments provide compelling evidence for the role of targets in retrogradely specifying the neurotransmitter properties of the sympathetic neurons that innervate them. Not only the expression of traditional transmitters but the expression of neuropeptides is affected. Cross-innervation studies of neuropeptide expression in sensory neurons indicate that target regulation of transmitter phenotype may be a common strategy. Cutaneous nerves that normally contain SP-IR lost this property when forced to innervate muscle; conversely, when muscle afferents innervated skin, they acquired SP (McMahon and Gibson, 1987). Further, since these later studies were done in adult rats, they suggest that plasticity is not restricted to developing neurons. Such observations raise the possibility that at least some of the numerous instances in which restriction of neuropeptide expression to a subpopulation of peripheral neurons is correlated with innervation of a particular target arise because of retrograde specification from the target (Lundberg *et al.*, 1982a; Horn *et al.*, 1987; Morris and Gibbins, 1987; Leblanc and Landis, 1988).

V. Molecules That Specify Neurotransmitter Phenotype

Studies of sympathetic neurons developing in cell culture have provided an excellent system for the dissection of the cellular and molecular mechanisms that influence transmitter choice. When neurons are dissociated from the superior cervical ganglia of newborn rats, all of them initially synthesize and store catecholamines (Patterson and Chun, 1977; Landis, 1980). If the neurons are grown in the absence of other cell types (Patterson and Chun, 1977), particularly in defined medium or under chronically depolarizing conditions, the sympathetic neurons continue to differentiate noradrenergically (Walicke *et al.*, 1977; Iacovitti *et al.*, 1982; Wolinsky and Patterson, 1985; Raynaud *et al.*, 1987). However, if they are grown in the presence of certain types of nonneuronal cells or in medium conditioned by nonneuronal cells, the neurons acquire cholinergic function and decrease their expression of noradrenergic properties (Patterson and Chun, 1977; Swerts *et al.*, 1983; Wolinsky and Patterson, 1983; Raynaud *et al.*, 1987). In heart or skeletal muscle cells, the induction of cholinergic properties does not require direct contact but can occur through the release of a soluble cholinergic inducing activity into the medium. The effect of this conditioned medium or cholinergic differentiation factor (CDF) is blocked by growth under conditions that are thought to mimic neuronal activity, for example, elevated potassium (Walicke *et al.*, 1977). That the cholinergic factor produced by nonneuronal cells induces neurons that have already begun to differentiate along a noradrenergic pathway to become cholinergic has been demonstrated unequivocally in studies of neuron–heart microcultures in which the changing transmitter properties of single neurons were followed over time (Potter *et al.*, 1986).

Initially, studies of the mechanism of cholinergic induction in cultured sympathetic neurons focused on CDF, the cholinergic factor in heart-cell-conditioned medium. The purified factor is a relatively heat-stable 45 kDa glycoprotein with at least five glycosylation sites (Fukada, 1985). Removal of the carbohydrate yields a 22 kDa protein that retains biological activity. Antisera raised against a partial peptide sequence obtained for CDF immuno-precipitate both the 45 kDa protein and the cholinergic inducing activity (Yamamori *et al.*, 1989). Most recently, structural analysis and biological assays have shown that CDF is identical to leukemia inhibitory factor (LIF), a hematopoeitic factor that was characterized based on its ability to induce differentiation in a myeloid cell line (Yamamori *et al.*, 1989). It is of interest that this molecule influences differentiation decisions in both the nervous and immune systems.

It is now clear, however, that a number of more-or-less well-characterized environmental signals can induce cholinergic function in cultured sympathetic neurons. Ciliary neurotrophic factor (CNTF), first identified because it supports the survival of ciliary neurons in culture, induces ChAT and decreases TH activity in cultured rat sympathetic neurons (Saadat *et al.*, 1989). In addition, CNTF increases the number of VIP-IR (and presumably cholinergic) neurons and decreases the number of TH-immunoreactive neurons in cultures of chick sympathetic ganglia (Ernsberger *et al.*, 1989). Two membrane associated molecules that induce cholinergic function in cultured rat sympathetic neurons have recently been partially purified from spinal cord (Wong and Kessler, 1987; Adler *et al.*, 1989). Examination of the biological and immunological properties of the three best-characterized factors—CDF, CNTF, and MANS (membrane-associated neurotransmitter-stimulating factor; Wong and Kessler, 1987)—indicate that CDF is different from CNTF and MANS (Rao *et al.*, 1990), a conclusion confirmed by comparison of the recently published sequences for CDF (Yamamori *et al.*, 1989) and CNTF (Lin *et al.*, 1989; Stockli *et al.*, 1989). Having defined the presence of several factors that alter the transmitter phenotype of cultured sympathetic neurons, it will be important to determine the roles these proteins play in transmitter specification during normal development. The cholinergic sympathetic innervation of sweat glands described earlier provides an excellent system in which to address this question.

It is of interest to speculate why there might be several different molecules that cause cholinergic induction. One possibility is that the functional roles of the proteins are segregated in space or time. For example, each could influence the development of a distinct population of cholinergic neurons, including sympathetic and parasympathetic neurons in the periphery and motor and basal forebrain neurons in the central nervous system. Since CDF, CNTF, and MANS influence not only classical transmitter expression but also neuropeptide expression (see below; Wong and Kessler, 1987; Ernsberger *et al.*, 1989; Nawa and Sah, 1990a,b), they and other phenotype-specifying factors could also act on neurons in a combinatorial fashion to produce the exceedingly large variety of neurotransmitter and neuropeptide combinations found in the nervous system.

Although environmental factors influence the choice of traditional neurotransmitters by cultured sympathetic neurons, several studies have described effects on the expression of neuropeptides as well. For example, co-culture with ganglionic nonneuronal cells or with the membrane-associated cholinergic factors increases the expression of SP whereas culture under growth conditions that mimic activity decreases it (Kessler, 1985; Wong and Kessler, 1987; Adler *et al.*, 1989). Co-culture with nonneuronal cells from different autonomic targets or in medium conditioned by these tissues has differential effects on neuropeptide expression by sympathetic neurons (Kessler, 1984, 1985). Fractionation of heart-cell-conditioned medium has revealed the existence of several distinct peptidergic factors (Nawa and Sah, 1990b); CDF increases the expression of VIP, SP, and somatostatin but other factors specifically increase only VIP or somatostatin.

It is of interest to determine the molecular nature of the signal between the sweat glands and the neurons that innervate them. Since axons never come in direct cell contact with sweat glands but are always separated by a basal lamina (Landis and Keefe, 1983), it seems likely that a soluble factor is involved. We have found that soluble extracts of footpads contain cholinergic activity when tested on cultured sympathetic neurons (Rao and Landis, 1990). The extracted activity not only induces ChAT activity, but also induces VIP expression and reduces catecholamine synthesis and NPY. Thus, its effects on the cultured neurons mimic those of the footpad transplants *in vivo* and in the anterior chamber studies. The activity appears in the footpad as early as P5 and increases to adult levels by P21, parallelling the transmitter conversion observed in sweat gland innervation (Landis and Keefe, 1983; Leblanc and Landis, 1986; Landis *et al.*, 1988). This activity is not found in soluble extracts of liver, hairy skin, or parotid gland, consistent with the inability of the two latter tissues to induce the cholinergic conversion *in vivo* (Schotzinger and Landis, 1988; Schotzinger and Landis, 1990a).

The activity that can be extracted from footpads is a reasonable candidate for mediator of the target effects on transmitter choice. Studies are in progress to determine whether the activity corresponds to either CDF/LIF or CNTF. The size and charge of the footpad activity differ from those of CDF/LIF (M. Rao and S. Landis, unpublished observations). Further, anti-CDF/LIF antiserum does not precipitate the cholinergic activity from footpad extracts (Rao and Landis, 1990). Recent studies using a reverse transcriptase polymerase chain reaction (RT-PCR) method, however, have disclosed the presence of MRNA for CDF/LIF in the footpad, raising the possibility that CDF/LIF might be present as a minor component (Yamamori, 1991). The major footpad cholinergic activity and CNTF are quite similar in physical properties. The partially purified footpad factor contains ciliary neurotrophic activity, and an antiserum produced against recombinant CNTF can precipitate 80% of the cholinergic activity in footpad extracts, 50% of the VIP-inducing activity, and 20% of the NPY-suppressing activity (M. Rao and S. Landis, unpublished observations). No signal, however, is detected in immunoblots of footpads using two different anti-CNTF antisera that yield strong signals in immunoblots of sciatic nerve. Moreover, analysis of CNTF mRNA by Northern blots and *in situ* hybridization were negative for footpads and positive for sciatic nerve (M. Rao and S. Landis, unpublished observations). At this time, the best summary of these results appears to be that the major cholinergic activity in footpads resides in a CNTF-like protein. The minor cholinergic factor, accounting for the activity not precipitated by the anti-CNTF antibodies, could be a CDF/LIF-like protein. Further experiments are required to determine which component is required for the transmitter switch *in situ*.

VI. Transient Catecholaminergic Cells of the Gut Also Change Their Phenotype

The neurotransmitter plasticity displayed by the developing sweat gland innervation is not unique. Examination of the development of neurotransmitter properties has disclosed a number of examples of altered expression of transmitter synthetic enzymes and neuropeptides. Such findings suggest that qualitative as well as quantitative changes in transmitter expression may be common. The most thoroughly studied example is the population of transient catecholaminergic (TC) cells of the gut (Rothman *et al.*, 1978; Teillet *et al.*, 1978; Cochard *et al.*, 1979; Jonakait *et al.*, 1985). In the guts of embryonic but not postnatal rats, cells are present that express TH-IR, DBH-IR, and catecholamine histofluorescence. In addition to these noradrenergic properties, the TC cells of the gut express a number of neuronal markers (Baetge and Gershon, 1989; Baetge *et al.*, 1990). At least some of the TC cells represent neuronal precursor cells, since they take up tritiated thymidine (Teitelman *et al.*, 1981). It is now clear that these cells do not die but acquire a different transmitter phenotype. This has been established in a series of immunocytochemical studies that document the presence of markers in the TC cells, including DBH, the low affinity NGF receptor, and NPY, that are maintained by mature enteric neurons (Baetge *et al.*, 1990). Thus, the TC cells give rise to at least serotonin-, SP-, and VIP-containing neurons of the gut. In contrast to the specification of neurotransmitter phenotype in cholinergic sympathetic neurons and of neuropeptide phenotype in some sensory neurons, it seems likely that, in the case of the gut, the local environment rather than the target provides instructive cues.

VII. Effects of the Alteration in Transmitter Properties on Target Function

The development and maintenance of secretory responsiveness in sweat glands appear to depend on the presence of cholinergic innervation and, therefore, on the target-dependent induction of cholinergic function in the sweat gland innervation (Fig. 3). Functional transmission first becomes detectable at 14 days and, even in developing animals whose sweat gland innervation still contains catecholamines, nerve-evoked sweat secretion is mediated by acetylcholine (Stevens and Landis, 1987). It is of interest that the onset of nerve- and agonist-induced sweating lags behind the development of cholinergic properties in the sweat gland innervation and that glands that do not respond to nerve stimulation in developing rats are also unresponsive to agonists. These observations raise the possibility that secretory responsiveness of the gland cells is induced by acetylcholine released from the gland innervation. Consistent with this hypothesis is the finding that glands of adult animals sympathetically denervated at birth do not sweat in response to cholinergic agonists (Stevens and Landis, 1987). In addition, when the innervation of the sweat glands is delayed, the development of responsiveness to exogenous ligands is also delayed and linked temporally to the onset of secretion following nerve stimulation (Stevens and Landis, 1988). Finally, when glands are acutely denervated by sciatic nerve section, they become unresponsive to cholinergic agonists; thus, maintenance of secretory responsiveness is dependent on cholinergic innervation (Kennedy and Sakuta, 1984).

To determine whether acetylcholine itself regulates the development and maintenance of secretory function, we utilized three experimental paradigms (M. Grant and S. Landis, unpublished observations). First, we treated developing rat pups with atropine, a muscarinic antagonist from postnatal days 11–18, the period in which cholinergic function is first expressed in the developing innervation (Leblanc and Landis, 1986; Stevens and Landis, 1987). This resulted in a significant delay in the onset of secretory function; it was not until postnatal day 27 that secretion reached levels seen in control animals. In a second series of experiments, adult rats were treated with a similar dose of atropine for 7 days. This resulted in a striking loss of secretory function that persisted for 3 days; normal function was not restored for 1 wk. In contrast, several other cholinergic autonomic responses were fully restored within 24 hr of the cessation of atropine treatment. Finally, muscarinic stimulation was replaced by administration of pilocarpine in adult rats after cutting the sciatic nerve. In this case, the loss of gland function that normally follows denervation was almost entirely prevented. These results indicate that acetylcholine acting via a muscarinic receptor is directly responsible for promoting the development and maintenance of secretory function in this system. This seems most likely to be because of regulation of transcription of one or more genes required for secretion.

We have examined the expression of muscarinic ligand binding sites in sweat glands as a first step in determining how the innervation regulates secretory responsiveness in the target (Grant and Landis, 1991; Grant *et al.*, 1991). Ligand binding, competition, and autoradiographic studies reveal that mature innervated glands possess typical glandular receptors, the m3 molecular subtype. There is no correlation, however, between the presence of muscarinic binding sites and the ability of the glands to secrete in response to cholinergic agonists. During development, muscarinic binding sites appear well before secretory responsiveness and are expressed at nearly normal levels on both uninnervated and acutely denervated glands that are nonresponsive. Thus, the expression of muscarinic binding sites is intrinsically programmed in this target tissue. However, one of the several steps required to couple muscarinic ligand binding to sweat secretion is innervation dependent. Since receptors in both responsive and nonresponsive glands are coupled to phospholipase C and increased turnover of phophoinositide, regulation appears to occur at a step distal to signal transduction across the cell membrane, possibly at the level of channel expression or modulation of channel function.

VIII. Summary and Conclusions

Analysis of sympathetic neurons developing in cell culture demonstrated that noradrenergic neurons can be induced to become cholinergic under the influence of soluble factors released by nonneuronal cells. Similarly, the neurons that innervate developing sweat glands are noradrenergic at the time of innervation but, as the sweat glands and their innervation mature, both cholinergic and peptidergic properties appear. It will be of interest to determine whether this developmental history is common to all cholinergic sympathetic neurons. Although no other cholinergic sympathetic systems have been identified yet in the rat, the presence of catecholamine-negative and ChAT-IR neurons in sympathetic ganglia that do not provide innervation to footpads makes it clear that other cholinergic sympathetic neurons exist. The changes in neurotransmitter phenotype observed in the sweat gland innervation are retrogradely specified by interactions with the target tissue and are required for the final functional maturation of the sweat gland cells. Thus, complex developmental interactions can underlie the establishment of functional transmission in the autonomic nervous system.

The developmental strategy employed in this system, initial noradrenergic differentiation that is subsequently suppressed and the acquisition of a second set of cholinergic and peptidergic functions that are maintained, appears at first to be an unwieldy mechanism for the establishment of a functionally appropriate match between neurotransmitters used by a population of neurons and the target of those neurons. The explanation may lie in the early developmental history of sympathetic neurons described above. Sympathetic precursors acquire noradrenergic neurotransmitter properties early in development; as soon as neural crest cells aggregate to form sympathetic ganglia, noradrenergic properties are expressed (DeChamplain *et al.*, 1970; Cochard *et al.*, 1979; Teitelman *et al.*, 1979; Rothman *et al.*, 1980). Although most sympathetic neurons are noradrenergic in the mature animal, a minority population is cholinergic. This minority could, in principle, be generated either through the failure to induce adrenergic properties in the entire population of presumptive sympathetic neuroblasts or through the secondary induction of cholinergic properties in a subset of adrenergic neurons. Our studies of the development of cholinergic sympathetic neurons indicate that the second strategy is used. It is possible that this strategy is a common one; the commitment of a neuroblast to a particular class of neuron may involve the acquisition of a transmitter phenotype that represents a "default" state that is maintained in the absence of other cues. With environmental instruction, however, this "default" phenotype could be modulated through the induction of a different or additional classical transmitter or neuropeptide. Such instructive signals could come from target tissues, as is the case for cholinergic sympathetic neurons, from afferent innervation, or from the local glial or neuronal environment.

The finding that targets can retrogradely specify the transmitter phenotype of neurons that innervate them provides additional insight into the roles that neuronal targets can play in development. That targets can determine the final number of neurons surviving during development of the vertebrate nervous system is well established. In addition to the experiments summarized here, recent studies in several other systems demonstrate that targets not only decide neuron number but can also influence the phenotypic properties of the neurons that survive. For example, the size of sympathetic neuron cell bodies and the extent and branching of their dendritic arbors is influenced by the size of the target that they innervate during development (Purves *et al.*, 1988; Voyvodic, 1989). Peripheral targets of sensory neurons, cutaneous or muscle, may determine the nature and specificity of their central connections (Smith and Frank, 1987) or the neuropeptide that they contain (McMahon and Gibson, 1987). In the leech, the morphology and central connections of Retzius cells in the reproductive system differ from those of Retzius cells in other segments; this difference develops after target contact and is dependent on innervation of the reproductive organs (Macagno *et al.*, 1986; Jellies *et al.*, 1987; Loer *et al.*, 1987; Loer and Kristan, 1989). The notion of retrograde specification of neuronal properties is not a new one; nearly 50 years ago, Weiss argued that the specificity of central sensory connections had its origin in the periphery (Weiss, 1942). The application of modern experimental approaches to this question is likely to define exactly when and where this strategy is used in the developing nervous system and to elucidate the cellular and molecular mechanisms responsible for it.

Acknowledgments

The work summarized in this chapter was supported in part by NIH NS 23678 and HD 25681 and by the American Heart Association.

References

Adler, J. E., Schleifer, L. S., and Black, I. B. (1989). Partial purification and characterization of a membrane-derived factor regulating neurotransmitter phenotypic expression. *Proc. Natl. Acad. Sci.* **86,** 1080–1083.

Anderson, D. L., and Axel, R. (1986). A bipotential neuroendocrine precursor whose choice of cell fate is determined by NGF and glucocorticoids. *Cell* **47,** 1079–1090.

Baetge, G., and Gershon, M. D. (1989). Transient catecholaminergic (TC) cells in the vagus nerves and bowel of fetal mice: Relationship to the development of enteric neurons. *Dev. Biol.* **132,** 189–211.

Baetge, G., Pintar, J. E., and Gershon, M. D. (1990). Transiently catecholaminergic (TC) cells in the bowel of the fetal rat: Precursors of noncatecholaminergic enteric neurons. *Dev. Biol.* **141,** 353–380.

Buckley, G., Consolo, S., Giacobini, E., and Sjoqvist, F. (1967). Cholinacetylase in innervated and denervated sympathetic ganglia and ganglion cells of the cat. *Acta Physiol. Scand.* **71,** 348–357.

Buckley, N. M., Brazeau, P., Frazier, I. D., and Gootman, P. (1981). Femoral circulatory responses to lumbar nerve stimulation in developing swine. *Am. J. Physiol.* **240,** H505–511.

Cochard, P. M., Goldstein, M., and Black, I. B. (1979). Initial development of the noradrenergic phenotype in autonomic neuroblasts of the rat embryo *in vivo. Dev. Biol.* **71,** 100–114.

Cohen, A. M. (1972). Factors directing the expression of sympathetic nerve traits in cells of neural crest origin. *J. Exp. Zool.* **97,** 167–182.

Dale, H. H., and Feldberg, W. (1934). The chemical transmission of secretory impulses to the sweat glands of the cat. *J. Physiol. (London)* **82,** 121–134.

DeChamplain, J., Malmfors, T., Olson, L., and Sachs, C. (1970). Ontogenesis of peripheral adrenergic neurons in the rat: Pre- and postnatal observations. *Acta Physiol. Scand.* **80,** 276–288.

Eranko, L. (1972). Ultrastructure of the developing sympathetic nerve cell and the storage of catecholamines. *Brain Res.* **46,** 159–175.

Eranko, L., and Eranko, O. (1971). Effects of guanethidine on nerve cells and small intensely fluorescent cells in the sympathetic ganglia of newborn and adult rats. *Acta Pharmacol. Toxicol.* **30,** 403–412.

Ernsberger, U., Sendtner, M., and Rohrer, H. (1989). Proliferation and differentiation of embryonic chick sympathetic neurons: Effects of ciliary neurotrophic factor. *Neuron* **2,** 1275–1284.

Finch, L., Haeusler, G., and Thoenen, H. (1973). A comparison of the effects of chemical sympathectomy by 6-hydroxydopamine in newborn and adult rats. *Br. J. Pharmacol.* **47,** 249–260.

Foster, K. G., and Weiner, J. S. (1970). Effects of cholinergic and adrenergic blocking agents on the activity of eccrine sweat glands. *J. Physiol. (London)* **210**, 883–897.

Fukada, K. (1985). Purification and partial characterization of a cholinergic differentiation factor. *Proc. Natl. Acad. Sci. U.S.A.* **82**, 8795–8799.

Grant, M. P., and Landis, S. C. (1991). Developmental expression of muscarinic cholinergic receptors and coupling to phospholipase C in rat sweat glands is independent of innervation. *J. Neurosci.* **11** (in press).

Grant, M. P., Landis, S. C., and Siegel, R. E. (1991). The molecular and pharmacological properties of muscarinic cholinergic receptors expressed by rat sweat glands are unaltered by denervation. *J. Neurosci.* **11** (in press).

Grzanna, R., and Coyle, J. T. (1978). Dopamine-β-hydroxylase in rat submandibular ganglion cells which lack norepinephrine. *Brain Res.* **152**, 206–212.

Hamberger, B., Norberg, K.-A., and Sjoqvist, F. (1963). Correlated studies of monoamines and acetylcholinesterase in sympathetic ganglia, illustrating the distribution of adrenergic and cholinergic neurons. *2d Int. Pharmacol. Mtg.* 41–55.

Hand, A. R. (1972). Adrenergic and cholinergic nerve terminals in the rate parotid gland. Electron microscopic observations on permanganate-fixed glands. *Anat. Rec.* **173**, 131–140.

Hayashi, H., and Nakagawa, T. (1963). Functional activity of the sweat glands of the albino rat. *J. Invest. Dermatol.* **41**, 365–367.

Hendry, I. A. (1977). Cell division in the developing sympathetic nervous system. *J. Neurocytol.* **6**, 299–313.

Hokfelt, T., Elfvin, L. G., Elde, R., Schultzberg, M., Goldstein, M., and Luft, R. (1977). Occurrence of somatostatin-like immunoreactivity in some peripheral sympathetic noradrenergic neurons. *Proc. Natl. Acad. Sci. U.S.A.* **74**, 3587–92.

Hokfelt, T., Johansson, O., Ljungdahl, A., Lundberg, J. M., and Schultzberg, M. (1980). Peptidergic neurons. *Nature (London)* **284**, 515–521.

Horn, J. P., Stoffer, W. D., and Fatherazi, S. (1987). Neuropeptide Y-like immunoreactivity in bullfrog sympathetic ganglion is restricted to C cells. *J. Neurosci.* **7**, 1717–1727.

Howard, M. J., and Bronner-Fraser, M. (1985). The influence of neural tube-derived factors on the differentiation of neural crest cells *in vitro*. I. Histochemical study on the appearance of adrenergic cells. *J. Neurosci.* **5**, 3302–3309.

Howard, M. J., and Bronner-Fraser, M. (1986). Neural tube-derived factors influence differentiation of neural crest cells *in vitro*: Effects on activity of neurotransmitter biosynthetic enzymes. *Dev. Biol.* **117**, 45–54.

Iacovitti, L., Johnson, M. I., Joh, T. J., and Bunge, R. P. (1982). Biochemical and morphological characterization of sympathetic neurons grown in a chemically defined medium. *Neurosci.* **7**, 2225–2239.

Itoh, W., Obata, K., Yanaihara, N., and Okamoto, H. (1983). Human mepro-vasoactive intestinal polypeptide (VIP) mRNA contains the coding sequence for a novel PHI-27-like peptide, PHM-27. *Nature (London)* **304**, 547–549.

Janig, W., Sundlof, G., and Wallin, B. G. (1983). Discharge patterns of sympathetic neurons supplying skeletal muscle and skin in man and cat. *J. Auton. Nervous System* **7**, 239–248.

Jarvi, R., Helen, P., Pelto-Huikko, M., and Hervonen, A. (1986). Neuropeptide Y-like immunoreactivity in rat sympathetic neurons and small granule containing cells. *Neurosci. Lett.* **67**, 223–227.

Jellies, J., Loer, C. M., and Kristan, W. B. (1987). Morphological changes in leech Retzius neurons after target contact during embryogenesis. *J. Neurosci.* **7**, 2618–2629.

Jonakait, G. M., Markey, K., Goldstein, M., Dreyfus, C. F., and Black, I. B. (1985). Selective expression of high affinity uptake of catecholamines by transiently catecholaminergic cells of the rat embryo: Studies *in vivo* and *in vitro*. *Dev. Biol.* **108**, 6–19.

Kennedy, W. R., and Sakuta, M. (1984). Collateral reinnervation of sweat glands. *Ann. Neurol.* **15,** 73–85.

Kessler, J. A. (1984). Non-neuronal cell conditioned medium stimulates peptidergic expression in sympathetic and sensory neurons *in vitro*. *Dev. Biol.* **106,** 61–73.

Kessler, J. A. (1985). Differential regulation of peptide and catecholamine characters in cultured sympathetic neurons. *Neurosci.* **1,** 827–839.

Landis, S. C. (1980). Developmental changes in the neurotransmitter properties of dissociated sympathetic neurons: A cytochemical study of the effects of medium. *Dev. Biol.* **7,** 348–361.

Landis, S. C., and Keefe, D. (1983). Evidence for neurotransmitter plasticity *in vivo*: Developmental changes in the properties of cholinergic sympathetic neurons. *Dev. Biol.* **98,** 349–372.

Landis, S. C., Fredieu, J. R., and Yodlowski, M. (1985). Neonatal treatment with nerve growth factor antiserum eliminates cholinergic sympathetic innervation of rat sweat glands. *Dev. Biol.* **112,** 222–229.

Landis, S. C., and Fredieu, J. R. (1986). Coexistence of calcitonin gene-related peptide and vasoactive intestinal peptide in cholinergic sympathetic innervation of rat sweat glands. *Brain Res.* **377,** 177–181.

Landis, S. C., Jackson, P. C., Fredieu, J. R., and Thibault, J. (1987). Catecholaminergic properties of cholinergic neurons and synapses in adult rat ciliary ganglion. *J. Neurosci.* **7,** 3574–3588.

Landis, S. C., Schwab, M., and Siegel, R. E. (1988). Evidence for neurotransmitter plasticity *in vivo*. II. Immunocytochemical studies of rat sweat gland innervation. *Dev. Biol.* **126,** 129–138.

Langley, J. N. (1891). On the course and connections of the secretory fibers supplying the sweat glands of the feet of the cat. *J. Physiol. (London)* **12,** 347–363.

Langley, J. N. (1894). Further observations on the secretory and vaso-motor fibres of the foot of the cat, with notes on other sympathetic nerve fibres. *J. Physiol. (London)* **17,** 296–310.

Langley, J. N. (1922). The secretion of sweat. Part I. Supposed inhibitory nerve fibres on the posterior nerve roots. Secretion after denervation. *J. Physiol. (London)* **56,** 110–145.

Leblanc, G., and Landis, S. C. (1986). Development of choline acetyltransferase activity in the cholinergic sympathetic innervation of sweat glands. *J. Neursci.* **6,** 260–265.

Leblanc, G. G., and Landis, S. C. (1988). Target specificity of neuropeptide Y-immunoreactive cranial parasympathetic neurons. *J. Neurosci.* **8,** 146–155.

Lee, Y., Takami, K., Kawai, Y., Girgis, S., Hillyard, C. J., MacIntyre, I., Emson, P. C., and Tohyama, M. (1985). Distribution of calcitonin gene-related peptide in the rat peripheral nervous system with reference to its coexistence with substance P. *Neurosci.* **15,** 1227–1237.

Lin, L. H., Mismer, D., Lile, J. D., Armes, L., Butler, E. T., Vannice, J. L., and Collins, F. (1989). Purification, cloning, and expression of ciliary neurotrophic factor (CNTF). *Science* **246,** 1023–1025.

Lindh, B., Lundberg, J. M., and Hokfelt, T. (1989). NPY-, galanin-, VIP/PHI-, CGRP-, and Substance P-immunoreactive neuronal subpopulations in cat autonomic and sensory ganglia and their projections. *Cell Tissue Res.* **256,** 259–273.

Loer, C. M., Jellies, J., and Kristan, W. B. (1987). Segment-specific morphogenesis of leech Retzius neurons requires particular peripheral targets. *J. Neurosci.* **7,** 2630–2638.

Loer, C. M., and Kristan, W. B. (1989). Peripheral target choice by homologous neurons during embryogenesis of the medicinal leech. II. Innervation of ectopic reproductive tissue by nonreproductive Retzius neurons. *J. Neurosci.* **9,** 528–538.

Lundberg, J. M., Hokfelt, T., Schultzberg, M., Uvnas-Wallensten, K., Kohler, C., and Said, S. I. (1979). Occurrence of vasoactive intestinal polypeptide(VIP)-like immunoreactivity in certain cholinergic neurons of the cat: Evidence from combined immunohistochemistry and acetylcholinesterase staining. *Neurosci.* **4,** 1539–1559.

Lundberg, J. M., Angaard, A., Fahrenkrug, J., Hokfelt, T., and Mutt, V. (1980). Vasoactive intestinal polypeptide in cholinergic neurons of exocrine glands: Functional significance of coexisting transmitters fo vasodilation and secretion. *Proc. Natl. Acad. Sci. USA* **77,** 1651–1655.

Lundberg, J. M., Hokfelt, T., Angaard, A., Terenius, L., Elde, R., Markey, K., and Goldstein, M. (1982a). Organization principles in the peripheral nervous system: Subdivisions by coexisting peptides (somatostatin, avian pancreatic polypeptide, and vasoactive intestinal peptide-like materials). *Proc. Natl. Acad. Sci. U.S.A.* **79,** 1303–1307.

Lundberg, J. M., Terenius, L., Hokfelt, T., Martling, C., Tatemoto, K., Mutt, V., Polak, J., Bloom, S., and Goldstein, M. (1982b). Neuropeptide Y(NPY)-like immunoreactivity in peripheral noradrenergic neurons and effects of NPY on sympathetic function. *Acta Physiol. Scand.* **116,** 477–480.

Lundberg, J. M., Terenius, L., Hokfelt, T., and Goldstein, M. (1983). High levels of neuropeptide Y in peripheral noradrenergic neurons in various mammals including man. *Neurosci. Lett.* **42,** 167–172.

Lundberg, J. M., and Hokfelt, T. (1986). Multiple coexistence of peptides and classical neurotransmitters in peripheral autonomic and sensory neurons—Functional and pharmacological implications. *In* "Progress in Brain Research" (T. Hokfelt, K. Fuxe, and B. Pernow, eds.), Vol. 68. (pp. 241–262). Amsterdam: Elsevier.

Macagno, E. R., Peinado, A., and Stewart, R. R. (1986). Segmental differentiation in the leech nervous system: Specific phenotypic changes associated with ectopic targets. *Proc. Natl. Acad. Sci. U.S.A.* **83,** 2746–2750.

McMahon, S. B., and Gibson, S. (1987). Peptide expression is altered when afferent nerves reinnervate inappropriate tissue. *Neurosci. Lett.* **7,** 9–15.

Morris, J. L., and Gibbins, I. L. (1987). Neuronal colocalization of peptides, catecholamines, and catecholamine-synthesizing enzymes in guinea pig paracervical ganglia. *J. Neurosci.* **7,** 3117–3130.

Morris, J. L., and Gibbins, I. L. (1989). Co-localization and plasticity of transmitters in peripheral autonomic and sensory neurons. *Int. J. Dev. Neurosci.* **7,** 521–531.

Nawa, H., and Sah, D. W. (1990a). Different biological activities in conditioned media control the expression of a variety of neuropeptides in cultured sympathetic neurons. *Neuron* **4,** 279–287.

Nawa, H., and Sah, D. W. Y. (1990b). Distinct factors in conditioned media control the expression of a variety of neuropeptides in cultured sympathetic neurons. *Neuron* **4,** 279–287.

Nishizawa, M., Hayakawa, Y., Yanahara, N., and Okamoto, H. (1985). Nucleotide sequence divergence and functional constraint in VIP precursor mRNA evolution between human and rat. *Fed. Eur. Biochem. Soc.* **183,** 55–63.

Norberg, K., and Olson, L. (1965). Adrenergic innervation of the salivary glands in the rat. *Z. Zellforsch.* **68,** 183–189.

Norr, S. (1973). *In vitro* analysis of sympathetic neuron differentiation from chick neural crest cells. *Dev. Biol.* **34,** 16–38.

Patterson, P. H., and Chun, L. L. Y. (1977). Induction of acetylcholine synthesis in primary cultures of dissociated rat sympathetic neurons. I. Effects of conditioned medium. *Dev. Biol.* **56,** 263–280.

Patton, H. D. (1948). Secretory innervation of the cat's footpad. *J. Neurophysiol.* **11,** 217–229.

Potter, D. D., Landis, S. C., Matsumoto, S. G., and Furshpan, E. J. (1986). Synaptic functions in rat sympathetic neurons in microcultures. II. Adrenergic/cholinergic dual status and plasticity. *J. Neurosci.* **6,** 1080–1090.

Purves, D., Snider, W., and Voyvodic, J. T. (1988). Trophic regulation of nerve cell morphology and innervation in the autonomic nervous system. *Nature (London)* **336,** 123–128.

Rao, M., and Landis, S. C. (1990). Characterization of a target-derived neuronal cholinergic differentiation factor. *Neuron* **5,** 899–910.

Rao, M., Landis, S. C., and Patterson, P. H. (1990). The cholinergic neuronal differentiation factor from heart cell conditioned medium is different from the cholinergic factors in sciatic nerve and spinal cord. *Dev. Biol.* **139,** 65–74.

Raynaud, B., Clarous, D., Vidal, S., Ferrand, C., and Weber, M. J. (1987). Comparison of the effects of elevated K^+ ions and muscle-conditioned medium on the neurotransmitter phenotype of cultured sympathetic neurons. *Dev. Biol.* **121,** 548–558.

Ring, J. R., and Randall, W. C. (1947). The distribution and histological structure of sweat glands in the albino rat and their response to prolonged nervous stimulation. *Anat. Rec.* **99,** 7–16.

Rohrer, H., and Thoenen, H. (1987). Relationship between differentiation and terminal mitosis: Chick sensory and ciliary neurons differentiate after terminal mitosis of precursor cells, whereas sympathetic neurons continue to divide after differentiation. *J. Neurosci.* **7,** 3739–3751.

Rosenfeld, M. G., Mermod, J. J., Amara, S. G., Swanson, L. W., Sawchenko, P. E., Rivier, J., Vale, W. W., and Evans, R. H. (1983). Production of a novel neuropeptide encoded by the calcitonin gene via tissue-specific RNA processing. *Nature (London)* **304,** 129–135.

Rothman, R. P., Gershon, M. D., and Holtzer, H. (1978). The relationship of cell division to the acquisition of adrenergic characteristics by developing sympathetic ganglion cell precursors. *Dev. Biol.* **65,** 322–335.

Rothman, R. P., Specht, L. A., Gershon, M. D., Joh, T. H., Teitelman, G., Pickel, V. M., and Reis, D. J. (1980). Catecholamine biosynthetic enzymes are expressed in replicating cells of the peripheral but not the central nervous system. *Proc. Natl. Acad. Sci. U.S.A.* **77,** 6221–6225.

Rubin, E. (1985a). Development of the rat superior cervical ganglion: Ganglion cell maturation. *J. Neurosci.* **5,** 673–684.

Rubin, E. (1985b). Development of the rat superior cervical ganglion: Ingrowth of preganglionic axons. *J. Neurosci.* **5,** 685–696.

Rubin, E. (1985c). Development of the rat superior cervical ganglion: Initial stages of synapse formation. *J. Neurosci.* **5,** 697–708.

Saadat, S., Sendtner, M., and Rohrer, H. (1989). Ciliary neurotrophic factor induces cholinergic differentiation of rat sympathetic neurons in culture. *Cell Biol.* **108,** 1807–1816.

Schon, R., Allen, J. M., Yeats, J. C., Allen, Y. D., Ballesta, J., Polak, J., Kelly, J. S., and Bloom, S. R. (1985). Neuropeptide Y innervation of the rodent pineal gland and cerebral vessels. *Neurosci. Lett.* **57,** 65–71.

Schotzinger, R., and Landis, S. C. (1988). Cholinergic phenotype developed by noradrenergic sympathetic neurons after innervation of a novel cholinergic target *in vivo. Nature (London)* **335,** 637–639.

Schotzinger, R., and Landis, S. C. (1990a). Acquisition of cholinergic and peptidergic properties by the sympathetic innervation of rat sweat glands requires interaction with normal target. *Neuron* **5,** 91–100.

Schotzinger, R., and Landis, S. C. (1990b). Postnatal development of autonomic and sensory innervation of thoracic hairy skin in the rat: A histochemical, cytochemical and radioenzymatic study. *Cell Tissue Res.* **260,** 575–587.

Schultzberg, M., Hokfelt, T., Terenius, L., Elfvin, L. -G., Lundberg, J. M., Brandt, J., Elde, R. P., and Goldstein, M. (1979). Enkephalin immunoreactive nerve fibers and cell bodies in sympathetic ganglia of the guinea-pig and rat. *Neurosci.* **4,** 249–270.

Sjoqvist, F. (1963). The correlation between the occurrence and localization of acetylcholinesterase-rich cell bodies in the stellate ganglion and the outflow of cholinergic sweat secretory fibers to the forepaw of the cat. *Acta Physiol. Scand.* **57,** 339–349.

Smith, C. L., and Frank, E. (1987). Peripheral specification of sensory neurons transplanted to novel locations along the neuraxis. *J. Neurosci.* **7,** 1537–1549.

Stevens, L. M., and Landis, S. C. (1987). Development and properties of the secretory response in rat sweat glands: Relationship to the induction of cholinergic function in sweat gland innervation. *Dev. Biol.* **123,** 179–190.

Stevens, L. M., and Landis, S. C. (1988). Developmental interactions between sweat glands and the sympathetic neurons which innervate them: Effects of delayed innervation on neurotransmitter plasticity and gland maturation. *Dev. Biol.* **130,** 703–720.

Stevens, L. M., and Landis, S. C. (1990). Target influences on transmitter choice by sympathetic neurons developing in the anterior chamber of the eye. *Dev. Biol.* **137,** 109–124.

Stockli, K. A., Lottspeich, F., Sendtner, M., Masiakowski, P., Carroll, P., Gotz, R., Lindholm, D., and Thoenen, H. (1989). Molecular cloning, expression and regional distribution of rat ciliary neurotrophic factor. *Nature (London)* **342,** 920–923.

Swerts, J. P., Le Van Thai, A., Vigny, A., and Weber, M. J. (1983). Regulation of enzymes responsible for neurotransmitter synthesis and degradation in cultured rat sympathetic neurons. *Dev. Biol.* **100,** 1–11.

Takami, K., Kawai, Y., Shiosaka, S., Lee, Y., Girgis, S., Hillyard, C., MacIntyre, I., Emson, P., and Tohyama, M. (1985). Immunohistochemical evidence for the coexistence of calcitonin gene-related peptide- and choline acetyltransferase-like immunoreactivity in neurons of the rat hypoglossal, facial, and ambiguous nuclei. *Brain Res.* **328,** 386–395.

Teillet, M. A., Cochard, P., LeDourain, N. M. (1978). Relative roles of the mesenchymal tissues and of the complex neural tube–notochord on the expression of adrenergic metabolism in neural crest cells. *Zoon.* **6,** 115–122.

Teitelman, G., Baker, H., Joh, T. H., and Reis, D. J. (1979). Appearance of catecholamine synthesizing enzymes during development of the rat nervous system: Possible role of tissue environment. *Proc. Natl. Acad. Sci. U.S.A.* **76,** 509–513.

Teitelman, G., Gershon, M. D., Rothman, T. P., Joh, T. H., and Reis, D. J. (1981). Proliferation and distribution of cells that transiently express a catecholaminergic phenotype during development in mice and rats. *Dev. Biol.* **86,** 348–357.

Uvnas, B. (1966). Cholinergic vasodilator nerves. *Fed. Proc.* **25,** 1618–1624.

Voyvodic, J. T. (1989). Peripheral target regulation of dendritic geometry in the rat superior cervical ganglion. *J. Neurosci.* **9,** 1997–2010.

Walicke, P. A., Campenot, R. B., and Patterson, P. H. (1977). Determination of transmitter function by neuronal activity. *Proc. Natl. Acad. Sci. U.S.A.* **74,** 3767–3771.

Weiss, P. (1942). Lid-closure reflex from eyes transplanted to atypical locations in *Triturus torosus. J. Comp. Neurol.* **77,** 131–169.

Wolinsky, E., and Patterson, P. H. (1983). Tyrosine hydroxylase activity decreases with induction of cholinergic properties in cultured sympathetic neurons. *J. Neurosci.* **3,** 1495–1500.

Wolinsky, E., and Patterson, P. H. (1985). Rat serum contains a developmentally regulated cholinergic inducing activity. *J. Neurosci.* **5,** 1509–1512.

Wong, V., and Kessler, J. A. (1987). Solubilization of a membrane factor that stimulates levels of Substance P and choline acetyltransferase in sympathetic neurons. *Proc. Natl. Acad. Sci. U.S.A.* **84,** 8726–8729.

Yamamori, T. (1991). Localization of CDF/LIF mRNA in the rat brain and peripheral tissues. *Proc. Natl. Acad. Sci. U.S.A.* **88,** 7298–7302.

Yamamori, T., Fukada, K., Aebersold, R., Korsching, S., Fann, M. J., and Patterson, P. H. (1989). The cholinergic neuronal differentiation factor from heart cells is identical to leukemia inhibitory factor. *Science* **246,** 1412–1416.

Yamauchi, A., and Lever, J. D. (1971). Correlations between formol fluorescence and acetylcholinesterase staining in the superior cervical ganglion of normal rat, pig and sheep. *J. Anat.* **110,** 435–443.

Yamauchi, A., Lever, J. D., and Kemp, K. W. (1973). Catecholamine loading and depletion in the rat superior cervical ganglion. A formal fluorescence and enzyme histochemical study with numerical assessments. *J. Anat.* **114,** 271–280.

Yardley, C. P., and Hilton, S. M. (1987). Vasodilatation in hind-limb skeletal muscle evoked as part of the defense reaction in the rat. *J. Auton. Nervous System* **19,** 127–137.

Yodlowski, M. L., Fredieu, J. R., and Landis, S. C. (1984). Neonatal 6-hydroxydopamine treatment eliminates cholinergic sympathetic innervation and induces sensory sprouting in rat sweat glands. *J. Neurosci.* **4,** 1535–1548.

Index